EVIDENCE-BASED NURSING

A Guide to Clinical Practice

ALBA DiCENSO, RN, PhD
CHSRF/CIHR Chair in Advanced Practice Nursing;
Professor, Nursing and Clinical Epidemiology & Biostatistics
Faculty of Health Sciences, McMaster University
Hamilton, Ontario, Canada

GORDON GUYATT, MD, MSc
Chair, Evidence-Based Medicine Working Group;
Professor, Clinical Epidemiology & Biostatistics and Medicine
Faculty of Health Sciences, McMaster University
Hamilton, Ontario, Canada

DONNA CILISKA, RN, PhD
Professor, Nursing, Faculty of Health Sciences, McMaster University;
Consultant, Hamilton Public Health Research, Education, and Development Program
Hamilton, Ontario, Canada

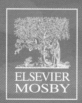

ELSEVIER
MOSBY

ELSEVIER
MOSBY

11830 Westline Industrial Drive
St. Louis, MO 63146

NOTICE

Nursing is an ever-changing field. Standard safety precautions must be followed, but as new research and clinical experience broaden our knowledge, changes in treatment and drug therapy may become necessary or appropriate. Readers are advised to check the most current product information provided by the manufacturer of each drug to be administered to verify the recommended dose, the method and duration of administration, and contraindications. It is the responsibility of the licensed prescriber, relying on experience and knowledge of the patient, to determine dosages and the best treatment for each individual patient. Neither the publisher nor the authors assume any liability for any injury and/or damage to persons or property arising from this publication.

The Publisher

Portions of this book have been reprinted or adapted from Guyatt G and Rennie D, eds. *Users' Guides to the Medical Literature: A Manual for Evidence-Based Clinical Practice,* © 2002, American Medical Association, by permission of the American Medical Association.

ISBN-13 978-0-323-02591-1
ISBN-10 0-323-02591-9

Vice President, Publishing Director: *Sally Schrefer*
Executive Publisher: *Barbara Nelson Cullen*
Managing Editor: *Robin Levin Richman*
Publishing Services Manager: *John Rogers*
Project Manager: *Doug Turner*
Senior Designer: *Amy Buxton*

Printed in the United States of America

Last digit is the print number: 9   8   7   6   5

Ai miei genitori, NICOLINA E FRANCESCO DICENSO, con eterna gratitudine per i loro immensi sacrifici, che mi hanno permesso di raggiungere importanti traguardi nel corso della mia vita.

To BRIAN HUTCHISON, my husband, colleague, and best friend, whose positive spirit, unfailing love, and wise counsel sustain me.

To my precious son, WILL MITCHELL, with love and gratitude for making parenting such a joy.

To two special young men, PAUL AND EVAN HUTCHISON, for their gentle encouragement and support.

To GORDON GUYATT, my professional mentor and friend, for so generously sharing his original work on which this book heavily relies.

AD

To ALBA DICENSO, for allowing me the temporary role of honorary nurse.

To THE AUTHORS of the *Users' Guides to the Medical Literature*, whose contributions formed the basis of this book.

To ROBYN GUYATT, who keeps me humble by justly wondering, since evidence-based health care is so obviously necessary, why I think it is such a big idea.

GG

To STUDENTS—undergraduate, graduate and postgraduate—who have inspired me to find different ways of learning and teaching this content.

DC

Contributors

Donna Ciliska, RN, PhD
Professor
School of Nursing
Faculty of Health Sciences
McMaster University
Hamilton, Ontario
Canada

Seana Collins, MA, MLIS
AHFMR Librarian
John W Scott Health Sciences Library
University of Alberta
Edmonton, Alberta
Canada

Nicky Cullum, RN, PhD
Professor and Director
Centre for Evidence-Based Nursing
Department of Health Sciences
University of York
York, North Yorkshire
United Kingdom

Catherine Demers, MD, MSc
Assistant Professor
Department of Medicine
Faculty of Health Sciences
McMaster University
Hamilton, Ontario
Canada

Alba DiCenso, RN, PhD
Professor
Nursing and Clinical
  Epidemiology & Biostatistics
Faculty of Health Sciences
McMaster University
Hamilton, Ontario
Canada

Maureen Dobbins, RN, PhD
Assistant Professor
School of Nursing
Faculty of Health Sciences
McMaster University
Hamilton, Ontario
Canada

Dawn Dowding, RN, PhD
*Senior Lecturer in Clinical Decision
  Making*
Department of Health Sciences
  and Hull York Medical School
University of York
York, North Yorkshire
United Kingdom

Nancy Edwards, RN, PhD
Professor
School of Nursing
University of Ottawa
Ottawa, Ontario
Canada

Carole Estabrooks, RN, PhD
Associate Professor
Faculty of Nursing
University of Alberta
Edmonton, Alberta
Canada

David Gregory, RN, PhD
Professor
Faculty of Nursing
University of Manitoba
Winnipeg, Manitoba
Canada

Jeremy Grimshaw, MBChB, PhD
Professor
Department of Medicine
University of Ottawa
Ottawa, Ontario
Canada

Gordon Guyatt, MD, MSc
Professor
Clinical Epidemiology & Biostatistics
 and Medicine
Faculty of Health Sciences
McMaster University
Hamilton, Ontario
Canada

Sarah Hayward RN, MPH
Director
Applied Health Research Programs
Alberta Heritage Foundation
 for Medical Research
Edmonton, Alberta
Canada

Brian Hutchison, MD, MSc
Professor
Family Medicine and Clinical
 Epidemiology & Biostatistics
Faculty of Health Sciences
McMaster University
Hamilton, Ontario
Canada

Andrew Jull, RN, MA
Research Fellow
Clinical Trials Research Unit
School of Population Health
University of Auckland
Auckland, New Zealand

Cathy Kessenich, ARNP, DSN
Professor
Nursing Department
University of Tampa
Tampa, Florida
United States

Deborah Marshall, PhD
Assistant Professor
Department of Clinical Epidemiology
 & Biostatistics
Faculty of Health Sciences
McMaster University
Hamilton, Ontario
Canada

Bernie O'Brien, PhD[†]
Professor
Department of Clinical Epidemiology
 & Biostatistics
Faculty of Health Sciences
McMaster University
Hamilton, Ontario
Canada

Annette O'Connor, RN, PhD
Professor
School of Nursing and Department
 of Epidemiology & Community
 Medicine
University of Ottawa
Ottawa, Ontario
Canada

Jenny Ploeg, RN, PhD
Associate Professor
School of Nursing
Faculty of Health Sciences
McMaster University
Hamilton, Ontario
Canada

Cynthia Russell, RN, PhD
*Associate Professor & Assistant Dean
 for Distributive Programs*
College of Nursing
The University of Tennessee Health
 Science Center
Memphis, Tennessee
United States

[†]Deceased.

Dawn Stacey, RN, MScN
PhD Candidate
Institute of Population Health
University of Ottawa
Ottawa, Ontario
Canada

Carl Thompson, RN, DPhil
Senior Lecturer
Department of Health Sciences
University of York
York, North Yorkshire
United Kingdom

Peter Tugwell, MD, MSc
Professor
Institute of Population Health
   and Faculty of Medicine
University of Ottawa
Ottawa, Ontario
Canada

Tanya Voth, BA, MLIS
Program Manager
Centre for Health Evidence
University of Alberta
Edmonton, Alberta
Canada

Editorial Board

Contributors to *Users' Guides to the Medical Literature,* Edited by Guyatt and Rennie

John Attia, MD, PhD
Clinical Epidemiology & Biostatistics
Royal Newcastle Hospital
Newcastle, New South Wales
Australia

Alexandra Barratt, MBBS, PhD
*Public Health & Community
 Medicine*
University of Sydney
Sydney, New South Wales
Australia

Eric Bass, MD, MPH
Internal Medicine
Johns Hopkins University School
 of Medicine
Baltimore, Maryland
United States

Patrick Bossuyt, PhD
Clinical Epidemiology & Biostatistics
University of Amsterdam
Amsterdam, The Netherlands

Heiner Bucher, MD, MPH
Internal Medicine
University Hospital Basel
Basel, Switzerland

Deborah Cook, MD, MSc
*Clinical Epidemiology & Biostatistics
 and Medicine*
McMaster University
Hamilton, Ontario
Canada

Jonathan Craig, MBChB, PhD
Public Health & Community Medicine
University of Sydney
Sydney, New South Wales
Australia

Robert Cumming, MBBS, PhD
Public Health & Community Medicine
University of Sydney
Sydney, New South Wales
Australia

Antonio Dans, MD, MSc
Clinical Epidemiological Unit
University of the Philippines
Manila, Philippines

Leonila Dans, MD, MSc
Clinical Epidemiological Unit
University of the Philippines
Manila, Philippines

Alan Detsky, MD, PhD
Medicine
University of Toronto
Toronto, Ontario
Canada

P J Devereaux, MD, BSc
*Clinical Epidemiology & Biostatistics
 and Medicine*
McMaster University
Hamilton, Ontario
Canada

Michael Drummond, DPhil
Centre for Health Economics
University of York
York, North Yorkshire
United Kingdom

Mita Giacomini, PhD
Clinical Epidemiology & Biostatistics
McMaster University
Hamilton, Ontario
Canada

Paul Glasziou, MBBS, PhD
Centre for Evidence Based Medicine
University of Oxford
Oxford, United Kingdom

Lee Green, MD, MPH
Family Medicine
University of Michigan
Ann Arbor, Michigan
United States

Trisha Greenhalgh, MD, MA
*Unit for Evidence-Based Practice
 and Policy*
Royal Free and University College
 Medical School
London, United Kingdom

Gordon Guyatt, MD, MSc
*Clinical Epidemiology & Biostatistics
 and Medicine*
McMaster University
Hamilton, Ontario
Canada

Ted Haines, MD, MSc
*Clinical Epidemiology & Biostatistics
 and Occupational Health*
McMaster University
Hamilton, Ontario
Canada

David Haslam, MD, MSc
*Psychiatry, Family Medicine, and
 Epidemiology & Biostatistics*
University of Western Ontario
London, Ontario
Canada

Rose Hatala, MD, MSc
Medicine
University of British Columbia
Vancouver, British Columbia
Canada

Brian Haynes, MD, PhD
*Clinical Epidemiology & Biostatistics
 and Medicine*
McMaster University
Hamilton, Ontario
Canada

Robert Hayward, MD, MPH
Centre for Health Evidence
University of Alberta
Edmonton, Alberta
Canada

Daren Heyland, MD, MSc
*Medicine and Community Health
 & Epidemiology*
Queen's University
Kingston, Ontario
Canada

Anne Holbrook, MD, PharmD, MSc
Centre for Evaluation of Medicines
McMaster University
Hamilton, Ontario
Canada

Dereck Hunt, MD, MSc
Medicine
McMaster University
Hamilton, Ontario
Canada

Les Irwig, MBBCh, PhD
Public Health & Community Medicine
University of Sydney
Sydney, New South Wales
Australia

Roman Jaeschke, MD, MSc
Medicine
McMaster University
Hamilton, Ontario
Canada

Regina Kunz, MD, PhD
Nephrology
Charite Humboldt-University
Berlin, Germany

Christina Lacchetti, MHSc
*Clinical Epidemiology & Biostatistics
and Medicine*
McMaster University
Hamilton, Ontario
Canada

Andreas Laupacis, MD, MSc
*Institute for Clinical Evaluative
Sciences*
Toronto, Ontario
Canada

Hui Lee, MD, MSc†
Medicine
McMaster University
Hamilton, Ontario
Canada

Luz Letelier, MD
Internal Medicine
Pontificia Universidad Catolica de
Chile
Santiago, Chile

Raymond Leung, MDCM
Cardiac Science
Royal Alexandra Hospital
Edmonton, Alberta
Canada

Mitchell Levine, MD, MSc
Clinical Epidemiology & Biostatistics
McMaster University
Hamilton, Ontario
Canada

Jeroen Lijmer, MD
Clinical Epidemiology & Biostatistics
University of Amsterdam
Amsterdam, The Netherlands

Finlay McAlister, MD, MSc
Medicine
University of Alberta
Edmonton, Alberta
Canada

Thomas McGinn, MD
Primary Care Medicine
Mount Sinai Medical Center
New York, New York
United States

Ann McKibbon, MLS
Clinical Epidemiology & Biostatistics
McMaster University
Hamilton, Ontario
Canada

Maureen Meade, MD, MSc
*Clinical Epidemiology & Biostatistics
and Medicine*
McMaster University
Hamilton, Ontario
Canada

Victor Montori, MD, MSc
Medicine
Mayo Clinic College of Medicine
Rochester, Minnesota
United States

Virginia Moyer, MD, MPH
Pediatrics
University of Texas
Houston, Texas
United States

---

†Deceased.

David Naylor, MD, DPhil
Medicine
University of Toronto
Toronto, Ontario
Canada

Thomas Newman, MD, MPH
Epidemiology & Biostatistics,
 Pediatrics and Laboratory Medicine
University of California, San Francisco
San Francisco, California
United States

Jim Nishikawa, MD, MSc
Medicine
University of Ottawa
Ottawa, Ontario
Canada

Bernie O'Brien, PhD†
Clinical Epidemiology & Biostatistics
McMaster University
Hamilton, Ontario
Canada

Andrew Oxman, MD, MSc
Health Services Research Unit
National Institute of Public Health
Oslo, Norway

Peter Pronovost, MD, PhD
Anesthesiology and Critical Care
 Medicine
Johns Hopkins University
Baltimore, Maryland
United States

Adrienne Randolph, MD, MSc
Pediatrics
Children's Hospital
Boston, Massachusetts
United States

Drummond Rennie, MD
Institute for Health Policy Studies
University of California, San Francisco
San Francisco, California
United States

Scott Richardson, MD
Medicine
Wright State University
Dayton, Ohio
United States

Holger Schünemann, MD, PhD
Medicine and Social & Preventative
 Medicine
University at Buffalo
Buffalo, New York
United States

Jack Sinclair, MD
Clinical Epidemiology & Biostatistics
 and Pediatrics
McMaster University
Hamilton, Ontario
Canada

Martin Stockler, MBBS, MSc
Medicine
University of Sydney
Sydney, New South Wales
Australia

Sharon Straus, MD, MSc
Medicine
University of Toronto and Mount Sinai
 Hospital
Toronto, Ontario
Canada

---

†Deceased.

Peter Tugwell, MD, MSc
*Institute of Population Health
and Faculty of Medicine*
University of Ottawa
Ottawa, Ontario
Canada

Stephen Walter, PhD
Clinical Epidemiology & Biostatistics
McMaster University
Hamilton, Ontario
Canada

Bruce Weaver, MSc
Psychology
Lakehead University
Thunder Bay, Ontario
Canada

George Wells, PhD
*Clinical Epidemiology Unit
and Departments of Medicine
and Epidemiology*
University of Ottawa
Ottawa, Ontario
Canada

Mark Wilson, MD, MPH
Medicine
University of Iowa College of Medicine
Iowa City, Iowa
United States

Jeremy Wyatt, PhD
Knowledge Management Centre
University College London
London, United Kingdom

Peter Wyer, MD
Medicine
Columbia University College of
Physicians and Surgeons
Pelham, New York
United States

Foreword

The words *evidence-based nursing* (EBN) are on the lips and in the minds of nurses around the world. They ask, "What is it?" "How is it practiced?" and "When will I know I'm acting on solid evidence that will benefit patients?" Nurses also query about tools, resources, and services to improve their knowledge, competency, and skills in order to fully engage in EBN.

The EBN era is upon us in health care, and nurses need not wait any longer for solutions to their inquiries about it! This much needed book, *Evidence-Based Nursing: A Guide to Clinical Practice,* provides answers and how-to's for practitioners, faculty, and students, enabling them to frame clinical questions in a way that supports finding and using evidence. It illustrates how to identify and distinguish between strong and weak evidence, clearly understand study results, weigh the risks and benefits of clinical management options, and apply the evidence to individual patient needs and preferences in order to improve outcomes.

Written by world-renowned leaders in the EBN field, this resource also brings together the best thinking on EBN through its editors, contributors, and editorial board members. This team from 13 countries creates and presents a comprehensive, cutting-edge resource that will help nurses implement evidence-based care around the world. Its unique approach provides nurses with tools for using and evaluating nursing literature, clinical scenarios, and case presentations that stimulate critical thinking toward problem resolution, appropriate interventions, and desired outcomes.

Sigma Theta Tau International made a commitment to being a leading source of knowledge and resources that foster EBN practice globally, and in 2003 the Honor Society issued the following position statement on EBN:

> The Honor Society of Nursing, Sigma Theta Tau International, defines EBN as an integration of the best evidence available, nursing expertise, and the values and preferences of the individuals, families, and communities who are served. This assumes that optimal nursing care is provided when nurses and health care decision-makers have access to a synthesis of the latest research, a consensus of expert opinion, and are thus able to exercise their judgment as they plan and provide care that takes into account cultural and personal values and preferences. This approach to nursing care bridges the gap between the best evidence available and the most appropriate nursing care of individuals, groups, and populations with varied needs.

To underscore this commitment, the Honor Society formed strategic partnerships with international organizations centered on EBN; launched a peer-reviewed, quarterly journal, *Worldviews on Evidence-Based Nursing;* and produced and distributed multiple on-line courses and resources. Providing knowledge resources on EBN fulfills the Honor Society's goal to develop, disseminate, and promote knowledge use for service of others.

This text is an excellent resource that fosters and promotes EBN practice, and the Honor Society commends it to nurses around the world as a valuable asset for enhancing the health of all people.

Enjoy, read, and expand your knowledge—for soon EBN will not just be on nurses' lips and minds, but in these nurses' every action and the resulting outcomes.

Nancy Dickenson-Hazard

Nancy Dickenson-Hazard, RN, MSN, FAAN
Chief Executive Officer
Honor Society of Nursing, Sigma Theta Tau International

Preface

The term *evidence-based nursing* (EBN) was coined only 10 or so years ago; yet, in this short time, the concept has become central to the nursing profession around the world. Major international nursing organizations such as Sigma Theta Tau International have incorporated the promotion of evidence-based practice into their strategic plan. Centers for EBN have sprung up around the world. The journal, *Evidence-Based Nursing,* first published in 1998, and its associated Web site enjoy a high subscription rate. EBN courses are being developed and incorporated into many nursing education programs. Health care agencies have struck EBN committees, and governments around the world are encouraging evidence-based practice. We are pleased to contribute to this growing movement by offering this book.

As we will discuss in more detail in Chapter 1, Introduction to Evidence-Based Nursing, evidence-based practice is the integration of best research evidence with clinical expertise and patient values to facilitate clinical decision making. While research has repeatedly shown that nurses are highly motivated to be evidence-based practitioners, it has also shown that most nurses, especially those educated more than 10 years ago, lack the skills to discriminate high quality research from that which is flawed and to interpret the results of research studies. This book is designed to help readers learn these skills.

HOW DID THIS BOOK COME ABOUT?

Between 1993 and 2000 the Evidence-Based Medicine Working Group, led by Gordon Guyatt, produced a series of 25 "Users' Guides to the Medical Literature" that were published in *JAMA*. This series, which outlined criteria to identify high-quality research, proved very popular not only in medicine but also in other health professions. At McMaster University, many of these guides formed the foundation for the Critical Appraisal of Data undergraduate nursing course. In 2002, Guyatt and his colleagues updated these guides and incorporated them into a book entitled *Users' Guides to the Medical Literature: A Manual for Evidence-Based Clinical Practice.*

Even as Guyatt and his colleagues prepared the *Users' Guides* book, we began to discuss the possibility of adapting their book to create a much needed nursing version. As with the *Users' Guides* book, *Evidence-Based Nursing* is available in both print and electronic format. Robert Hayward has taken primary responsibility for translation of the material into CD-ROM format. Rob and his team have done a magnificent job with the electronic version.

WHO SHOULD READ THIS BOOK?

Any nurse who wishes to understand the health care literature, and to use it more effectively in solving patient problems, will benefit from this book. Those who wish to develop a core knowledge of basic concepts will read Part I of the book thoroughly and delve into Part II only for issues that catch their particular interest. Most undergraduate nursing students and clinical nurses will likely be satisfied with this level of understanding. They will find Part I filled with case scenarios and clinical examples that facilitate their understanding, and they will also uncover tips for finding the best information and applying it to their practice.

Those who wish to reach a higher level of proficiency in using the health care literature in patient care, administration, and teaching will find the in-depth discussions in Part II useful. Nurses involved in delivering continuing nursing education, nursing faculty, and graduate nursing students will wish to master the concepts we present in Part II.

A NOTE ABOUT AUTHORSHIP

As noted above, many of the book chapters were adapted from chapters that originally appeared in the *Users' Guides* book. The contributors to this nursing text are the editors or colleagues who took responsibility for making the required modifications to the original chapters. Upon completion, most chapters were sent to members of the editorial board for review. We acknowledge those who provided input immediately below the chapter author byline. Below this line, we acknowledge those who wrote the original version of the chapter for the *Users' Guides* book, and thank them for kindly consenting to the adaptation of their original chapter for inclusion in this text.

A number of chapters that do not appear in the *Users' Guides* book were identified as important to a text on EBN. These included Chapter 1, Introduction to Evidence-Based Nursing; Chapter 11, Changing Nursing Practice in an Organization; and Chapter 17, Health Services Interventions.

Grounding nursing practice in evidence, rather than tradition, is necessary to (1) provide high quality nursing care, (2) meet nursing's social obligation of accountability, (3) gain and maintain credibility among other health disciplines, and (4) build a nursing knowledge base that can be used to influence policy in both health care organizations and government. Using this book, nurses can acquire the necessary knowledge and skills to become evidence-based practitioners.

Alba DiCenso, RN, PhD
Gordon Guyatt, MD, MSc
Donna Ciliska, RN, PhD
McMaster University

Acknowledgments

We thank our students who through their motivation for advanced knowledge strive to improve health care delivery. They helped us to clarify our ideas and provided encouragement and support during the preparation of this book. We are also grateful to the authors of the original chapters that appeared in the *Users' Guides to the Medical Literature: A Manual for Evidence-Based Clinical Practice*, edited by Gordon Guyatt and Drummond Rennie. They kindly provided permission for the adaptation of their work for this nursing text. We thank those who contributed chapters to this book, often under tight time constraints. Many colleagues on our editorial board read chapters and provided their reactions and suggestions; for all of this we are most thankful. Marielle Layton and Tanya Voth worked efficiently behind the scenes to translate the material into an electronic format. Thank you both for your important contribution.

Barbara Nelson Cullen, Robin Levin Richman, and Doug Turner at Elsevier deserve enormous thanks for patiently supporting us through the preparation of the chapters and review of copyedits. And finally, deepest thanks to Rose Vonau for providing superb administrative support throughout the preparation of this book, Susan Marks for her meticulous copyediting and page proofing, and Monique Lloyd for her careful review of the text.

How to Use This Book

Like evidence-based nursing (EBN), this book is about clinical decision making. In particular, our objective is to make efficient use of the published literature to help with patient care. What does the published literature comprise? Our definition is broad. Evidence may be published in a wide variety of sources, including original journal articles, reviews and synopses of primary studies, practice guidelines, and traditional and innovative nursing textbooks. Increasingly, clinicians can most easily access many of these sources through the Internet.

PART I: THE BASICS: USING THE NURSING LITERATURE

Part I of the book covers the basics: what every nursing student and practicing nurse should know about reading the health care literature. We kept this part as succinct as possible. From an instructor's point of view, Part I constitutes a curriculum for a course to teach nursing students how to use the literature; it is also appropriate for a continuing education program for practicing nurses.

Part I of this book teaches a systematic approach that involves three steps to using an article from the health care literature. Nurses should ask whether the study is of sufficiently high quality that the study findings are likely to be true, what the study findings are, and how this information can be used in their nursing practice. In the first step, the nurse considers the likelihood of bias in the way the study was carried out. In the second and third steps, the nurse comes to understand the results and to apply those results to practice. To help demonstrate the clinical relevance of this approach, we begin each chapter with a clinical scenario, demonstrate a search for relevant literature, and present a table that summarizes criteria for the three steps.

A wide array of preprocessed (or prefiltered) evidence-based resources already exist, and most are easily accessed by computer. The number and quality of these resources are certain to increase dramatically during the next few years. Chapter 2, Finding the Evidence, will teach you how to identify the right databases—ones providing evidence that is both valid and applicable to your practice—and to efficiently find the information you want within them. The remaining chapters in Part I will teach you how to make optimal use of what you find to address clinical problems. A challenge that faces nurses once they have identified strong evidence for a change in nursing practice is mobilizing that change in their work environment. To assist with this, the last chapter in Part I, Changing Nursing Practice in an Organization, describes a framework for adopting an evidence-based innovation in the workplace.

Mastering the concepts in Part I will help you to ensure that your practice is evidence-based. From Part I, you will learn the following:

- How research evidence fits into clinical decision making
- How to efficiently find the best evidence
- How to distinguish stronger evidence from weaker evidence
- How to conduct a detailed critical appraisal, summarize the evidence, and balance the benefits and risks that should precede clinical decisions
- How to apply evidence from the literature to your nursing practice and, in particular, how to individualize the application to each unique patient
- How to change nursing practice in an organization

You need not read all of Part I. The book is designed so that each chapter is largely self-contained. If all you need is guidance on formulating and carrying out searches, read only Chapter 2. If the only original articles you are interested in are primary studies that seek to evaluate a nursing intervention and systematic reviews of those studies, read only Chapter 4, Health Care Interventions and Chapter 9, Summarizing the Evidence Through Systematic Reviews. We avoided excessive redundancy, so there are times when rather than repeating a concept common to two or more chapters, we refer you to the original chapter in which it is described. You will find such instances clearly denoted.

PART II: BEYOND THE BASICS: USING AND TEACHING THE PRINCIPLES OF EVIDENCE-BASED NURSING

Part II of this book is directed to nurses who want to practice EBN at a more sophisticated level. Reading Part II will deepen your understanding of study methodology, statistical issues, and effective use of the numbers that emerge from health care research in helping patients make the best health care choices. We wrote Part II mindful of an additional audience: those who teach evidence-based practice.

You need not read Part II from beginning to end in the order presented. Our intent is for you to read sections of Part II as the need arises when considering issues that emerge in critical appraisal and application of articles that may guide your clinical nursing practice. How should you use Part II? Many of the chapters include more detailed discussion of concepts introduced in Part I. For instance, in Part I, Chapter 4, Health Care Interventions, we introduce the concepts of intention-to-treat and number needed to treat. For those interested in more detailed discussion of these concepts, Part II includes chapters specifically focused on these concepts (Chapter 15, The Principle of Intention to Treat, and Chapter 32, Number Needed to Treat).

Thus, we anticipate that clinicians may be selective in their reading of both parts of this book. On the first read, you may choose only a few chapters that interest you. If, as you use the health care literature, you find the need to expand your understanding of specific concepts, you can return to the relevant chapter to familiarize or reacquaint yourself with the issues.

Throughout the book, we have used clinical examples to illustrate the concepts. As much as possible, we have used examples of direct relevance to nursing practice. However, there were times when the concepts were best illustrated using examples that were more medically focused. While these examples may not have direct relevance to all nurses, they do often have relevance to advanced practice nurses in primary health care and acute care settings. As nursing research continues to grow and develop, it will be easier to find illustrations that are more broadly applicable to nursing practice.

Some may find the CD-ROM version more convenient to use as the core content of the textbook is rendered to a format suitable for viewing, browsing, and searching on personal computers. All illustrations and tables are in a form suitable for electronic display, and there is a consistent navigational, iconographic, and graphical interface. Hypertext links allow you to quickly move from one section to another and to access glossary definitions and reference abstracts as you read. Interactive tools such as wizards, calculators, and worksheets allow you to work with the materials in ways that are not possible with the printed textbook and provide alternative ways for learning key concepts. We hope that this organization and functionality is well suited to the needs of any nurse who is eager to achieve an evidence-based practice.

Contents

PART I THE BASICS: USING THE NURSING LITERATURE

1 Introduction to Evidence-Based Nursing, *3*
2 Finding the Evidence, *20*
3 Health Care Interventions and Harm: An Introduction, *44*
4 Health Care Interventions, *48*
5 Harm, *71*
6 Diagnosis, *87*
7 Prognosis, *108*
8 Qualitative Research, *120*
9 Summarizing the Evidence Through Systematic Reviews, *137*
10 Moving From Evidence to Action Using Clinical Practice Guidelines, *154*
11 Changing Nursing Practice in an Organization, *172*

PART II BEYOND THE BASICS: USING AND TEACHING THE PRINCIPLES OF EVIDENCE-BASED NURSING

Unit I Health Care Interventions
12 Quality of Life, *205*
13 Surrogate Outcomes, *222*
14 Surprising Results of Randomized Controlled Trials, *235*
15 The Principle of Intention to Treat, *245*
16 When to Believe a Subgroup Analysis, *251*

Unit II Health Services Research
17 Health Services Interventions, *265*
18 Economic Evaluation, *298*
19 Computer Decision Support Systems, *318*

Unit III Diagnosis
20 Clinical Manifestations of Disease, *339*
21 Differential Diagnosis, *349*
22 Clinical Prediction Rules, *359*

Unit IV   Summarizing the Evidence Through Systematic Reviews
  23   Publication Bias, *373*
  24   Evaluating Differences in Study Results, *381*
  25   Fixed-Effects and Random-Effects Models, *388*

Unit V   Understanding the Results
  26   Bias and Random Error, *397*
  27   Measures of Association, *407*
  28   Hypothesis Testing, *423*
  29   Confidence Intervals, *432*
  30   Measuring Agreement Beyond Chance, *446*
  31   Regression and Correlation, *455*

Unit VI   Moving From Evidence to Action
  32   Number Needed to Treat, *469*
  33   Applying Results to Individual Patients, *481*
  34   Incorporating Patient Values, *490*
  35   Interpreting Levels of Evidence and Grades of Health Care
        Recommendations, *508*
  36   Recommendations About Screening, *526*

Appendix, *542*
Glossary, *547*

The Basics: Using the Nursing Literature

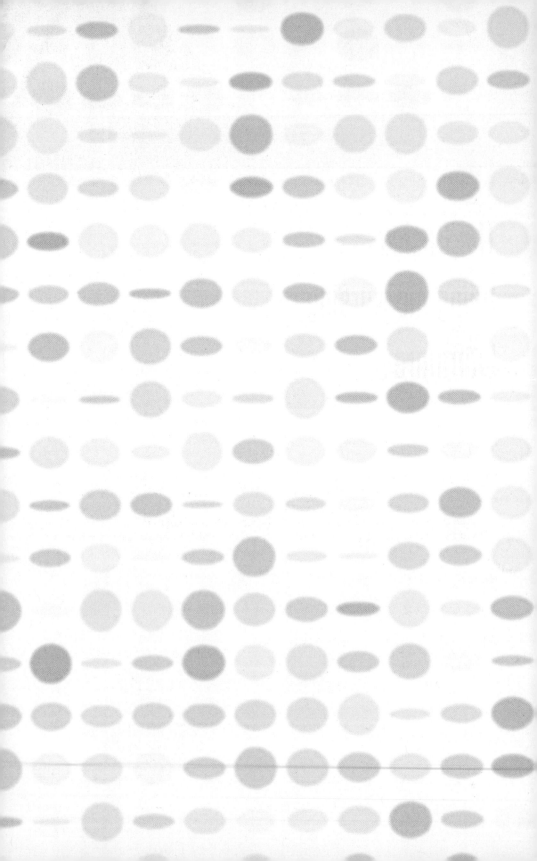

1

Introduction to Evidence-Based Nursing

Alba DiCenso, Donna Ciliska, and Gordon Guyatt

The following Editorial Board members also made substantive contributions to this chapter: Carole Estabrooks, Ellen Fineout-Overholt, Annette Flanagin, Kate Flemming, Sarah Hayward, Cathy Kessenich, Susan Marks, Dorothy McCaughan, Bernadette Melnyk, Mark Newman, Pauline Raynor, Kate Seers, Carl Thompson, and Margaret Wallace.

In This Chapter

What Is Evidence-Based Nursing?

Clinical Skills, Humanism, Social Responsibility, and Evidence-Based Nursing

Misconceptions About Evidence-Based Nursing
    Evidence-Based Nursing Ignores Patient Preferences and Values
    Evidence-Based Nursing Is Atheoretical
    Evidence-Based Nursing Is Only About Quantitative Research
    Evidence-Based Nursing Overemphasizes Randomized Controlled Trials and
        Systematic Reviews

Hierarchy of Evidence

Does Evidence-Based Nursing Make a Difference?

Barriers to Evidence-Based Nursing
    Strategies to Overcome Organization-Related Barriers to Evidence-Based
        Nursing

Two students in a graduate nursing program were reviewing the outline of a new course entitled "Evidence-Based Health Care." "That's a course I would like to take," said one student enthusiastically. She remarked that although she did not know anything about evidence-based nursing (EBN), she had heard that this shift toward evidence-based practice could revolutionize health care delivery. Her colleague looked skeptically at her and said that although this could be the right direction for medicine, it was not for nursing. He explained that he had heard that EBN did not support patient-centered care and that it was inconsistent with the values and interests of patients.

The differing viewpoints expressed by these two graduate students are commonly heard in nursing circles. Is there a place for EBN in the nursing profession? To answer this question, let's examine the definition of EBN, identify common misconceptions about EBN, consider whether EBN improves nursing practice, and identify barriers to EBN.

WHAT IS EVIDENCE-BASED NURSING?

Evidence-based practice is the integration of best research evidence with clinical expertise and patient values to facilitate clinical decision making.[1] Figure 1-1 depicts a model for evidence-based clinical decisions that builds on this definition. Evidence-based clinical decision making should incorporate consideration of the patient's *clinical state, the clinical setting, and clinical circumstances.*[2] For example, patients living in remote areas may not have access to the same diagnostic or treatment options that are available to patients living near tertiary care medical centers. Patients' clinical circumstances (e.g., severity of illness) will influence their response to a nursing intervention.

Identification and consideration of *patient preferences and actions* are central to evidence-based decision making. Patients may have no views or very strong views about their health care options depending on factors such as their condition, personal values and experiences, degree of aversion to risk, health care insurance and resources, accuracy of information at hand, and family.[2] Regardless of what their preferences may be, patients' actions may differ from both their preferences and their clinicians' advice. For example, patients may choose to quit smoking or to increase their physical activity, but they may then find it difficult to change these behaviors.

In nursing, *best research evidence* refers to methodologically sound, clinically relevant research about the effectiveness and safety of nursing interventions, the accuracy and precision of nursing assessment measures, the power of prognostic markers, the strength of causal relationships, the cost-effectiveness of nursing interventions, and the meaning of illness or patient experiences. Evidence-based practice posits a hierarchy of evidence to guide clinical decision making (discussed in more detail later in this chapter). A key element of evidence-based clinical decision making is personalizing the evidence to fit a specific patient's circumstances.[2]

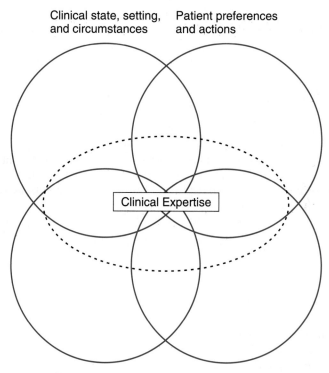

Clinical state, setting,   Patient preferences
and circumstances   and actions

Clinical Expertise

Research evidence   Health care resources

Figure 1-1. A model for evidence-based clinical decisions. *(Modified and reproduced with permission of the American College of Physicians from Haynes RB, Devereaux PJ, Guyatt GH. Clinical expertise in the era of evidence-based medicine and patient choice.* ACP J Club. *2002;136:A11-14.)*

We know that most decisions in health care have *resource implications* that nurses must consider. Occasions arise when decision makers may conclude that the potential benefits of an intervention are not worth the costs. Decision makers must always weigh the benefits and risks, inconvenience, and costs associated with alternative management strategies and, in doing so, consider the patient's values.[3]

Clinical expertise is overlaid as the means to integrate the other four components, thus constituting a fifth element in the model.[2] Clinical expertise refers to our ability to use clinical skills and past experience to identify the health state of patients or populations, their risks, their preferences and actions, and the potential benefits of interventions; to communicate information to patients and their families; and to provide them with an environment they find comforting and supportive.

Since the late 1970s, research utilization has been the focus of numerous articles in the nursing literature. Is EBN the same as research utilization? Estabrooks[4] defines research utilization as "the use of research findings in any and all aspects of one's work as a registered nurse" (p 19). EBN is much broader than research utilization because it encompasses not only research findings, but also other dimensions of clinical decision making such as clinical expertise, patient values, and resources.[1] The skills necessary for evidence-based practice include the ability to define a patient problem precisely and ascertain what information is required to resolve the problem, to conduct an efficient search of the literature, to select the best of the relevant studies, to apply rules of evidence to determine their validity, to extract the clinical message, to determine how the patient's values affect the balance between advantages and disadvantages of the available management options, to involve the patient appropriately in the decision, and to implement and evaluate the management plan.

Estabrooks[4] conducted a survey of 1500 randomly selected staff nurses drawn from the Alberta (Canada) Association of Registered Nurses membership list in 1996 to identify the frequency with which they used various sources of information. The respondents most frequently used experiential information sources (patient data, personal experience), followed by basic nursing education programs, in-service programs and conferences, policy and procedure manuals, physician sources, intuition, and "what has worked for years." Articles published in nursing research journals ranked second to last in frequency of usage (fifteenth of 16 ranked sources). Estabrooks identified several troubling issues from these data including the reliance on nonscientific knowledge and on basic nursing education, even though these nurses had graduated from their nursing education programs an average of 18 years earlier.

All too often we find it easier simply to rely on our formal, but increasingly dated, basic nursing education despite a full awareness that more recent research findings may inform changes in the way we do things. For example, many of us were taught to swab umbilical cords with alcohol; now we know from a randomized controlled trial (RCT) that swabbing the umbilical cord with sterile water shortens the time to cord separation without increasing infections.[5] Until recently, nursing students were taught sterile techniques for insulin injections; now we know that patients with diabetes can safely inject insulin through clothing.[6] There is an increased emphasis on early discharge from hospital with follow-up care in the community. From an RCT, we know, for example, that prompt hospital discharge with home care improves physical health and community reintegration and reduces initial length of hospital stay after acute stroke in comparison with usual care (discharge planning and clinician referral to follow-up services).[7]

CLINICAL SKILLS, HUMANISM, SOCIAL RESPONSIBILITY, AND EVIDENCE-BASED NURSING

The essential skills of assessing a patient or a population and the astute formulation of the health problem come only with thorough background training and extensive experience. Nurses make use of reasoning to interpret the results of the history, physical examination, or needs assessment. Clinical expertise is further required to define the relevant intervention options before one examines the evidence regarding the expected benefits and risks of those options.

Nurses also rely on their expertise to define features that influence the generalizability or relevance of study findings to their individual patients or population. They attempt to generalize results obtained in study patients to the individual patient before them. Nurses must judge the extent to which differences in intervention characteristics (local clinical expertise or the possibility of patient nonadherence, for instance) or patient characteristics (such as age, comorbidity, or concomitant treatment) may affect the benefits and risks that a patient can expect from an intervention.

Knowing the tools of evidence-based practice is necessary but not sufficient for delivering the highest-quality patient care. In addition to clinical knowledge, nurses require compassion, sensitive listening skills, and broad perspectives from the humanities and social sciences. These attributes allow understanding of patients' illnesses in the context of their experiences, personalities, and cultures.

Ideally, nurses are effective advocates for their patients both in the direct context of the health system in which they work and in broader health policy issues. Most nurses see their role as focusing on specific health care interventions for individual patients. Even when they consider preventive therapy, they often focus on individual patient behavior. However, we consider this focus to be too narrow. Nurses have a responsibility to consider their role in influencing the health of the society. Observational studies have consistently documented the inverse relationship between income and health.[8] There are numerous determinants of societal health, only one of which is the health care system. As well as delivering health care, nurses can play a crucial role in influencing public health policy to address determinants of health such as poverty and the environment. For example, observational studies have shown a strong and consistent association between pollution levels and respiratory and cardiovascular health.[9] Clinicians seeing patients with chronic obstructive pulmonary disease will suggest that they stop smoking. However, should they also be concerned with the polluted air that patients are breathing? We believe they should.

This book deals primarily with decision making at the level of the individual patient. Evidence-based approaches can also inform health policy making,[10] day-to-day decisions in public health, and systems-level decisions such as those facing hospital managers. In each of these arenas, EBN can support the appropriate goal of gaining the greatest health benefit from limited resources. Conversely, evidence—in support of an ideology, rather than a focus for reasoned debate—has been used as a justification for many agendas in health care, ranging from crude cost cutting to the promotion of extremely expensive technologies with minimal marginal returns.

In the policy arena, dealing with differing values poses even more challenges than in the arena of individual patient care. Should we restrict ourselves to alternative resource allocation within a fixed pool of health care resources, or should we trade off health care services against, for instance, lower tax rates for individuals or corporations? How should we deal with the large body of observational studies suggesting that social and economic factors may have a larger effect than health care delivery on the health of populations? How should we deal with the tension between what may be best for a person and what may be optimal for the society of which that person is a member? The debate about such issues is at the heart of evidence-based health policy making, but, inevitably, it has implications for decision making at the individual patient level.

MISCONCEPTIONS ABOUT EVIDENCE-BASED NURSING

There are four common misconceptions about EBN:
- Evidence-based nursing ignores patient preferences and values
- Evidence-based nursing is atheoretical
- Evidence-based nursing is only about quantitative research
- Evidence-based nursing overemphasizes randomized controlled trials and systematic reviews

Evidence-Based Nursing Ignores Patient Preferences and Values

A fundamental principle of EBN is that research evidence alone is never sufficient to make a clinical decision. Clinicians must always trade the benefits and risks, inconvenience, and costs associated with alternative management strategies and, in doing so, consider the patient's values.[2]

An RCT has shown that the addition of coping skills training provided by a nurse practitioner to a diabetes management program improved metabolic control and quality of life in adolescents with insulin-dependent, poorly controlled diabetes mellitus.[11] The intervention comprised intensive diabetes management that included three or more daily insulin injections or continuous subcutaneous insulin infusion, self-monitoring of blood glucose levels four or more times daily, monthly outpatient visits, interim telephone contact, and participation in a coping skills training program consisting of six weekly 1- to 1.5-hour small group sessions and monthly follow-up visits for 12 months. The small group sessions focused on developing coping skills around social problem solving, social skills training, cognitive behavior modification, and conflict resolution through role playing, with feedback and modeling of appropriate coping behavior by the nurse practitioner.[11]

Although the study results indicate that this program is effective, both patient preferences and costs may influence whether the intervention is practical and cost-effective. Many adolescents may be too shy or embarrassed to participate in small group sessions or may not be willing to invest the considerable time that this intervention would require. Of 105 adolescents who met the eligibility criteria for the coping skills training study, 77 (73%) agreed to participate; the major reason for refusal to participate was the amount of time it would take to be involved in the study.[11] From the perspective of cost-focused health care institutions, some may not be willing to fund this resource-intensive intervention.

The terms *patient values* and *preferences* refer to the underlying assumptions and beliefs that are involved when clinicians, along with patients, weigh what they will gain—or lose—when making a management decision. The explicit enumeration and balancing of benefits and risks that are central to EBN bring into bold relief the underlying value judgments involved in making management decisions.

Sensitive understanding of the patient connects to evidence-based practice in several ways. For some patients, incorporating their values in major decisions will mean a full enumeration of the possible benefits, risks, and inconveniences associated with alternative management strategies. Sometimes this discussion will involve their families. For other problems—the discussion of breast feeding with young mothers, for instance—attempts to involve family members may violate strong cultural norms.

Other patients are uncomfortable with an explicit discussion of benefits and risks, and they object to having what they perceive as excessive responsibility for decision making placed on them.[12] For such patients who want the health care team to make the decision on their behalf, the team's responsibility is to develop insight to ensure that choices will be consistent with patients' values and preferences. Understanding and implementing the decision-making process that patients desire and effectively communicating the information they need require clinicians to take the time to learn the extent to which patients want to be involved and to respond accordingly.[13]

Although we acknowledge that values play a role in every important patient care decision, our understanding of how to elicit and incorporate societal and individual values is limited. Health economists have played a major role in developing the science of measuring patient preferences.[14,15] Some decision aids incorporate patient values indirectly. If patients truly understand the potential risks and benefits, their decisions will likely reflect their preferences.[16] These developments in measuring patient preferences constitute a promising start. Nevertheless, there remain many unanswered questions about how to elicit patient preferences and how to incorporate them in clinical encounters already subject to crushing time pressures. Addressing these issues will be a challenge for EBN. We discuss these issues in more detail in Chapter 34, Incorporating Patient Values.

Evidence-Based Nursing Is Atheoretical

Some nurses believe that the "current call for evidence-based nursing practice has set the debate in a conventional, atheoretical, medically dominated, empirical model of evidence, which threatens the foundation of nursing's disciplinary perspective on theory-guided practice."[17] This concern is based on a perception that even though multiple patterns of knowing exist in nursing, EBN focuses only on empirical knowing and even more narrowly on RCTs as the only legitimate source of knowledge.[18] This misconception about RCTs is addressed later in this chapter but for now, let us examine the perception of EBN's exclusive focus on empirical knowing. Carper identified four ways of knowing in nursing: empirical, ethical, personal, and aesthetic.[19,20] Carper's work was significant because it highlighted the centrality of empirically derived theoretical knowledge but also recognized the equal importance of knowledge gained through clinical practice.[21] If we keep in mind the components of clinical decision making described earlier that included both research evidence and clinical experience, one can quickly see that EBN does indeed recognize the importance of clinical experience, patient preferences and values, and resource considerations.

To explore further the issue of whether EBN is atheoretical, let us examine the definition of theory. The word *theory* comes from the Greek word, *theoria*, which means "to see," that is, to reveal phenomena previously hidden from our awareness and attention.[22] Fawcett expanded this meaning to define theory as a way of seeing through "a set of relatively concrete and specific concepts and the propositions that describe or link those concepts."[23] Fawcett and colleagues[18] proposed that evidence must extend beyond the current emphasis on empirical research to the kinds of evidence generated from ethical theories, personal theories, and aesthetic theories. Ethical theories focus on the identification, analysis, and clarification of moral obligations and values. Personal theories focus on the interpersonal relationships in nursing, and aesthetic theories focus on understanding the patient's behavior and on the "artful" performance of manual and technical skills.[18] None of these are inconsistent with EBN as we defined it earlier. As long as we incorrectly interpret EBN as a synonym for research utilization and research-based practice,[24] Mitchell's criticisms of EBN may be justified: "(it) obstructs nursing process, human care, and professional accountability" (p 30); "restrains nurses from defining the values and theories that guide the nurse-person process" (p 31); and "does not support the shift to patient-centered care, is inconsistent with the values and interests of consumers"(p 34).[25] The more accurate view of EBN is that research use and research-based practice are subsets within the broader domain of EBN. Once seen in the context of the clinical decision-making process, EBN is consistent with all four patterns of knowing in nursing as described earlier.

Evidence-Based Nursing Is Only About Quantitative Research

The purpose of formal inquiry is to build knowledge in a discipline. Inquiry about clinical practice issues generally takes one of two paths. One path tests hypotheses and leads to quantitative findings numerically presented for the purpose of generalizing to a population and making predictions. The other path generates meaning or identifies patterns and leads to qualitative data for the purpose of describing. Both quantitative and qualitative data build nursing knowledge.[26]

For many years there has been an unfortunate tension between quantitative and qualitative researchers in nursing. This tension has created a polarity that some would say has been destructive to the advancement of nursing knowledge. More recently, however, there has been a shift to recognizing that both quantitative and qualitative methods are crucial to informing nursing practice.[27]

Some nurses also see the benefits of a critical nursing science that combines stories and numbers.[28] Wolfer noted "that arguments for the need for, or the superiority of, some methodologies over others (usually cast as quantitative vs. qualitative approaches) have essentially boiled down to a recognition that basically different types of problems require different methods" (p 141).[29]

Multiple paradigms of nursing science indicate a healthy scientific community because they encourage creativity, stimulate debate and exchange of ideas, provide diversity of views, promote productivity, and keep open avenues of inquiry.[30] Qualitative and quantitative modes of inquiry are complementary. Qualitative methods can describe phenomena of interest in nursing and can generate theories that propose relationships between identified concepts. Quantitative methods can test the relationships in qualitatively developed theories and can suggest whether the theories should be accepted or revised.[30]

Because quantitative methods have been the foundation of most biomedical research and because the concept of evidence-based practice evolved from applying the results of quantitative studies to clinical practice, many nurses incorrectly conclude that EBN is only about quantitative research. EBN involves the application of best research evidence in clinical decision making. The best research evidence can be quantitative or qualitative depending on the question asked. Quantitative designs are best for evaluating the effectiveness and safety of nursing interventions, the accuracy and precision of nursing assessment measures, the power of prognostic markers, the strength of causal relationships, and the cost-effectiveness of nursing interventions. Qualitative designs are best for understanding the meaning of illness or patient experiences, attitudes, and beliefs. Results of intervention studies may inform nurses about the optimal effects of an intervention in a sample of patients, but they do not explore and explain the barriers to patient adherence with the intervention, how the intervention affects the patient's everyday life, the meaning of illness to the patient, or the adjustment required to accommodate a lifelong treatment regimen. A key issue in EBN is whether the best design has been used to answer the question posed.

Examples of types of questions relevant to nursing practice are found in Table 1-1.

Table **1-1**   Examples of Research Questions of Relevance to Nursing

Effectiveness of Nursing Interventions

Can a multicomponent, senior center (day hospital) program led by a nurse practitioner reduce disability, increase activity, and improve management of chronic disease in older adults?[31]

Diagnosis (Nursing Assessment or Screening)

Can visual inspection of urine specimen clarity be used to exclude a diagnosis of urinary tract infection?[32]

Prognosis

In young children, is middle ear disease associated with subsequent behavior and cognitive problems?[33]

Harm (Causation or Etiology)

Are children who were exposed to antenatal corticosteroids and had birth weights ≤ 1500 gr at increased risk of adverse growth, cognitive, and lung function outcomes at age 14 years?[34]

Quality Improvement

For patients who require oral anticoagulation, is a nurse-led clinic that uses on-site blood testing and a computerized decision support system as effective as routine hospital care for maintaining appropriate international normalized ratios?[35]

Economic Evaluation

Is an in-hospital smoking cessation program for a general population of adult patients cost-effective?[36]

Clinical Prediction Guide

Are there demographic, perinatal, and psychosocial risk factors that can be used to develop a predictive index for postpartum depression?[37]

Understanding Meaning of Illness or Patient's Experiences, Beliefs, or Attitudes

What are parents' experiences of obtaining a diagnosis of cancer in their children?[38]

Evidence-Based Nursing Overemphasizes Randomized Controlled Trials and Systematic Reviews

Evidence-based practitioners search out the best available evidence to inform their clinical decision making. As can be seen from Table 1-1, nursing practice generates numerous questions, only a few of which are best addressed with an RCT. The RCT is the most appropriate design for evaluating the effectiveness and safety of a nursing intervention, such as whether protocol-directed sedation by nurses reduces the duration of mechanical ventilation in critically ill patients with acute respiratory failure.[39] The RCT is the most appropriate research design to address this type of question because through random assignment of patients to comparison groups, known and unknown determinants of outcome are most likely to be distributed evenly between the groups, a method ensuring that any difference in outcome is the result of the intervention being evaluated.

There are numerous examples of interventions both in nursing and in medicine that initially appeared beneficial, but when they were evaluated using randomized trials, they were shown to be of doubtful value or even harmful. Examples include the use of cover gowns by nurses when caring for healthy newborns in the nursery[40] and shaving of patients before surgical procedures.[41] Few of us would want to begin a drug regimen that had not been proved safe and effective in an RCT.

Different study designs best address other questions of importance to nursing practice. For example, observational studies are often best for questions of prognosis or harm. Qualitative designs are best to understand patients' experiences, attitudes, and beliefs. EBN is about the application of the best research to practice, be it an RCT to evaluate a nursing intervention, a cohort study to examine a question of prognosis, a case-control study to examine a causal association (when an RCT or cohort study is not possible), or a qualitative study to learn more about the meaning of illness.

Whenever possible, scientifically sound systematic reviews of the literature should be used instead of single studies. Given the play of chance, any single study, even a methodologically rigorous RCT, may arrive at a false conclusion. In a systematic review, all studies that address a specific research question are identified, relevant studies are critically appraised, data are extracted and summarized either quantitatively or nonquantitatively, and conclusions are drawn. When possible, data from the individual studies included in a systematic review are statistically combined (or pooled) to, in effect, create one large study. This process, known as *meta-analysis,* results in a more precise estimate of effect than can be obtained from any individual study included in the meta-analysis. Systematic reviews can be used to address all the questions listed in Table 1-1, including questions best addressed by qualitative studies. We describe systematic reviews in more detail in Chapter 9, Summarizing the Evidence Through Systematic Reviews.

HIERARCHY OF EVIDENCE

What is the nature of the evidence in EBN? We suggest a broad definition: any observation about the apparent relation between events constitutes potential evidence. Thus, the unsystematic clinical observations of an individual nurse constitute one source of evidence, and the results of physiologic experiments comprise another source.

Unsystematic observations can lead to important insights, and experienced nurses develop a healthy respect for the insights of their senior colleagues in issues of clinical observation and relations with patients and colleagues. Some of these insights can be taught, yet they rarely appear in the nursing literature.

At the same time, unsystematic clinical observations are limited by small sample size and, more important, by deficiencies in human processes of making inferences.[42] Predictions about intervention effects on clinically important outcomes based on physiologic experiments usually are correct, but occasionally they are disastrously wrong. We provide some examples of just how wrong predictions based on physiologic rationale can be in Chapter 14, Surprising Results of Randomized Controlled Trials.

Given the limitations of unsystematic clinical observations and physiologic rationale, EBN suggests a hierarchy of evidence. Table 1-2 presents a hierarchy of study designs to address questions about evaluations of nursing interventions; different hierarchies are necessary for questions about assessment, causation, or prognosis. Clinical research goes beyond unsystematic clinical observation in providing strategies that avoid or minimize erroneous results.

When considering research evidence about interventions, nurses generalize from results in other people to patients in their practice, an approach that inevitably weakens inferences about the impact of the intervention and introduces complex issues of how trial results apply to individual patients. Inferences may nevertheless be very strong if results come from a systematic review of high-quality RCTs with consistent results. However, inferences generally will be somewhat weaker if only a single RCT is being considered, unless it is very large and has enrolled a diverse patient population (see Table 1-2). Because observational studies may overestimate the effects of an intervention in an unpredictable fashion,[43,44] their results are far less trustworthy than those of randomized trials. Physiologic studies and unsystematic clinical observations provide the weakest inferences about intervention effects.

This hierarchy is not absolute. If intervention effects are sufficiently large and consistent, for instance, observational studies may provide more compelling evidence than most RCTs. By way of example, observational studies have allowed extremely strong inferences about the efficacy of insulin in diabetic ketoacidosis or that of hip replacement in patients with debilitating hip osteoarthritis. At the same time, instances in

Table 1-2   A Hierarchy of Strength of Evidence for Treatment Decisions

- Systematic reviews of randomized trials
- Single randomized trial
- Systematic review of observational studies addressing patient-important outcomes
- Single observational study addressing patient-important outcomes
- Physiologic studies (e.g., studies of blood pressure, cardiac output, exercise capacity, bone density)
- Unsystematic clinical observations

which RCT results contradict consistent findings from observational studies reinforce the need for caution. For example, observational studies have shown a significant benefit of adolescent pregnancy prevention interventions, whereas RCTs have not.[43] Defining the extent to which nurses should temper the strength of their inferences when only observational studies are available remains one of the important challenges for EBN. The challenge is particularly important given that much of the evidence regarding the harmful effects of treatments or interventions comes from observational studies.

This hierarchy of evidence implies a clear course of action for nurses considering alternative interventions to address patients' problems: nurses should look for the highest level of available evidence from the hierarchy of study designs relevant to their clinical question. The hierarchy makes clear that there always exists some form of evidence about the effect of a particular treatment or intervention. The evidence may be extremely weak—it may be the unsystematic observation of a single nurse or a generalization from physiologic studies that are related only indirectly—but there is always evidence.

DOES EVIDENCE-BASED NURSING MAKE A DIFFERENCE?

We do not have convincing studies showing that patients of clinicians who use evidence-based practices are better off than those of clinicians who do not; no one has done an RCT of evidence-based practice with patient outcomes as the measure of success. Such a trial would be impossible because the control group could not be effectively isolated from the research that evidence-based practice is attempting to transfer, and it would be regarded as unethical to attempt to do so.[45] However, in a meta-analysis designed to determine the contribution of research-based nursing practice to patient outcomes published in 1988, Heater and colleagues pooled results from 84 nurse-conducted research studies involving 4146 patients. The investigators reported that patients who received research-based nursing care made "sizeable gains" in behavioral, knowledge, physiologic, and psychosocial outcomes compared with those who received routine, procedural nursing care. Based on their review, the authors concluded that research-based nursing practice offers patients better outcomes than routine, procedural nursing care.[46]

Grounding nursing practice in evidence, rather than in tradition, is necessary to meet nursing's social obligation of accountability, to gain and maintain credibility among other health disciplines, and to build a nursing knowledge base that can be used to influence policy at agency and government levels.[47] Governments around the world are encouraging evidence-based practice. In Canada, the National Health Forum, a federally funded group charged with making health care recommendations, stated that "a key objective for the health sector should be to move rapidly toward the development of an evidence-based health system, in which decisions are made by health care providers, administrators, policy makers, patients and the public on the basis of appropriate, balanced and high quality evidence."[48] In the United Kingdom, the Department of Health stipulated that, to enhance the quality of patient care, nursing, midwifery, and health visiting, practice needs to be evidence based.[49]

In the United States, the Agency for Healthcare Research and Quality (AHRQ), formerly the Agency for Health Care Policy and Research (AHCPR), leads national efforts in the use of evidence to guide health care decisions through funding of evidence-based practice centers that undertake systematic reviews on selected clinical topics, sponsoring a National Guideline Clearinghouse of abstracts of evidence-based practice guidelines (*http://www.guideline.gov*), and funding studies that evaluate strategies for effectively disseminating research findings to practitioners and policy makers.[50]

BARRIERS TO EVIDENCE-BASED NURSING

Most nurses have a positive attitude about evidence-based practice.[51] However, there are substantial barriers to EBN, at both individual and organizational levels. At the individual level, nurses lack skill in evaluating the quality of research,[52] they are isolated from knowledgeable colleagues with whom to discuss research,[53] and they lack confidence to implement change.[52,54]

Organizational characteristics of health care settings are overwhelmingly the most significant barriers to research use among nurses.[52-55] Nurses have noted that they have insufficient time to go to the library to read or to implement findings from research.[51,53-56] Related to this problem is the inadequacy of library holdings in health care institutions, many of which lack nursing research journals.[57] Mitchell and colleagues found that health care institutions that reported making changes based on the research process were more likely to have at least one nursing research committee and to have access to nurses with expertise in nursing research.[57]

Nurses identified a lack of organizational support for EBN and noted lack of interest, lack of motivation, lack of leadership, and lack of vision, strategy, and direction among managers.[52] However, this organizational support is crucial in situations in which nurses do not believe they have the authority or autonomy to implement changes in patient care.[52-55] For example, a physician may read about the effectiveness of a new pain medication and can begin prescribing it immediately; nurses who identify a new effective nursing intervention for pain management must often obtain approval from nursing administration before implementing it.

Strategies to Overcome Organization-Related Barriers to Evidence-Based Nursing

One of the biggest challenges to evidence-based practice is time limitation. Fortunately, new resources for efficient searching of the literature are available, and the pace of innovation is rapid. One can consider a hierarchy of preprocessed information sources that comes with a mnemonic device, 5S: systems, synopses of syntheses (systematic reviews), syntheses (systematic reviews), synopses of single studies, and single studies. By *preprocessed,* we mean that someone has reviewed the literature and filtered out the flawed studies and included only the methodologically strongest studies.[58]

Systems include practice guidelines, clinical pathways, or evidence-based textbook summaries that integrate evidence-based information about specific clinical problems and provide regular updating (for details about practice guidelines, see Chapter 10, Moving from Evidence to Action Using Clinical Practice Guidelines). When no evidence-based information system exists for a clinical problem, then synopses of syntheses (systematic reviews) constitute the next best source. *Synopses of syntheses* encapsulate the key methodological details and results of a systematic review that are required to apply the evidence to individual patient care. Moving down the hierarchy, *syntheses* provide clinicians with a summary of all the evidence addressing a focused clinical question. When a systematic review does not exist on a topic, the next best source of evidence-based information is a *synopsis of a single study,* which summarizes the methodological details about the study and often addresses the clinical applicability of the study findings. At the bottom of the hierarchy are preprocessed *single studies,* which have been selected because they are both highly relevant and characterized by study designs that minimize bias and thus permit a high strength of inference[58] (Table 1-3) (see Chapter 2, Finding the Evidence).

Ciliska and colleagues[59] suggested numerous strategies to facilitate organizational support for EBN. These include the following: allowing nurses time for activities that foster EBN, such as going to the library, learning how to conduct electronic searches, and holding journal club meetings; establishing nurse researcher positions and formalizing nursing research committees; linking staff nurses and advanced practice nurses with university nurse faculty researchers; ensuring that the health care institution library has print or online subscriptions to nursing research journals; and making preprocessed evidence resources, such as *Clinical Evidence, Cochrane Library,* and abstraction journals, for example, *Evidence-Based Nursing,* available (see Chapter 2, Finding the Evidence).

One case study of nurses in acute care settings revealed that human sources such as clinical nurse specialists, physicians, and experienced clinical colleagues were seen as more

Table 1-3 A Hierarchy of Preprocessed Evidence

Systems	Practice guidelines, clinical pathways, or evidence-based textbook summaries of a clinical area provide the clinician with much of the information needed to guide the care of individual patients.
Synopses of syntheses (systematic reviews)	Synopses of systematic reviews encapsulate the key methodological details and results required to apply the evidence to individual patient care.
Syntheses (systematic reviews)	Systematic reviews provide clinicians with an overview of all the evidence addressing a focused clinical question.
Synopses of single studies	Synopses of individual studies encapsulate the key methodological details and results required to apply the evidence to individual patient care.
Single studies	Preprocessing involves selecting only those studies that are both highly relevant and characterized by study designs that minimize bias and thus permit a high strength of inference.

Modified and reproduced with permission of the BMJ Publishing Group from Haynes RB. Of studies, summaries, synopses, and systems: the "4S" evolution of services for finding current best evidence. Evid Based Ment Health. 2001;4:37-39.

accessible sources of research-based knowledge than were text-based or electronic resources.[60] The authors recommended that organizations may want to consider how persons in these roles could act as conduits through which research-based messages for practice, and information for clinical decision making, could flow.[60,61]

Evaluation of interventions to promote the implementation of research findings has been done predominantly in medicine,[62] and it has shown that simple dissemination of information is usually insufficient to change professional practice. Effective strategies include one-to-one sessions between experts, such as nurse facilitators, and individual staff members to explain the desired practice change; manual and computerized reminders to prompt behavior change; educational meetings in which learners actively participate; and audit and feedback, in which clinical performance is assessed through chart reviews or direct observation of practice, and feedback is provided. Multifaceted interventions that use more than one of these strategies are likely to be more effective than single interventions. Ineffective strategies include didactic continuing education workshops and conferences and written materials. For more details, see Chapter 11, Changing Nursing Practice in an Organization.

Centers for EBN have been established in Australia, New Zealand, Hong Kong, the United States, Germany, the United Kingdom, and Canada to educate nurses through workshops or formal courses on the use of EBN in clinical practice, to conduct systematic reviews, and to design and evaluate strategies for disseminating and using research to support EBN.[63]

CONCLUSION

Most criticisms of EBN are based on a different understanding of its philosophy than the one we offer. An accurate understanding of EBN is growing in the nursing community, and with this growth, enthusiasm for EBN increases. We must now address the challenges to evidence-based practice and teaching by facilitating efficient access to the evidence, helping clinicians apply that evidence to patient care, and discovering better ways to integrate patient values into the process of health care provision.

REFERENCES

1. Sackett DL, Straus SE, Richardson WS, Rosenberg WMC, Haynes RB. *Evidence-based Medicine: How to Practice and Teach EBM.* London: Churchill Livingstone; 2000.
2. Haynes RB, Devereaux PJ, Guyatt GH. Clinical expertise in the era of evidence-based medicine and patient choice. *ACP J Club.* 2002;136:A11-14.
3. DiCenso A, Cullum N, Ciliska D. Implementing evidence-based nursing: some misconceptions. *Evid Based Nurs.* 1998;1:38-40.
4. Estabrooks CA. Will evidence-based nursing practice make practice perfect? *Can J Nurs Res.* 1998;30:15-36.
5. Medves JM, O'Brien BA. Cleaning solutions and bacterial colonization in promoting healing and early separation of the umbilical cord in healthy newborns. *Can J Public Health.* 1997;88:380-382.
6. Fleming DR, Jacober SJ, Vandenberg MA, et al. The safety of injecting insulin through clothing. *Diabetes Care.* 1997;20:244-247.
7. Mayo NE, Wood-Dauphinee S, Cote R, et al. There's no place like home: an evaluation of early supported discharge for stroke. *Stroke.* 2000;31:1016-1023.
8. Evans R. Interpreting and addressing inequalities in health: from Black to Acheson to Blair to…? UK Office of Health Economics; 2002. Available at: *http://www.ohe.org.* Accessed November 7, 2002.
9. Dockery DW, Brunekreef B. Longitudinal studies of air pollution effects on lung function. *Am J Respir Crit Care Med* 1996;154(suppl):250-256.

10. Muir Gray JA, Haynes RB, Sackett DL, Cook DJ, Guyatt GH. Transferring evidence from research into practice, 3: developing evidence-based clinical policy. *ACP J Club*. 1997;126:A14-16.

11. Grey M, Boland EA, Davidson M, Li J, Tamborlane WV. Coping skills training for youth with diabetes mellitus has long-lasting effects on metabolic control and quality of life. *J Pediatr*. 2000;137:107-113.

12. Sutherland HJ, Llewellyn-Thomas HA, Lockwood GA, Tritchler DL, Till JE. Cancer patients: their desire for information and participation in treatment decisions. *J R Soc Med*. 1989;82:260-263.

13. Paterson B. Myth of empowerment in chronic illness. *J Adv Nurs*. 2001;34:574-581.

14. Drummond MF, Richardson WS, O'Brien B, Levine M, Heyland DK, for the Evidence-Based Medicine Working Group. Users' Guides to the Medical Literature, XIII: how to use an article on economic analysis of clinical practice. A. Are the results of the study valid? *JAMA*. 1997;277:1552-1557.

15. Feeny DH, Furlong W, Boyle M, Torrance GW. Multi-attribute health status classification systems: health utilities index. *Pharmacoeconomics*. 1995;7:490-502.

16. O'Connor AM, Rostom A, Fiset V, et al. Decision aids for patients facing health treatment or screening decisions: systematic review. *BMJ*. 1999;319:731-734.

17. Walker PH, Redmond R. Theory-guided, evidence-based reflective practice. *Nurs Sci Q*. 1999;12:298-303.

18. Fawcett J, Watson J, Neuman B, Walker PH, Fitzpatrick JJ. On nursing theories and evidence. *J Nurs Scholarsh*. 2001;33:115-119.

19. Carper B. Fundamental patterns of knowing in nursing. *ANS Adv Nurs Sci*. 1978;1:13-23.

20. Carper BA. Fundamental patterns of knowing in nursing. In: Polifroni EC, Welch M, eds. *Perspectives on Philosophy of Science in Nursing: An Historical and Contemporary Anthology*. Philadelphia: JB Lippincott; 1999:12–19.

21. Stein KF, Corte C, Colling KB, Whall A. A theoretical analysis of Carper's Ways of Knowing using a model of social cognition....including commentary by Higgins P. *Schol Inq Nurs Pract*. 1998;12:43-64.

22. Watson J. *Postmodern Nursing and Beyond*. New York, NY: Churchill Livingstone; 1999.

23. Fawcett J. *The Relationship of Theory and Research*. 3rd ed. Philadelphia: FA Davis; 1999.

24. Mowinski Jennings B, Loan LA. Misconceptions among nurses about evidence-based practice. *J Nurs Scholarsh*. 2001;33:121-127.

25. Mitchell GJ. Evidence-based practice: critique and alternative view. *Nurs Sci Q*. 1999;12:30-35.

26. Parse RR. Building knowledge through qualitative research: the road less traveled. *Nurs Sci Q*. 1996;9:10-16.

27. Hawley P, Young S, Pasco AC. Reductionism in the pursuit of nursing science: (in)congruent with nursing's core values? *Can J Nurs Res*. 2000;32:75-88.

28. Berman H, Ford-Gilboe M, Campbell JC. Combining stories and numbers: a methodologic approach for a critical nursing science. *ANS Adv Nurs Sci*. 1998;21:1-15.

29. Wolfer J. Aspects of "reality" and ways of knowing in nursing: in search of an integrating paradigm. *Image J Nurs Sch*. 1993;25:141-146.

30. Monti EJ, Tingen MS. Multiple paradigms of nursing science. *ANS Adv Nurs Sci*. 1999;21:64-80.

31. Leveille SG, Wagner EH, Davis C, et al. Preventing disability and managing chronic illness in frail older adults: a randomized trial of a community-based partnership with primary care. *J Am Geriatr Soc*. 1998;46:1191-1198.

32. Bulloch B, Bausher JC, Pomerantz WJ, Connors JM, Mahabee-Gittens M, Dowd MD. Can urine clarity exclude the diagnosis of urinary tract infection? *Pediatrics*. 2000;106:E60.

33. Bennett KE, Haggard MP. Behaviour and cognitive outcomes from middle ear disease. *Arch Dis Child*. 1999;80:28-35.

34. Doyle LW, Ford GW, Rickards AL, et al. Antenatal corticosteroids and outcome at 14 years of age in children with birth weight less than 1501 grams. *Pediatrics*. 2000;106:E2.

35. Fitzmaurice DA, Hobbs FD, Murray ET, Holder RL, Allan TF, Rose PE. Oral anticoagulation management in primary care with the use of computerized decision support and near-patient testing: a randomized, controlled trial. *Arch Intern Med*. 2000;160:2343-2348.

36. Meenan RT, Stevens VJ, Hornbrook MC, et al. Cost-effectiveness of a hospital-based smoking cessation intervention. *Med Care*. 1998;36:670-678.

37. Nielsen Forman D, Videbech P, Hedegaard M, et al. Postpartum depression: identification of women at risk. *Br J Obstet Gynaecol*. 2000;107:1210-1217.

38. Dixon-Woods M, Findlay M, Young B, Cox H, Heney D. Parents' accounts of obtaining a diagnosis of childhood cancer. *Lancet.* 2001;357:670-674.

39. Brook AD, Ahrens TS, Schaiff R, et al. Effect of a nursing-implemented sedation protocol on the duration of mechanical ventilation. *Crit Care Med.* 1999;27:2609-2615.

40. Rush J, Fiorino-Chiovitti R, Kaufman K, Mitchell A. A randomized controlled trial of a nursery ritual: wearing cover gowns to care for healthy newborns. *Birth.* 1990;17:25-30.

41. Hoe NY, Nambiar R. Is preoperative shaving really necessary? *Ann Acad Med Singapore.* 1985;14:700-704.

42. Nisbett R, Ross L. *Human Inference.* Englewood Cliffs, NJ: Prentice-Hall; 1980.

43. Guyatt GH, DiCenso A, Farewell V, Willan A, Griffith L. Randomized trials versus observational studies in adolescent pregnancy prevention. *J Clin Epidemiol.* 2000;53:167-174.

44. Kunz R, Oxman AD. The unpredictability paradox: review of empirical comparisons of randomised and non-randomised clinical trials. *BMJ.* 1998;317:1185-1190.

45. Haynes RB. What kind of evidence is it that evidence-based medicine advocates want health care providers and consumers to pay attention to? *BMC Health Serv Res* [serial online]. 2002;2:3. Available at: *http://www.biomedcentral.com/1472-6963/2/3.* Accessed November 7, 2002.

46. Heater BS, Becker AM, Olson RK. Nursing interventions and patient outcomes: a meta-analysis of studies. *Nurs Res.* 1988;37:303-307.

47. Rafael ARF. Evidence-based practice: the good, the bad, the ugly, part 1. *Regist Nurs J.* 2000;12:5-6, 9.

48. National Forum on Health. *Canada Health Action: Building on the Legacy.* Vol. 1. Ottawa: National Forum on Health; 1997:3-43.

49. UK Department of Health. Making a difference: strengthening the nursing, midwifery and health visiting contribution to health and healthcare. 1999. Available at: *http://www.doh.gov.uk/nurstrat.htm.* Accessed November 7, 2002.

50. Titler MG. Use of research in practice. In: LoBiondo-Wood G, Haber J, eds. *Nursing Research.* 5th ed. St. Louis: Mosby-Year Book; 2002:411–444.

51. Upton D. Attitudes towards, and knowledge of, clinical effectiveness in nurses, midwives, practice nurses and health visitors. *J Adv Nurs.* 1999;29:885-893.

52. Parahoo K. Barriers to, and facilitators of, research utilization among nurses in Northern Ireland. *J Adv Nurs.* 2000;31:89-98.

53. Nilsson Kajermo K, Nordstrom G, Krusebrant A, Bjorvell H. Barriers to and facilitators of research utilization, as perceived by a group of registered nurses in Sweden. *J Adv Nurs.* 1998;27:798-807.

54. Rodgers S. An exploratory study of research utilization by nurses in general medical and surgical wards. *J Adv Nurs.*1994;20:904-911.

55. Retsas A. Barriers to using research evidence in nursing practice. *J Adv Nurs.* 2000;31:599-606.

56. Retsas A, Nolan M. Barriers to nurses' use of research: an Australian hospital study. *Int J Nurs Stud.* 1999;36:335-343.

57. Mitchell A, Janzen K, Pask E, Southwell D. Assessment of nursing research utilization needs in Ontario health agencies. *Can J Nurs Admin.* 1995;8:77-91.

58. Haynes RB. Of studies, summaries, synopses, and systems: the "4S" evolution of services for finding current best evidence. *Evid Based Ment Health.* 2001;4:37-39.

59. Ciliska DK, Pinelli J, DiCenso A, Cullum N. Resources to enhance evidence-based nursing practice. *AACN Clin Issues.* 2001;12:520-528.

60. Thompson C, McCaughan D, Cullum N, Sheldon TA, Mulhall A, Thompson DR. The accessibility of research-based knowledge for nurses in United Kingdom acute care settings. *J Adv Nurs.* 2001;36:11-22.

61. Thompson C, McCaughan D, Cullum N, Sheldon TA, Mulhall A, Thompson DR. Research information in nurses' clinical decision-making: what is useful? *J Adv Nurs.* 2001;36:376-388.

62. Bero LA, Grilli R, Grimshaw JM, Harvey E, Oxman AD, Thomson MA. Closing the gap between research and practice: an overview of systematic reviews of interventions to promote the implementation of research findings: the Cochrane Effective Practice and Organization of Care Review Group. *BMJ.* 1998;317:465-468.

63. Ciliska D, DiCenso A, Cullum N. Implementation forum: centres of evidence-based nursing: directions and challenges. *Evid Based Nurs.* 1999;2:102-104.

2

Finding the Evidence

Seana Collins, Tanya Voth, Alba DiCenso, and Gordon Guyatt

The following Editorial Board members also made substantive contributions to this chapter: Lazelle Benefield, Phyllis Brenner, Olga Cortes, Rien de Vos, Kate Flemming, and Karen Smith.

We gratefully acknowledge the work of Ann McKibbon, Dereck Hunt, Scott Richardson, Robert Hayward, Mark Wilson, Roman Jaeschke, Brian Haynes, Peter Wyer, and Jonathan Craig on the original chapter that appears in the Users' Guides to the Medical Literature, *edited by Guyatt and Rennie.*

In This Chapter

Ways of Using the Health Care Literature
    Background and Foreground Questions
    Keeping Up To Date
    Informing Clinical Decision Making

Framing the Question
    Example 1: Smoking Cessation
    Example 2: Hand Washing
    Example 3: Menopause and Hormone Replacement Therapy
    Example 4: Caregiver Stress
    Example 5: Organ Transplant Follow-up

Searching for the Answer
    Determining Question Type
    Quantitative Studies
    Qualitative Studies
    Systematic Reviews

Sources of Evidence
    Selecting the Best Nursing Information Resources
    Using Preprocessed Nursing Information Resources
    Using Unprocessed Nursing Information Resources

Evidence-based practice challenges nurses to integrate best research evidence with clinical expertise, patient circumstances and values, and resource considerations to facilitate clinical decision making, but how do nurses locate the best evidence when the sheer volume of nursing literature is more than any nurse can manage? *Ulrich's Periodicals Directory* on-line lists more than 800 nursing journals.[1] To compound this problem further, many studies of relevance to nursing are published in periodicals other than nursing journals (e.g., medical journals, social science journals, allied health literature). Once nurses locate studies of interest, they face the daunting task of discriminating sound studies from fatally flawed investigations. The advent of the Internet has resulted in access to huge volumes of information, some of high quality and some of questionable worth, which only further confuses and complicates the integration of quality evidence into clinical decision making. Work settings have historically presented obstacles or failed to provide expertise and supportive environments to facilitate evidence-based nursing.[2-4] Examples of obstacles include the absence of nursing research journals in the libraries of health care settings, insufficient time for nurses to locate and read research reports, and lack of support and leadership from nurse managers to implement evidence-based findings.

All health care providers face the task of managing an overwhelming amount of information. There is rarely time during the work day to sit down, let alone to skim articles and search for evidence relevant to one's practice. Nurses are highly motivated to be evidence-based practitioners, but one of the major barriers is their lack of skill in efficiently locating high-quality research evidence.[4,5] In this chapter, we help you to refine these skills. We outline the reasons nurses access the health care literature, describe how to frame a research question, review quantitative and qualitative research designs to address various types of research questions, and describe resources that are most likely to lead nurses efficiently to high-quality relevant research evidence.

WAYS OF USING THE HEALTH CARE LITERATURE

This book is about using the health care literature to keep up to date and to inform your clinical decision making.

Background and Foreground Questions

Initially, the primary interest of nursing students is in understanding normal human physiology and the pathophysiology associated with a patient's condition or problem. When presented with a patient problem, nurses' first questions are likely to include, for example, what is a pressure ulcer, why did this patient develop it, and how can we manage it?

By contrast, experienced nurses ask different sorts of questions. They are interested less in the diagnostic approach to a presenting problem and more in how to interpret a specific diagnostic test, less in the general prognosis of a disease and more in a particular patient's prognosis, less in the management strategies that could be applied to a patient's problems and more in the risks and benefits of a particular intervention compared with an alternative management strategy. Experienced nurses are also more interested in the meaning of illness or patient experiences.

Think of the first set of questions, those of nursing students, as background questions; think of the second set as foreground questions. In most situations, clinicians need to understand the background thoroughly before it makes sense to address issues in the foreground.

On his or her first day on the ward or unit, a nursing student will still need to acquire a great deal of background knowledge. However, in deciding how to manage the first patient seen, the nursing student may also need to address a foreground issue. A seasoned nurse, although well versed in issues that represent the background of his or her clinical practice, may nevertheless occasionally require background information. This may happen when new conditions or medical syndromes appear (consider that as recently as 20 years ago, experienced clinicians were asking, "What is the acquired immunodeficiency syndrome?") or when new diagnostic tests or treatment modalities are introduced into the clinical arena. At every stage of training and experience, clinicians' grasp of the relevant background issues of health problems informs their ability to identify and formulate the most pertinent foreground questions for individual patients (or families or communities).

Figure 2-1 represents the evolution of the questions we ask as we progress from being novices (who pose almost exclusively background questions) to being experts (who pose

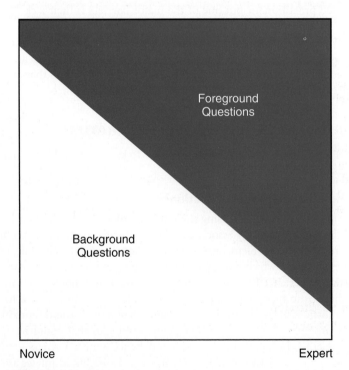

Figure 2-1. Asking questions.

almost exclusively foreground questions). This book is devoted to how nurses can use the health care literature to solve their foreground questions.

Keeping Up To Date

We need only to read a newspaper to know that investigators are continually reporting new research findings. In an effort to stay current with scientific developments in their specialty area, many nurses subscribe to journals, have tables of contents sent to them by email, or scan various Web sites and on-line resources. Most nurses are likely to skim or browse these resources quickly, or if they do not have sufficient time to browse, they may feel overwhelmed by the magnitude of the reading pile. Compounding this is the problem that only a few of the studies published in core health care journals are both of high quality and clinically useful. In this chapter, we offer some solutions on how to keep up efficiently with high-quality research of relevance to nursing practice.

If keeping up to date with developments in your specialty area is your goal, perhaps the most efficient strategy is to restrict your browsing to secondary journals. A secondary journal does not publish original research but rather includes synopses of published research studies that meet criteria of both clinical relevance and methodological quality. *Evidence-Based Nursing* (www.evidencebasednursing.com) summarizes high-quality studies of relevance to nursing that are identified through review of each issue of more than 100 health care journals. We describe this secondary journal in more detail later in this chapter. Depending on your specialty area, other secondary journals may be of interest, such as *Evidence-Based Medicine, Evidence-Based Mental Health, Evidence-Based Cardiovascular Medicine,* and *ACP Journal Club.*

Informing Clinical Decision Making

Another way for nurses to deal with the overwhelming amount of published research is to use a problem-solving mode. Here, nurses define specific questions raised in caring for patients and then consult the literature to resolve these questions. Whether you are operating in the browsing mode to keep up to date or the problem-solving mode to inform clinical decision making, this book can help you to judge the validity of the information in the articles you are examining, gain a clear understanding of their results, and apply them to patient care. Each chapter is devoted to a nursing topic and takes you through the steps of assessing clinical problems, searching for evidence, appraising the literature, and applying research results to your practice. When you have learned the skills, you will be surprised at the small proportion of research studies to which you need to attend and the efficiency with which you can identify them.

FRAMING THE QUESTION

Searches of the literature are most likely to be successful if they are based on well-formulated questions. Clinical questions often spring to clinicians' minds in a form that makes finding answers in the health care literature a challenge. Dissecting a question into its component parts to facilitate finding the best evidence is a fundamental skill of evidence-based practitioners.[6,7] The searchable question requires focus to avoid complicated and time-consuming searches that retrieve irrelevant material. The nature of the question will determine whether it is likely to be addressed by a quantitative study or a qualitative study. Quantitative studies are most appropriate when answering questions of "how many" or "how much." Qualitative studies are more appropriate when answering questions about how people "feel about" or "experience" certain situations and conditions.[8] We can divide most quantitative questions into three parts:

1. **The population.** Who are the patients or clients? Are they individual persons, families, communities, or groups? Is there a particular age or sex grouping? What is their specific health care problem?

2. **The interventions or exposures.** For issues of health care or health services interventions, what preventive, therapeutic, or health services interventions are we interested in knowing more about? What are the management strategies we are interested in comparing? For issues of harm, what potentially harmful *exposure* are we concerned about? In such studies, there will usually two or more parts: the intervention or exposure and a control or alternative intervention or exposure.

3. **The outcome.** What are the patient-relevant consequences of the intervention or exposure in which we are interested?

Most qualitative questions can be divided into two parts:

1. **The population.** Who are the patients or clients? Are they individual persons, families, communities, or groups? Is there a particular age or sex grouping? What is their specific health care problem?

2. **The situation.** What circumstances, conditions, or experiences are we interested in knowing more about?

We now provide examples of the transformation of unstructured clinical questions into structured questions that facilitate use of the health care literature. Once we formulate the structured question, we can extract keywords from the question to guide the search process.

Example 1: Smoking Cessation

You are a school nurse at a large high school in your community. You have just completed a day of information sessions on the harmful effects of smoking and have offered to meet with students who are interested in quitting smoking. The next day you are visited in your office by an 18-year-old girl who has smoked half a pack of cigarettes a day for the past year. She has tried unsuccessfully to quit smoking. She asks you whether "the patch" works.

Type of Study: Quantitative

Initial Question: Is the nicotine patch effective?

Digging Deeper: One limitation of the formulation of this question is that it does not specify the population. The effectiveness of the nicotine patch may differ in adolescents versus adults, in women versus men, in those who smoke many cigarettes versus those who smoke fewer cigarettes per day, as well as in those who have smoked for many years versus a few years. Another limitation of this question is the absence of an outcome, which we know to be smoking cessation.

Improved (Searchable) Question: A searchable question would specify the relevant patient population, the management strategy, and the patient-relevant consequences of that intervention, as follows:

Population: Young women who are moderate smokers
Intervention: Nicotine replacement therapy
Outcome: Smoking cessation

Formulated Question: Among young women who are moderate smokers, does nicotine replacement therapy increase the probability of smoking cessation?

Example 2: Hand Washing

You are a staff nurse who has been asked to join an infection control committee in the hospital to address the issue of hand washing in light of the recent outbreak of severe acute respiratory syndrome in neighboring communities. The committee has decided that all persons entering the hospital must wash their hands, but committee members disagree on how best to implement this recommendation. Some committee members believe that antiseptic soap must be used, and others believe that a waterless, alcohol-based solution would be preferable. You offer to seek out studies that could help the committee to make a final decision.

Type of Study: Quantitative
Initial Question: Is a waterless, alcohol-based solution an effective agent for hand washing?
Digging Deeper: Although this question identifies a waterless, alcohol-based solution as the intervention of interest, it fails to provide additional necessary details. It does not include specific information about the population, the alternative intervention, or the outcome that we are interested in achieving.
Improved (Searchable) Question: A searchable question would specify the relevant patient population, the management strategy, and the patient-relevant consequences of that strategy, as follows:

Population: All persons entering the hospital
Intervention: Waterless, alcohol-based solution versus antiseptic soap
Outcome: Bacterial hand contamination

Formulated Question: For persons entering a health facility, is hand rubbing with a waterless, alcohol-based solution as effective as standard hand washing with antiseptic soap for reducing hand contamination?

Example 3: Menopause and Hormone Replacement Therapy

A 51-year-old woman who has had a total hysterectomy presents to the nurse practitioner in a primary health care clinic with signs and symptoms of menopause. She is experiencing hot flashes, night sweats, and disturbed sleep. She is a healthy, active woman with no family history of breast cancer or cardiovascular disease. She has been reluctant to consider hormone replacement therapy (HRT) because she heard about a study that was stopped early because women taking HRT had a higher risk of breast cancer and heart attacks. However, the menopause symptoms are seriously affecting her quality of life, and she feels she has to do something about them.

Type of Study: Quantitative

Initial Question: Is it safe to prescribe HRT for this woman?

Digging Deeper: The initial question gives us little idea of where to look in the literature for an answer. We can break down the issue by noting that the woman has had a total hysterectomy and therefore will require estrogen only, rather than the combination of estrogen and progestin. We recall that although the study of combination HRT has been completed, the study of estrogen alone is continuing, and the results are not yet available. We also note that the patient is 51 years old and will be taking estrogen for relief of menopausal symptoms on a short-term basis compared with women in the past, who had taken HRT over a long period. The patient has no family history of breast cancer or heart disease.

What outcomes are important to this woman? Certainly, alleviation of menopausal symptoms is important, but given her concerns about the link between HRT and breast cancer and between HRT and heart disease, she will need information about these relationships to make an informed decision.

Improved (Searchable) Question: A searchable question would specify the relevant patient population, the management strategy and exposure, and the patient-relevant consequences of that exposure, as follows:

Population: Middle-aged women with symptoms of menopause
Intervention/Exposure: Estrogen
Outcomes: Development of new breast cancer, myocardial infarction, angina, stroke, and cardiovascular death

Formulated Question: Among healthy middle-aged women, does estrogen increase the incidence of breast cancer, ischemic cardiovascular disease, cardiovascular death, or stroke?

Example 4: Caregiver Stress

You are a public health nurse who has been visiting an elderly man with Alzheimer's disease who is living at home. His daughter is his primary caregiver. As his condition deteriorates, she is increasingly worried about his safety and finds the situation physically and emotionally draining. The daughter is experiencing anguish and guilt as she realizes that her father will soon need to be placed in a special care unit. She asks you whether others in this situation have similar feelings and what she can expect to feel once he is placed in the special care unit.

Type of Study: Qualitative

Initial Question: What is it like to place a relative in special care?

Digging Deeper: Limitations of this formulation of the question include failure to specify the population and insufficient detail about the situation.

Improved (Searchable) Question: A searchable question would specify the relevant patient population and situation, as follows:

Population: Caregivers
Situation: Placing a relative with Alzheimer's disease in a special care unit

Formulated Question: How do caregivers describe their experiences of deciding to place a relative with Alzheimer's disease in a special care unit?

Example 5: Organ Transplant Follow-up

You are a nurse practitioner working in a multiorgan adult transplant follow-up clinic. At the age of 18 years, patients who had organ transplants as children transfer their care from the pediatric transplant center to the adult transplant center where you work. You have noticed that these young people have difficulties adapting to the new health care setting and team. Many of them make frequent visits to the emergency department, are admitted to hospital, are noncompliant with medication, and have depression, violent episodes, and family problems. You are considering developing a transition program to help these young people adjust to the adult transplant program but do not feel that you fully understand what they experience.

Type of Study: Qualitative
Initial Question: What is it like to have care transferred from a pediatric center to an adult clinic?
Digging Deeper: Limitations of this formulation of the question include failure to specify the population and to provide sufficient detail about the situation.
Improved (Searchable) Question: A searchable question would specify the relevant patient population and situation, as follows:

Population: Young adult transplant recipients
Situation: Transition from a pediatric transplant program to an adult transplant program

Formulated Question: How do young adult transplant recipients experience the process of transition from a pediatric transplant program to an adult transplant program?

These examples illustrate that constructing a searchable question that allows clinicians to use the health care literature to generate an answer is often no simple matter. It requires an in-depth understanding of the clinical issues involved in patient management. The five foregoing examples illustrate that each patient may trigger a large number of clinical questions, and clinicians must give careful thought to what they really want to know. Bearing the structure of the question in mind is extremely helpful in arriving at an answerable question.

Once the question is posed, the next step is translating the question into an effective search strategy. Developing a search strategy is easier if you first identify the components of the question.

SEARCHING FOR THE ANSWER

In this section, we demonstrate how the careful definition of a quantitative or qualitative research question can help you to develop a workable search strategy. However, you must also consider a fourth component. What type of study do you hope to find? By type of study, we mean the way the study is organized or constructed, the *study design*.

Determining Question Type

In nursing, as in other health professions, we ask different types of research questions. We ask about the prevention, treatment, assessment, cause, course, economics, and meaning of health problems managed by nurses. Part I of this book addresses issues of study design. The following is a brief introduction:

Health Care Interventions (or Treatment, Prevention, Therapy): Determining the effect of different interventions on improving patient function or avoiding adverse events

Harm (or Causation, Etiology): Ascertaining the effects of potentially harmful agents on patient function, morbidity, and mortality

Prognosis: Estimating the future course of a patient's disease or condition

Diagnosis (or Assessment): Establishing the power of a diagnostic tool to differentiate between persons with and persons without a target condition or disease

Meaning: Describing, exploring, and explaining phenomena being studied (focus on process rather than outcome)

Economics: Studying the economic efficiency of health care programs or interventions

Once you have determined the type of question you are asking, you will be better equipped to search the literature for evidence. The next section provides an overview of quantitative and qualitative study designs.

Quantitative Studies

To evaluate nursing interventions, we identify studies in which a process analogous to flipping a coin determines participants' receipt of an experimental or standard treatment, the so-called *randomized controlled trial* (see Chapter 4, Health Care Interventions). Once investigators allocate participants to treatment or control groups, they follow them forward in time to determine whether they experience an *outcome* of interest, such as reduced hospital stay, pain relief, or wound healing (Figure 2-2).

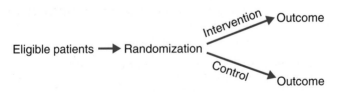

Figure 2-2. Randomized controlled trial.

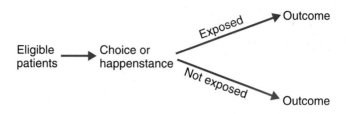

Direction of data collection: assessment of exposure →
presence of outcome

Figure 2-3. Observational study (cohort study).

Ideally, we would also look to randomized trials to address issues of harm. However, for many potentially harmful exposures, randomly allocating patients is neither practical nor ethical. For instance, one could not suggest to potential study participants that an investigator will decide by the flip of a coin whether or not they smoke during the next 20 years. For exposures such as smoking, the best one can do is to identify studies in which personal choice, or happenstance, determines whether people are exposed or not exposed to potential harm. These are called *observational studies,* and they provide weaker evidence than do randomized trials.

Figure 2-3 depicts a common observational study design in which patients with and without the exposure of interest are followed forward in time to determine whether they experience the outcome of interest. The specific term for this particular observational study is *cohort study.*

Figure 2-4 depicts another observational study design in which investigators identify patients with and without the target outcome and look back in time to determine whether they have had exposure to the potentially harmful agent. The specific term for this observational study is *case-control study.* We use the relationship between smoking and lung cancer to illustrate the differences between these two types of observational studies.

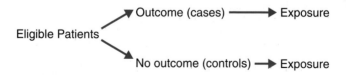

Direction of data collection: presence of outcome →
assessment of exposure

Figure 2-4. Observational study (case-control study).

In a cohort study, the investigator identifies smokers and nonsmokers and follows them forward in time to monitor the occurrence of lung cancer in each group. In a case-control study, the investigator identifies a group of people who have lung cancer (cases) and a group of people who do not have lung cancer (controls) but who are reasonably similar to those with lung cancer with respect to important determinants of outcome such as age, sex, and concurrent medical conditions. The investigator then asks the cases and controls about their smoking history.

A third type of observational study examines patients' prognosis and may identify factors that modify that prognosis. Here, investigators identify one group of patients (e.g., pregnant women, patients undergoing surgery, or children with middle ear infection) and follow them forward in time. Investigators collect data about factors that may modify their prognosis (e.g., age, comorbidity). At the end of the follow-up period, investigators identify those patients who experience the target outcome and compare them with those who do not experience the target outcome. For example, having followed up a group of pregnant women, investigators determine how many of the women have a premature delivery and compare these women with those who did not have a premature delivery to identify factors that influenced the outcome (e.g., age of mother, parity). In the case of patients undergoing surgery, investigators may follow them up to identify how many patients develop a postoperative infection and then, by comparing them with those who do not develop an infection, identify the factors that contributed to the infection. Finally, investigators may follow up a group of children who had middle ear infection and determine how many later develop behavior problems and, by comparing them with the group of children who do not develop behavior problems, identify factors that distinguish the two groups (Figure 2-5).

To establish how well a diagnostic test works (what we call its *properties* or *operating characteristics*), we need yet another study design. In diagnostic test studies, investigators

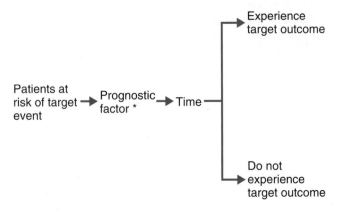

* Also known as *determinant of outcome.*

Figure 2-5. Observational study to assess prognosis.

identify a group of patients who may or may not have the disease or condition of inter-est (e.g., tuberculosis, depression, or iron-deficiency anemia), which we will call the *target condition.* Investigators begin by collecting a group of patients whom they suspect may have the target condition. These patients undergo both the new diagnostic test and a *gold standard* (i.e., the test considered to be the diagnostic standard for a particular dis-ease or condition; synonyms include *criterion standard, diagnostic standard,* or *reference standard*). Investigators evaluate the diagnostic test by comparing its classification of patients with that of the gold standard (Figure 2-6).

One of the clinician's tasks in searching the health care literature is to identify correctly the category of study that will address the question. For example, if you look for a randomized controlled trial to inform you of the properties of a diagnostic test (as opposed to whether patients benefit from its application), you are unlikely to find the answer you seek because the study design does not match the research question.

Think back to the questions we identified in the previous section. Determining the impact of nicotine replacement therapy on smoking cessation is a treatment (or inter-vention) issue for which we would seek a randomized trial in which people are allocated to a patch that contains nicotine replacement therapy or a patch that contains a placebo (see Figure 2-2). Determining the impact of waterless, alcohol-based hand rubbing on hand contamination is also an intervention (or prevention) issue for which we would want a randomized controlled trial that allocated people to a waterless, alcohol-based solution or antiseptic soap.

Considering the third example we presented, we can formulate the question in two ways. Determining whether estrogen relieves menopausal symptoms is clearly a treat-ment issue. However, we are also interested in whether estrogen causes breast cancer,

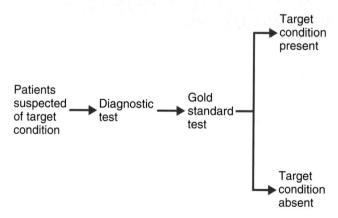

Figure 2-6. Study design to assess a diagnostic test.

ischemic cardiovascular disease, cardiovascular death, or stroke, which are questions of harm. Again, we would seek a randomized controlled trial in which women are allocated to estrogen or placebo (see Figure 2-2).

Qualitative Studies

The most common qualitative study designs in published health care research include case studies, ethnography, grounded theory, and phenomenology. In a *case study*, some cases are studied in depth to inquire into the phenomenon of interest. Individual cases, which may be similar or dissimilar, are chosen because it is believed that understanding them will lead to a better understanding about a still larger collection of cases.[9]

The goal of *ethnography* is to learn about a culture from the people who actually live in that culture.[10] The process of ethnography is characterized by intensive, ongoing, face-to-face involvement with participants of the culture and by participation in their settings and social worlds during a period of fieldwork.

The purpose of a *grounded theory* approach to qualitative research is to discover the meanings that humans assign to people and objects with whom and with which they interact and to develop a theory that accounts for behavioral variation.[11] Both observation and interviews are commonly used for data collection.

The aim of a *phenomenologic approach* to qualitative research is to gain a deeper understanding of the nature or meaning of the everyday "lived" experience of people.[12] Because the primary source of data is the life world of the individual being studied, in-depth interviews are the most common means of data collection from which themes emerge.

These qualitative study designs are described in more detail in Chapter 8, Qualitative Research. Think back to the questions we identified in the previous section. The qualitative design most likely to inform us about how caregivers describe their experiences of deciding to place a relative with Alzheimer's disease in a special care unit would be phenomenology, using in-depth interviews. To learn about how young adult transplant recipients experience the process of transition from a pediatric transplant program to an adult transplant program, investigators could use a case study approach in which they study certain cases in depth.

Systematic Reviews

A *systematic review* is a rigorous method of summarizing the findings of studies that address a focused clinical question. Most commonly, investigators have used this approach with quantitative studies, but researchers have begun to summarize the results of qualitative studies into *metasyntheses*. In a systematic review, extensive efforts are made to locate, appraise, and synthesize research studies. Some systematic reviews of quantitative studies lend themselves to *meta-analysis*, the statistical combination of the results of more than one study. This strategy effectively increases the sample size and results in a more precise estimate of effect than can be obtained from any of the individual studies included in the meta-analysis.[13] Chapter 9, Summarizing the Evidence Through Systematic Reviews, describes systematic reviews in more detail.

When one is searching for the best evidence, high-quality systematic reviews of the literature are preferred to single studies. These reviews address targeted clinical questions using strategies that decrease the likelihood of bias.

SOURCES OF EVIDENCE

The health care literature is continually and rapidly expanding; the task of keeping up with relevant health care information is daunting for all health care professionals. Strategies to facilitate access to research evidence include formulating a clear and concise clinical question, identifying the research design that would best answer the question, and identifying the most appropriate place to look for studies that answer the question.

The remainder of this chapter focuses on online rather than print resources because they are generally easier to search and more current than print resources. For further study, the article by Morrisey and DeBourgh about refining literature searching skills may prove helpful.[14] If you are experiencing any difficulties using online resources, it may be useful to solicit the assistance of a professional health sciences librarian. The health sciences librarian is well versed in all the online resources used by clinicians to answer clinical questions and is usually available for personal consultations and tutorial sessions.

Selecting the Best Nursing Information Resources

What are the optimal nursing information resources? To a large extent, it depends on the type of question you are asking, how much time you have, and the resources available to you. It is important to match your question to the source of information that will likely provide the most appropriate answer. To take extreme examples, the Cumulative Index to Nursing and Allied Health Literature (CINAHL) is not the best source of information on gross anatomy, and the hospital information system is the best place to access laboratory data for a specific patient.

Practical resources to support evidence-based health care decisions are rapidly evolving.[15] To answer focused foreground questions, the most efficient approach is to begin with a prefiltered or preprocessed resource. By *preprocessed,* we mean that someone has reviewed the literature and has chosen only the methodologically strongest studies. The authors of these products have designed them to make searching easy. The sources are updated regularly—from months to a couple of years—with methodologically sound and clinically important studies.

Figure 2-7 illustrates a hierarchy of preprocessed sources of evidence.[15] Information seekers should begin by looking at the highest-level resource available for the problem that prompted their search. At the top of the hierarchy, *systems* include practice guidelines, clinical pathways, or evidence-based textbook summaries that integrate evidence-based information about specific clinical problems and provide regular updating. When no evidence-based information system exists for a clinical problem, then *synopses of syntheses (systematic reviews)* constitute the next best source. *Synopses* encapsulate the key methodological details and results of a review that are required to apply the evidence to individual patient care. Moving down the hierarchy, *syntheses* provide clinicians with a systematic review of all the evidence addressing a focused clinical question. Next we have *synopses of single studies,* and at the bottom of the hierarchy are *preprocessed single studies,* which have been selected because they are both highly relevant and characterized by study designs that minimize bias and thus permit a high strength of inference. We next describe preprocessed databases for accessing current best evidence at the systems, synopses, syntheses, and study levels.

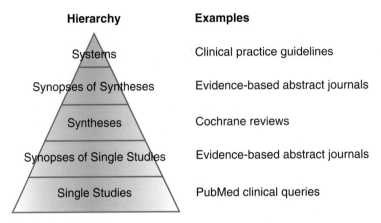

Hierarchy	Examples
Systems	Clinical practice guidelines
Synopses of Syntheses	Evidence-based abstract journals
Syntheses	Cochrane reviews
Synopses of Single Studies	Evidence-based abstract journals
Single Studies	PubMed clinical queries

Figure 2-7. A hierarchy of preprocessed evidence. *(Modified and reproduced with permission of the BMJ Publishing Group from Haynes RB. Of studies, summaries, synopses, and systems: the "4S" evolution of services for finding current best evidence.* Evid Based Ment Health. *2001;4:37–39.)*

Using Preprocessed Nursing Information Resources

Certain preprocessed resources can be very useful to nurses. At the systems level, there is *Clinical Evidence;* at the synopses level, there is *Evidence-Based Nursing;* at the syntheses level, there is the *Cochrane Library;* and at the studies level, there is PubMed (Table 2-1) We review each of these resources and illustrate their use in addressing the following question: Among persons who smoke, do nursing interventions increase the probability of smoking cessation?

Well-developed clinical practice guidelines and computer decision support systems can also be resources at the systems level. *Clinical practice guidelines* are systematically developed statements to assist practitioner and patient decisions about appropriate health care for specific clinical circumstances. Two sources of clinical practice guidelines of relevance to nursing include the National Guidelines Clearinghouse (*www.guideline.gov*) and the Registered Nurses Association of Ontario (RNAO) Best Practice Guidelines Project *(www.rnao.org). Computer decision support systems* are designed to aid directly in clinical decision making about individual patients. In computer decision support systems, detailed individual patient data are entered into a computer program and are sorted and matched to programs or algorithms in a computerized database, resulting in the generation of patient-specific assessments or recommendations for clinicians. These two resources are described in detail in separate chapters in this book (see Chapter 10, Moving From Evidence to Action Using Clinical Practice Guidelines, and Chapter 19, Computer Decision Support Systems).

Clinical Evidence

Clinical Evidence is published by the BMJ Publishing Group. It summarizes the best available evidence on the effects of common medical and nursing interventions. *Clinical*

Table **2-1**   On-line Nursing Information Resources

Resource	Internet Address	Estimated Annual Cost*
Preprocessed Databases		
Clinical Evidence	*www.clinicalevidence.com*	$145 individual; institution rate varies by number of users
Evidence-Based Nursing	*www.evidencebasednursing.com*	$127 individual; institution rate varies by number of users
Evidence-Based Mental Health	*http://ebmh.bmjjournals.com/*	$126 individual; institution rate varies by number of users
Cochrane Library	*www.cochrane.org*	$245 individual $460 institution (Access to abstracts of Cochrane Systematic Reviews is free via PubMed Clinical Queries)
PubMed Clinical Queries	*www.pubmed.gov*	Free
Unprocessed Databases		
CINAHL	*www.cinahl.com*	$20 individual; institution rate varies by number of users
MEDLINE (National Library of Medicine resource; includes: MEDLINE, Pre-Medline, and HealthStar)	*www.pubmed.gov*	Free
EMBASE	*www.embase.com*	Costs vary by number of users

Continued

Table 2-1   On-line Nursing Information Resources—cont'd

Resource	Internet Address	Estimated Annual Cost*
Clinical Practice Guidelines		
National Guidelines Clearinghouse	www.guideline.gov	Free
RNAO Best Practice Guidelines	www.rnao.org	Free
Other Evidence-Based Resources		
ScHARR Netting the Evidence	www.shef.ac.uk/scharr/ir/netting	Free
Centre for Evidence-Based Nursing (York, UK)	www.york.ac.uk/healthsciences/centres/evidence/cebn.htm	Free
Joanna Briggs Institute	www.joannabriggs.edu.au	Free
German Centre for Evidence-Based Nursing	www.pflegeforschung.de	Free
Sarah Cole Hirsh Institute	http://fpb.cwru.edu/HirshInstitute	Free
EBM Toolkit	www.med.ualberta.ca/ebm/ebm.htm	Free
Centre for Evidence-Based Medicine (Oxford, UK)	www.cebm.net	Free
Centre for Evidence-Based Medicine (Toronto, CN)	www.cebm.utoronto.ca	Free

*Costs in 2004 U.S. Dollars.

Evidence provides a concise account of the current state of knowledge about the prevention and treatment of a wide range of clinical conditions. It also highlights areas of uncertainty in which evidence is lacking. This resource does not aim to make recommendations, nor does it judge clinical effectiveness or cost-effectiveness. Both beneficial and harmful effects of interventions are presented, but clinicians are left to translate these effects into recommendations for individual patients. Searches initially focus on high-quality systematic reviews and, failing this, go on to well-designed single studies. Each section begins with a list of the questions addressed, some key points, and a list of interventions categorized according to their effectiveness (beneficial, likely to be beneficial, of unknown effectiveness, and likely to be ineffective or harmful). It is published biannually with weekly updates on-line.

Example of a *Clinical Evidence* Search. We accessed *Clinical Evidence* on-line *(www.clinicalevidence.com)* and entered "smoking cessation intervention" in the search box. This search returned 18 results. From the choices, we selected the topic "Changing Behaviour." This took us to the "Cardiovascular, Changing Behaviour" section of the text and a listing of potential interventions. The intervention that appeared to be most relevant was "Advice from physicians and trained counselors to quit smoking." In reading this section, we found that one systematic review had been identified, which concluded that advice from a nurse increased the rate of quitting smoking.[16]

Evidence-Based Nursing Journal

The Royal College of Nursing Publishing Company and the BMJ Publishing Group publish the *Evidence-Based Nursing* journal on a quarterly basis. This journal, like its counterparts *ACP Journal Club, Evidence-Based Medicine, Evidence-Based Cardiovascular Medicine,* and *Evidence-Based Mental Health,* is a secondary publication in which studies published in any of more than 100 health care journals are identified, critically appraised, and summarized in brief abstracts. Because these journals include only articles that reviewers have decided meet basic standards of methodological quality, they include a substantially smaller set of articles than health care literature databases. The relatively high methodological quality of the articles compensates for this limitation. The most successful results are produced by conducting a global keyword search against the entire *Evidence-Based Nursing* collection. Through the *Evidence-Based Nursing Online (www.evidencebasednursing.com)* Web site, subscribers can search all issues of *Evidence-Based Nursing* published since 1998 for abstracts, commentaries, and editorials and can often link to the full text of the original article. They can search for other high-quality studies that passed the rigorous *Evidence-Based Nursing* selection criteria but were not abstracted because, in the judgment of the editors, they were not as widely applicable to nursing practice or covered a topic that was recently addressed in another abstract.

Example of an *Evidence-Based Nursing* Journal Search. We accessed *Evidence-Based Nursing Online* and conducted a search using the following keywords: "smoking cessation" AND "intervention." This yielded 33 citations, five of which were reviews. On close examination of the abstract headings, two reviews focused on nursing interventions and smoking cessation rates. One of the reviews was from the *Cochrane Library* and looked specifically at nursing interventions and their effectiveness in increasing smoking cessation rates.[17]

Cochrane Library

The Cochrane Collaboration, an international organization that prepares, maintains, and disseminates systematic reviews of health care interventions, offers an electronic resource for locating high-quality information quickly. They publish a series of on-line resources referred to as the *Cochrane Library* that focuses primarily on systematic reviews of controlled trials of therapeutic interventions. These summaries are based on a rigorous search for evidence, explicit scientific review of the studies uncovered in the search, and systematic assembly of the evidence to provide as clear a signal about the effects of a health care intervention as the evidence will allow.[15] Although the *Cochrane Library* has an increasingly important role in informing clinicians about effective interventions, it provides little help in addressing other aspects of health care, such as the value of a new diagnostic test or a patient's prognosis. The *Cochrane Library* abstracts of reviews can be accessed at no charge through the Internet *(www.cochrane.org)*. It is updated quarterly, and access to full-text articles on-line or on CD-ROM requires an annual subscription.

The *Cochrane Library* contains numerous databases, three of which are most useful to clinicians in answering clinical questions. The first of these, the *Cochrane Database of Systematic Reviews,* includes completed and proposed systematic reviews; these reviews have been peer-reviewed to ensure that they meet rigorous standards of methodology and are updated regularly. The second database, the *Database of Abstracts of Reviews of Effectiveness,* includes systematic reviews that have been published outside the Cochrane Collaboration. The third database, the *Cochrane Controlled Trials Registry,* contains a growing list of hundreds of thousands of references to clinical trials that Cochrane investigators have found by searching a wide range of sources.

Example of a *Cochrane Library* Search.　To locate information about smoking cessation interventions in the *Cochrane Library,* we entered the following search terms: "smoking cessation program" AND "nursing," using the 2003 version of the *Cochrane Library* (issue 3). This yielded 10 completed reviews and no protocols in the *Cochrane Database of Systematic Reviews,* one abstract in the *Database of Abstracts of Reviews of Effectiveness,* and eight references in the *Cochrane Controlled Trials Registry.* A Cochrane review entitled "Nursing interventions for smoking cessation"[18] appeared promising. Double-clicking on this item, we found an entire Cochrane Collaboration systematic review, including information on the methodology for the review, the inclusion and exclusion criteria, the results, and a discussion.

PubMed

PubMed is an on-line, Internet-based, free version of MEDLINE, the bibliographic database produced by the United States National Center for Biotechnology Information and the United States National Library of Medicine (NLM). In addition to providing access to MEDLINE, PubMed *(www.pubmed.gov)* also offers a user-friendly approach to evidence-based searching called Clinical Queries. Users do not need to be familiar with the Medical Subject Heading (MeSH) terms that are the basis of MEDLINE searching. PubMed contains a sophisticated search engine that maps terms for you. In addition, the Clinical Queries feature uses preset research methodology filters that enable searchers to locate relevant methodologically sound studies that meet evidence-based standards for four types of research: therapy (or interventions), diagnosis, etiology (or harm), and prognosis. Searches can be more sensitive (retrieving larger numbers of relevant citations, but including those that are less relevant) or more specific (retrieving fewer citations, but including those more likely to be relevant).[19] The most recent enhancement to the PubMed Clinical Queries is the addition of a systematic review filter. When the systematic review filter is selected, relevant systematic reviews indexed in PubMed, including those in the *Cochrane Database of Systematic Reviews,* are retrieved.

Example of a PubMed Search. We accessed PubMed on the Internet, clicked on the Clinical Queries feature found in the navigation bar on the left side of the screen, and typed in the following keywords: "nursing interventions smoking cessation." We then selected the following options on the screen: "therapy," "sensitivity," and "systematic review." Our search resulted in six citations, two of which were different versions of the same Cochrane systematic review by Rice and Stead about nursing interventions for smoking cessation[18] and one of which was a meta-analysis on the same topic.[16]

Using Unprocessed Nursing Information Resources

If a search of *Clinical Evidence,* secondary journals, the *Cochrane Library,* and PubMed does not provide a satisfactory answer to a focused clinical question, it is time to turn to CINAHL, MEDLINE, and EMBASE (see Table 2-1). These unprocessed databases are very large; CINAHL includes more than 2.5 million citations from more than 924 journals, MEDLINE includes more than 12 million citations from more than 4600 biomedicine or life sciences journals, and EMBASE includes more than 9.5 million citations from more than 3800 journals. These databases consist largely of original studies, the methodological quality of which may be excellent or very poor. Only a few of the studies are immediately useful in answering clinical questions. To retrieve the highest level of evidence for a particular question, you may need to add methodology filters to subject terms. This means that you must create a more complex search strategy to replace the simple text word strategy appropriate for a small preprocessed resource. In the following subsections, we review the unprocessed resources suitable for answering our clinical question about nursing interventions and smoking cessation rates, this time defining our population as adolescents.

CINAHL

CINAHL *(www.cinahl.com)* is the largest bibliographic database specifically related to nursing, allied health disciplines, health sciences librarianship, and consumer health. It is a commercial product maintained by Information Systems and is updated quarterly. CINAHL is useful primarily to answer focused foreground questions related to nursing and allied health practice.

The database includes many features such as full-text articles, clinical practice guidelines, bibliographies of major articles, research instruments, government publications, comments, book reviews, evaluations of multimedia and computer software and systems, and patient education materials. CINAHL subject headings are used to index the literature contained in the database. These subject headings were developed to reflect the terminology used by nurses and allied health professionals. Search terms cannot necessarily be used universally across the various health sciences databases. For example, the term "bed sore" is indexed under the subject heading "pressure ulcer" in CINAHL, "decubitus ulcer" in MEDLINE, and "decubitus" in EMBASE.

Example of a CINAHL Search. We accessed CINAHL from our office computer and entered the subject heading "smoking cessation," yielding more than 1400 citations. We then entered the subject heading "adolescence" and combined this with "smoking cessation," yielding approximately 140 citations. We then considered the type of study design that we would like to assess. Understanding the importance of finding a recent systematic review rather than a single study, we limited this search to publication type "systematic review" and to publication dates in 2001 to 2003. This was done by entering the text word "systematic review" and combining it with the subject search and then limiting the result to the publication dates. Of the 26 resulting citations, we chose one that dealt with mass media interventions for preventing smoking in youth.[20]

MEDLINE

The United States National Library of Medicine maintains this impressive bibliographic database. A complementary database, known as PreMEDLINE, includes citations and abstracts for studies that have been published recently but not yet indexed. MEDLINE is an essential resource for finding clinical information because of its comprehensive coverage of health care journals and because it is readily accessible—anyone with Internet access can search MEDLINE free of charge using PubMed. In addition, most health sciences or hospital libraries provide access to MEDLINE through a commercial vendor such as OVID, Knowledge Finder, or Silver Platter.

These positive features are balanced with a disadvantage that relates to MEDLINE's size and to the range of publications that it encompasses. Searching MEDLINE effectively often requires careful thought, along with a thorough knowledge of how the database is structured and how publications are indexed. Understanding how to use Medical Subject Headings (MeSH) is essential, as are text word searching, exploding, and use of the *logical operators* AND and OR to combine different search results. If you are unfamiliar with MEDLINE searching techniques, an article by Greenhalgh[21] presents a good introduction.

Example of a MEDLINE Search. To search for information on smoking cessation and adolescents, we used the National Library of Medicine's PubMed MEDLINE searching system and accessed this from our office. We began by entering the term "smoking cessation." This yielded a total of 8588 citations dating back to 1966. The PubMed system processes a search request by executing a text word search and a MeSH term search simultaneously across both MEDLINE and PreMEDLINE to provide a more comprehensive search result. PubMed automatically *explodes* the MeSH terms entered; this means that all the subheadings and related terms are included in the search result.

We then searched using the term "adolescent," which yielded 990,500 references. To combine these two searches, we clicked on the "History" button, which displayed a numbered summary of all the searches executed; these are referred to as *search sets*. In our search, we entered two separate terms: #1, "smoking cessation," and #2, "adolescent."

To answer our original question, we had to find the cross-section of literature that focused on both these topics by combining our search sets using the logical operator "AND" (in this case, #1 AND #2). The logical operator "AND" in the strategy asked MEDLINE to identify publications that focused on both smoking cessation and adolescents.

The list of publications on smoking cessation and adolescents included 1391 references. This large yield prompted us to take advantage of other searching options designed to help us focus or limit our search results. Combining our previous strategy with a publication-type term such as "meta-analysis" or using the "Limits" function of PubMed to limit our search results to a specific publication type (e.g., meta-analysis) yielded a list of nine publications that focused on our original search topic.

EMBASE

EMBASE (Excerpta Medica Database) is a comprehensive bibliographic database covering the worldwide literature on biomedical and pharmaceutical fields. It is produced by Elsevier Science, the world's largest publisher of scientific information, and it indexes a large proportion of the European biomedical and science literature. As with MEDLINE, the size and complexity of EMBASE make searching somewhat more difficult and time consuming. It is useful primarily for answering focused foreground questions. Searching EMBASE effectively often requires careful thought, along with a thorough knowledge of how the database is structured and how publications are indexed. EMBASE uses EMTREE, a hierarchically ordered controlled vocabulary, which contains 38,000 preferred terms and more than 150,000 synonyms. EMTREE terms are different from MeSH terms, and they should not be confused when performing searches.

Example of an EMBASE Search. We accessed EMBASE from our office computer and entered "smoking cessation" in the search box, to yield 8177 citations. We then entered the term "adolescent," which yielded 267,503 citations, and combined this with "smoking cessation," yielding 39 citations. We then considered the type of study design that we would like to access. EMBASE does provide a "Limit" function for publication type; however, publication types do not include systematic review, meta-analysis, or randomized controlled trial. To limit an EMBASE search to evidence-based study designs, we had to combine our subject search with the search term "evidence-based medicine." We entered the search term "evidence-based medicine," yielding 125,920 citations. We then combined our previous search terms with "evidence-based medicine," (e.g., "smoking cessation AND adolescent AND evidence-based medicine") yielding 20 citations. Of the resulting citations, we chose a randomized controlled trial that dealt with smoking cessation interventions for adolescents.[22]

The World Wide Web

The World Wide Web is rapidly becoming an important source of health care information for both health care professionals and consumers. Although the thousands of sites provide increased access to health care information, the potential for harm from inaccurate information is substantial.[23] As a result, it is important to evaluate the quality of Web-based materials on the Internet. Holloway and colleagues[24] wrote a useful chapter (in *Internet Resources for Nurses,* edited by Fitzpatrick and Montgomery) on evaluating health care information on the Internet. In their chapter, they cited the White Paper, which provides a robust set of criteria that can be used to judge the quality of health information on the Internet. The target audience for the White Paper includes the general public, policy makers, health professionals, and providers of Web-based information. A detailed description of the seven broad categories of criteria used in the White Paper (credibility, content, disclosure, links, design, interactivity, and caveats) can be found at *http://hitiweb.mitretek.org/docs/policy.pdf.*

To facilitate access to the myriad of health information resources, many Web sites act as portals by providing a collection of links to health care information sites. Many Internet portals employ specific criteria when selecting links for their Web sites. Some examples of evidence-based Internet resources include the following: Netting the Evidence *(www.shef.ac.uk/scharr/ir/netting)*, Bandolier *(www.jr2.ox.ac.uk/bandolier/)*, and the TRIP Database *(www.tripdatabase.com)*. The World Wide Web also provides access to many different evidence-based educational resources, including the Centre for Evidence-Based Nursing *(www.york.ac.uk/healthsciences/centres/evidence/cebn.htm)* and the Agency for Healthcare Research and Quality *(www.ahrq.gov/)*. Nurses can also use the Internet to access nursing journals such as *Evidence-Based Nursing Online (www.evidencebasednursing.com)* and clinical practice guidelines such as the National Guidelines Clearinghouse *(www.guideline.gov)* and the RNAO Best Practice Guidelines Project *(www.rnao.org)*.

CONCLUSION

The health sciences literature is enormous and continues to expand rapidly. To the extent that this reflects ongoing research and the identification of potential improvements for patient care, this scope is very promising. At the same time, however, it makes the task of locating the best and most current evidence more challenging. The emergence of new information resources specifically designed to provide ready access to high-quality, clinically relevant, and current information is timely and encouraging.

REFERENCES

1. Ulrich's Periodicals Directory. Available at: *http://www.ulrichsweb.com.* Accessed September 15, 2003.
2. Royle J, Blythe J, Ciliska D, Ing D. The organizational environment and evidence-based nursing. *Can J Nurs Leader.* 2000;13:31-37.
3. Hicks C. Barriers to evidence-based care in nursing: historical legacies and conflicting cultures. *Health Serv Manag Res.* 1998;11:137-147.
4. Parahoo K. Barriers to, and facilitators of, research utilization among nurses in Northern Ireland. *J Adv Nurs.* 2000;31:89-98.
5. Royle JA, Blythe J, DiCenso A, Baumann A, Fitzgerald D. Do nurses have the information resources and skills for research utilization? *Can J Nurs Adm.* 1997;10:9-30.
6. Flemming K. Asking answerable questions. *Evid Based Nurs.* 1998;1:36-37.
7. Richardson WS, Wilson MC, Nishikawa J, Hayward RSA. The well-built clinical question: a key to evidence-based decisions. *ACP J Club.* 1995;123:A12.
8. McKibbon A, Eady A, Marks S. *PDQ Evidence-Based Principles and Practice.* Hamilton, Ontario, Canada: Decker; 1999.
9. Keen J, Packwood T. Case study evaluation. In: Mays N, Pope C, eds. *Qualitative Research in Healthcare.* London, UK: BMJ Publishing Group; 1996:59-67.

10. Atkinson P, Coffey A, Delamont S, Lofland J, Lofland L, eds. *Handbook of Ethnography.* London, UK: Sage Publications; 2001.

11. Strauss A, Corbin J. *Basics of Qualitative Research: Grounded Theory Procedures and Techniques.* Newbury Park, CA: Sage Publications; 1990.

12. Van Manen M. *Researching Lived Experience: Human Science for an Action Sensitive Pedagogy.* London, Ontario, Canada: Althouse Press; 1990.

13. Ciliska D, Cullum N, Marks S. Evaluation of systematic reviews of treatment or prevention interventions. *Evid Based Nurs.* 2001;4:100-103.

14. Morrisey LJ, DeBourgh GA. Finding evidence: refining literature searching skills for the advanced practice nurse. *AACN Clin Issues.* 2001;12:560-77.

15. Haynes RB. Of studies, summaries, synopses, and systems: the "4S" evolution of services for finding current best evidence. *Evid Based Ment Health.* 2001;4:37-39.

16. Rice VH. Nursing intervention and smoking cessation: a meta-analysis. *Heart Lung,* 1999;28:438-454.

17. Review: nursing interventions increase smoking cessation rates in adults [abstract]. *Evid Based Nurs.* 2000;3:47. Abstract of: Rice VH, Stead LF. Nursing interventions for smoking cessation. *Cochrane Database Syst Rev.* 2001;CD001188.

18. Rice VH, Stead LF. Nursing interventions for smoking cessation. *Cochrane Database Syst Rev.* 2001; CD001188.

19. Zaroukian MH. PubMed clinical queries. *Evid Based Med.* 2001;6:8.

20. Sowden AJ, Arblaster L. Mass media interventions for preventing smoking in young people. *Cochrane Database Syst Rev.* 2000;CD001006.

21. Greenhalgh T. How to read a paper: the Medline database. *BMJ.* 1997;315:180-183.

22. Maguire TA, McElnay JC, Drummond A. A randomized controlled trial of a smoking cessation intervention based in community pharmacies. *Addiction.* 2001;96:325-331.

23. Jadad A, Gagliardi A. Rating health information on the Internet: navigating to knowledge or to Babel? *JAMA.* 1998;279:611-614.

24. Holloway N, Kripps B, Koepke K, Skiba DJ. Evaluating health care information on the Internet. In: Fitzpatrick JJ, Montgomery KS, eds. *Internet Resources for Nurses.* New York, NY: Springer; 2000:197-213.

3

Health Care Interventions and Harm: An Introduction

Nicky Cullum and Gordon Guyatt

In This Chapter

Three Steps in Using an Article From the Health Care Literature

Health Care Interventions and Harm: Study Designs
    Randomized Controlled Trials to Evaluate Nursing Interventions
    Observational Studies to Assess Harm

Applying Appropriate Criteria

Nurses frequently have to choose among alternative interventions for patients. For example, should we advise new mothers to swab their infants' umbilical cords with water or with alcohol? Should we introduce telephone-based peer support to help primiparous mothers breast-feed longer or should we continue with usual care? If we teach relaxation techniques to patients with chronic pain, will they experience more pain relief than if they use conventional pain medications alone? Will exercise or dietary change reduce the risk of developing diabetes? What are the benefits of screening patients for pressure ulcer development or prostate cancer or of instituting a smoking cessation program? What benefit may people with asthma or diabetes anticipate from learning self-management techniques? Equally important, what short-term or long-term adverse effects could they expect as a result of these interventions?

These questions address two related issues. First, when we implement an intervention, does it result in the intended outcome? For example, do primiparous mothers breast-feed longer when they receive telephone-based peer support? This is an issue of *treatment*. Throughout this book we will use the terms *treatment, therapy, nursing intervention,* and *health care intervention* interchangeably to mean those maneuvers that we, as nurses, engage in (usually in collaboration with others), with the aim of benefiting patients and their families, populations, or communities. Second, what adverse consequences do individuals experience either as unintended deleterious effects of treatment (e.g., increased risk of breast cancer with hormone replacement therapy) or as a result of exposure to a harmful agent (e.g., smoking)? This is an issue of *harm*.

When we address questions of either harm or treatment, we are confronting issues of causation. For example, in healthy men or women, is there a causal relationship between an exposure (e.g., long flight on an airplane) and a particular anticipated outcome (e.g., deep vein thrombosis) or between an intervention (e.g., compression stockings) and an unanticipated outcome (e.g., toe ischemia resulting from an ill-fitting compression stocking in a person with undiagnosed peripheral vascular disease)?

These questions have underlying true answers. If our inferences about the underlying truth are wrong, the consequences may be disastrous. Consider how many lives must have been lost over the course of several hundred years when physicians were convinced that bloodletting was an effective treatment for a wide variety of illnesses. Consider how many postoperative infections occurred when nurses were convinced that preoperative shaving was preventing those very infections.

Why has the health care community made such disastrous blunders, and what can we do to prevent them in the future? The answer lies in health care professionals, including nurses, learning rules of evidence that allow them to differentiate misleading research reports from valid ones. This book provides a practical approach to determining when you can believe study results and when you cannot.

THREE STEPS IN USING AN ARTICLE FROM THE HEALTH CARE LITERATURE

When using the health care literature to answer a clinical question, approach the study using three discrete steps.

1. In the first step, ask "**Are the results of the study valid?**" This question has to do with the believability or credibility of the results. Whether the study provides valid

results depends on whether it was designed and conducted well enough that the study findings accurately represent the direction and magnitude of the underlying true effect. Another way to state this question is: "Are the study methods sufficiently rigorous to ensure that the study results represent an unbiased estimate of the true effect, or are the study methods sufficiently biased to lead to a false conclusion?" If the study methods are rigorous, then the results are worth examining further.

2. In the second step, ask "**What are the results?**" This question considers the size and precision of the estimate of effect. The best estimate of that effect will be the study findings themselves; the precision of the estimate may be superior in larger studies.

3. Once you understand the results, ask yourself the third question: "**How can I apply these results to patient care?**" This question has two parts. First, can you apply the results to patients in your clinical setting? For instance, you should hesitate to provide an intervention if the patient in your setting is too dissimilar from those who participated in the trial. Second, if the results are generalizable to patients in your setting, what is the net impact of the intervention? Have the investigators measured all outcomes of importance to patients? The impact depends on both benefits and risks (adverse effects) of the intervention and the consequences of withholding it. Thus, even an effective intervention may be withheld if a patient's prognosis is already good without it, especially if the intervention is accompanied by important adverse effects.

HEALTH CARE INTERVENTIONS AND HARM: STUDY DESIGNS

Randomized Controlled Trials to Evaluate Nursing Interventions

Researchers have much more control when investigating whether an intervention is effective than when exploring whether an agent causes harm. For instance, they can determine who receives the experimental intervention and who receives the alternative (e.g., no intervention or an inert substance called a placebo). Ideally, they will allocate patients to groups according to a process analogous to a coin flip, called *randomization*, and they will conduct a randomized controlled trial. Through the process of randomization, the investigators aim to create groups that are similar in all respects except exposure to the intervention. In this way, at the end of the study, any differences between the groups can be attributed to the intervention.

Observational Studies to Assess Harm

By contrast, researchers looking at issues of harm generally do not have this sort of control. They cannot randomly allocate people to smoke or not smoke or to live in high- or low-pollution environments or in spacious or overcrowded settings. As a result, investigators use observational study designs. In one type of observational study design called a *cohort study*, the investigators follow groups of study participants who, as a result of preference or circumstances, either have or have not been exposed to a harmful stimulus. Investigators follow the study participants forward in time to determine how many in each group experience the outcome of interest or target outcome (e.g., follow up a group of laborers who work near coke ovens and a group of laborers who do not for 20 years to compare the occurrence of genitourinary cancer). Alternatively, researchers may conduct a *case-control study*, in which they select persons who have already suffered the target outcome and persons who have not suffered the target outcome and compare the extent to which the two groups were exposed to the agent suspected of causing harm (e.g., select two groups of men, one with genitourinary cancer and one without, and compare their past exposure to coke ovens) (see Chapter 5, Harm).

APPLYING APPROPRIATE CRITERIA

The conclusions or inferences we can draw from studies investigating harm are generally much weaker than those drawn from studies of health care interventions. As a user of the nursing and health care literature, you must apply different criteria to studies evaluating nursing interventions from those investigating potentially harmful exposures. We therefore provide separate chapters on the issues of treatment (Chapter 4, Health Care Interventions) and harm (Chapter 5, Harm).

There are exceptions to this general rule. Sometimes the harmful exposure may be a health care intervention, such as a piece of equipment (e.g., a pressure-relieving bed) or a drug, and researchers will perceive the suspected harmful effect as occurring quickly and frequently. Under these circumstances, investigators may be able to use the study design usually associated with treatment (i.e., randomized controlled trial) to determine whether a causal relation exists between an intervention and an adverse effect. This was the case in the recent randomized controlled trial that was stopped early because combined hormone replacement therapy was found to increase the risk of breast cancer.[1] Similarly, there may be no randomized trials available—or even feasible—that evaluate a particular health care intervention. Investigations of rare conditions, community interventions, care delivered in different hospitals (see Chapter 17, Health Services Interventions), or the quality of care within a hospital (see Chapter 10, Moving From Evidence to Action Using Clinical Practice Guidelines) do not easily lend themselves to randomized trials. For example, randomizing health care systems to rely more on nurse practitioners or clinical nurse specialists seems improbable, at least for the foreseeable future.

In situations when nurses find that randomized trials of certain nursing interventions are unavailable, they need to rely on cohort and case-control studies—the strongest evidence available. In doing so, nurses must apply the appropriate criteria for the evaluation of these studies, criteria that ordinarily would be associated with investigations of potentially harmful exposures. When relying on cohort or case-control studies to address issues of therapeutic benefit, however, nurses must bear in mind that the strength of any inferences about the causal relation between an intervention and an outcome is much weaker than when evidence comes from a randomized trial.

REFERENCE

1. Rossouw JE, Anderson GL, Prentice RL, et al. Risks and benefits of estrogen plus progestin in healthy postmenopausal women: principal results from the Women's Health Initiative randomized controlled trial. *JAMA.* 2002;288:321-333.

4

Health Care Interventions

Alba DiCenso and Gordon Guyatt

The following Editorial Board members also made substantive contributions to this chapter: Rien de Vos, Paola DiGiulio, Kate Flemming, Andrew Jull, Mark Newman, and Jenny Ploeg.

We gratefully acknowledge the work of Deborah Cook, P. J. Devereaux, Maureen Meade, and Sharon Straus on the original chapter that appears in the Users' Guides to the Medical Literature, *edited by Guyatt and Rennie.*

In This Chapter

Finding the Evidence

Are the Results Valid?
    Were Patients Randomized?
    Was Randomization Concealed?
    Were Patients Analyzed in the Groups to Which They Were Randomized?
    Were Groups Shown to be Similar in All Known Determinants of Outcome, or
        Were Analyses Adjusted for Differences?
    Were Patients Aware of Group Allocation?
    Were Clinicians Aware of Group Allocation?
    Were Outcome Assessors Aware of Group Allocation?
    Was Follow-up Complete?

What Are the Results?
    How Large Was the Intervention Effect?
    How Precise Was the Estimate of the Intervention Effect?
    When Authors Do Not Report the Confidence Interval

How Can I Apply the Results to Patient Care?
    Were the Study Patients Similar to the Patients in My Clinical Setting?
    Were All Important Outcomes Considered?
    Are the Likely Intervention Benefits Worth the Potential Harm and Costs?

What Needle Should Nurses Use to Vaccinate Infants?

You are one of a group of nurses working in a large primary care practice. One of your responsibilities is vaccinating infants. Various needles are available in the clinic, and in chatting with your colleagues you find that choice of needles differs. Some of you use a larger-bore, longer needle (23 gauge, 25 mm) and some a smaller-bore, shorter needle (25 gauge, 16 mm). Based on data collected from parents about infants' reactions to vaccinations, all the nurses believe that their rates of reaction are less than 50%. Advocates of the larger needle argue that one can be more certain it reaches the target, the muscle, whereas the shorter needle may only reach the subcutaneous tissue, with a higher likelihood of a reaction. Those using the smaller needle argue that a smaller bore is likely to result in less tissue trauma. You and your colleagues decide to see whether there is any high-quality evidence to resolve the conflicting views.

FINDING THE EVIDENCE

You begin by formulating your question: In infants receiving vaccinations, do the length and bore of the needle influence reactions to the injection, including redness, swelling, and tenderness?

You recently attended a workshop on the best strategies to find research evidence and recall a hierarchy that progresses from the most to the least evolved preprocessed evidence-based information sources. The hierarchy begins with *systems* as the highest level resource, followed by *synopses of syntheses, syntheses* (systematic reviews), *synopses of single studies,* and, finally, *single studies* (see Chapter 2, Finding the Evidence, for details about this hierarchy). Following this framework, you begin by searching *Clinical Evidence,* a systems-level, regularly updated, Web-based and print publication that integrates evidence-based information about specific clinical problems. Your search fails to identify any information on needle length and routine immunizations. At the synopses level, you search the secondary journal, *Evidence-Based Nursing* (for more information about secondary journals, see Chapter 2, Finding the Evidence). You type in the following terms: "immunisation" (this is a British publication, and therefore you must use British spelling where applicable) and "needle" and get one result, entitled "Routine primary immunisation using a longer needle resulted in fewer local reactions in infants."[1] This is an abstract of a published article entitled: "Effect of needle length on incidence of local reactions to routine immunisation in infants aged 4 months: randomised controlled trial."[2]

Although you expect that *Evidence-Based Nursing* would have included any recent syntheses on the topic, you do a final search of the *Cochrane Library,* a synthesis-level resource, to determine whether a systematic review exists on needle length and routine immunizations; however, your search does not reveal a review on this topic. You decide to retrieve and review the randomized trial summarized in *Evidence-Based Nursing.*

The article reports a trial in which investigators randomized 119 infants to receive their third dose of primary immunization (diphtheria, pertussis, and tetanus vaccine and *Haemophilus influenzae* type B vaccine) with a 23-gauge, 25-mm needle or a 25-gauge, 16-mm needle. The investigators instructed nurses in eight general practices, both by demonstration and in writing, to use the technique of injecting into the patient's antero-lateral thigh, by stretching the skin taut and inserting the needle at a 90-degree angle to the skin. Parents recorded redness, swelling, and tenderness in a diary for 3 days after the injection. You and your colleagues decide to review the trial carefully.

Although this chapter discusses the critical appraisal of studies that evaluate health care interventions (interchangeable with the terms therapy and treatment), we emphasize that our definition of an intervention is broad. The principles apply to the following: interventions designed to promote the health of the public (e.g., physical activity programs for healthy, sedentary adults); interventions designed to reduce symptoms or improve outcomes in those who are acutely or chronically ill (e.g., débridement using hydrogel for healing diabetic foot ulcers); interventions designed to prevent future events in patients with known underlying disease (e.g., compression stockings to prevent leg ulceration for people with venous insufficiency); interventions designed to prevent morbidity and mortality in those at risk but without current evident illness (e.g., treatment of high blood pressure); interventions designed to improve patient outcome by improving the process of care (see Chapter 19, Computer Decision Support Systems); and the combination of diagnostic testing and subsequent treatment that make up screening programs (e.g., mammography in women older than 50 years of age) (see Chapter 36, Recommendations About Screening). In each of these types of interventions, you risk doing more harm than good when you intervene. Before acting, therefore, ascertain the benefits and risks of the health care intervention and seek assurance that the societal resources (usually valued in dollars) consumed in the intervention are warranted given the incremental benefits of the intervention (see Chapter 18, Economic Evaluation).

ARE THE RESULTS VALID?

As described in Chapter 3, Health Care Interventions and Harm: An Introduction, we suggest a three-step approach to using an article from the health care literature to guide patient care. We recommend that you first determine whether the study provides valid results, then review the results, and, finally, consider how the results can be applied to patients in your care (Table 4-1).

Whether the study will provide valid results depends on whether it was designed and conducted in a way that justifies claims about the benefits or risks of the intervention. Tests of study methods break down into two sets of four questions. The first set helps you to decide whether persons exposed to the experimental intervention had a similar prognosis to patients exposed to a control intervention at the beginning of the study. The second set helps you to confirm that the two groups were still similar with respect to prognostic factors (also known as determinants of outcome) throughout the study.

Table 4-1   Users' Guides for an Article Evaluating a
            Health Care Intervention

Are the Results Valid?

Did intervention and control groups begin the study with a similar prognosis?
- Were patients randomized?
- Was randomization concealed?
- Were patients analyzed in the groups to which they were randomized?
- Were groups shown to be similar in all known determinants of outcome, or were analyses adjusted for differences?

Did intervention and control groups retain a similar prognosis after the study started?
- Were patients aware of group allocation?
- Were clinicians aware of group allocation?
- Were outcome assessors aware of group allocation?
- Was follow-up complete?

What Are the Results?
- How large was the intervention effect?
- How precise was the estimate of the intervention effect?

How Can I Apply the Results to Patient Care?
- Were the study patients similar to the patients in my clinical setting?
- Were all important outcomes considered?
- Are the likely intervention benefits worth the potential harm and costs?

Were Patients Randomized?

Whenever possible, the most rigorous way to evaluate a health care intervention is to randomize patients to receive or not receive the intervention. Randomization is a process analogous to flipping a coin, and its advantage is that, when done correctly it leaves the determination of who receives the intervention to chance rather than to patient or clinician preference. For example, if investigators chose which patients should receive the intervention, they could consciously or unconsciously choose patients who they believe have a higher likelihood of responding favorably to the intervention.

The power of randomization is that intervention and control groups are likely to be similar in all respects except receipt of the intervention. The groups are balanced with respect to both the known and unknown determinants of outcome. An outcome is a change in health status that may occur after exposure to an intervention, for example, pain reduction. A determinant of outcome (or prognostic factor) is a characteristic of study participants that confers increased or decreased likelihood of experiencing the outcome. Characteristics such as a patient's age, sex, underlying severity of illness, and presence of comorbid conditions are examples of determinants. Because such factors can also influence the occurrence of the outcome, it is important that they be balanced in the comparison groups so that any difference between groups in outcome can be correctly attributed to the intervention. If the determinants of outcome—either those we know about or those we do not know about—prove unbalanced between intervention and control groups, a study's outcome will be biased, either underestimating or overestimating the intervention's effect (see Chapter 26, Bias and Random Error).

In a randomized controlled trial (RCT), the groups are likely to be similar with respect to known and unknown determinants of outcome, and therefore, we can be more confident that any observed differences in outcome are due to the intervention. In a *cohort study* (a type of *observational study*), patient or clinician preference, rather than randomization, determines whether a patient is allocated to the intervention or control group. In the absence of randomization, there is a greater risk of imbalance in both the known and unknown determinants of outcome, and consequently any observed differences in outcome might be unrelated to the intervention but due to differences between groups at baseline. As a result, the strength of inference from a cohort study will always be less than that of a rigorously conducted randomized trial.

For many years, nurses helped to prepare patients for surgery by shaving body hair from the operative site. Nurses were instructed, and believed, that preoperative shaving reduced the risk of postoperative wound infections. However, to everyone's surprise, RCTs in which patients were randomized to shaving or hair clipping demonstrated that preoperative shaving increased rather than decreased wound infections in the immediate postsurgical period.[3,4]

Findings of RCTs often contradict the results of less rigorous studies; for example, the demonstration that modern, occlusive wound dressings do not heal venous leg ulcers more quickly than simple nonadherent dressings,[5] that hormone replacement therapy does not reduce coronary heart disease in healthy postmenopausal women,[6] and that educational and community interventions do not reduce rates of adolescent pregnancy.[7] Such surprises occur frequently (see Chapter 14, Surprising Results of Randomized Controlled Trials) when interventions are assigned by random allocation, rather than by the conscious decisions of clinicians and patients.

Typically, observational studies tend to show larger intervention effects than do RCTs,[8-11] although systematic underestimation of intervention effects also may occur.[12] Observational studies can theoretically match patients, either in selecting patients for study or in the subsequent statistical analysis, for known determinants of outcome (see Chapter 5, Harm; and see Chapter 26, Bias and Random Error).

Randomization does not always succeed in its goal of achieving similar groups. Investigators may make mistakes that compromise randomization—if those who determine eligibility are aware of the group to which patients will be allocated or if patients are not analyzed in the group to which they were allocated—or they may encounter bad luck.

Was Randomization Concealed?

The success of randomization depends on two interrelated processes.[13-15] The first entails generating a sequence by which participants in a trial are allocated to intervention groups. To ensure unpredictability of the allocation sequence, investigators should generate it by a random process (e.g., computer-generated numbers, random number tables, or coin flipping). The second process, *allocation concealment*, shields those involved in a trial from knowing upcoming assignments in advance.[16] Without this protection, investigators have been known to manipulate who receives the next assignment, thus compromising the balance in treatment and control groups.[17]

Suppose, for example, that an investigator creates an adequate allocation sequence using a random number table. However, the investigator then affixes the list of that sequence to a bulletin board, with no allocation concealment. Those responsible for admitting participants could ascertain the upcoming treatment allocations and then route participants with better prognoses to the experimental group and those with poorer prognoses to the control group, or vice versa. Bias would result. Inadequate allocation concealment also exists, for example, when assignment to groups depends on whether a participant's hospital number is odd or even or depends on translucent envelopes that allow discernment of assignments when they are held up to the light. The following surgical trial illustrates this pitfall.

Some years ago, a group of Australian investigators undertook a randomized trial of open versus laparoscopic appendectomy.[18] The trial ran smoothly during the day. At night, however, the attending surgeon's presence was required for the laparoscopic procedure but not for the open one, and limited operating room availability made the longer laparoscopic procedure an annoyance. Reluctant to call in a consultant, and particularly reluctant with specific senior colleagues, the residents sometimes adopted a practical solution. When an eligible patient appeared, the residents checked the attending staff and the lineup for the operating room and, depending on the personality of the attending surgeon and the length of the lineup, held the translucent envelopes containing orders up to the light. As soon as they found one that dictated an open procedure, they opened that envelope. The first eligible patient in the morning would then be allocated to a laparoscopic appendectomy group according to the passed-over envelope (D. Wall, written communication, June 9, 2000). If patients who presented at night were sicker than those who presented during the day, the residents' behavior would bias the results against the open procedure.

This story demonstrates that if those making the decision about patient eligibility are aware of the group to which a patient will be allocated—that is, if randomization is unconcealed (unblinded or unmasked)—they may systematically enroll sicker, or less sick, patients to either intervention or control groups. This behavior will defeat the purpose of randomization, and the study will yield a biased result.[17,19]

Studies have shown that poorly designed RCTs and poorly reported RCTs yield biased results. For example, in a study of 250 controlled trials from 33 meta-analyses in pregnancy and childbirth, investigators found that alleged RCTs with inadequate and unclear allocation concealment yielded larger estimates of treatment effects (on average, 41% and 33%, respectively) than trials in which authors reported adequate concealment.[17] Investigators found similar results for trials in digestive diseases, circulatory diseases, mental health, and stroke.[19] Trials that used inadequate or unclear allocation concealment yielded, on average, 37% larger estimates of effect than trials that used adequate concealment. These exaggerated estimates of intervention effects reveal meaningful levels of bias.

Careful investigators will ensure that randomization is concealed through, for example, (1) remote randomization, in which the individual recruiting patients calls a central coordinating office to discover the group to which a patient is allocated; (2) preparation of study medication in a pharmacy and storage in numbered bottles or containers; or

(3) ensuring that the envelope containing the code is opaque, sealed, and sequentially numbered.

Were Patients Analyzed in the Groups to Which They Were Randomized?

Investigators can also corrupt randomization by systematically omitting the results of patients who do not receive their assigned intervention. Readers may initially agree that patients who did not actually receive their assigned intervention should be excluded from the results. Their exclusion, however, will bias the results. We need to know the outcomes of all individual patients in a trial—including those in the experimental group who do not adhere to the intervention—and we need to include the outcome data for these nonadherent patients in the analysis to arrive at an unbiased estimate of the intervention effect.

The reasons people do not receive their assigned intervention are often related to prognosis. Some patients randomized to an intervention may never receive it because they are too sick or because they suffer the outcome of interest before they receive the intervention. For example, in an RCT comparing usual care with weekly home visits by a nurse for women at risk of postpartum depression, some of the women may be rehospitalized with postpartum depression in the first week after discharge before they receive a home visit. If investigators include such patients in the control arm but not in the home visits arm of a trial, even a useless intervention will appear to be effective. However, the apparent effectiveness of home visits will come not from the benefit to those who have weekly home visits, but from the systematic exclusion of those with the poorest prognosis from the home visit group.

Patients may choose not to adhere to a study intervention; for example, in an RCT of a 10-week smoking cessation program, some persons randomized to the program may choose not to attend after the first week. Excluding nonadherent patients from the analysis leaves those who may be destined to have a better outcome and destroys the unbiased comparison provided by randomization. If nonadherent persons were destined to do better than other members of their group and were excluded from the analysis, this would result in a misleading underestimate of the true intervention effect. If, as is more often the case, members of the nonadherent group were more likely to have an adverse outcome (i.e., failure to stop smoking), their omission would lead to a misleading overestimate of the benefit of the intervention.

The principle that dictates that we count all events in all randomized patients, regardless of whether they received the intended intervention, is the *intention-to-treat principle*. When investigators adhere to the intention-to-treat principle, they analyze outcomes based on the group to which patients were randomized, rather than on the intervention they actually received. This strategy preserves the value of randomization: determinants of outcome that we know about—and those we do not know about—will be, on average, equally distributed in the two groups, and the effect we see will result simply from the intervention assigned.

In conclusion, when reviewing a report of an RCT, look for evidence that the investigators analyzed all patients in the groups to which they were randomized, regardless of whether patients received their assigned intervention or not (see Chapter 15, The Principle of Intention-to-Treat).

Were Groups Shown to be Similar in All Known Determinants of Outcome, or Were Analyses Adjusted for Differences?

The purpose of randomization is to create groups with a similar prognosis in terms of outcome. Sometimes, through bad luck, randomization fails to achieve this goal. The smaller the sample size is, the more likely the groups in a trial will be imbalanced in the determinants of outcome.

Picture a trial testing a new nursing intervention that enrolls patients with New York Heart Association functional class III and class IV heart failure. Patients in class IV have a much worse prognosis than those in class III. The trial is small, with only eight patients. One would not be terribly surprised if, by chance, all four class III patients were allocated to the intervention group and all four class IV patients were allocated to the control group. Such a result of the allocation process would seriously bias the study in favor of the intervention. If the trial enrolled 800 patients, one would be startled if randomization placed all 400 class III patients in the intervention arm. The larger the sample size is, the more likely randomization will be to achieve its goal of balancing determinants of outcome.

Investigators can check how well randomization has done its job by examining the distribution of all determinants of outcome in intervention and control groups. Readers should look for a display of the characteristics of intervention and control patients at the beginning of the study—the baseline or entry determinants of outcome. Although we never will know whether similarity exists for unknown prognostic factors, we are reassured when known prognostic factors are well balanced.

The issue is not whether comparison groups have statistically significant differences in known determinants of outcome (i.e., in a randomized trial, one knows in advance that any differences that occur will happen by chance, making the frequently cited P values unhelpful), but, rather, the size of these differences. If the differences are large, then the validity of the study may be compromised. The stronger the relationship is between the determinants and outcome, and the greater the differences in distribution between groups, the more the differences will weaken the strength of any inference about treatment effect (i.e., you will have less confidence in the study results).

All is not lost if the intervention and control groups are not similar at baseline. Statistical techniques permit adjustment of study results for baseline differences. Accordingly, readers should look for similarity in relevant baseline characteristics; if substantial differences exist, they should note whether the investigators conducted an analysis that adjusted for those differences. When both unadjusted and adjusted analyses generate the same conclusion, readers justifiably gain confidence in the validity of the study result.

Were Patients Aware of Group Allocation?

Patients who receive an intervention that they believe is efficacious may feel and perform better than those who do not, even if the intervention has no biologic action. Although we know relatively little about the magnitude and consistency of this *placebo effect*,[20] its possible presence can mislead clinicians interested in determining the biologic effect of an intervention. Even in the absence of placebo effects, patients may respond differently, depending on whether they believe they are receiving an active intervention.

The best way to avoid these problems is to ensure that patients are unaware of whether they are receiving an experimental intervention (also known as *blinding or masking* of patients). The most common trials in which patients are unaware of group allocation are trials of a new drug in which control group patients receive an inert tablet or capsule that is identical in color, taste, and consistency to the active medication given to treatment group patients. These placebos can ensure that control group patients benefit from placebo effects to the same extent as actively treated patients. For example, in the Women's Health Initiative RCT, postmenopausal women were randomized to one daily tablet of conjugated equine estrogen (0.625 mg) combined with medroxyproges-terone acetate (2.5 mg) or a matching placebo.[6]

However, nursing interventions often involve patient education or behavior modification strategies that are difficult to duplicate in an inert form. Most often, investigators compare new nursing interventions with standard care, for example, a breast-feeding promotion intervention compared with standard care to determine its effect on duration and exclusivity of breast-feeding.[21] Alternatively, investigators compare two interventions, for example, home-based health checks by a practice nurse combined with an offer for influenza vaccination compared with a personal letter encouraging attendance at an influenza vaccination clinic for older people.[22] In each of these types of comparisons, patients are usually aware of their group allocation.

A review of the secondary journal, *Evidence-Based Nursing* (see Chapter 2, Finding the Evidence, for a description of secondary journals), revealed very few nondrug trials in which patients were blinded to their group allocation. Examples include randomization of malnourished postsurgical patients to treatment with an oral nutritional supplement or routine nutritional management,[23] randomization of patients in a coronary care unit to intercessory prayers or usual care (patients were unaware of others' prayers on their behalf),[24] allocation of men with incontinence after radical prostatectomy to pelvic-floor re-education or a placebo including electrotherapy that was applied to the abdomen and thighs but that could not affect pelvic-floor function,[25] and randomization of infants with colic to spinal manipulation by a chiropractor or being held by the nurse for 10 minutes (to keep parents blind to group allocation, a nurse was responsible for taking the infant to the chiropractor or holding the infant).[26]

Given the difficulty of blinding patients to group allocation in nursing intervention studies, it is important that outcome assessors (sometimes referred to as data collectors) and, when possible, clinicians be blinded.

Were Clinicians Aware of Group Allocation?

If randomization succeeds, intervention and control groups begin with a very similar prognosis. However, randomization provides no guarantees that the two groups will remain similar. Differences in patient care other than the intervention under study can *bias* the results. For example, imagine a trial comparing the effects of larval therapy with moist wound dressings for sloughy, sacral pressure ulcers. It is simply not possible to blind either nurses or patients to who is receiving the larval therapy. Although pressure relief is of paramount importance in healing any pressure ulcer, it becomes doubly important when lying on the sacrum may kill the fly larvae. One can imagine that patients in the larval treatment group would receive far greater attention to their pressure relief than their control group counterparts. The results would yield an overestimate of the intervention effect. The reason is that the *cointervention* of pressure relief will itself promote ulcer healing.

Clinicians gain greatest confidence in study results when investigators document that all cointerventions that may plausibly affect the outcome are administered more or less equally in intervention and control groups. The absence of such documentation is a less serious problem if clinicians are blinded to whether patients are receiving an active intervention or are part of a control group. Effective blinding eliminates the possibility of either conscious or unconscious differential administration of effective interventions to the comparison groups.

However, as discussed earlier, because clinicians often deliver the intervention (e.g., patient education or behavior modification strategies), it is difficult, if not impossible, to blind clinicians in many studies of nursing interventions.

Were Outcome Assessors Aware of Group Allocation?

If either intervention or control group participants receive closer follow-up, target outcome events may be reported more frequently in that group. In addition, unblinded study personnel who measure or record outcomes such as psychometric tests, clinical status, or quality of life may provide different interpretations of marginal findings or may offer differential encouragement during performance tests, either of which can distort results.[27] Study personnel assessing outcomes can almost always be blinded to group allocation, even if patients and health care providers cannot. Investigators can take additional precautions by constructing a blinded adjudication committee to review clinical data and decide on outcome-related issues. For example, the committee can review photographs of wounds to determine whether a wound has healed or can evaluate study data to determine whether a patient has had a postoperative complication. The more judgment required in determining whether a patient has had a target outcome, the more important blinding becomes. For example, blinding is less crucial in studies in which the outcome is all-cause mortality.

Was Follow-up Complete?

Ideally, at the conclusion of a trial, investigators will know the status of each patient with respect to the target outcome. We often refer to patients whose status is unknown as *lost to follow-up*. The greater the number of patients who are lost to follow-up, the more a study's validity is potentially compromised. The reason is that patients who are lost to follow-up often have different prognoses from those who are retained; these patients may disappear because they experience adverse outcomes (even death) or because they are doing well (and so did not return to be assessed). The situation is analogous to the reason for the necessity for an intention-to-treat analysis: patients who withdraw from an intervention or treatment program may be less or (usually) more likely to suffer the target adverse event of interest.

When does loss to follow-up seriously threaten validity? Rules of thumb (you may run across thresholds such as 20%) are misleading. Consider two hypothetical randomized trials, each of which enrolls 1000 patients into both intervention and control

Table **4-2**   When Does Loss to Follow-up Seriously Threaten Validity?

	Trial A		Trial B	
	Intervention	*Control*	*Intervention*	*Control*
Number of patients randomized	1000	1000	1000	1000
Number (%) lost to follow-up	30 (3%)	30 (3%)	30 (3%)	30 (3%)
Number (%) of readmissions	200 (20%)	400 (40%)	30 (3%)	60 (6%)
Relative risk reduction: not counting patients lost to follow-up	0.2/0.4 = 0.50		0.03/0.06 = 0.50	
Relative risk reduction: worst-case scenario*	0.17/0.4 = 0.43		0.00/0.06 = 0	

The worst-case scenario assumes that all patients allocated to the intervention group and lost to follow-up were readmitted, and all patients allocated to the control group and lost to follow-up were not readmitted.

groups, of whom 30 (3%) are lost to follow-up (Table 4-2). In trial *A*, treated patients are readmitted to hospital at half the rate of the control group (200 versus 400), a reduction in relative risk of 50%. To what extent does the loss to follow-up potentially threaten our inference that the intervention reduces the hospital readmission rate by half? If we assume the worst, that is, that all treated patients lost to follow-up were readmitted, the number of hospital readmissions in the experimental group would be 230 (23%). If there were no readmissions among the control patients who were lost to follow-up, our best estimate of the effect of the intervention in reducing the risk of hospital readmission would drop from 200 out of 400, or 50%, to (400 minus 230) or 170 out of 400, or 43%. Thus, even assuming the worst makes little difference in the best estimate of the magnitude of the intervention effect. Our inference is therefore secure.

Contrast this with trial *B*. Here, the reduction in the relative risk of hospital readmission is also 50%. In this case, however, the total number of readmissions is much lower: 30 patients who receive the intervention are readmitted to hospital, and 60 control patients are readmitted. In trial *B*, if we make the same worst-case assumption about the fate of the patients lost to follow-up, the results would change markedly. If we assume that all patients initially allocated to the intervention—but subsequently lost to follow-up—are readmitted, the number of readmissions among treated patients rises from 30 to 60, which is equal to the number of control group readmissions. Let us assume that this assumption is accurate. Because we would have 60 readmissions in both intervention and control groups, the effect of the intervention drops to zero. Because of this dramatic change in the intervention effect (i.e., 50% relative risk reduction [RRR] if we ignore those lost to follow-up; 0% RRR if we assume all patients in the intervention group who were lost to follow-up were readmitted), the 3% loss to follow-up in trial *B* threatens our inference about the magnitude of the RRR.

Of course, this worst-case scenario is unlikely. When a worst-case scenario, if true, substantially alters the results, you must judge the plausibility of a markedly different outcome *event rate* in intervention and control group patients who have not been followed-up. Demonstration that patients lost to follow-up are similar with respect to important determinants of outcome, such as age and disease severity, reduces, but does not eliminate, the possibility of a different rate of target events.

In conclusion, loss to follow-up potentially threatens a study's validity. If assuming a worst-case scenario does not change the inferences arising from study results, then loss to follow-up is not a problem. If such an assumption would significantly alter the results, validity is compromised. The extent of that compromise remains a matter of judgment and will depend on the likelihood that intervention patients lost to follow-up did poorly whereas control patients lost to follow-up did well.

USING THE GUIDE

How well did the study of alternative needle lengths for routine immunization in infants aged 4 months achieve the goal of creating groups with similar determinants of outcome? The investigators tell us the study was randomized, with 58 infants allocated to the long-needle group and 61 to the short-needle group. The authors explicitly addressed the issue of concealment and noted that "allocations were concealed in sequentially numbered opaque envelopes opened once written parental consent was obtained."

They documented the two groups' similarity with respect to weight, age at vaccination, sex, site of injection, and vaccine type. Of these variables, only sex showed substantial imbalance (36% girls in the long-needle group and 47% in the short-needle group). It seems implausible, however, that boys and girls would have systematically different reactions to vaccine injection.

As is the usual case with evaluations of nursing interventions, clinicians were not blinded to group allocation. The investigators noted, however, that parents were not told of the needle length. Furthermore, the investigators commented that if bias was introduced by unblinding, it could more plausibly go against, rather than for, the longer needle. The investigators did not include nine of the randomized infants in the analysis, five in the long-needle group and four in the short-needle group, and therefore did not do an intention-to-treat analysis. Of these nine infants, eight parents did not return the diary, whereas the ninth was mistakenly included in the study at the second vaccination. No infants were lost to follow-up, and all were accounted for at the end of the study.

The final assessment of validity is never a yes/no decision. Rather, think of validity as a continuum ranging from strong studies that are very likely to yield an accurate estimate of an intervention effect to weak studies that are very likely to yield a biased estimate of effect. Inevitably, the judgment about where a study lies along this continuum involves some subjectivity. In this case, uncertainty arises from the imbalance in sex, the lack of blinding of clinicians, and the nine patients randomized but not included in the analysis. Our judgment is that none of these limitations is likely to introduce major bias in the results. We would therefore put the study high on the continuum between very low and very high validity.

WHAT ARE THE RESULTS?

How Large Was the Intervention Effect?

Frequently, RCTs carefully monitor how often patients experience some adverse event or outcome. Examples of these *dichotomous outcomes* (yes/no outcomes—ones that either happen or do not happen) include hospital readmissions, postoperative infections, and development of pressure ulcers. Patients either do or do not suffer an event, and the authors report the proportion of patients who develop such events. Consider, for example, a study in which 20% of control group patients were readmitted to hospital, but only 15% of those receiving a new intervention were readmitted. How might these results be expressed?

One way would be as the absolute difference (known as the *absolute risk reduction* or risk difference) between the proportion of patients who were readmitted in the control group (x) and the proportion of patients who were readmitted in the intervention group (y), or $x - y = 0.20 - 0.15 = 0.05$. Another way to express the impact of an intervention would be as a *relative risk:* the risk of hospital readmissions among patients receiving the new intervention, relative to that risk among patients in the control group, or $y/x = 0.15/0.20 = 0.75$.

The most commonly reported measure of dichotomous intervention effects is the complement of this relative risk, the *RRR*. It is expressed as a percentage: $(1 - y/x) \times 100 = (1 - 0.75) \times 100 = 25\%$. An RRR of 25% means that the new intervention reduced the risk of hospital readmission by 25% relative to that occurring among control patients; and the greater the RRR, the more effective is the intervention. Investigators may compute the relative risk over time, as in a *survival analysis,* and call it a *hazard ratio* (see Chapter 27, Measures of Association). When people do not specify whether they are talking about RRR or absolute risk reduction (e.g., "Intervention X was 30% effective in reducing the risk of hospital readmission" or "The efficacy of the vaccine was 92%"), they are almost invariably talking about RRR. Advertisements for drugs and devices, whether they make it explicit or not, almost invariably cite relative risk. See Chapter 27, Measures of Association, for more detail about how the RRR results in a subjective impression of a larger intervention effect than do other ways of expressing intervention effects.

The terms *absolute risk reduction* and *RRR* are appropriate when we are interested in reducing harmful events such as death, readmissions, and pain. However, these terms are not useful when we are interested in increasing beneficial events such as breastfeeding duration and wound healing. In these cases, the corresponding terms are *absolute benefit increase* and *relative benefit increase.* Table 4-3 illustrates the relationships between event rates in control and intervention groups when the outcome is harmful versus beneficial, as well as the associated terminology. You may also see more generic terms such as *absolute difference* and *relative difference.*

Sometimes, particularly in studies of nursing interventions, authors express results in terms of mean or median differences in a continuous variable (one that can take a wide range of values). Often, the meaning of these results is quite clear. For instance, in an RCT of the effect of preoperative smoking interventions on postoperative complications, the median length of hospital stay was 11 days in the intervention group and 13 days in

Table 4-3   Interpreting Harmful and Beneficial Outcomes

	Outcome	
	Harmful *(e.g., premature death)*	*Beneficial* *(e.g., wound healing)*
Terms used	Absolute risk reduction Relative risk reduction	Absolute benefit increase Relative benefit increase
Result favors intervention	x>y	x<y
Result favors control	x<y	x>y

x, *Control group event rate; y, intervention group event rate.*

the control group.[28] In other instances, one requires specialized knowledge to interpret differences in continuous outcomes. A trial of insulin adjustment by a diabetes nurse educator found that the control group had a decrease in hemoglobin A_{1c} levels of 0.005, and the treatment group had a decrease of 0.018.[29] One would need to know something about usual levels of hemoglobin A_{1c} in people with diabetes to know whether this difference was trivial or large.

How Precise Was the Estimate of the Intervention Effect?

Realistically, the true risk reduction can never be known. The best we have is the estimate provided by rigorous controlled trials, and the best estimate of the true intervention effect is that observed in the trial. This estimate is called a *point estimate,* a single value calculated from observations of the sample that is used to estimate a population value or parameter. Although the point estimate approximates the true value, it is unlikely to be precisely correct. Investigators often tell us the limits within which the true effect likely lies by calculating *confidence intervals,* a range of values within which one can be confident that the true value is situated.[30]

We usually (although arbitrarily) use the 95% confidence interval (see Chapter 29, Confidence Intervals). You can consider the 95% confidence interval as defining the range that includes the true RRR 95% of the time. You will seldom find the true RRR toward the extremes of this interval, and you will find the true RRR beyond these extremes only 5% of the time, a property of the confidence interval that relates closely to the conventional level of statistical significance of $P < 0.05$ (see Chapter 28, Hypothesis Testing). We illustrate the use of confidence intervals in the following examples.

Example 1. If a trial to prevent pressure ulcers randomized 100 patients each to intervention and control groups, and 20 pressure ulcers developed in the control group and 15 pressure ulcers developed in the intervention group, the authors would calculate a point estimate for the RRR of 25% (x = 20/100 or 0.20, y = 15/100 or 0.15, and $1 - y/x = 1 - \{0.15/0.20\} \times 100 = 25\%$). You could guess, however, that the true RRR may be much smaller or much greater than this 25%, based on a difference of only 5 pressure ulcers. In fact, you could surmise that the intervention may provide no benefit (an RRR of 0%) or may even do harm (a negative RRR), and you would be correct. In fact, these results are consistent with both an RRR of −38% (i.e., patients given the new intervention may be 38% *more* likely to develop a pressure ulcer than control patients) and an RRR of nearly 59% (i.e., patients receiving the new intervention may have a risk of developing a pressure ulcer almost 60% *less* than that of those who do not receive the intervention). In other words, the 95% confidence interval around this RRR is −38% to 59%, and the trial really has not helped us decide whether to offer the new intervention.

Example 2. What if the trial enrolled 1000 patients per group rather than 100 patients per group, and the same event rates were observed as before, so there were 200 pressure ulcers in the control group ($x = 200/1000 = 0.20$) and 150 pressure ulcers in the intervention group ($y = 150/1000 = 0.15$)? Again, the point estimate of the RRR is 25% ($1 - y/x = 1 - \{0.15/0.20\} \times 100 = 25\%$). In this larger trial, you could think that the true reduction in risk is much closer to 25% and, again, you would be correct. The 95% confidence interval around the RRR for this result is entirely on the positive side of zero and runs from 9% to 41%.

These examples show that the larger the sample size of a trial is, the larger the number of outcome events will be, and the greater our confidence will be that the true RRR (or any other measure of efficacy) is close to what we have observed. In the second example mentioned earlier, the lowest plausible value for the RRR was 9%, and the highest value was 41%. The point estimate—in this case, 25%—is the one value most likely to represent the true RRR. As one considers values farther and farther from the point estimate, they become less and less consistent with the observed RRR. By the time one crosses the upper or lower boundaries of the 95% confidence interval, the values are extremely unlikely to represent the true RRR, given the point estimate (i.e., the observed RRR).

Figure 4-1 represents the confidence intervals around the point estimate of a RRR of 25% in these two examples, with a risk reduction of zero representing no intervention effect. In both scenarios, the point estimate of the RRR is 25%, but the confidence interval is far narrower in the second scenario and, therefore, the estimate of effect is more precise.

It is evident that results based on larger sample sizes and a greater number of outcome events will be associated with narrower confidence intervals. When is the sample size big enough[31] (see Chapter 29, Confidence Intervals)? In a *positive study,* a study in which the authors conclude that the intervention is effective, one can look at the lower boundary of the confidence interval. In the second example, this lower boundary was +9%. If this RRR (the lowest RRR that is consistent with the study results) is still important (i.e., it is large enough for you to recommend the intervention to the patient), then the investigators have enrolled sufficient patients. Conversely, if you do not consider an RRR of 9% important, then the study cannot be considered definitive, even if its results are statistically significant (i.e., they exclude a risk reduction of zero). Keep in mind that the probability that the true value is less than the lower boundary of the confidence interval is only 2.5%, and a different criterion for the confidence interval (e.g., a 90% confidence interval) may be as or more appropriate.

The confidence interval also helps us interpret *negative studies,* in which the authors have concluded that the experimental intervention is no better than the control

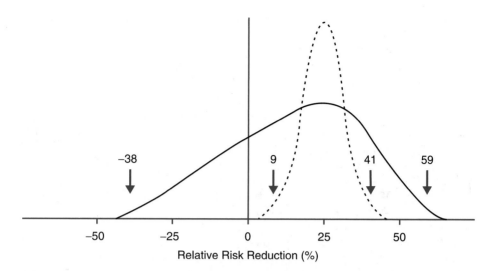

Figure 4-1. Confidence intervals around relative risk reduction. Two studies with the same point estimates, a 25% relative risk reduction, but different sample sizes and correspondingly different confidence intervals. The *solid line* represents the confidence interval around the first example, in which there were 100 patients per group and the numbers of events in intervention and control groups were 15 and 20, respectively. The *broken line* represents the confidence interval around the second example, in which there were 1000 patients per group, and the numbers of events in intervention and control groups were 150 and 200, respectively.

intervention. All we need to do is look at the upper boundary of the confidence interval. If the RRR at this upper boundary would, if true, be clinically important, the study has failed to exclude an important intervention effect. Consider Example 1 presented earlier, the study with 100 patients in each group. This study does not exclude the possibility of harm (indeed, it is consistent with a 38% increase in relative risk), the associated P value would be greater than 0.05, and the study would be considered negative in that it failed to show a convincing intervention effect (see Figure 4-1). Recall, however, that the upper boundary of the confidence interval was an RRR of 59%. Clearly, if this large RRR represented the truth, the benefit of the intervention would be substantial. We can conclude that, although the investigators failed to prove that the experimental intervention was better than standard treatment, they also failed to prove that it was not; they did not exclude a large, positive intervention effect. Once again, you must bear in mind the proviso that the choice of a 95% confidence interval is arbitrary. A reasonable alternative, a 90% confidence interval, would be somewhat narrower.

The 95% confidence intervals also help us to interpret studies using continuous outcomes. For instance, a randomized trial showed that home visitation after childbirth increased the length of time between the first and second child from a mean of 26.6 months to 30.3 months, a difference of 3.7 months. The 95% confidence interval tells us that the true effect may range from 1.2 to 6.1 months.[32]

When Authors Do Not Report the Confidence Interval

What can you do if the *confidence interval* around the RRR is not reported in the article? The easiest approach is to examine the *P* value. If it is exactly 0.05, then the lower bound of the 95% confidence limit for the RRR has to lie exactly at zero (a relative risk of 1), and you cannot exclude the possibility that the intervention has no effect. As the *P* value decreases to less than 0.05, the lower bound of the 95% confidence limit for the RRR increases above zero. For instance, in the trial of preoperative smoking interventions,[28] the *P* value associated with the difference between the median values of 11 days in the hospital for the intervention group and 13 days for the control group was 0.41; if the confidence interval was calculated, it would include an effect favoring the control group as well as the intervention group. Conversely, the difference in hemoglobin A_{1c} levels in the trial of insulin adjustment by a diabetes nurse educator[29] was associated with a *P* value of 0.01, a finding telling you that the entire confidence interval would lie in the region favoring the intervention group.

A second approach involves calculating the confidence intervals yourself[33] or asking the help of someone else (e.g., a statistician) to do so. Once you obtain the confidence intervals, you will know how high and low the RRR could be (i.e., you know the precision of the estimate of the intervention effect) and can interpret the results as described earlier.

Not all randomized trials have dichotomous outcomes, nor should they. For example, many studies report changes in length of hospital stay, quality of life, blood pressure, or pain with an intervention. In a study of respiratory-muscle training for patients with chronic airflow limitation, one primary outcome measured how far patients could walk in 6 minutes in an enclosed corridor.[34] This 6-minute walk improved from an average of 406 to 416 m (an increase of 10 m) in the experimental group receiving respiratory-muscle training and from 409 to 429 m (an increase of 20 m) in the control group. The point estimate for improvement in the 6-minute walk resulting from respiratory-muscle training therefore was negative, at −10 m (or a 10 m difference in favor of the control group).

Here, too, you should look for the 95% confidence intervals around the difference in changes in exercise capacity and consider their implications. The investigators tell us that the lower boundary of the 95% confidence interval was −26 m (i.e., the results are consistent with a difference of 26 m in favor of the control intervention), and the upper boundary was +5 m. Even in the best of circumstances, adding 5 m to the 400 m recorded at the start of the trial would not be important to the patient, and this result effectively excludes an important benefit of respiratory muscle training as applied in this study. Having determined the magnitude and precision of the intervention effect, readers can turn to the final question of how to apply the article's results to patients in their clinical practice.

The investigators in the trial of alternative needle length asked parents to measure redness, swelling, and tenderness at the injection site at 6 hours and at 1, 2, and 3 days after the injection. The worst redness and swelling occurred on day 1, and we focus on results at that point. The investigators found a nonsignificant trend in tenderness in favor of the long-needle (4/53; 8%) versus the short-needle group (8/57; 14%) (relative risk, 0.54; 95% confidence interval, 0.17 to 1.68; $P = 0.3$). Differences in redness and swelling favoring the long-needle group were larger, with far narrower confidence intervals and impressive P values. On day 1, parents found redness in 15 of 53 (28%) infants in the long-needle group compared with 36 of 57 (63%) in the short-needle group (relative risk, 0.45; 95% confidence interval, 0.28 to 0.72; $P = 0.0002$). The results for swelling were identical: 15 of 53 (28%) infants in the long-needle group and 36 of 57 (63%) in the short-needle group (relative risk, 0.45; 95% confidence interval, 0.28 to 0.72; $P = 0.0002$).

HOW CAN I APPLY THE RESULTS TO PATIENT CARE?

Were the Study Patients Similar to the Patients in My Clinical Setting?

Often, your patient has different attributes or characteristics from those enrolled in the trial. He or she may be older, sicker, or may have comorbid disease that would have excluded him or her from participation in the research study. If the patient had qualified for enrollment in the study (i.e., if the patient had met all *inclusion criteria* and had violated none of the *exclusion criteria*), you could apply the results with considerable confidence.

Even here, however, there is a limitation. Interventions are not uniformly effective in every individual patient. Typically, some patients respond extremely well, whereas others achieve no benefit whatsoever. RCTs estimate average intervention effects. Applying these average effects means that clinicians will likely expose some patients to the cost, inconvenience, and potential side effects of an intervention without benefit.

What if the patient in your setting does not meet a study's inclusion criteria? The study result would probably apply even if, for example, he or she were 2 years too old for the study, had more severe disease, had previously been treated with a different intervention, or had a comorbid condition. A better approach than rigidly applying a study's inclusion and exclusion criteria is to ask whether there is some compelling reason that the results should *not* be applied to the patient. A compelling reason usually will not be found, and often you can generalize the results to the patient in your setting with confidence (see Chapter 33, Applying Results to Individual Patients).

A related issue has to do with the extent to which we can generalize findings from a study using a particular intervention to another closely (or not so closely) related intervention. This question frequently arises in relation to drug treatments, but it also pertains to other types of health care interventions, including equipment and devices. For example, if one brand of hydrocolloid dressings is effective in healing grade 2 pressure ulcers, are we safe in assuming that all hydrocolloid dressings are similarly effective?

A final issue arises when a patient fits the features of a subgroup of patients in the trial report. In articles reporting the results of a trial (especially when the intervention does not appear to be effective for the average patient), the authors may have examined a number of subgroups, such as patients at different stages of illness, or with different comorbid conditions, or of different ages. Often, these subgroup analyses were not planned ahead of time, and the data are simply dredged to see what may be revealed. Investigators may over-interpret these data-dependent analyses as demonstrating that an intervention really has different effects in various subgroups of patients. For example, authors may say that older or sicker patients benefit substantially more or less than other subgroups of patients.

We encourage you to be skeptical of subgroup analyses[35] (see Chapter 16, When to Believe a Subgroup Analysis). An intervention is likely to benefit a subgroup more or less than other patients only if the difference in the effects of the intervention in the subgroups is large and very unlikely to occur by chance. Even when these conditions apply, results may be misleading if investigators did not specify their hypotheses before the study began, if they had a large number of hypotheses, or if other studies fail to replicate the finding.

Were All Important Outcomes Considered?

Interventions are indicated when they have been shown to provide important benefits. Demonstrating that an adolescent pregnancy prevention program improves knowledge and attitudes about birth control or that a lipid-lowering agent improves lipid profiles does not necessarily provide a sufficient reason for recommending these interventions. What is required is evidence that the interventions improve outcomes that are important to patients, such as reducing the number of adolescent pregnancies or decreasing the risk of myocardial infarction. We can consider knowledge and attitudes about birth control and lipid profiles as substitute or *surrogate end points* or outcomes (see Chapter 13, Surrogate Outcomes). In other words, investigators have chosen to substitute these variables for those that patients would consider important, usually because to confirm benefits on the latter, they would have had to enroll many more patients and follow them up for far longer periods.

Currently, the most striking examples of the danger of using surrogate end points relate to medication trials. Because antiarrhythmic drugs after myocardial infarction were shown to reduce abnormal ventricular depolarizations (the surrogate end points) in the short term, it made sense that they would reduce the occurrence of life-threatening arrhythmias in the long term. A group of investigators conducted randomized trials on three agents (encainide, flecainide, and moricizine) previously shown to be effective in suppressing the surrogate end point of abnormal ventricular depolarizations to determine whether these drugs reduced mortality in patients with asymptomatic or mildly symptomatic arrhythmias after myocardial infarction. The investigators had to stop the trials when they discovered that mortality was substantially higher in patients receiving antiarrhythmic treatment than in those receiving placebo.[36,37] Clinicians relying on the surrogate end point of arrhythmia suppression would have continued to administer the three drugs, to the considerable detriment of their patients.

Even when investigators report favorable effects of an intervention on one clinically important outcome, you must consider the possibility of deleterious effects on other outcomes. For instance, patients who had pressure bandages applied to their legs after coronary angiography had less bleeding but more nausea, urinary discomfort, and pain in the groin, back, and leg.[38] Cancer chemotherapy can lengthen life but may decrease its quality (see Chapter 12, Quality of Life). The most common limitation of RCTs with regard to reporting important outcomes is the omission of documentation of adverse effects.

Another long-neglected outcome is the resource implications of alternative management strategies. Few randomized trials measure either direct costs, such as intervention or program expenses and health care worker salaries, or indirect costs, such as patients' loss of income from illness. Nevertheless, the increasing resource constraints that health care systems face mandate careful attention to *economic analysis,* particularly of resource-intense interventions (see Chapter 18, Economic Evaluation).

Are the Likely Intervention Benefits Worth the Potential Harm and Costs?

If you can apply the study's results to a patient, and its outcomes are important, the next question concerns whether the probable benefits of the intervention are worth the effort that you and the patient must expend. A 25% reduction in the relative risk of a postoperative infection, for example, may sound quite impressive, but its impact on the patient and your practice may nevertheless be minimal. This notion is illustrated using a concept called *number needed to treat* (NNT), the number of patients who must receive an intervention during a specific period to prevent one adverse outcome or produce one positive outcome.[39,40]

The impact of an intervention is related not only to its RRR, but also to the risk of the adverse outcome it is designed to prevent. One large trial suggests that tissue plasminogen activator (tPA) administration reduces the relative risk of death after myocardial infarction by approximately 12% compared with streptokinase.[41] Table 4-4 considers two patients presenting with acute myocardial infarction associated with ST segment elevations on their electrocardiograms.

In the first case, a 40-year-old man presents with electrocardiographic findings suggesting an inferior myocardial infarction. You find no signs of heart failure, and the patient is in normal sinus rhythm with a rate of 90 beats per minute. This patient's risk

Table **4-4**   Considerations in the Decision to Treat Two Patients With Myocardial Infarction With Tissue Plasminogen Activator or Streptokinase

	Risk of Death at 1 Year After Myocardial Infarction		
	Streptokinase	tPA (Absolute Risk Reduction)	Number Needed to Treat
40-year-old man, with small MI	2%	1.76% (0.24% or 0.0024)	417
70-year-old man, large MI and heart failure	40%	35.2% (4.8% or 0.048)	21

MI, *Myocardial infarction;* tPA, *tissue plasminogen activator.*

of death in the first year after infarction may be as low as 2%. Compared with streptokinase, tPA would reduce this risk by 12% to 1.76%, an absolute risk reduction of 0.24% (0.0024). The inverse of this absolute risk reduction (i.e., 1 divided by the absolute risk reduction) is equal to the number of such patients we would need to treat to prevent one event (in this case, to prevent one death after a mild heart attack in a low-risk patient)—the NNT. In this case, we would have to treat approximately 417 such patients to save a single life (1/0.0024 = 417). Given the small increased risk of intracerebral hemorrhage associated with tPA, and its additional cost, many clinicians might prefer streptokinase in this patient.

In the second case, a 70-year-old man presents with electrocardiographic signs of anterior myocardial infarction with pulmonary edema. His risk of dying in the next year is approximately 40%. Compared with streptokinase, tPA would reduce this risk by 12% to 35.2%, thus generating an absolute risk reduction of 4.8% (0.048), and we would need to treat only 21 such patients to avert a premature death (1/0.048 = 20.8). Many clinicians would consider tPA the preferable agent for this man.

The actual calculation of NNT warrants a note here. NNT can be calculated in any of three ways. Earlier we calculated the inverse of the absolute risk reduction by using proportions: 1/0.048 = 20.8. Alternatively, we could have calculated it by using percentages; in this case, we use 100% as our numerator and the absolute risk reduction as a percentage (i.e., 4.8% resulting in 100/4.8 = 20.8). The third way is to divide the absolute risk reduction as a percentage into 1 but then multiply by 100: $1/4.8 \times 100 = 20.8$. All three ways of calculating the NNT yield the same value; it is simply a matter of preference.

A key element of the decision to implement an intervention, therefore, is to consider a patient's risk of an adverse event if the condition is left untreated. For any given RRR, the higher the probability that a patient will experience an adverse outcome if we do not intervene, the more likely the patient will benefit from the intervention and the fewer such patients we would need to treat to prevent one adverse outcome (see Chapter 27, Measures of Association). Knowing the NNT helps clinicians in the process of weighing the benefits and risks associated with management options (see Chapter 33, Applying Results to Individual Patients). Chapter 32, Number Needed to Treat, presents NNTs associated with clearly defined risk groups in some common therapeutic situations.

Trading off benefits and risks requires an accurate assessment of the adverse effects associated with an intervention. RCTs with relatively small sample sizes are unsuitable for detecting rare but catastrophic adverse effects of treatment. Although RCTs are the correct vehicle for reporting commonly occurring adverse effects, study reports usually do not include these outcomes. Clinicians must look to other sources of information— often characterized by weaker methodologies—to obtain estimates of the adverse effects of an intervention.

Individual patient preferences or values determine the correct choice when weighing benefits and risks. Clinicians should attend to the growing literature on patients' response to illness (see Chapter 8, Qualitative Research). Uncertainty remains about how best to communicate information to patients and how to incorporate their values into clinical decision making. Vigorous investigation of this frontier of evidence-based decision making is underway (see Chapter 34, Incorporating Patient Values).

CLINICAL RESOLUTION

The investigators enrolled all infants who were receiving vaccines, and the results are therefore widely generalizable. Redness, swelling, and tenderness are key reactions to a vaccination that may be attributable to needle length or bore. The effect was impressive, with a reduction of more than 50% in the proportion of infants with redness and swelling. In absolute terms, the reduction in both redness and swelling was 35%. Thus, one would need to use the longer needle in about three infants (100/35 or 1/0.35) to prevent a single infant from experiencing redness and swelling. You and your colleagues agree that in future, clinic policy will be to use the longer needle for infant vaccination.

REFERENCES

1. Routine primary immunisation using a longer needle resulted in fewer local reactions in infants. *Evid Based Nurs.* 2001;4:41. Abstract of: Diggle L, Deeks J. Effect of needle length on incidence of local reactions to routine immunisation in infants aged 4 months: randomised controlled trial. *BMJ.* 2000;321:931-933.

2. Diggle L, Deeks J. Effect of needle length on incidence of local reactions to routine immunisation in infants aged 4 months: randomised controlled trial. *BMJ.* 2000;321:931-933.

3. Alexander JW, Fischer JE, Boyajian M, et al. The influence of hair removal methods on wound infections. *Arch Surg.* 1983;118:347-352.

4. Hoe NY, Nambiar R. Is preoperative shaving really necessary? *Ann Acad Med Singapore.* 1985;14:700-704.

5. Backhouse CM, Blair SD, Savage AP, et al. Controlled trial of occlusive dressings in healing chronic venous ulcers. *Br J Surg.* 1987;47:626-627.

6. Rossouw JE, Anderson GL, Prentice RL, et al. Risks and benefits of estrogen plus progestin in healthy postmenopausal women: principal results from the Women's Health Initiative randomized controlled trial. *JAMA.* 2002;288:321-333.

7. Guyatt GH, DiCenso A, Farewell V, Willan A, Griffith L. Randomized trials versus observational studies in adolescent pregnancy prevention. *J Clin Epidemiol.* 2000;53:167-174.

8. Sacks HS, Chalmers TC, Smith H Jr. Sensitivity and specificity of clinical trials: randomized v historical controls. *Arch Intern Med.* 1983;143:753-755.

9. Chalmers TC, Celano P, Sacks HS, Smith H Jr. Bias in treatment assignment in controlled clinical trials. *N Engl J Med.* 1983;309:1358-1361.

10. Colditz GA, Miller JN, Mosteller F. How study design affects outcomes in comparisons of therapy. I. Medical. *Stat Med.* 1989;8:441-454.

11. Emerson JD, Burdick E, Hoaglin DC, et al. An empirical study of the possible relation of treatment differences to quality scores in controlled randomized clinical trials. *Control Clin Trials.* 1990;11:339-352.

12. Kunz R, Oxman AD. The unpredictability paradox: review of empirical comparisons of randomised and non-randomised clinical trials. *BMJ.* 1998;317:1185-1190.

13. Schulz KF. Subverting randomization in controlled trials. *JAMA.* 1995;274:1456-1458.

14. Schulz KF. Randomized trials, human nature, and reporting guidelines. *Lancet.* 1996;348:596-598.

15. Schulz KF. Assessing allocation concealment and blinding in randomised controlled trials: why bother? *Evid Based Nurs.* 2001;4:4-6.

16. Schulz KF, Chalmers I, Grimes DA, et al. Assessing the quality of randomization from reports of controlled trials published in obstetrics and gynecology journals. *JAMA.* 1994;272:125-128.

17. Schulz KF, Chalmers I, Hayes RJ, Altman DG. Empirical evidence of bias, dimensions of methodological quality associated with estimates of treatment effects in controlled trials. *JAMA.* 1995;273:408-412.

18. Hansen JB, Smithers BM, Schache D, Wall DR, Miller BJ, Menzies BL. Laparoscopic versus open appendectomy: prospective randomized trial. *World J Surg.* 1996;20:17-20.

19. Moher D, Jones A, Cook DJ, et al. Does quality of reports of randomised trials affect estimates of intervention efficacy reported in meta-analyses? *Lancet*. 1998;352:609-613.

20. Kaptchuk TJ. Powerful placebo: the dark side of the randomised controlled trial. *Lancet*. 1998;351:1722-1725.

21. Kramer MS, Guo T, Platt RW, et al for the PROBIT Study Group. Breastfeeding and infant growth: biology or bias? *Pediatrics*. 2002;110:343-347.

22. Arthur AJ, Matthews RJ, Jagger C, et al. Improving uptake of influenza vaccination among older people: a randomised controlled trial. *Br J Gen Pract*. 2002;52:717-722.

23. Beattie AH, Prach AT, Baxter JP, et al. A randomised controlled trial evaluating the use of enteral nutritional supplements postoperatively in malnourished surgical patients. *Gut*. 2000;46:813-818.

24. Harris WS, Gowda M, Kolb JW, et al. A randomized, controlled trial of the effects of remote, intercessory prayer on outcomes in patients admitted to the coronary care unit. *Arch Intern Med*. 1999;159:2273-2278.

25. Van Kampen M, DeWeerdt W, Van Poppel H, et al. Effect of pelvic-floor re-education on duration and degree of incontinence after radical prostatectomy: a randomised controlled trial. *Lancet*. 2000;355:98-102.

26. Olafsdottir E, Forshei S, Fluge G, et al. Randomised controlled trial of infantile colic treated with chiropractic spinal manipulation. *Arch Dis Child*. 2001;84:138-141.

27. Guyatt GH, Pugsley SO, Sullivan MJ, et al. Effect of encouragement on walking test performance. *Thorax*. 1984;39:818-822.

28. Moller AM, Villebro N, Pedersen T, Tonnesen H. Effect of preoperative smoking intervention on postoperative complications: a randomised clinical trial. *Lancet*. 2002;359:114-117.

29. Thompson DM, Kozak SE, Sheps S. Insulin adjustment by a diabetes nurse educator improves glucose control in insulin-requiring diabetic patients: a randomized trial. *Can Med Assoc J*. 1999;161:959-962.

30. Altman DG, Gore SM, Gardner MJ, Pocock SJ. Statistical guidelines for contributors to medical journals. In: Gardner MJ, Altman DG, eds. *Statistics With Confidence: Confidence Intervals and Statistical Guidelines*. London, UK: BMJ Publishing Group; 1989:83-100.

31. Detsky AS, Sackett DL. When was a "negative" trial big enough? How many patients you needed depends on what you found. *Arch Intern Med*. 1985;145:709-715.

32. Kitzman H, Olds DL, Sidora K, et al. Enduring effects of nurse home visitation on maternal life course: a 3-year follow-up of a randomized trial. *JAMA*. 2000;283:1983-1989.

33. Sackett DL, Haynes RB, Guyatt GH, Tugwell P. *Clinical Epidemiology: A Basic Science for Clinical Medicine*. 2nd ed. Boston, MA: Little, Brown; 1991:218.

34. Guyatt G, Keller J, Singer J, Halcrow S, Newhouse M. Controlled trial of respiratory muscle training in chronic airflow limitation. *Thorax*. 1992;47:598-602.

35. Oxman AD, Guyatt GH. A consumer's guide to subgroup analysis. *Ann Intern Med*. 1992;116;78-84.

36. Echt DS, Liebson PR, Mitchell LB, et al. Mortality and morbidity in patients receiving encainide, flecainide, or placebo: the Cardiac Arrhythmia Suppression Trial. *N Engl J Med*. 1991;324:781-788.

37. Cardiac Arrhythmia Suppression Trial II Investigators. Effect of the antiarrhythmic agent moricizine on survival after myocardial infarction. *N Engl J Med*. 1992;327:227-233.

38. Botti M, Williamson B, Steen K, et al. The effect of pressure bandaging on complications and comfort in patients undergoing coronary angiography: a multicenter randomized trial. *Heart Lung*. 1998;27:360-373.

39. Laupacis A, Sackett DL, Roberts RS. An assessment of clinically useful measures of the consequences of treatment. *N Engl J Med*. 1988;318:1728-1733.

40. DiCenso A. Clinically useful measures of the effects of treatment. *Evid Based Nurs*. 2001;4:36-39.

41. The GUSTO Investigators. An international randomized trial comparing four thrombolytic strategies for acute myocardial infarction. *N Engl J Med*. 1993;329:673-682.

Harm

5

Nicky Cullum and Gordon Guyatt

The following Editorial Board members also made substantive contributions to this section: Lazelle Benefield, Paola DiGiulio, and Kate Seers.

We gratefully acknowledge the work of Mitchell Levine, David Haslam, Stephen Walter, Robert Cumming, Hui Lee, Ted Haines, Anne Holbrook, and Virginia Moyer on the original chapter that appears in the Users' Guides to the Medical Literature, *edited by Guyatt and Rennie.*

In This Chapter

Finding the Evidence

Are the Results Valid?
    Were Groups Shown to be Similar in All Known Determinants of Outcome, or Were Analyses Adjusted for Differences?
    Were Exposed People Equally Likely to Be Identified in the Two Groups?
    Were Outcomes Assessed Uniformly in the Comparison Groups?
    Was Follow-up Sufficiently Complete?

What Are the Results?
    How Strong Was the Association Between Exposure and Outcome?
    How Precise Was the Estimate of the Risk?

How Can I Apply the Results to Patient Care?
    Were the Study Participants Similar to the People in My Clinical Setting?
    Was the Duration of Follow-up Adequate?
    What Was the Magnitude of the Risk?
    Should I Attempt to Stop the Exposure?

Does the Combined Measles-Mumps-Rubella Vaccination Cause Autism?

You are a community health nurse whose role is health promotion for children and families. Childhood immunizations are part of your responsibility, and the combined measles-mumps-rubella (MMR) vaccine is given to children at around 1 year, with a booster given before children start school at 4 years. Recently, there has been a great deal of media interest in the safety of the MMR vaccine, particularly focusing on research that purports a link between MMR vaccine and the development of autism.[1] You have become increasingly confused about the best way to proceed. Several groups are calling for single vaccines to be made available alongside the combined MMR vaccine. The government maintains that there is no evidence of a link between the MMR vaccine and autism and that single vaccines expose children to greater risk. Parents arriving at your child health clinic are extremely anxious, and many are now declining the MMR vaccine. Your medical colleagues are concerned that the practice's immunization rate for MMR is now falling below target; you share their concern but worry that by continuing to advocate and administer MMR vaccine to these very young children you may be contributing to the development of autism in some of them. You resolve to review the best evidence on this topic before the next child health clinic.

FINDING THE EVIDENCE

You formulate the following focused question: Do children immunized using the MMR vaccine have an increased risk of developing autism or autistic-spectrum disorder compared with those not immunized?

Because you are interested in the very latest information, you go to the PubMed version of MEDLINE and PreMEDLINE (*www.pubmed.gov*). For optimum search efficiency, you click on "Clinical Queries" under "PubMed Services," a specialized search with built-in filters to identify only studies that meet specified methodological standards (see Chapter 2, Finding the Evidence). You enter "MMR" and "autism" for the subject search terms and click on "etiology" for study category and "sensitivity" for emphasis. Your MEDLINE search (from 1966 through 2002) identifies 26 citations, the first of which is a recent epidemiologic study assessing the association between MMR and autism.[2] You review the abstract and decide that because the study appears to address the question you are interested in answering, you will retrieve a copy of the article from the library.

ARE THE RESULTS VALID?

Nurses often encounter patients who are facing potentially harmful exposures, either to health care interventions or environmental agents, and important questions arise. Are pregnant women at increased risk of miscarriage if they work in front of video display terminals? Do secondhand crib mattresses cause crib death? Are women who take oral contraceptives at increased risk of thrombosis? Does smoking cause decreased bone mineral density in postmenopausal women? When examining these questions, readers must evaluate the validity of the data, the strength of the association between the assumed causal factor and the adverse outcome, and the relevance to patients in their care.

As when answering any clinical question, the first goal is to identify a systematic review that can provide an objective summary of all available evidence on the topic (see Chapter 9, Summarizing the Evidence Through Systematic Reviews). However, interpreting a systematic review that addresses an issue of harm requires an understanding of the rules of evidence for observational (nonrandomized) studies. The tests for judging the validity of observational study results, like the validity tests for randomized controlled trials (RCTs), help you to decide whether comparison groups began the study with a similar prognosis and whether similarity with respect to determinants of outcome persisted after the study began (Table 5-1).

Were Groups Shown to be Similar in All Known Determinants of Outcome, or Were Analyses Adjusted for Differences?

Studies of potentially harmful exposures will yield biased results if the group exposed to the suspected harmful agent and the unexposed group begin with a different prognosis. Let's say that we are interested in the impact of hospitalization on mortality rate. To investigate this question, we compare mortality in hospitalized patients with that in

Table **5-1** Users' Guides for an Article About Harm

Are the Results Valid?

Did comparison groups begin the study with a similar prognosis?
- Were groups shown to be similar in all known determinants of outcome, or were analyses adjusted for differences?
- Were exposed people equally likely to be identified in the two groups (in case-control studies)?

Did comparison groups retain a similar prognosis after the study started?
- Were outcomes assessed uniformly in the comparison groups (in cohort studies)?
- Was follow-up sufficiently complete?

What Are the Results?
- How strong was the association between exposure and outcome?
- How precise was the estimate of the risk?

How Can I Apply the Results to Patient Care?
- Were the study participants similar to the people in my clinical setting?
- Was the duration of follow-up adequate?
- What was the magnitude of the risk?
- Should I attempt to stop the exposure?

people of similar age and sex in the community. Although an examination of the results would lead us to stay clear of hospitals, few would take these results seriously. The reason for skepticism is that people are admitted to hospitals because they are sick and therefore are at greater risk of dying. This higher risk results in a spurious (i.e., non-causal) association between exposure (hospitalization) and outcome (death). In general, people who seek health care or who take medications are sicker than people who do not. However, these spurious associations are not always as easy to spot as in this example; if readers miss them, they risk making inaccurate inferences about causal relations between health care interventions (e.g., hormone replacement therapy) and adverse effects or suspected harmful agents (e.g., smoking) and adverse effects.

How can investigators ensure that their comparison groups start with a similar like-lihood of the target outcome? RCTs provide less biased estimates of potentially harmful effects than other study designs because randomization is the best way to ensure that groups are balanced at baseline with respect to both known and unknown determinants of outcome (see Chapter 4, Health Care Interventions). Although investigators conduct RCTs to determine whether health care interventions are beneficial, RCTs can also demonstrate harm. The unexpected results of some randomized trials (e.g., interventions expected to show benefit may be associated with increased morbidity or mortality) illustrate the potential of this study design for demonstrating harm (see Chapter 14, Surprising Results of Randomized Controlled Trials). For example, although bed rest is widely used as a therapeutic intervention for everything from suspected myocardial infarction to headache prophylaxis after a lumbar puncture, a systematic review of RCTs of bed rest identified a lack of benefit and evidence of increased harm.[3] An RCT of estrogen and progestin was stopped early (at a mean of 5.2 years instead of the expected 8.5 years) because the investigators found that women who received combination hormone replacement therapy had a greater incidence of coronary heart disease, stroke, and venous thromboembolism than did women who received placebo.[4]

Usually, there are two reasons that we cannot find RCTs to help us determine whether a potentially harmful agent truly has deleterious effects. First, we consider it unethical to randomize patients to exposures that may be harmful. Imagine trying to randomize people to smoke or to eat a high-fat, high-salt diet! Second, we are often concerned about rare and serious adverse effects that occur over prolonged periods—ones that become evident only after tens of thousands of patients have received an intervention or have followed a particular lifestyle. For instance, even a very large randomized trial[5] failed to detect an association between clopidogrel and thrombotic thrombocytopenic purpura, an association that was detected by a subsequent observational study.[6] RCTs specifically addressing side effects may be feasible for adverse event rates as low as 1%[7,8] and meta-analyses may be helpful when event rates are low.[9] The RCTs needed to explore harmful events that occur in less than one in 100 exposed patients—trials characterized by huge sample sizes and lengthy follow-up—are logistically difficult, prohibitively expensive, and currently unheard of in nursing.

Given that clinicians will not find RCTs to answer most questions about harm, they must understand alternative strategies for ensuring a balanced prognosis in the groups being compared. This understanding requires familiarity with observational study designs, which we now describe (Table 5-2).

Table **5-2**   Directions of Inquiry and Key Methodological Strengths
and Weaknesses for Different Study Designs

Design	Starting Point	Assessment	Strengths	Weaknesses
Cohort	Exposure status	Outcome event status	Feasible when randomization of exposure not possible	Susceptible to bias, limited validity
Case-Control	Outcome event status	Exposure status	Overcomes temporal delays, may only require small sample size	Susceptible to bias, limited validity
Randomized controlled trial	Exposure status	Adverse event status	Has low susceptibility to bias	Limited feasibility, generalizability

Cohort Studies

In a *cohort study,* the investigator identifies exposed and nonexposed groups of people, each a cohort, and follows them forward in time to monitor the occurrence of the outcome of interest. In one such study, for example, investigators assessed cardiovascular outcomes among women who used oral contraception compared with other forms of contraception.[10] The investigators found that among heavy smokers, use of oral contraceptives was associated with a fourfold increase in myocardial infarction compared with use of other forms of contraception.

Investigators may rely on cohort designs when harmful outcomes occur infrequently. For example, clinically apparent upper gastrointestinal hemorrhage occurs approximately 1.5 times per 1000 person-years of exposure in patients using nonsteroidal anti-inflammatory drugs (NSAIDs), compared with 1.0 per 1000 person-years in those not taking NSAIDs.[11] Because the event rate in unexposed patients is so low (0.1%), a randomized trial to study a 50% increase in risk would require huge numbers of patients (sample size calculations suggest about 75,000 patients per group) for adequate power to test the hypothesis that NSAIDs cause additional bleeding.[12] Such a randomized trial would not be feasible, but a cohort study, which uses information from large administrative databases, would be possible.

The danger in using observational studies to assess possible harmful exposures is that exposed and unexposed people may begin with different risks of the target outcome. For instance, in the association between NSAIDs and the increased risk of upper gastrointestinal bleeding, age may be associated both with exposure to NSAIDs and with gastrointestinal bleeding. In other words, because patients taking NSAIDs are older and because older patients are more likely to bleed, this *confounding variable* makes attribution of an increased risk of bleeding to NSAID exposure problematic.

There is no reason to expect that people who self-select (or are selected by their clinician) for exposure to a potentially harmful agent should be similar to nonexposed patients, with respect to other important determinants of outcome. Indeed, there are many reasons to expect that they will not be similar. Physicians and nurses are reluctant to prescribe medications or other interventions that they perceive will put patients at risk and so they selectively prescribe low-risk alternatives.

The prescription of benzodiazepines to elderly patients provides an example of the way that selective prescribing practices can lead to a different distribution of risk in patients receiving particular medications. This situation is referred to as the *channeling effect*.[13,14] Ray and colleagues[15] found an association between long-acting benzodiazepines and the risk of falls (relative risk [RR], 2.0; 95% confidence interval [CI], 1.6 to 2.5) in data from 1977 to 1979, but not in data from 1984 to 1985 (RR, 1.3; 95% CI, 0.9 to 1.8). The most plausible explanation for the change is that patients at high risk of falls (those with dementia and anxiety or agitation) selectively received benzodiazepines during the earlier period. Reports of associations between benzodiazepine use and falls led to greater caution, and the apparent association disappeared when clinicians began to avoid benzodiazepine use in patients at high risk of falling.

Therefore, investigators must document the characteristics of exposed and non-exposed participants and either demonstrate their comparability or use statistical techniques to adjust for differences. Effective adjustment for baseline differences in determinants of outcome requires the accurate measurement of those determinants. Although large administrative databases provide a sample size that allows ascertainment of rare events, they sometimes have limited quality of data concerning relevant patient characteristics. For example, Phipps and colleagues[16] combined data from the comprehensive 1996 and 1997 United States Birth/Infant Death data sets, which include all recorded births in the United States during those 2 years, to determine whether full-term, healthy infants born to adolescents 15 years old and younger were at a higher risk of postneonatal death compared with infants born to adult mothers. This database allowed the investigators to identify postneonatal deaths in infants of more than 1.8 million mothers aged 12 to 29 years. The authors acknowledged, however, that although the use of vital statistics data gave them enormous analytic power, they did not have information on important determinants of outcome such as socioeconomic status.

Even if investigators document the comparability of potentially confounding variables in exposed and nonexposed cohorts and even if they use statistical techniques to adjust for differences, important determinants that they do not know about or have not measured may be unbalanced between groups and thus may be responsible for differences in outcome. Returning to our earlier example, for instance, it may be that the illnesses that require NSAIDs, rather than the NSAIDs themselves, are responsible for the increased risk of bleeding. Given this potential for imbalance between groups with respect to unknown determinants of outcome, the strength of inference from a cohort study will always be less than that of a rigorously conducted RCT because randomization is the best way to ensure that groups are balanced at baseline with respect to both known and unknown determinants of outcome.

Case-Control Studies

Rare outcomes, or those that take a long time to develop, threaten the feasibility of cohort studies. An alternative design relies on the initial identification of *cases,* that is, persons who have already developed the target outcome. The investigators then choose *controls*—persons who, as a group, are reasonably similar to the cases with respect to important determinants of outcome (e.g., age, sex, and concurrent medical conditions) but have not experienced the target outcome. Using this *case-control* design, investigators assess the relative frequency of exposure to the suspected harmful agent in the cases and controls and then adjust for differences in the known and measured determinants of outcome. This design permits the simultaneous exploration of multiple exposures that have a possible association with the target outcome.

For example, investigators used a case-control design to demonstrate the association between diethylstilbestrol (DES) ingestion by pregnant women and the development of vaginal adenocarcinomas in their daughters many years later.[17] An RCT or prospective cohort study designed to test this cause-and-effect relationship would have required at least 20 years from the time when the association was first suspected until the completion of the study. Furthermore, given the infrequency of the disease, either an RCT or a cohort study would have required hundreds of thousands of participants. By contrast, using a case-control strategy, the investigators identified two groups of young women. Those who had the outcome of interest (vaginal adenocarcinoma) were designated as cases (n = 8), and those who did not experience the outcome were designated as controls (n = 32). Then, working backward in time, the investigators determined exposure rates to DES for the two groups. The investigators found a strong association between in utero DES exposure and vaginal adenocarcinoma that was extremely unlikely to be attributable to the play of chance ($P < 0.00001$). The investigators found their answer without a delay of 20 years and by studying outcomes in only 40 women.

In another example, investigators used a case-control design to investigate the possible relationship between residential exposure to magnetic fields from power lines and the development of childhood acute lymphoblastic leukemia.[18] They included 463 case-control pairs from nine states in the United States in a matched analysis; the cases were diagnosed with leukemia before the age of 15 years, and the controls were children matched for age, race, and the first eight digits of their telephone number. Technicians, who were blinded to the case and control status of the participants, measured magnetic fields for a 24-hour period in homes in which the children had lived for at least 70% of the 5 years before the date of diagnosis. The technicians also assessed residential wire code categories. The investigators adjusted risk estimates for the child's age at diagnosis, sex, mother's educational level, and family income and found a nonsignificant trend toward an increased risk of childhood leukemia with magnetic field exposure (odds ratio [OR], 1.53; 95% CI, 0.91 to 2.56).

As with cohort studies, case-control studies are susceptible to unmeasured confounding variables, particularly when exposures vary over time. Furthermore, choice of controls may inadvertently create spurious associations. For instance, in a study that examined the association between coffee and pancreatic cancer, the investigators chose control patients from the practices of the physicians who were looking after the patients with pancreatic cancer.[19] These control patients had various gastrointestinal problems, some of which were exacerbated by coffee ingestion. The control patients had learned to avoid coffee; as a result, the investigators found an association between coffee (which the patients with pancreatic cancer consumed at general population levels) and cancer. Subsequent investigations, using more appropriate controls, refuted the association.[20,21] These problems illustrate why clinicians can draw inferences of only limited strength from the results of observational studies, even after adjustments are made for known determinants of outcome.

Case Series and Case Reports

Case series (descriptions of a series of patients) and *case reports* (descriptions of individual patients) do not provide any comparison group and are therefore unable to satisfy the requirement that comparison groups share a similar prognosis. Descriptive studies occasionally demonstrate dramatic findings mandating an immediate change in clinician behavior (e.g., recall the consequences when thalidomide was linked to birth defects[22]). However, potentially undesirable consequences may occur when actions are taken in response to weak evidence. Consider the case of the drug Bendectin (a combination of doxylamine, pyridoxine, and dicyclomine used as an antiemetic in pregnancy), whose manufacturer withdrew it from the market as a result of case reports suggesting that it was teratogenic.[23] Later, even though some comparative studies demonstrated the drug's relative safety,[24] these investigations could not eradicate the prevailing litigious atmosphere, which prevented the manufacturer from reintroducing Bendectin. Thus, many pregnant women who potentially could have benefited from the drug's availability were denied the symptomatic relief it could have offered.

In general, clinicians should not draw conclusions about cause-and-effect relationships from case series but, rather, should recognize that the results may generate questions for regulatory agencies and clinical investigators to address.

Design Issues: Summary

Just as is true for the resolution of questions of the effectiveness of health care interventions, readers should look first for randomized trials to resolve issues of harm. They will often be disappointed in this search and must make use of studies of weaker design. Regardless of the design, however, readers should look for an appropriate control population before they make strong inferences about potentially harmful agents. For RCTs and cohort studies, the control group should have a similar baseline risk of outcome, or investigators should use statistical techniques to adjust or correct for differences. Similarly, in case-control studies the exposed and nonexposed groups should be similar with respect to determinants of outcome other than the exposure under study. Alternatively, investigators should use statistical techniques to adjust for differences. Even when investigators have taken all the appropriate steps to minimize bias, readers should bear in mind that residual differences between groups may always bias the results of observational studies.[25] Because health care decisions in the real world are informed not just by research evidence but also by professional judgment and patient preferences, people offered interventions or exposures in nonrandomized studies are liable to differ in many ways (some related to outcome) from persons who are not offered interventions or exposures (*channeling bias* or effect).

Were Exposed People Equally Likely to Be Identified in the Two Groups?

In case-control studies, ascertainment of the exposure is a key issue. For example, when the parents of children with leukemia are asked about prior exposure to high-voltage electricity, such as power lines, they may be more likely to recall exposure than would control group members, either because of increased motivation (*recall bias*) or because of greater probing by an interviewer (*interviewer bias*). Readers should note whether investigators used bias-minimizing strategies such as blinding participants and interviewers to the hypothesis of the study. For example, a case-control study found a twofold increase in risk of hip fracture associated with psychotropic drug use. In this study, investigators established drug exposure by examining computerized claims files of the Michigan Medicaid program, a strategy that avoided both recall and interviewer bias.[26] The study of residential exposure to magnetic fields from power lines and its association with the development of childhood acute lymphoblastic leukemia relied on technicians, who were blinded to the case and control status of the study participants, to measure magnetic fields.[18] In both cases, the assurance of unbiased identification of exposure status increases our confidence in the findings.

Were Outcomes Assessed Uniformly in the Comparison Groups?

In RCTs and cohort studies, ascertainment of outcome is a key issue. For example, investigators have reported a threefold increase in the risk of malignant melanoma in persons who work with radioactive materials. One possible explanation for some of the increased risk could be that clinicians, aware of a possible risk, search more diligently and therefore detect disease in exposed patients that would otherwise go unnoticed (or they may detect disease earlier). This could cause the exposed cohort to have an apparent, but spurious, increase in risk—a situation we refer to as *surveillance* or *detection bias*.[27]

Was Follow-up Sufficiently Complete?

As we point out in Chapter 4, Health Care Interventions, loss to follow-up can introduce bias because patients who are lost to follow-up may have very different outcomes from those still available for assessment. The longer the required follow-up period, the greater the possibility that the follow-up will be incomplete.

For example, in a well-executed study, investigators determined the vital status of 1235 of 1261 white men (98%) employed in a chrysotile asbestos textile operation between 1940 and 1975.[28] The relative risk of lung cancer death over time increased from 1.4 to 18.2 in direct proportion to the cumulative exposure among asbestos workers with at least 15 years since first exposure. Because the 2% missing data were unlikely to affect the results, the loss to follow-up does not threaten the validity of the inference that asbestos exposure causes lung cancer deaths.

USING THE GUIDE

The study[2] examining the impact of the MMR vaccine on autism used a population-based cohort design and included all children born in Denmark between 1991 and 1998 (537,303 children representing 2,129,864 person-years) of whom 440,655 (82%) had received the MMR vaccine. The investigators obtained data

Continued

from existing national databases. They identified the children through the national birth registry and determined vaccination status from a national database maintained on an ongoing basis from mandatory reports by general practitioners. It appears, therefore, that both exposed (vaccinated) and unexposed (unvaccinated) children were equally likely to be identified in the birth cohort. The major strength of the use of large databases for this study is that it eliminates the possibility of biased assessment of exposure. If the data had been collected from parents instead, it is possible that those with children who developed autism might recall vaccination-related information differently than those whose children did not develop autism *(recall bias)* or interviewers may have probed more or less depending on whether the child had autism *(interviewer bias)*.

The investigators ascertained the main outcome of interest—a diagnosis of autism or autistic-spectrum disorder—from the Danish Psychiatric Central Register in which all such diagnoses are routinely registered. They identified 316 children with a diagnosis of autistic disorder and 422 with a diagnosis of other autistic-spectrum disorders. It seems likely that vaccinated children were no more or less likely to be assessed for autism than unvaccinated children because most of the adverse publicity around the MMR vaccine has happened since 1999; however, it is possible that some of the diagnosing psychiatrists were attuned to a suspected link and therefore may have looked more carefully for signs of autism in those children whom they knew had received the MMR vaccine, a state of affairs known as *surveillance or detection bias*. As a check on this, the authors of the study performed an extensive review of the records of 40 children (13% of all the children with autistic disorder) diagnosed with autism. The diagnosis was validated in 37 of these cases; the three children who did not meet the criteria for autistic disorder were all classified as having other autistic-spectrum disorders. Furthermore, any heightened awareness of the possibility of autism among the clinicians would bias the results in favor of a spurious association between autism and vaccine exposure.

The authors followed each child from 1 year of age until the diagnosis of autism or an associated condition, emigration, death, or the end of 1999, whichever occurred first. Given that children born between January 1, 1991 and December 31, 1998 were included in the study, the minimum follow-up period was 1 year, and the maximum was 9 years. Any events that occurred before vaccination were attributed to the nonvaccinated group. After children were vaccinated, all events were attributed to the vaccinated group. The data from 5028 children (0.9%) were censored as a result of death or emigration.

The investigators obtained information on potential confounders from the Danish Medical Birth Registry, the National Hospital Registry, and Statistics Denmark. These confounders, which included age, sex, birth weight, gestational age, mother's education, and the socioeconomic status of the family, were controlled for in the analysis.

The number lost to follow-up is small in percentage terms (less than 1% of the total population). This still leaves us uncomfortable because the absolute number lost to follow-up (5028) is much larger than the number of children who developed autism or related disorders (738).

In summary, even though the study has the limitation inherent in any observational study—that exposed (vaccinated) and unexposed (unvaccinated) children may differ in prognosis at baseline—and despite the loss to follow-up that is relatively large in relation to the number of outcome events, this study has many strengths and warrants a review of the results.

WHAT ARE THE RESULTS?

How Strong Was the Association Between Exposure and Outcome?

We describe the alternatives for expressing the association between an exposure and an outcome, *relative risk* and *odds ratio,* in other sections of this book (see Chapter 4, Health Care Interventions, and Chapter 27, Measures of Association). In a cohort study assessing the long-term effects of alcohol consumption on mortality in men, 38 of 1833 nondrinking men died of stroke, compared with 17 of 503 men who drank more than 35 units of alcohol per week. The relative risk of mortality from stroke, (17/503)/ (38/1833), was 1.6.[29] When adjusted for age, this relative risk became 2.3. The relative risk tells us that death from stroke occurs more than twice as often in men who drink at least 35 units of alcohol per week than in men who do not drink alcohol.

The estimate of relative risk depends on the availability of samples of exposed and unexposed people in which the proportion of people with the outcome of interest can be determined. The relative risk is therefore not applicable to case-control studies in which the number of cases and controls—and, therefore, the proportion of persons with the outcome—is determined a priori by the investigator based on the sample size required for the study. For case-control studies, instead of using a ratio of risks (*relative risk*), we use a ratio of odds (*odds ratio*): the odds of exposure of a case patient divided by the odds of exposure of a control patient (see Chapter 27, Measures of Association).

When considering both study design and strength of association, we may be ready to interpret a small increase in risk as representing a true harmful effect when the study design is strong, such as an RCT. A much higher increase in risk may be required of weaker designs, such as cohort or case-control studies, because subtle findings are more likely to be caused by the inevitably higher risk of bias. Very large values of relative risk or odds ratio represent strong associations that are less likely to be caused by confounding variables or bias.

In addition to showing a large magnitude of relative risk or odds ratio, a second finding will strengthen an inference that we are dealing with a true harmful effect. If, as the quantity or the duration of exposure to the putative harmful agent increases, the risk of the adverse outcome also increases (i.e., the data suggest a *dose-response gradient*), we are more likely to be dealing with a causal relationship between exposure and outcome. The finding that the risk of dying from lung cancer in male physicians who smoke increases by 50%, 132%, and 220% for 1 to 14, 15 to 24, and 25 or more cigarettes smoked per day, respectively, strengthens our inference that cigarette smoking causes lung cancer.[30]

How Precise Was the Estimate of the Risk?

Readers can evaluate the precision of the estimate of risk by examining the confidence interval around that estimate (see Chapter 4, Health Care Interventions, and Chapter 29, Confidence Intervals). In a study in which investigators have shown an association between an exposure and an adverse outcome, the lower limit of the estimate of relative risk associated with the adverse exposure provides a minimal estimate of the strength of the association. By contrast, in a study in which investigators fail to demonstrate an association (a negative study), the upper boundary of the confidence interval around the relative risk tells the clinician just how great an adverse effect may still be present, despite the failure to show a statistically significant association (see Chapter 29, Confidence Intervals).

USING THE GUIDE

The investigators calculated the relative risk of autism in children immunized with MMR vaccine versus those not immunized. The investigators found no association between MMR vaccination and autism (adjusted RR, 0.92; 95% CI, 0.68 to 1.24). The relative risk of other autistic-spectrum disorders was 0.83 (95% CI, 0.65 to 1.07). There was no association between age at time of vaccination, time since vaccination, or date of vaccination and development of autistic disorder.

HOW CAN I APPLY THE RESULTS TO PATIENT CARE?

Were the Study Participants Similar to the People in My Clinical Setting?

If possible biases in a study are not sufficient to dismiss the study out of hand, you must consider the extent to which they may apply to the people in your community or the patients in your care. Is the person in your setting similar to those described in the study with respect to morbidity, age, sex, race, or other potentially important factors? If not, is the biology of the harmful exposure likely to differ in the patient you are attending (see Chapter 33, Applying Results to Individual Patients)? Are there important differences in the treatments or exposures between the patients you see and the patients studied? For example, the risk of thrombophlebitis associated with oral contraceptive use described in the 1970s may not be applicable to patients in the 1990s because of the lower estrogen dose in oral contraceptives used in the 1990s. Similarly, increases in uterine cancer secondary to postmenopausal estrogen replacement do not apply to women who are also taking concomitant progestins tailored to produce monthly withdrawal bleeding with long-term, noncyclic use.

Was the Duration of Follow-up Adequate?

Let us return for a moment to the study that showed that workers employed in a chrysotile asbestos textile operation between 1940 and 1975 showed an increased risk of lung cancer death, a risk that increased from 1.4 to 18.2 in direct relation to cumulative exposure among asbestos workers with at least 15 years since first exposure.[28] Because the follow-up was sufficiently long to capture a large proportion of the lung cancers destined to occur, the results enhance our confidence in application of the results to patients in our practice. By contrast, excessively short follow-up may fail to detect harmful effects that emerge with longer observation.

What Was the Magnitude of the Risk?

The relative risk and the odds ratio do not tell us how frequently a problem occurs; they tell us only that the observed effect occurs more or less often in the exposed group compared with the unexposed group. Thus, we need a method for assessing clinical importance. In our discussion of evaluation of health care interventions (see Chapter 4, Health Care Interventions, and Chapter 27, Measures of Association), we describe a way to calculate the number of patients who must be treated to prevent an adverse event. When the issue is harm, we can use data from a randomized trial or a cohort study, but not a case-control study, to make an analogous calculation to determine how many people must be exposed to the harmful agent to cause an adverse outcome.

For example, investigators studied the relationship between MMR vaccination and seizures in a large birth cohort as part of the Vaccine Safety Datalink project[31] and found that children vaccinated with MMR vaccine were significantly more likely to experience febrile convulsions within 1 to 2 weeks of immunization than were unvaccinated children of the same age. After adjustment for age, sex, health maintenance organization, calendar time, and receipt of diphtheria-tetanus-pertussis vaccine, administration of MMR vaccine was associated with a relative risk of febrile seizures between 8 and 14 days after vaccination of 2.83 (95% CI, 1.44 to 5.55). When compared with seizure rates in unvaccinated children, the *absolute risk increase* was 0.025%, the reciprocal of which tells us that, on average, for every 4000 children we immunize with MMR vaccine, we will cause one excess febrile seizure. None of the children with febrile seizures after vaccination went on to experience further nonfebrile seizures or to develop epilepsy. In contrast, studies of antibiotic use for otitis media in children found that for every 17 children treated with antibiotics, one child experienced an adverse event (usually vomiting, diarrhea, or skin rash).[32]

Should I Attempt to Stop the Exposure?

After evaluating the evidence that an exposure is harmful and after establishing that the results are potentially applicable to the people in your care, determining subsequent actions may not be simple. At least three factors should be considered in making a clinical decision. First, how strong was the inference in the study or studies that demonstrated harm in the first place? Second, what is the magnitude of the risk to patients if exposure to the harmful agent continues? Third, what are the adverse consequences of reducing or eliminating exposure to the harmful agent, that is, what is the magnitude of the benefit that patients will no longer receive?

Clinical decision making is simple when both the likelihood of harm and its magnitude are great. Because the evidence of increased morbidity from bed rest came from randomized trials,[3] we can be more confident of the causal connection. The clinical decision is also made easier when an acceptable alternative for avoiding the risk is available. For example, beta blockers prescribed for the treatment of hypertension can result in a symptomatic increase in airway resistance in patients with asthma or chronic airflow limitation. This risk mandates the use of an alternative drug, such as a thiazide diuretic, in susceptible patients.[33]

Even if the evidence is relatively weak, the availability of an alternative can result in a clear decision. Early case-control studies demonstrating an association between aspirin use and Reye's syndrome, for example, were relatively weak and left considerable doubt about the causal relationship. Although the strength of inference was not great, the availability of a safe, inexpensive, and well-tolerated alternative, acetaminophen, justified use of this alternative agent in children who were at risk of Reye's syndrome.[34]

In contrast to early studies of aspirin and Reye's syndrome, multiple well-designed cohort and case-control studies have consistently demonstrated an association between NSAIDs and upper gastrointestinal bleeding; therefore, the inference about harm has been relatively strong. However, the risk of an upper gastrointestinal bleeding episode is quite low, and, until recently, safer and equally efficacious antiinflammatory alternatives have not been available. Clinicians have probably been correct in continuing to prescribe NSAIDs for appropriate clinical conditions. Depending on both their safety profile after longer experience and cost-effectiveness considerations, NSAIDs that inhibit cyclooxygenase 2 may prove to be an appropriate alternative class of agents.

CLINICAL RESOLUTION

The MMR vaccine and autism study was based on a large database-derived birth cohort. Even though the study suffers from the limitation inherent in any observational study— that exposed (vaccinated) and unexposed (unvaccinated) children may differ in prognosis at baseline—and despite the loss to follow-up that is relatively large in relation to the number of outcome events, this study has many strengths, including objective assessment of exposure to the MMR vaccine (rather than relying on self-report and the possibility of recall bias), identification and adjustment for relevant baseline differences, and accurate diagnosis of autism or autistic-spectrum disorders. Furthermore, any possible ascertainment bias is likely to have led to an increase in autism diagnosis in the exposed children versus the unexposed children. The investigators found no association between MMR vaccine and autism or MMR vaccine and other autistic-spectrum disorders.

In focusing on an individual study, we have neglected to consider how the results fit in with other evidence. A search of *Clinical Evidence* reveals a summary,[35] which had a search date of November 2001 and included a systematic review,[36] an RCT comparing short-term effects of MMR vaccine in twins[37] and two population-based studies[38,39] that assessed harm. These studies, individually and together, found no evidence that MMR vaccine was associated with developmental regression or autism compared with placebo or no vaccine. Similarly, large cross-sectional time series studies have consistently found no association between rates of MMR vaccine uptake and rates of autism. Thus, the results of other studies are consistent with the findings of the study we have reviewed in detail here. You decide that the strength of the study and the volume of related evidence, matched against the known consequences of measles infection, strengthen your conviction that MMR vaccine is safe and is an important part of your health promotion role.

Finally, and most important, having scrutinized this research evidence, you feel equipped to help parents participate in decisions about vaccinating their children. You also feel better able to identify the inadequacies of the original research that first suggested a link between autism and MMR vaccine. This study[1] was a case series of 12 children with developmental disorders. In eight of these children, the onset of behavioral problems had been attributed by parents to MMR vaccination. Such a

CLINICAL RESOLUTION—CONT'D

study design meets none of the criteria for demonstrating a causal link because there was no comparison group of unvaccinated children. In other words, only very weak evidence supports the link whereas stronger evidence suggests no causal relation.

REFERENCES

1. Wakefield AJ, Murch SH, Anthony A, et al. Ileal-lymphoid-nodular hyperplasia, non-specific colitis and pervasive developmental disorder in children. *Lancet.* 1998;351:637-641.

2. Madsen KM, Hviid A, Vestergaard M, et al. A population-based study of measles, mumps, and rubella vaccination and autism. *N Engl J Med.* 2002;347:1477-1482.

3. Allen C, Glasziou P, Del Mar C. Bed rest: a potentially harmful treatment needing more careful evaluation. *Lancet.* 1999;354:1229-1233.

4. Rossouw JE, Anderson GL, Prentice RL, et al. Risks and benefits of estrogen plus progestin in healthy postmenopausal women: principal results from the Women's Health Initiative randomized controlled trial. *JAMA.* 2002;288:321-333.

5. CAPRIE Steering Committee. A randomised, blinded, trial of clopidogrel versus aspirin in patients at risk of ischaemic events (CAPRIE). *Lancet.* 1996;348:1329-1339.

6. Bennett CL, Connors JM, Carwile JM, et al. Thrombotic thrombocytopenic purpura associated with clopidogrel. *N Engl J Med.* 2000;342:1773-1777.

7. Silverstein FE, Graham DY, Senior JR, et al. Misoprostol reduces serious gastrointestinal complications in patients with rheumatoid arthritis receiving nonsteroidal anti-inflammatory drugs: a randomized, double-blind, placebo-controlled trial. *Ann Intern Med.* 1995;123:241-249.

8. Merck and Co. VIGOR Study Summary. Paper presented at: Digestive Disease Week Congress; May 24, 2000; San Diego, CA.

9. Langman MJ, Jensen DM, Watson DJ, et al. Adverse upper gastrointestinal effects of rofecoxib compared with NSAIDs. *JAMA.* 1999;282:1929-1933.

10. Mant J, Painter R, Vessey M. Risk of myocardial infarction, angina and stroke in users of oral contraceptives: an updated analysis of a cohort study. *Br J Obstet Gynaecol.* 1998;105:890-896.

11. Carson JL, Strom BL, Soper KA, et al. The association of nonsteroidal anti-inflammatory drugs with upper gastrointestinal tract bleeding. *Arch Intern Med.* 1987;147:85-88.

12. Walter SD. Determination of significant relative risks and optimal sampling procedures in prospective and retrospective comparative studies of various sizes. *Am J Epidemiol.* 1977;105:387-397.

13. Joseph KS. The evolution of clinical practice and time trends in drug effects. *J Clin Epidemiol.* 1994;47:593-598.

14. Leufkens HG, Urquhart J. Variability in patterns of drug usage. *J Pharm Pharmacol.* 1994;46(suppl 1): 433-437.

15. Ray WA, Griffin MR, Downey W. Benzodiazepines of long and short elimination half-life and risk of hip fracture. *JAMA.* 1989;262:3303-3307.

16. Phipps MG, Blume JD, DeMonner SM. Young maternal age associated with increased risk of postneonatal death. *Obstet Gynecol.* 2002;100:481-486.

17. Herbst AL, Ulfelder H, Poskanzer DC. Adenocarcinoma of the vagina: association of maternal stilbestrol therapy with tumor appearance in young women. *N Engl J Med.* 1971;284:878-881.

18. Linet MS, Hatch EE, Kleinerman RA, et al. Residential exposure to magnetic fields and acute lymphoblastic leukemia in children. *N Engl J Med.* 1997;337:1-7.

19. MacMahon B, Yen S, Trichopoulos D, Warren K, Nardi G. Coffee and cancer of the pancreas. *N Engl J Med.* 1981;304:630-633.

20. Baghurst PA, McMichael AJ, Slavotineck AH, Baghurst KI, Boyle P, Walker AM. A case-control study of diet and cancer of the pancreas. *Am J Epidemiol.* 1991;134:167-179.

21. Zheng W, McLaughlin JK, Gridley G, et al. A cohort study of smoking, alcohol consumption and dietary factors for pancreatic cancer. *Cancer Causes Control.* 1993;4:477-482.

22. Lenz W. Epidemiology of congenital malformations. *Ann NY Acad Sci.* 1965;123:228-236.

23. Soverchia G, Perri PF. Two cases of malformation of a limb in infants of mothers treated with an antiemetic in a very early phase of pregnancy. *Pediatr Med Chir.* 1981;3:97-99.

24. Holmes LB. Teratogen update: Bendectin. *Teratology.* 1983;27:277-281.

25. Kellermann AL, Rivara FP, Rushforth NB, et al. Gun ownership as a risk factor for homicide in the home. *N Engl J Med.* 1993;329:1084-1091.

26. Ray WA, Griffin MR, Schaffner W, et al. Psychotropic drug use and the risk of hip fracture. *N Engl J Med.* 1987;316:363-369.

27. Hiatt RA, Fireman B. The possible effect of increased surveillance on the incidence of malignant melanoma. *Prev Med.* 1986;15:652-660.

28. Dement JM, Harris RL Jr, Symons MJ, Shy CM. Exposures and mortality among chrysotile asbestos workers, II: mortality. *Am J Ind Med.* 1983;4:421-433.

29. Hart CL, Davey Smith G, Hole DJ, Hawthorne VM. Alcohol consumption and mortality from all causes, coronary heart disease, and stroke: results from a prospective cohort study of Scottish men with 21 years of follow up. *BMJ.* 1999;318:1725-1729.

30. Doll R, Hill AB. Mortality in relation to smoking: ten years' observation of British doctors. *BMJ.* 1964;1:1399-1410, 1460-1467.

31. Barlow WE, Davis RL, Glasser JW, et al. The risk of seizures after receipt of whole-cell pertussis or measles, mumps and rubella vaccine. *N Engl J Med.* 2001;345:656-661.

32. O'Neill P. Acute otitis media. *Clin Evid.* 2002;7:236-243.

33. Ogilvie RI, Burgess ED, Cusson JR, Feldman RD, Leiter LA, Myers MG. Report of the Canadian Hypertension Society Consensus Conference, 3: Pharmacologic treatment of essential hypertension. *Can Med Assoc J.* 1993;149:575-584.

34. Soumerai SB, Ross-Degnan D, Kahn JS. Effects of professional and media warnings about the association between aspirin use in children and Reye's syndrome. *Milbank Q.* 1992;70:155-182.

35. Donald A, Muthu V. Measles. *Clin Evid.* 2002;7:331-340.

36. Stratton K, Gable A, Shetty P, McCormick M, eds. *Immunization Safety Review: Measles-Mumps-Rubella Vaccine and Autism.* Washington, DC: National Academies Press; 2001.

37. Vitanen M, Peltola H, Paunio M, Heinonen OP. Day-to-day reactogenicity and the healthy vaccinee effect of measles-mumps-rubella vaccination. *Pediatrics.* 2000;106:E62.

38. Taylor B, Miller E, Farrington CP, et al. Autism and measles, mumps, and rubella vaccine: no epidemiological evidence for a causal association. *Lancet.* 1999;353:2026-2029.

39. Patja A, Davidkin I, Kurki T, Kallio MJ, Valle M, Peltola H. Serious adverse events after measles-mumps-rubella vaccination during a fourteen-year prospective follow-up. *Pediatr Infect Dis J.* 2000;19:1127-1134.

6

Diagnosis

Alba DiCenso, Andrew Jull, and Gordon Guyatt

The following Editorial Board members also made substantive contributions to this chapter: Rien de Vos, Teresa Icart Isern, and Mary van Soeren.

We gratefully acknowledge the work of Scott Richardson, Mark Wilson, Roman Jaeschke, and Jeroen Lijmer on the original chapters that appear in the Users' Guides to the Medical Literature, edited by Guyatt and Rennie.

In This Chapter

The Diagnostic Process
    Choices in the Diagnostic Process
    Diagnostic and Therapeutic Thresholds
    Using Systematic Research to Aid in the Diagnostic Process

Diagnostic Tests

Finding the Evidence

Are the Results Valid?
    Was the Diagnostic Test Evaluated in a Spectrum of Patients With a Low to
        High Probability of Having the Target Disorder?
    Was There a Blind Comparison With an Independent Reference (Gold)
        Standard Applied Similarly to All Patients?
    Did the Results of the Test Being Evaluated Influence the Decision to Perform
        the Reference (Gold) Standard?

What Are the Results?
    What Likelihood Ratios Were Associated With the Range of Possible Test Results?

How Can I Apply the Results to Patient Care?
    Will the Reproducibility of the Test Result and Its Interpretation Be Satisfactory
        in My Clinical Setting?
    Are the Results Applicable to the Patients in My Clinical Setting?

Continued

Will the Results Change My Management Strategy?
Will Patients Be Better off as a Result of the Test?

THE DIAGNOSTIC PROCESS

Nurses make a variety of diagnoses in their daily practice including dehydration, skin breakdown, electrolyte imbalance, and wound infection. Nurse practitioners also diagnose common acute conditions such as ear, vaginal, urinary, and respiratory tract infections; chronic illnesses; physical and substance abuse; and common psychiatric illnesses. Making a diagnosis is a complex cognitive task that involves both logical reasoning and pattern recognition.[1,2] Although the process happens largely at an unconscious level, there are two essential steps.

Step 1. In the first step, we identify possible diagnoses and estimate their relative likelihood.[3] Possible diagnoses may be of biological, psychological, or sociological origins and are the object of the *differential diagnosis.* A differential diagnosis considers the active alternatives that can plausibly explain a patient's presentation (see Chapter 21, Differential Diagnosis).

Step 2. In the second step of the diagnostic process, we incorporate new information to change the relative probabilities, rule out some of the possibilities, and, ultimately, choose the most likely diagnosis. The additional information increases or decreases the likelihood of each possible diagnosis. Thus, with each new finding, we move, albeit intuitively and implicitly, from the pretest probability, to the posttest probability. *Pretest probability* is the probability of the target condition being present *before* the results of a diagnostic test are available. *Posttest probability* is the probability of the target condition being present *after* the results of a diagnostic test are available.

If we know the properties of each piece of information, we can be highly quantitative in our sequential move from pretest to posttest probability. Later in this chapter, we will learn how. Because the properties of the individual components of the history and physical examination often are not available, we must rely on clinical experience and intuition to predict the extent to which findings from the various components will modify our differential diagnosis.

Choices in the Diagnostic Process

How can we decide which disorders to pursue when considering a patient's differential diagnosis? If we were to consider all known causes to be equally likely and test for them all simultaneously (the possibilistic approach), the patient would undergo unnecessary testing. Instead, experienced clinicians are selective and consider first those disorders that are more likely (a probabilistic approach), more serious if left undiagnosed and untreated (a prognostic approach), or more responsive to treatment (a pragmatic approach).

Wisely selecting a patient's differential diagnosis involves all three considerations (probabilistic, prognostic, and pragmatic). Our single best explanation for the patient's clinical problem can be termed the *leading hypothesis* or *working diagnosis.* A few (usually one to five) other diagnoses, termed *active alternatives,* may be worth considering at the time of initial work-up because of their likelihood, seriousness if undiagnosed and untreated, or responsiveness to treatment. Additional causes of the clinical problem, termed *other hypotheses,* may be too unlikely to consider at the time of initial diagnostic work-up, but they remain possible and could be considered further if the working diagnosis and active alternatives are later disproved.

Diagnostic and Therapeutic Thresholds

Consider a patient who presents with a painful eruption of grouped vesicles in the distribution of a single dermatome. In an instant, an experienced clinician would make a diagnosis of herpes zoster (shingles) and would consider whether to offer the patient treatment. In other words, given the hallmark clinical signs, the probability of herpes zoster is so high (near 100%) that it is above a threshold at which no further testing is required.

Next, consider a previously healthy athlete who presents with lateral rib cage pain after being accidentally struck by an errant baseball pitch. Again, an experienced clinician would recognize the clinical problem (posttraumatic lateral chest pain), identify a leading hypothesis (rib contusion) and an active alternative (rib fracture), and plan a test (radiograph) to exclude the latter. If asked, the clinician could also list disorders that are too unlikely to consider further (such as myocardial infarction). In other words, although not as likely as rib contusion, the probability of a rib fracture is above a threshold for testing, whereas the probability of myocardial infarction is below the threshold for testing.

These cases illustrate how we can estimate the probability of disease and then compare disease probabilities to two thresholds (Figure 6-1). The probability above which the diagnosis is sufficiently likely to warrant intervention defines the upper threshold. That is, if a clinician believes that the diagnosis is sufficiently likely that he or she is ready to

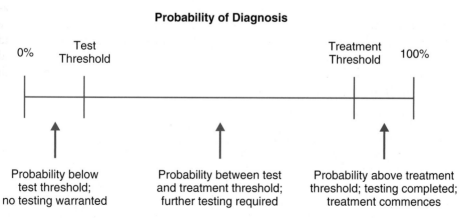

Probability of Diagnosis

0%   Test Threshold   Treatment Threshold   100%

Probability below test threshold; no testing warranted

Probability between test and treatment threshold; further testing required

Probability above treatment threshold; testing completed; treatment commences

Figure 6-1. Test and treatment thresholds in the diagnostic process.

recommend treatment, the upper threshold has been crossed. This threshold is termed the *treatment threshold.*[4] In the case of shingles described earlier, the clinician judged the diagnosis of herpes zoster to be above this treatment threshold of probability.

The probability below which a clinician decides a diagnosis warrants no further consideration defines the lower threshold. This threshold is termed the *no-test threshold* or the *test threshold.* In the case of posttraumatic lateral chest pain described earlier, the diagnosis of rib fracture fell above the test threshold, and the diagnosis of myocardial infarction fell below it.

For a disorder with a pretest probability above the treatment threshold, a confirming test that raises the probability further would not assist diagnostically. On the other end of the scale, for a disorder with a pretest probability below the test threshold, an exclusionary test that lowers the probability further would not help diagnostically. When a clinician believes that the pretest probability is high enough to test for, but not high enough to begin treatment without confirmation (i.e., when probability is between the two thresholds), testing will be diagnostically useful. It will be most valuable if it moves the probability across either threshold.

What determines the treatment threshold? The greater the adverse effects of treatment will be, the more we will be inclined to choose a high treatment threshold. For instance, because a diagnosis of pulmonary embolus involves long-term anticoagulation with appreciable risks of hemorrhage, we are very concerned about falsely labeling patients. The invasiveness of the next test we are considering will also affect our threshold. If the next test (such as a ventilation-perfusion scan) is without serious risk, we will be ready to choose a high treatment threshold. We will be more reluctant to institute an invasive test associated with risks to the patient, such as pulmonary angiogram, and this will drive our treatment threshold downward; that is, we will be more inclined to accept a risk of a *false-positive* diagnosis because a higher treatment threshold implies putting some patients through the test unnecessarily.

Similar considerations bear on the test threshold. The more serious a missed diagnosis is, the lower we will set our test threshold. Because a missed diagnosis of a pulmonary embolus could be fatal, we would be inclined to set our diagnostic threshold low. However, this is again counterbalanced by the risks associated with the next test we are considering. If the risks are low, we will be comfortable with our low diagnostic threshold. The higher the risks will be, the more it will push our threshold upward.

Using Systematic Research to Aid in the Diagnostic Process

How do clinicians generate differential diagnoses and arrive at pretest estimates of disease probability? They remember prior cases with the same clinical problem, so disorders diagnosed frequently have higher probabilities than diagnoses made less frequently. Remembered cases are easily and quickly available, and they are calibrated to our local practice setting. Yet our memories are imperfect, and the resulting probabilities are subject to bias and error.[5-7]

Two sorts of systematic investigations can inform the process of generating a differential diagnosis. One type of study addresses the presenting manifestations of a disease or condition (see Chapter 20, Clinical Manifestations of Disease). The second, and more important, type of study directly addresses the underlying causes of a presenting symptom, sign, or constellation of symptoms and signs (see Chapter 21, Differential Diagnosis).

Having generated an initial differential diagnosis with associated pretest probabilities, how can we incorporate additional information to arrive at an ultimate diagnosis? For each finding, we must implicitly ask the following question: How frequently will this result be seen in patients with one particular diagnostic possibility (or target condition) relative to the frequency with which it is seen in competing diagnostic conditions? Once again, we may intuitively refer to our own past experience. Alternatively, we can use data from research studies focusing on test properties.

DIAGNOSTIC TESTS

We now provide guidelines to assess the validity of studies that explore the properties of a diagnostic test. The validity will depend on the answers to questions about two key design features: did the investigators (1) enroll the appropriate group of patients and (2) undertake the appropriate investigations to determine the true diagnosis? A systematic review of all diagnostic test studies addressing a particular issue will provide the strongest inference (see Chapter 9, Summarizing the Evidence Through Systematic Reviews). To understand and interpret such reviews, we must use the principles of assessing primary diagnostic studies.

CLINICAL SCENARIO

How Accurate is Serum Ferritin for Diagnosing Iron-Deficiency Anemia in the Elderly?

As a new graduate of the nurse practitioner education program, you were recently hired to work in a primary health care clinic. Last week, you saw a 73-year-old patient who was new to the practice. His wife died last year, and he recently moved to this community to live with his daughter. The patient described feeling increasingly fatigued over the past few weeks and not having the energy he used to have. He reported needing to take frequent rests and a nap in the afternoon, which was unusual for him. You learned that he is a retired businessman who has enjoyed good health except for longstanding osteoarthritis in the left knee. He has been taking ibuprofen for relief of the knee pain. Clinical history and physical examination revealed nothing of note except the signs of arthritis in the left knee. You ordered a complete blood cell count and asked to see him again in 1 week. The test results came back today with a hemoglobin value of 10.0 g/dL and a mean cell volume of 82. You are scheduled to see the patient tomorrow.

Iron-deficiency anemia is the most likely diagnosis, and a probabilistic approach to diagnosis leads you to focus on this possibility. At the same time, the seriousness of competing diagnoses of multiple myeloma and a primary bone marrow problem such as myelodysplastic disorder leads you to keep these alternatives in the back of your mind. You are aware of certain tests purported to help with the diagnosis of iron-deficiency anemia and decide to review these tests to confirm which is most appropriate to use for this patient.

FINDING THE EVIDENCE

You begin by formulating your question. The patient is an older person with anemia and suspected iron deficiency; the exposure is the test for iron-deficiency anemia; and the outcome is the definitive diagnosis of anemia by bone marrow aspiration. Although you would not order bone marrow aspiration to diagnose anemia, you want to find a study that evaluates noninvasive tests for iron-deficiency anemia against this "ideal" but invasive test. You formulate the following question: in older persons, which noninvasive tests accurately diagnose iron-deficiency anemia? Past experience has taught you that many articles about diagnostic tests omit the key information that would be most valuable, the likelihood ratios associated with the tests of interest. You connect to the Internet and to MEDLINE at the United States National Library of Medicine Web site through PubMed. Using the Clinical Queries feature, with *diagnosis* as the category and *sensitivity* as the emphasis, and guided by the question you have formulated, you enter the terms "elderly," "iron-deficiency anemia tests," "bone marrow aspiration," and "likelihood." The search identifies two articles, but you rule out the first because it focuses on patients with liver cirrhosis. The second article, however, "Diagnosis of iron-deficiency anemia in the elderly," by Guyatt and colleagues,[8] seems highly applicable to your question. You decide to obtain a copy of this article from the library.

In this chapter, we focus on how to evaluate the validity, results, and applicability of studies examining the properties of diagnostic tests. Table 6-1 summarizes the criteria for evaluating a study about interpreting diagnostic test results.

Table **6-1** Users' Guides for an Article About Interpreting Diagnostic Test Results

Are the Results Valid?

- Was the diagnostic test evaluated in a spectrum of patients with a low to high probability of having the target disorder?
- Was there a blind comparison with an independent reference (gold) standard applied similarly to all patients?
- Did the results of the test being evaluated influence the decision to perform the reference (gold) standard?

What Are the Results?

- What likelihood ratios were associated with the range of possible test results?

How Can I Apply the Results to Patient Care?

- Will the reproducibility of the test result and its interpretation be satisfactory in my clinical setting?
- Are the results applicable to the patients in my clinical setting?
- Will the results change my management strategy?
- Will patients be better off as a result of the test?

ARE THE RESULTS VALID?

Was the Diagnostic Test Evaluated in a Spectrum of Patients With a Low to High Probability of Having the Target Disorder?

A diagnostic test is useful only to the extent that it distinguishes among conditions or disorders that could otherwise be confused. Almost any test can differentiate healthy persons from severely ill persons; this ability, however, tells us nothing about the clinical utility of a test. The true, pragmatic value of a test is established only in a study that closely resembles clinical practice. Another way to understand this point is to refer back to Figure 6-1. The population of interest comprises patients with pretest probabilities between test and treatment thresholds.

Tests are often developed by using an accessible population of patients known to have the target condition and a group of healthy controls. If an instrument does not discriminate between those with and without the condition at this stage of development, then it is unlikely to be clinically useful. The value of an assessment lies, however, in its ability to distinguish the full spectrum of patients with the condition (those with mild and severe symptoms) from those who have similar symptoms arising from different disorders. Diagnostically, it is easier to distinguish patients with florid presentation from those without the condition than it is to identify patients with a mild presentation. A test will only be useful if it can differentiate those likely to have the condition from those who do not.

Evaluations of new tests often omit the essential developmental stage of evaluation in a real clinical population. For example, the ankle-brachial pressure index (ABPI), a measure of the functional state of lower limb circulation, is used to assess patients with leg ulcers to rule out peripheral arterial disease. Compression bandaging of leg ulcers is contraindicated in patients with peripheral arterial disease. In the late 1960s, the normal values of an ABPI were established by testing 110 patients with known occlusive peripheral arterial disease and comparing their test values with those of 25 healthy controls.[9] In patients with angiographic evidence of occlusion, the ABPI was less than 1.0, and in healthy controls, the ABPI was greater than 1.0. However, until the mid-1990s, studies on the validity of the ABPI had been conducted in selected populations such as patients in vascular clinics. It is only recently that the utility of the ABPI has been tested in community populations similar to those in which it is commonly used by community nurses.[10] Stoffers and colleagues[10] concluded that if the mean of three ABPIs was less than 0.9, it was highly probable that peripheral arterial disease was present; if the mean of three ABPIs was greater than 1.0, it was highly probable that peripheral arterial disease could be ruled out; and if the mean of three ABPIs fell in the range of 0.9 to 1.0, this represented a small area of diagnostic uncertainty requiring further assessment. A study examining the influence of study quality on diagnostic accuracy for a given test found that studies evaluating tests in diseased populations and a separate control group overestimated the diagnostic performance compared with studies that used clinical populations.[11]

In the study of iron-deficiency anemia, the patient sample was appropriate because it comprised consecutive patients who were older than 65 years who presented with anemia. The study included both inpatients and outpatients at two community hospitals in whom a complete blood count demonstrated previously undiagnosed anemia (men: hemoglobin level less than 12 g/dL; women: hemoglobin level less than 11 g/dL).

Was There a Blind Comparison With an Independent Reference (Gold) Standard Applied Similarly to All Patients?

The accuracy of a diagnostic test is best determined by comparing it to the "truth." Accordingly, readers must assure themselves that an appropriate reference standard or gold standard (such as biopsy, surgery, autopsy, or long-term follow-up) was applied to every patient, along with the test under investigation.[12] For example, to determine whether the Hopkins Verbal Learning Test could be used to detect mild dementia in older people, scores on the test were compared with an independent assessment by a psychiatrist using criteria from the *Diagnostic and Statistical Manual of Mental Disorder*, fourth edition.[13] Similarly, to determine the accuracy of rapid diagnostic testing (urine dipstick or Gram stain of unspun urine) for diagnosing urinary tract infection in children, test results were compared with the reference standard of urine culture.[14] In the study of iron-deficiency anemia, bone marrow aspiration was the reference standard.

One way a reference or gold standard can go wrong is if the test is part of the gold standard. For instance, one study evaluated the utility of measuring both serum and urinary amylase to diagnose pancreatitis.[15] The investigators constructed a gold standard that relied on certain tests, including tests for serum and urinary amylase. The incorporation of the test into the gold standard is likely to inflate the estimate of the test's diagnostic power. Thus, clinicians should insist on the independence of the test and the gold standard.

In reading articles about diagnostic tests, if you cannot accept the reference standard (within reason, that is—after all, nothing is perfect), then the study is unlikely to provide valid results. If you do accept the reference standard, the next question to ask is whether the test results and the reference standard were assessed blindly (that is, by interpreters who were unaware of the results of the other investigation). Clinical experience demonstrates the importance of blinding. Prior knowledge of the presence or absence of a disorder could influence a clinician's assessment. This is referred to as *expectation bias*. Lijmer and colleagues found that unblinded assessments overestimated correct diagnoses by as much as 30% compared with blinded studies (relative diagnostic odds ratio, 1.3; 95% confidence interval, 1.0 to 1.9).[11]

The more likely it is that awareness of the reference standard result could influence the interpretation of a new test, the greater is the importance of the blinded interpretation. Similarly, the more susceptible the reference standard is to changes in interpretation as a result of awareness of the test results, the more important is the blinding of the reference standard interpreter. In the iron-deficiency study, a hematologist who was blinded to the results of the laboratory tests interpreted the bone marrow aspiration as iron absent, reduced, present, or increased.

Did the Results of the Test Being Evaluated Influence the Decision to Perform the Reference (Gold) Standard?

The properties of a diagnostic test will be distorted if its results influence whether patients undergo confirmation by the reference standard. This situation is sometimes called *verification bias*[16,17] or *work-up bias*.[18,19] Lijmer and colleagues[11] showed that studies in which different reference tests were used for positive and negative results of the test under study overestimated the diagnostic performance compared with studies using a single reference test for all patients.

To avoid verification or work-up bias, participants need to receive both the test under consideration and the reference standard, regardless of the outcome of the first test. In some instances, participants who have had a negative test result may decide not to have the reference standard, especially if it is an invasive procedure such as angiography. Rather than exclude these participants, investigators can follow them up over an appropriate period and monitor them for symptoms of the target disorder.

In the iron-deficiency anemia study, all 259 patients had bone marrow aspiration and the following laboratory tests: hemoglobin, mean red cell volume, red cell distribution width, serum iron, iron-binding capacity, serum ferritin, and red cell protoporphyrin. Bone marrow aspiration proved uninterpretable in 24 patients, leaving a relevant group of 235 patients.

USING THE GUIDE

Thus far, we have established that the patients in the iron-deficiency anemia study[8] represented a spectrum of patients with low and high probability of having iron-deficiency anemia; there was blind comparison by a hematologist with an independent reference standard (bone marrow aspiration); and all patients had both bone marrow aspiration and the laboratory tests.

WHAT ARE THE RESULTS?

What Likelihood Ratios Were Associated With the Range of Possible Test Results?

The starting point of any diagnostic process is the patient presenting with a constellation of signs and symptoms. Consider two patients with fatigue who are found to be anemic (hemoglobin 10 g/dL). The first is the 73-year-old man who takes a nonsteroidal anti-inflammatory agent and has no signs of another underlying disease. The second is a similar patient with active rheumatoid arthritis, rheumatoid nodules, and an erythrocyte sedimentation rate of 80. Our clinical hunches about the likelihood of iron-deficiency anemia are very different in these two patients. In the first patient, the likelihood is quite high. In the second patient, because of the very high likelihood of anemia of chronic disease, the probability of iron-deficiency anemia is much lower. With the same intermediate serum ferritin result, the posttest probability of iron-deficiency anemia will be very different in these two patients.

This line of reasoning reveals that, regardless of the results of the serum ferritin test, the tests do not tell us whether anemia is present. What they do accomplish is to modify the pretest probability of that condition, thus yielding a new posttest probability. The direction and magnitude of the change from pretest to posttest probability are determined by the test's properties, and the most useful property is the *likelihood ratio.*

Table **6-2** Test Properties of Serum Ferritin

Serum Ferritin Results (mcg/L)	Iron-Deficiency Anemia Present		Absent		Likelihood Ratio*
	Number	Proportion	Number	Proportion	
≤18	47	47/85 = 0.553	2	2/150 = 0.013	42.5
> 18 ≤ 45	23	23/85 = 0.271	13	13/150 = 0.087	3.11
> 45 ≤ 100	7	7/85 = 0.082	27	27/150 = 0.18	0.46
> 100	8	8/85 = 0.094	108	108/150 = 0.72	0.13
Total	85		150		

*Likelihood ratio: relative likelihood that a specific serum ferritin level would be expected in a patient with (as opposed to without) iron-deficiency anemia. For example, for serum ferritin of ≤18 mcg/L,

the likelihood ratio would be as follows: $\frac{(47/85)}{(2/150)} = \frac{0.553}{0.013} = 42.5$

A serum ferritin level of 18 mcg/L or less is 42.5 times more likely to occur in a patient with (as opposed to without) iron-deficiency anemia.

The study of the diagnosis of iron-deficiency anemia revealed that serum ferritin was the most useful test. Consequently, the remainder of our discussion focuses on the ferritin results. As depicted in Table 6-2, which was constructed from the results of the iron-deficiency anemia study, there were 85 people with anemia as determined by bone marrow aspiration and 150 people whose bone marrow aspiration excluded that diagnosis. For all patients, serum ferritin levels were classified into four categories: up to 18 mcg/L; greater than 18 and up to 45 mcg/L; greater than 45 and up to 100 mcg/L; and, greater than 100 mcg/L. How likely is a serum ferritin level of 18 mcg/L or less among people who have iron-deficiency anemia? Table 6-2 shows that 47 of 85 patients (or 0.553) had serum ferritin levels of 18 mcg/L or less. How often is the same test result, a serum ferritin level of 18 mcg/L or less, found among people in whom iron-deficiency anemia was suspected but excluded? The answer is 2 of 150 (or 0.013). The ratio of these two likelihoods is called the likelihood ratio; for a serum ferritin level of 18 mcg/L or less, it equals 0.553 divided by 0.013 (or 42.5). In other words, a serum ferritin level of 18 mcg/L or less is 42.5 times more likely to occur in a patient with, as opposed to without, iron-deficiency anemia.

Similarly, we can calculate the likelihood ratio for each level of the diagnostic test results. Each calculation involves answering two questions: First, how likely is a given test result (say, a serum ferritin level greater than 18 and up to 45 mcg/L) among people with the target disorder (iron-deficiency anemia)? Second, how likely is the same test result among people without the target disorder? For a serum ferritin level greater than 18 and up to 45 mcg/L, these likelihoods are 23/85 (0.271) and 13/150 (0.087), respectively, and their ratio (the likelihood ratio for a serum ferritin level greater than 18 and up to 45 mcg/L) is 3.11. Table 6-2 provides the results of calculations for other serum ferritin results.

What do all these numbers mean? The likelihood ratios indicate by how much a given diagnostic test result will raise or lower the pretest probability of the target disorder. A likelihood ratio of 1 means that the posttest probability is exactly the same as the pretest probability. Likelihood ratios greater than 1 increase the probability that the target disorder is present, and the higher the likelihood ratio, the greater is this increase. Conversely, likelihood ratios less than 1 decrease the probability of the target disorder, and the smaller the likelihood ratio, the greater is the decrease in probability and the smaller is its final value. The *likelihood ratio for a positive test result* (LR+) is the ratio of true-positive results (i.e., those in whom the test correctly identified the target disorder) to false-positive results (i.e., those in whom the test incorrectly identified the target disorder). The *likelihood ratio for a negative test result* (LR–) is the ratio of false-negative results (i.e., those in whom the test incorrectly identified the absence of the target disorder) to true-negative results (i.e., those in whom the test correctly identified the absence of the target disorder).

How big is a "big" likelihood ratio, and how small is a "small" one? Using likelihood ratios in your day-to-day practice will lead to your own sense of their interpretation, but consider the following a rough guide:

- Likelihood ratios greater than 10 or less than 0.1 generate large and often conclusive changes from pretest to posttest probability.
- Likelihood ratios of 5 to 10 and 0.1 to 0.2 generate moderate shifts in pretest to posttest probability.
- Likelihood ratios of 2 to 5 and 0.2 to 0.5 generate small (but sometimes important) changes in probability.
- Likelihood ratios of 1 to 2 and of 0.5 to 1 alter probability to a small (and rarely important) degree.

Having determined the magnitude and significance of the likelihood ratios, how do we use these ratios to go from pretest to posttest probability? We cannot combine likelihoods directly in the same way that we can combine probabilities or percentages. Their formal use requires converting the pretest probability to odds, multiplying the result by the likelihood ratio, and converting the consequent posttest odds into a posttest probability. Although it is not difficult (see Chapter 27, Measures of Association), this calculation can be tedious and off-putting; fortunately, there is an easier way.

A nomogram proposed by Fagan[20] (Figure 6-2) does the conversions and allows an easy transition from pretest to posttest probability. The left-hand column of the nomogram represents the pretest probability, the middle column represents the likelihood ratio, and the right-hand column shows the posttest probability. You obtain the posttest probability by anchoring a ruler at the pretest probability and rotating it until it lines up with the likelihood ratio for the observed test result.

Recall the patient in our scenario, the otherwise healthy 73-year-old man who takes nonsteroidal anti-inflammatory agents. Most clinicians would agree that the probability of iron deficiency as the explanation for this man's anemia is quite high, about 70%. This value then represents the pretest probability. Suppose that his serum ferritin level is 150 mcg/L. Figure 6-2 shows how you can anchor a ruler at his pretest probability of 70% and align it with the likelihood ratio of 0.13 associated with a serum ferritin level greater than 100 mcg/L. The result: his posttest probability is 23%. If, by contrast, his

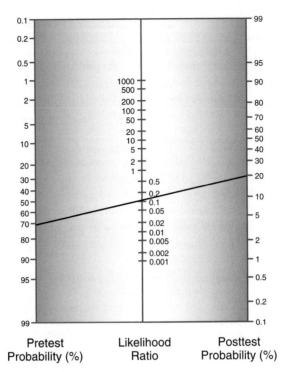

Figure 6-2. Likelihood ratio nomogram. *(Modified and reproduced with permission of the Massachusetts Medical Society from Fagan TJ. Nomogram for Bayes theorem [letter]. N Engl J. Med. 1975;293:257. Copyright © 1975, Massachusetts Medical Society. All rights reserved.)*

serum ferritin level is 30 mcg/L (likelihood ratio 3.11), then the probability of iron deficiency increases to 88%. A serum ferritin level of 15 mcg/L (likelihood ratio 42.5) moves the posttest probability to 99%.

The pretest probability is an estimate. We have already pointed out that the literature on differential diagnosis can help us in establishing the pretest probability. Clinicians can deal with residual uncertainty by examining the implications of a plausible range of pretest probabilities. Let us assume the pretest probability in this case is as low as 60% or as high as 80%. The posttest probabilities that would follow from these different pretest probabilities appear in Table 6-3.

We can repeat this exercise for our second patient, the 73-year-old man with active rheumatoid arthritis. Let us consider that his presentation is compatible with a 20% probability of iron deficiency. Using our nomogram (see Figure 6-2), the posttest probability with a serum ferritin level of 150 mcg/L (likelihood ratio 0.13) is 3%; with a ferritin level of 30 mcg/L (likelihood ratio 3.11), it is 44%; and with a serum ferritin level of 15 mcg/L (likelihood ratio 42.5), it is 91%. The pretest probability (with a range of possible pretest probabilities from 10% to 30%), likelihood ratios, and posttest probabilities associated with each of the four possible results also appear in Table 6-3.

Table **6-3**   Pretest Probabilities, Likelihood Ratios of Serum Ferritin Results, and Posttest Probabilities in Two Patients With Suspected Iron-Deficiency Anemia

Pretest Probability % (Range)*	Ferritin Result (Likelihood Ratio)	Posttest Probability % (Range)
73-Year-Old Healthy Man Taking Nonsteroidal Anti-inflammatory Agents		
70 (60–80)**	≤ 18 (42.5)	99 (98–99)
70 (60–80)	> 18 ≤ 45 (3.11)	88 (82–93)
70 (60–80)	> 45 ≤ 100 (0.46)	52 (41–65)
70 (60–80)	> 100 (0.13)	23 (16–34)
73-Year-Old Man With Active Rheumatoid Arthritis		
20 (10–30)	≤ 18 (42.5)	91 (82–95)
20 (10–30)	> 18 ≤ 45 (3.11)	44 (25–57)
20 (10–30)	> 45 ≤ 100 (0.46)	10 (5–17)
20 (10–30)	> 100 (0.13)	3 (1–5)

*The values in parentheses represent a plausible range of pretest probabilities; in the first case, the best guess of the pretest probability is 70%; values of 60% to 80% would also be reasonable estimates. In the second case, the best guess of the pretest probability is 20%; values of 10% to 30% would also be reasonable estimates.
**Sample calculation:
Pretest Probability = 70%

$$Odds = \frac{70\%}{100\% - 70\%} = \frac{0.70}{0.30} = 2.33$$

Likelihood Ratio: 42.5

$$Posttest\ Probability: \frac{Odds \times Likelihood\ Ratio}{1 + (Odds \times Likelihood\ Ratio)} = \frac{2.33 \times 42.5}{1 + (2.33 \times 42.5)} = \frac{99.025}{100.025} = 99\%$$

Having learned to use likelihood ratios, you may be curious about where to find easy access to the likelihood ratios of tests you use regularly in your clinical setting. The Rational Clinical Examination[21] is a series of systematic reviews of the diagnostic properties of the history and physical examination published in *JAMA*. Black and colleagues summarized much of the available information about diagnostic test properties in the form of a medical text.[22]

Sensitivity and Specificity

Readers who have followed the discussion to this point will understand the essentials of interpretation of diagnostic tests. It is also helpful to understand two other terms in the lexicon of diagnostic testing—*sensitivity* and *specificity*—because they remain in wide use. *Sensitivity* is the proportion of people with the target disorder in whom a test result is positive, and *specificity* is the proportion of people without the target disorder in whom a test result is negative. To use these concepts, we have to divide test results into normal and abnormal categories; in other words, we must create a table, two-rows by two-columns. Table 6-4 presents the general form of a two-by-two (2 × 2) table that we

Table 6-4 Comparison of the Results of a Diagnostic Test With the Results of the Reference Standard Using a 2 × 2 Table

	Reference Standard	
Test Results	Disease Present	Disease Absent
Disease present	True Positive (*a*)	False Positive (*b*)
Disease absent	False Negative (*c*)	True Negative (*d*)

Sensitivity (Sens) = $\dfrac{a}{a+c}$

Specificity (Spec) = $\dfrac{d}{b+d}$

Likelihood ratio for positive test (LR+) = $\dfrac{sens}{1 - spec} = \dfrac{a/(a+c)}{b/(b+d)}$

Likelihood ratio for negative test (LR–) = $\dfrac{1 - sens}{spec} = \dfrac{c/(a+c)}{d/(b+d)}$

use to understand sensitivity and specificity. We can transform a four-by-two table such as Table 6-2 into any of three such two-by-two tables, depending on what we call normal or abnormal (or depending on what we call negative and positive test results). Let us assume that we call serum ferritin values of 18 mcg/L or less abnormal (or positive).

Table 6-5 presents a two-by-two table comparing the results of serum ferritin levels with the results of bone marrow aspiration as a reference standard. To calculate sensitivity from the data in Table 6-5, we look at the number of people with proven iron-deficiency anemia (85) who were diagnosed as having the target disorder using the serum ferritin test (47). The sensitivity is a/(a+c) = 47/85 or 55.3%. To calculate specificity, we look at the number of people without the target disorder (150) whose serum ferritin test results were classified as normal (148). The specificity is d/(b + d) = 148/150 or 98.7%. We can also calculate likelihood ratios for the positive test result using the cut-point of 18 mcg/L: [a/(a + c)]/[b/(b + d)] = [47/(47 + 38)]/[2/(2 + 148)] = 42.5 (LR+) and for the negative test result using the same cut-point: [c/(a + c)]/[d/(b + d)] = [38/(47 + 38)]/[148/(2 + 148)] = 0.45 (LR–). Note that with this cut, we not only lose the diagnostic information associated with a varying serum ferritin greater than 18 mcg/L, but we also interpret serum ferritin results greater than 18 and up to 45 mcg/L as if they decrease the likelihood of iron deficiency (we attribute a likelihood ratio of 0.45 to all values greater than 18 mcg/L), when in fact they increase the likelihood (we have already seen that the likelihood ratio of ferritin of greater than 18 and up to 45 mcg/L is 3.11).

Let us see how the test performs if we decide to put the threshold of positive versus negative in a different place in the table. For example, let us define serum ferritin levels greater than 100 mcg/L as normal. As shown in Table 6-6, the sensitivity is now 77/85

Table **6-5** Comparison of the Results of a Diagnostic Test (Serum Ferritin) With the Results of the Reference Standard (Bone Marrow Aspiration), Assuming Only Values ≤18 mcg/L Are Positive (Truly Abnormal)

	Bone Marrow Aspiration	
Ferritin Results (mcg/L)	Iron-Deficiency Anemia Present	Iron-Deficiency Anemia Absent
≤18	47 (a)	2 (b)
>18	38 (c)	148 (d)
Total	85	150

$$Sensitivity = \frac{a}{a+c} = \frac{47}{85} = 55.3\%$$

$$Specificity = \frac{d}{b+d} = \frac{148}{150} = 98.7\%$$

$$Likelihood\ ratio\ of\ a\ positive\ test\ (LR+) = \frac{a/(a+c)}{b/(b+d)} = \frac{0.553}{0.013} = 42.5$$

$$Likelihood\ ratio\ of\ a\ negative\ test\ (LR-) = \frac{c/(a+c)}{d/(b+d)} = \frac{0.447}{0.987} = 0.45$$

or 90.6% (among 85 people with iron-deficiency anemia, 77 are diagnosed by bone marrow aspiration), but what has happened to specificity? Among 150 people without iron-deficiency anemia, only 108 had negative test results (specificity, 72%). The corresponding likelihood ratios are 3.24 and 0.13. With this cut, we not only lose the diagnostic information associated with varying serum ferritin levels of 100 mcg/L or less, but we also interpret serum ferritin levels of greater than 45 and up to 100 mcg/L as if they increase the likelihood of iron-deficiency anemia (we attribute a likelihood ratio of 3.24 to all values less than 100 mcg/L), when in fact they decrease the likelihood (we noted earlier that the likelihood ratio of a ferritin level of greater than 45 and up to 100 mcg/L is 0.46). You can generate the third two-by-two table by setting the cut-point in the middle. If your sensitivity and specificity values are 82.4% and 90%, respectively, and associated likelihood ratios of a positive and a negative test are 8.24 and 0.20, you have it right.

In using sensitivity and specificity, you must both discard important information and recalculate sensitivity and specificity for every cut-point. We recommend the likelihood ratio approach because it is simpler and more efficient and avoids the need to classify tests as "normal" and "abnormal".

USING THE GUIDE

Thus far, we have established that the results are likely true for the people who were included in the iron-deficiency anemia study, and we have ascertained the likelihood ratios associated with different test results. How useful is the test likely to be in our clinical practice?

Table 6-6   Comparison of the Results of a Diagnostic Test (Serum Ferritin) With the Results of the Reference Standard (Bone Marrow Aspiration), Assuming Only Values ≤100 mcg/L Are Positive (Truly Abnormal)

	Bone Marrow Aspiration	
Ferritin Results (mcg/L)	Iron-Deficiency Anemia Present	Iron-Deficiency Anemia Absent
≤ 100	77 (a)	42 (b)
> 100	8 (c)	108 (d)
Total	85	150

$$Sensitivity = \frac{a}{a+c} = \frac{77}{85} = 90.6\%$$

$$Specificity = \frac{d}{b+d} = \frac{108}{150} = 72.0\%$$

$$Likelihood\ ratio\ of\ a\ positive\ test\ (LR+) = \frac{a/(a+c)}{b/(b+d)} = \frac{0.906}{0.28} = 3.24$$

$$Likelihood\ ratio\ of\ a\ negative\ test\ (LR-) = \frac{c/(a+c)}{d/(b+d)} = \frac{0.094}{0.72} = 0.13$$

HOW CAN I APPLY THE RESULTS TO PATIENT CARE?

Will the Reproducibility of the Test Result and Its Interpretation Be Satisfactory in My Clinical Setting?

The value of any test depends on its ability to yield the same result when it is reapplied to the same patients whose clinical status has not changed. Poor reproducibility can result from problems with the test itself (e.g., variations in reagents in radioimmunoassay kits for determining hormone levels). A second cause of variable test results in these patients arises when a test requires interpretation (e.g., the extent of ST-segment elevation on an electrocardiogram). Ideally, an article about a diagnostic test will address the reproducibility of the test results using a measure that corrects for agreement by chance (see Chapter 30, Measuring Agreement Beyond Chance). This is especially important when expertise is required in performing or interpreting a test. You can confirm this by recalling the clinical disagreements that arise when you and one or more colleagues measure an infant's head circumference or a pregnant woman's fundal height or examine the same electrocardiogram or chest radiograph, even if all of you are experts.

If the reproducibility of a test in the study setting is mediocre and disagreement among observers is common, and yet the test still discriminates well between those with and without the target condition, it is very useful. Under these circumstances, the likelihood is good that the test can be readily applied to your clinical setting. If reproducibility of a diagnostic test is very high and observer variation is very low, either the test is simple and unambiguous or those interpreting it are highly skilled. If the latter applies, less skilled interpreters in your own clinical setting may not do as well.

The authors of the iron-deficiency anemia study[8] explained that the blood test was determined using a radioimmunoassay and provided a reference that could address its reproducibility. A laboratory would do well to conduct its own quality control program and run consistency checks on a periodic basis.

Are the Results Applicable to the Patients in My Clinical Setting?

Test properties may change with a different mix of disease severity or with a different distribution of competing conditions. When patients with the target disorder all have severe disease, likelihood ratios will move away from a value of 1.0 (sensitivity increases). If patients are all mildly affected, likelihood ratios move toward a value of 1.0 (sensitivity decreases). If patients without the target disorder have competing conditions that mimic the test results seen in patients who have the target disorder, the likelihood ratios will move closer to 1.0 and the test will appear less useful (specificity decreases). In a different clinical setting in which fewer of the disease-free patients have these competing conditions, the likelihood ratios will move away from 1.0 and the test will appear more useful (specificity increases).

The phenomenon of differing test properties in different subpopulations has been demonstrated most strikingly for exercise electrocardiography in the diagnosis of coronary artery disease. For instance, the more severe the coronary artery disease is, the larger are the likelihood ratios of abnormal exercise electrocardiography for angiographic narrowing of the coronary arteries.[23] Another example comes from the diagnosis of venous thromboembolism, in which compression ultrasound for proximal vein thrombosis has proved more accurate in symptomatic outpatients than in asymptomatic postoperative patients.[24]

Sometimes, a test fails in just the patients one hopes it will best serve. The likelihood ratio of a negative dipstick test for the rapid diagnosis of urinary tract infection is approximately 0.2 in patients with clear symptoms and thus a high probability of urinary tract infection, but is more than 0.5 in those with low probability,[25] a finding rendering the test of little help in ruling out infection in the latter situation.

If you practice in a setting similar to that of the investigation and if the patient in your setting meets all the study inclusion criteria and does not violate any of the exclusion criteria, you can be confident that the results are applicable. If not, judgment is required. As with health care interventions, you should ask whether there are compelling reasons why the results should not be applied to patients in your clinical setting, either because of the severity of disease or because the mix of competing conditions is so different that generalization is unwarranted. The issue of generalizability may be resolved if you can find a systematic review that pools the results of numerous studies.[26] For example, Gorelick and Shaw[14] conducted a systematic review of rapid diagnostic tests such as dipstick and Gram stain tests of unspun urine for diagnosing urinary tract infection in children.

The participants in the iron-deficiency anemia study[8] were a representative sample of men and women who were older than 65 years of age and were seen in one of two teaching hospitals. The study excluded groups such as institutionalized patients, those with recent blood transfusions or documented acute blood loss, and those who were too ill, dying, or severely demented. Such patients are likely to have had a different spectrum of competing conditions. The results of the study are readily applicable to most clinical practices in North America.

The patient before you, in whom the differential diagnosis includes iron-deficiency anemia, multiple myeloma, and a primary bone marrow problem such as myelodysplastic disorder, meets study eligibility criteria. Thus, you can be confident that the results will apply in his case.

Will the Results Change My Management Strategy?

It is useful, when making management decisions, to link them explicitly to the probability of the target disorder. As we have described, for any target disorder there are probabilities below which a clinician would dismiss a diagnosis and order no further tests—the test threshold. Similarly, there are probabilities above which a clinician would consider the diagnosis confirmed and would stop testing and initiate treatment—the treatment threshold. When the probability of the target disorder lies between the test and treatment thresholds, further testing is mandated.[27]

Once we decide on our test and treatment thresholds, posttest probabilities have direct treatment implications. Let us suppose that we are willing to treat patients with a probability of iron-deficiency anemia of 90% or higher (knowing that we will be treating 10% of them unnecessarily). Furthermore, let us suppose that we are willing to dismiss the diagnosis of iron-deficiency anemia in patients with a posttest probability of 10% or less. You may wish to apply different numbers here; the treatment and test thresholds are a matter of judgment, and they differ for different conditions depending on the risks of treatment (if it is risky, you want to be more certain of your diagnosis) and the danger of the disease if left untreated (if the danger of missing the disease is high, such as in pulmonary embolism, you want your posttest probability to be very low before abandoning the diagnostic search).

In the 73-year-old otherwise healthy man taking nonsteroidal anti-inflammatory agents, a serum ferritin level of 18 mcg/L or less would result in a posttest probability of 99% and would dictate treatment of iron deficiency and further investigation to determine its cause. A serum ferritin level greater than 18 and up to 45 mcg/L (88% posttest probability) would dictate further testing to determine whether the man has iron-deficiency anemia (perhaps a bone marrow aspiration or biopsy), as would a serum ferritin level higher than 100 mcg/L (posttest probability 23%). In the 73-year-old man with active rheumatoid arthritis, a serum ferritin level of 18 mcg/L or less would dictate treatment (91% posttest probability of iron-deficiency anemia), and an intermediate result of between 18 and 45 mcg/L (44% posttest probability) would require definitive diagnosis with bone marrow aspiration. A test result of more than 100 mcg/L (posttest probability of 3%) would allow the clinician to exclude a diagnosis of iron-deficiency anemia.

If most patients have test results with likelihood ratios near 1, the test will not be very useful. Thus, the usefulness of a diagnostic test is strongly influenced by the proportion of patients suspected of having the target disorder whose test results have very high or very low likelihood ratios. In the patients suspected of having iron-deficiency anemia, a review of Table 6-2 allows us to determine the proportion of patients with extreme results (either 18 mcg/L or less, with a likelihood ratio of 42.5, or greater than 100 mcg/L, with a likelihood ratio of 0.13). The proportion can be calculated as $(47 + 2 + 8 + 108)/235 = 165/235 = 70\%$. Thus, 70% of patients have extreme results, substantiating the test's usefulness.

A final comment has to do with the use of sequential tests. We have shown how each item of a history or each finding on physical examination represents a diagnostic test. We generate pretest probabilities that we modify with each new finding. In general, we can also use laboratory tests or imaging procedures in the same way. However, if two tests are very closely related, application of the second test may provide little or no additional information, and the sequential application of likelihood ratios will yield misleading results. For example, once one has the results of the most powerful laboratory test for iron-deficiency anemia, serum ferritin, additional tests such as serum iron or transferrin saturation add no further useful information.[28] *Clinical prediction rules* deal with the lack of independence of a series of tests that can be applied to a diagnostic dilemma and provide clinicians with a way of combining their results (see Chapter 22, Clinical Prediction Rules). For instance, the clinician in the scenario described earlier in this chapter could have used a rule that incorporated aspects of the history and physical examination to classify patients as having a high, medium, or low probability of iron-deficiency anemia.

Using the Guide

Given the extreme likelihood ratios of serum ferritin in elderly people with fatigue, serum ferritin levels are very likely to change management. For patients with a serum ferritin level of 18 mcg/L or less, investigation of the cause of the iron-deficiency anemia with colonoscopy and/or upper gastrointestinal endoscopy would be warranted for all but those with very low pretest probabilities. For other test results, the best course of action (bone marrow aspiration or biopsy, or investigation for blood loss) will differ depending on the posttest likelihood, which is determined by both the pretest likelihood and the test result.

Will Patients Be Better off as a Result of the Test?

The ultimate criterion for the usefulness of a diagnostic test is whether the benefits for patients are greater than the associated risks.[29] How can we establish the benefits and risks of applying a diagnostic test? The answer lies in thinking of a diagnostic test as a therapeutic maneuver (see Chapter 4, Health Care Interventions). Establishing whether a test does more good than harm will involve (1) randomizing patients to diagnostic strategies that include or do not include the test under investigation and (2) following patients in both groups forward in time to determine the frequency of important patient outcomes.

When is demonstrating accuracy sufficient to mandate the use of a test, and when does one require a randomized controlled trial? The value of an accurate test will be undisputed when the target disorder is dangerous if not diagnosed, the test has acceptable risks, and effective treatment exists. This is the case for the serum ferritin test that we have considered in this chapter. Depending on the pretest probability and the patient's relative aversion to bone marrow aspiration and biopsy or invasive tests to look for causes of iron deficiency, the appropriate interpretation of serum ferritin results will provide a clear course of action.

CLINICAL RESOLUTION

At his clinic visit, you explain to the patient that his hemoglobin value is 10.0 g/dL, which is lower than normal. You explain that you would like to do another blood test to help you determine whether he has iron-deficiency anemia. The patient is keen to learn more about why his hemoglobin is lower than it should be and agrees to have a serum ferritin test.

The next week, when the patient returns to the clinic, you inform him that his serum ferritin level is 15 mcg/L, a result with a likelihood ratio greater than 40, placing this patient's posttest probability of iron deficiency anemia well above 90%. You explain that the next step is to find out what is causing the iron deficiency. You have consulted with the family physician in the clinic, and she recommends an upper gastrointestinal endoscopy and colonoscopy. You tell the patient that an upper gastrointestinal endoscopy involves inserting a small, flexible device with a camera through the mouth and down the esophagus into the stomach and duodenum to identify possible sources of blood loss, and a colonoscopy is a similar procedure in which the device is inserted through the anus into the colon. The patient is worried but at the same time eager to find out what is causing him to feel so tired and agrees to the procedures.

REFERENCES

1. Sox HC, Blatt MA, Higgins MC, Marton KI. *Medical Decision Making.* Boston: Butterworth; 1988.
2. Glass RD. *Diagnosis: A Brief Introduction.* Melbourne: Oxford University Press; 1996.
3. Barondess JA, Carpenter CCJ, eds. *Differential Diagnosis.* Philadelphia: Lea & Febiger; 1994.
4. Pauker SG, Kassirer JP. The threshold approach to clinical decision making. *N Engl J Med.* 1980;302: 1109-1117.
5. Schmidt HG, Norman GR, Boshuizen HP. A cognitive perspective on medical expertise: theory and implication. *Acad Med.* 1990;65:611-621.
6. Bordage G. Elaborated knowledge: a key to successful diagnostic thinking. *Acad Med.* 1994;69:883-885.
7. Regehr G, Norman GR. Issues in cognitive psychology: implications for professional education. *Acad Med.* 1996;71:988-1001.
8. Guyatt GH, Patterson C, Ali M, et al. Diagnosis of iron-deficiency anemia in the elderly. *Am J Med.* 1990;88:205-209.
9. Yao ST, Hobbs JT, Irvine WT. Ankle systolic pressure measurements in arterial disease affecting the lower extremities. *Br J Surg.* 1969;56:676-679.
10. Stoffers HE, Kester AD, Kaiser V, Rinkens PE, Kitslaar PJ, Knottnerus JA. The diagnostic value of the measurement of the ankle-brachial systolic pressure index in primary health care. *J Clin Epidemiol.* 1996;49:1401-1405.

11. Lijmer JG, Mol BW, Heisterkamp S, et al. Empirical evidence of design-related bias in studies of diagnostic tests. *JAMA*. 1999;282:1061-1066.

12. Sackett DL, Haynes RB, Guyatt GH, Tugwell P. *Clinical Epidemiology: A Basic Science for Clinical Medicine*. 2nd ed. Boston: Little, Brown & Company; 1991:53-57.

13. Frank RM, Byrne GJ. The clinical utility of the Hopkins Verbal Learning Test as a screening test for mild dementia. *Int J Geriatr Psychiatry*. 2000;15:317-324.

14. Gorelick MH, Shaw KN. Screening tests for urinary tract infection in children: a meta-analysis. *Pediatrics* 1999;104:e54.

15. Kemppainen EA, Hedstrom JI, Puolakkainen PA, et al. Rapid measurement of urinary trypsinogen-2 as a screening test for acute pancreatitis. *N Engl J Med*. 1997;336:1788-1793.

16. Begg CB, Greenes RA. Assessment of diagnostic tests when disease verification is subject to selection bias. *Biometrics*. 1983;39:207-215.

17. Gray R, Begg CB, Greenes RA. Construction of receiver operating characteristic curves when disease verification is subject to selection bias. *Med Decis Making*. 1984;4:151-164.

18. Ransohoff DF, Feinstein AR. Problems of spectrum and bias in evaluating the efficacy of diagnostic tests. *N Engl J Med*. 1978;299:926-930.

19. Choi BC. Sensitivity and specificity of a single diagnostic test in the presence of work-up bias. *J Clin Epidemiol*. 1992;45:581-586.

20. Fagan TJ. Nomogram for Bayes theorem [letter]. *N Engl J Med*. 1975;293:257.

21. Sackett DL, Rennie D. The science and art of the clinical examination. *JAMA*. 1992;267:2650-2652.

22. Black ER, Bordley DR, Tape TG, Panzer RJ. *Diagnostic Strategies for Common Medical Problems*. 2nd ed. Philadelphia: American College of Physicians; 1999.

23. Hlatky MA, Pryor DB, Harrell FE. Factors affecting sensitivity and specificity of exercise electrocardiography. *Am J Med*. 1984;77:64-71.

24. Ginsberg JS, Caco CC, Brill-Edwards PA, et al. Venous thrombosis in patients who have undergone major hip or knee surgery: detection with compression US and impedance plethysmography. *Radiology*. 1991;181:651-654.

25. Lachs MS, Nachamkin I, Edelstein PH, et al. Spectrum bias in the evaluation of diagnostic tests: lessons from the rapid dipstick test for urinary tract infection. *Ann Intern Med*. 1992;117:135-140.

26. Irwig L, Tosteson AN, Gatsonis C, et al. Guidelines for meta-analyses evaluating diagnostic tests. *Ann Intern Med*. 1994;120:667-676.

27. Sackett DL, Haynes RB, Guyatt GH, Tugwell P. *Clinical Epidemiology: A Basic Science for Clinical Medicine*. 2nd ed. Boston: Little, Brown & Company; 1991:145-148.

28. Guyatt GH, Oxman A, Ali M, et al. Laboratory diagnosis of iron-deficiency anemia: an overview. *J Gen Intern Med*. 1992;7:145-153.

29. Guyatt GH, Tugwell PX, Feeny DH, Haynes RB, Drummond M. A framework for clinical evaluation of diagnostic technologies. *Can Med Assoc J*. 1986;134:587-594.

Prognosis

7

Alba DiCenso and Gordon Guyatt

The following Editorial Board members also made substantive contributions to this chapter: Heather Arthur and Andrea Nelson.

We gratefully acknowledge the work of Adrienne Randolph, Heiner Bucher, Scott Richardson, George Wells, and Peter Tugwell on the original chapter that appears in the Users' Guides to the Medical Literature, *edited by Guyatt and Rennie.*

In This Chapter

Finding the Evidence

Are the Results Valid?
  Was the Sample of Patients Representative?
  Were the Patients Sufficiently Homogeneous With Respect to Prognostic Risk?
  Was Follow-up Sufficiently Complete?
  Were Objective and Unbiased Outcome Criteria Used?

What Are the Results?
  How Likely Were the Outcomes Over Time?
  How Precise Were the Estimates of Likelihood?

How Can I Apply the Results to Patient Care?
  Were the Study Patients and Their Management Similar to Those in My Clinical Setting?
  Was Follow-up Sufficiently Long?
  Can I Use the Results in the Management of Patients in My Clinical Setting?

CLINICAL SCENARIO

A Child with Meningitis Before 1 Year of Age—What Is the Prognosis?

You are a pediatric nurse practitioner who has been caring for a 10-month-old infant who had an acute attack of meningococcal meningitis. The child was a term baby weighing 3500 g at birth who had been healthy before developing meningitis. The child's recovery has been uneventful, and she will be discharged in the next few days. Now that the immediate crisis of the illness has passed, the parents ask if she is likely to have any long-term consequences as a result of having had meningitis. In particular, they wonder if she is likely to have any significant disabilities. Because your knowledge about the prognosis of survivors of meningitis is limited, you tell the parents that you will search out specific information to address their concerns and report back to them.

FINDING THE EVIDENCE

During a break, you connect to the Internet and to MEDLINE at the United States National Library of Medicine Web site through PubMed. Using the Clinical Queries feature, with "prognosis" as the category and "sensitivity" as the emphasis, you enter the terms "meningitis," "infancy," and "health problems." The search identifies one article, "Meningitis in infancy in England and Wales: follow up at age 5 years," by Bedford and colleagues, and you obtain a copy from the library.[1]

Nurses require studies of patient *prognosis*—studies examining the possible outcomes of a disease and the probability with which they can be expected to occur—to give patients an indication of what the future is likely to hold. Although they strive to restore health, sometimes clinicians can offer only relief of discomfort and preparation for death or long-term disability by presenting the expected future course of the illness.

To estimate a patient's prognosis, we examine outcomes in groups of patients with a similar clinical presentation—infants who had meningitis before the age of 1 year, for example. We may then refine our question by looking at subgroups and deciding into which subgroup the patient falls. We may define these subgroups by demographic variables such as age (neonatal infants with meningitis may fare worse than postneonatal infants), disease-specific variables (infants' outcome may differ depending on the organism that caused the infection), or comorbid factors (infants with preexisting conditions, such as Down syndrome or cerebral palsy, may have worse outcomes). When these variables or factors really do predict which patients do better or worse, we call them *prognostic factors*.

Authors often distinguish between prognostic factors and *risk factors*, which are those patient characteristics associated with the development of the disease in the first place. For example, smoking is an important risk factor for the development of lung cancer, but it is not as important a prognostic factor as tumor stage in someone who has lung cancer. The issues in studies of prognostic factors and risk factors are identical in terms of assessing validity and using the results in patient care.

Determining a patient's prognosis can help clinicians and patients to know which outcomes could happen as a result of the condition, how likely they are to happen, and over what period they may occur. This information facilitates realistic planning for the future and may reduce anxiety if the prognosis is better than the patient or family feared. It also facilitates clinical decision making. Decisions to intervene may vary if a patient will get well anyway, is at low risk for adverse outcomes, is at high risk for adverse outcomes, or is destined to have poor outcomes despite whatever treatment is offered. For example, pressure area care to prevent skin breakdown is a low priority in a young adult bedridden for a week with a viral infection, a high priority for an elderly person bedridden with a stroke, and perhaps unjustified in a patient in the final stages of terminal illness when disturbing the patient to administer skin care is likely to cause discomfort.

Knowledge of prognosis is also useful for resolution of issues broader than the care of individual patients. Organizations may attempt to compare the quality of care across clinicians, or institutions, by measuring the outcomes of care. However, differences in outcome may be caused by the variability in the underlying severity of illness rather than by the treatments, clinicians, or health care institutions under study. For example, although it may be tempting to compare pressure ulcer incidence rates across inpatient units or even among hospitals, such comparisons are misleading if the underlying risk of pressure ulcer development differs between the units of comparison.[2] If we know patients' prognoses, we may be able to compare populations and adjust for differences in prognosis to obtain a more accurate indication of how management affects outcomes (see Chapter 17, Health Services Interventions).

In this chapter, we focus on how to use articles that may contain valid prognostic information that will be useful in counseling patients (Table 7-1). Using the same methodology as studies addressing issues of harm (see Chapter 5, Harm), investigators addressing issues of prognosis use *cohort* and *case-control* studies to explore the determinants of outcome. Implicitly, randomized controlled trials also address issues of prognosis. The results reported for both intervention and control groups provide prognostic information: the control group results tell us about the prognosis in patients who did

Table 7-1   Users' Guides for an Article About Prognosis

Are the Results Valid?

- Was the sample of patients representative?
- Were the patients sufficiently homogeneous with respect to prognostic risk?
- Was follow-up sufficiently complete?
- Were objective and unbiased outcome criteria used?

What Are the Results?

- How likely were the outcomes over time?
- How precise were the estimates of likelihood?

How Can I Apply the Results to Patient Care?

- Were the study patients and their management similar to those in my clinical setting?
- Was follow-up sufficiently long?
- Can I use the results in the management of patients in my clinical setting?

not receive treatment, and the intervention group results tell us about the prognosis in patients who received treatment. In this sense, each arm of a randomized trial represents a cohort study. If the randomized trial meets the criteria described in this chapter, it can provide extremely useful information about prognosis.

For questions of harm, the choice of appropriate treatment and control groups is crucial. For questions of prognosis, if there is a control group at all (if patients all have more or less the same prognosis, a control group may not be needed), it should include patients with different prognostic factors. In the same way that studies about diagnostic tests evaluate tests that distinguish between those with and without a target condition or disease, prognostic studies may suggest factors that differentiate between those at low and high risk for a target outcome or adverse event. Issues in evaluating prognostic studies, however, are sufficiently different from those related to harm or diagnosis that nurses may find the following guides helpful.

ARE THE RESULTS VALID?

Was the Sample of Patients Representative?

Bias has to do with systematic differences from the truth. A prognostic study is biased if it yields a systematic overestimate or underestimate of the likelihood of adverse outcomes in the patients under study. When a sample is systematically different from the underlying population—and is therefore likely to be biased because patients will have a better or worse prognosis than those in that population—that sample is considered *unrepresentative.*

How can you recognize an unrepresentative sample? First, look to see whether patients pass through some sort of filter before they enter the study. If they do, the result is likely to be from a sample that is systematically different from the underlying population of interest (e.g., infants who were premature, had low birth weights, or had congenital anomalies). One such filter is the sequence of referrals that leads patients from primary to tertiary centers. Tertiary centers often care for patients with rare and unusual disorders or severe illnesses. Research describing the outcomes of patients in tertiary centers may not be applicable to patients with the disorder receiving care in a primary care center.

For example, when a child is admitted to hospital with febrile seizures, the parents will want to know their child's risk of more seizures in the future. This risk is much lower in population-based studies (reported risks range from 1.5% to 4.6%) than in clinic-based studies (reported risks are 2.6% to 76.9%).[3] Patients in clinic-based studies may have other neurologic problems predisposing them to have higher rates of recurrence. For you to counsel parents adequately, you need to know how similar your patient is to the patients in the various samples. For example, results of a study based on patients in tertiary care centers are not likely to be applicable to patients in primary care but are very likely to be applicable to similar patients in other tertiary care centers.

Failure to define clearly the patients who entered a study increases the risk that the sample is unrepresentative. To help you decide about the representativeness of a sample, look for a clear description of which patients were included and excluded from a study. Investigators should specify the way the sample was selected, and they should use and describe objective criteria for diagnosing patients with the disorder.

Were the Patients Sufficiently Homogeneous With Respect to Prognostic Risk?

Prognostic studies are most useful if individual members of the entire group of patients being considered are similar enough that the outcome of the group is applicable to each group member. This will be true only if patients are at a similar, well-described point in their disease process. The point in the clinical course need not be early, but it does need to be consistent. For instance, in a study of the prognosis of children with acquired brain injury, researchers examined a subpopulation of children who remained unconscious after 90 days.[4]

After ensuring that the stage of the disease process is not a variable influencing outcome, it is important to consider other factors that could influence patient outcome. For instance, consider the example of acquired brain injury. A study that pools patients with and without head trauma but does not distinguish between them may not be useful if these two groups have different prognoses. If the overall mortality rate in a study is 50% but the patient population is made up of identifiable subgroups, one of which has a mortality rate near zero and the other of which has a mortality rate near 100%, the 50% estimate will be valid for the whole group but not valid for any individual in that group. If patients are heterogeneous with respect to risk of adverse outcomes, the study will be more useful if the investigators define subgroups that are at lower and higher risk than the overall group.

For example, Pincus and colleagues followed a cohort of patients with rheumatoid arthritis for 15 years.[5] These investigators separated patients into several cohorts depending on their demographic characteristics, disease variables, and functional status. They found that older patients and those with greater impairment of functional status (e.g., modified walking time and activities of daily living) died earlier than other patients. In another example, a study of children with acquired brain injury found that patients with posttraumatic injuries did much better than those with anoxic injuries. Of 36 patients with closed head trauma, 23 (64%) regained enough social function to be able to express their wants and needs, and nine (25%) eventually regained the capacity to walk independently. Of 13 children with anoxic injuries, none regained important social or cognitive function.[4]

Not only must investigators consider all important prognostic factors, but they must also consider them in relation to one another. Consider the Framingham study, in which investigators examined (among many other things) risk factors for stroke.[6] They reported that the rate of stroke in patients with atrial fibrillation and rheumatic heart disease was 41 per 1000 person-years, a rate that was very similar to the rate for patients with atrial fibrillation but without rheumatic heart disease. However, patients with rheumatic heart disease were, on average, much younger than those who did not have rheumatic heart disease. To understand the impact of rheumatic heart disease in these circumstances, investigators must consider separately (1) the relative risk of stroke in young people with and without rheumatic disease and (2) the risk of stroke in elderly people with and without rheumatic disease. We call this separate consideration an *adjusted analysis.* Once adjustments were made for age (and also for sex and hypertensive status), the investigators found that the rate of stroke was sixfold greater in patients with atrial fibrillation and rheumatic heart disease than in patients with atrial fibrillation who did not have rheumatic heart disease. If large numbers of variables have a major impact on prognosis, investigators should use sophisticated statistical techniques to determine the most powerful predictors (see Chapter 31, Regression and Correlation). Such an analysis may lead to a clinical decision rule that guides clinicians in simultaneously considering all the important prognostic factors (see Chapter 22, Clinical Prediction Rules).

How can you decide whether groups are sufficiently homogeneous with respect to risk? On the basis of your clinical experience and your understanding of the biology of the condition being studied, can you think of factors that the investigators have neglected that are likely to define subgroups with very different prognoses? To the extent that the answer is "yes," the validity of the study is compromised.

Was Follow-up Sufficiently Complete?

A high patient dropout rate threatens the validity of a study of prognosis. As the number of patients lost to follow-up increases, the likelihood of bias also increases (e.g., patients who are followed-up may be at systematically higher or lower risk than those not followed-up). When is the number of patients lost to follow-up too high? The answer depends on the relationship between the proportion of patients who are lost to follow-up and the proportion of patients who have the adverse outcome. The larger the number of patients whose fate is unknown relative to the number who have an event, the greater is the threat to a study's validity.

For example, let us assume that 30% of a particularly high-risk group (e.g., elderly patients with diabetes) experience an adverse outcome (e.g., cardiovascular death) during long-term follow-up. If 10% of patients are lost to follow-up, the true mortality rate may be as low as 27% (if 30% of the 90% followed-up group—27% of the total—had adverse outcomes, and none of the 10% lost to follow-up had adverse outcomes, then the total with adverse outcomes is 27%) or as high as 37% (if 30% of the 90% followed-up group—27% of the total—had adverse outcomes plus all those lost to follow-up, another 10% of the population). Across this range, the clinical implications would not change appreciably, and the loss to follow-up would not threaten the validity of the study. However, in a much lower-risk patient sample (e.g., otherwise healthy middle-aged men), the observed mortality rate may be 1%. In this case, if we assumed that all 10% of patients lost to follow-up died, the event rate of 11% could have very different implications.

A large loss to follow-up constitutes a more serious threat to study validity when the patients who are lost to follow-up may be different from those who are easier to find. In one study, for example, after much effort, 180 of 186 patients treated for neurosis were followed-up.[7] The death rate was 3% among the 60% who were easily traced. Among those who were more difficult to find, however, the death rate was 27%. If a differential fate for those followed-up and those lost to follow-up is plausible (and in most prognostic studies, it will be), loss to follow-up that is large relative to the proportion of patients with the adverse outcome constitutes an important threat to study validity.

Were Objective and Unbiased Outcome Criteria Used?

Outcome events can vary from those that are objective and easily measured (e.g., death), to those requiring some judgment (e.g., behavioral problems), to those that may require considerable judgment and are challenging to measure (e.g., disability or quality of life). Investigators should clearly specify and define their target outcomes before the study, and, if possible, they should base their criteria on objective measures. In addition, they should specify the intensity and frequency of monitoring. As the subjectivity of the outcome definition increases, it becomes more important that outcome assessors are blinded to the presence of prognostic factors.

The study of children with acquired brain injury mentioned earlier provides a good example of the issues involved in measuring outcome.[4] The examiners found that families frequently interpreted their children's social response as more developed than others might interpret it. The investigators therefore required that study personnel verify the development of a social response in the affected children.

USING THE GUIDE

In the article describing the prognosis of children who had had meningitis before the age of 1 year, the investigators prospectively enrolled all 1717 children in England and Wales who survived an acute attack of meningitis between 1985 and 1987.[1] Thus, patients were recruited at a common, early starting point. Because the study was community based, the population is representative of an unselected cohort of British children who survived an acute attack of meningitis before the age of 1 year. The authors noted that previous studies had relied on data from children referred to specialist centers, which by definition attract more serious cases.

Children, matched for sex and age from the same general practice as the child who had had meningitis, formed the control group. One could speculate that numerous factors could influence the risk of severe disabilities subsequent to meningitis, including age at infection, organism of infection, gestational age, and birth weight. The investigators analyzed these factors and found differences in prognosis across subgroups. They found that children who were infected as neonates had more health and developmental problems than those who had meningitis when they were older than 1 month ($\chi^2 = 4.5$, $P = 0.03$). They also found that the rate of disability differed widely in children infected with different organisms and in neonates with different gestational ages and birth weights. Infection with *Streptococcus pneumoniae* was associated with a higher rate of disability than was infection with *Haemophilus influenzae* and *Neisseria meningitidis*. Among children infected as neonates, a higher proportion of those who were less than 32 weeks of gestational age and those with very low birth weights (less than 1500 g) had moderate or severe disability.

The investigators followed 92% of the children who had had meningitis and 94% of the children in the control group to 5 years of age. General practitioners and parents completed questionnaires about each child's health and development to 5 years of age. Although it is likely that the general practitioners would be equally likely to identify major deficits in both groups, it is possible that subtle deficits such as middle ear disease, squint, and behavioral problems were overreported by parents of children who had had meningitis because of parental anxiety or close attention paid to these children. Detailed investigations using standardized procedures to examine all the children may have provided more objective data.

Continued

WHAT ARE THE RESULTS?

How Likely Were the Outcomes Over Time?

The quantitative results from studies of prognosis or risk are the number of events that occur over time. To illustrate this, we use the example of a man asking a nurse practitioner about the prognosis of his elderly mother who has dementia. The patient's son asks, "What are the chances that my mother will still be alive in 5 years?" A high-validity study of the prognosis of patients with dementia provides a simple and direct answer in absolute terms.[8] Five years after presentation to the clinic, about 50% of the patients had died. Thus, there is about a 50:50 chance that his mother will be alive in 5 years.

The patient's son then indicates that the only person he knows with Alzheimer's disease is a 65-year-old uncle who was diagnosed 10 years ago and is still living. He is surprised that his mother's chance of dying in the next 5 years is so high. This statement gives the nurse practitioner the opportunity to discuss some of the prognostic factors for death in patients with Alzheimer disease. The study suggested that older patients, those with more severe dementia, those with behavioral problems, and those with hearing loss died earlier.

The son then asks whether his mother's chance of survival will change over time. In other words, although she may be at low risk for the next 2 years, will the risk increase after that? Neither the absolute nor relative expressions of results address this question. For this answer, we turn to a *survival curve*, a graph of the number of events over time (or conversely, the chance of being free of these events over time) (see Chapter 27, Measures of Association). The events must be discrete (e.g., death, stroke, or recurrence of cancer), and the time at which they occur must be precisely known. The study of patients with dementia provided a survival curve that suggests that the chance of dying is more or less constant during the first 7 years after referral to the clinic for dementia.[8]

How Precise Were the Estimates of Likelihood?

The more precise the estimate of prognosis a study provides, the less uncertain we will be about the study results and the more useful they will be to us. Usually, risks of adverse outcomes are reported with associated 95% *confidence intervals*. If a study is valid, the 95% confidence interval defines the range of risks within which it is highly likely that the true risk lies (see Chapter 29, Confidence Intervals). For example, the study of the prognosis of patients with dementia provides the 95% confidence interval around the

49% estimate of survival at 5 years (i.e., 39% to 58%), meaning that the true survival rate can be as low as 39% or as high as 58%. The larger the sample size, the narrower the confidence interval, and therefore, the more precise the estimate of prognosis a study provides. In most survival curves, earlier follow-up periods usually include results from more patients than do the later periods (because of losses to follow-up and because patients are enrolled in the study at different times). This means that survival curves are more precise in earlier periods, and this should be indicated by narrower confidence bands around the left-hand parts of the curve. This is illustrated in a study that examined survival of patients with advanced-stage, low-grade follicular lymphoma over an 8-year period (Figure 7-1).[9] The survival curve starts at time 0 with all 157 patients (100%) alive. The number of patients at risk at each time point includes all those who have not yet died and whom the investigators have followed up for at least this duration of time. As the study progresses, prediction becomes less precise because there are fewer patients available to estimate the probability of survival. Confidence intervals around the survival rate at each time point capture the precision of the estimate.

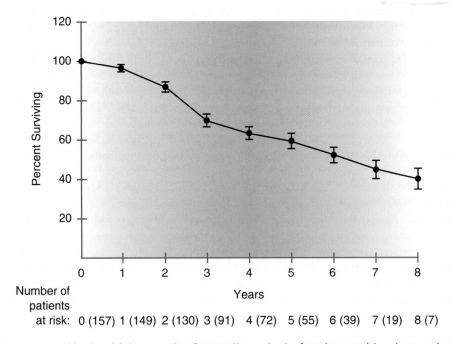

Figure 7-1. Kaplan-Meier graph of overall survival of patients with advanced-stage, low-grade follicular lymphoma over 8 years. Note: Confidence intervals around survival rates become wider (i.e., less precise) as the number of at-risk patients decreases. (*Modified and reproduced with permission of Wiley Liss, Inc., a subsidiary of John Wiley & Sons, Inc. from Wood LA, Coupland RW, North SA, Palmer MC. Outcome of advanced stage low grade follicular lymphomas in a population-based retrospective cohort. Cancer. 1999;85:1361-1368. Copyright © 1999. American Cancer Society.*)

Using the Guide

The authors of the meningitis study found a 10-fold increase in the risk of severe or moderate disability at 5 years of age among children who had had meningitis (relative risk, 10.3; 95% confidence interval, 6.7 to 16.0; $P < 0.001$). Of the children who had had meningitis, 15.6% had moderate or severe disability at 5 years of age compared with 1.5% of children in the control group (who had not had meningitis). This represents an absolute difference of 14.1%.

The investigators examined whether certain factors (i.e., age at infection, infecting organism, gestational age, and birth weight) influenced the risk of meningitis and found that they did. Children with neonatal meningitis (within the first month of life) were significantly more likely to have moderate disabilities than those with post-neonatal meningitis (18.2% vs 7.9%; $P < 0.001$; absolute difference, 10.3%), but the rate of severe disability was not significantly different between the groups (7.3% vs 5.5%). The rates of severe and moderate disability differed widely among children infected with different organisms. Infection with *Neisseria meningitidis* was associated with the lowest rate of severe and moderate disability (9.4% of those infected with the organism) compared with *Streptococcus pneumoniae*, which was associated with one of the highest rates of severe and moderate disability (23.6% of those infected with the organism). With respect to birth weight, among infants who weighed less than 1500 g at birth, 42.9% of those who had had meningitis had moderate or severe disability compared with none in the control group. Among those with a gestational age younger than 32 weeks, 43.2% who developed meningitis had moderate or severe disability compared with none in the control group.

HOW CAN I APPLY THE RESULTS TO PATIENT CARE?

Were the Study Patients and Their Management Similar to Those in My Clinical Setting?

The authors should describe the study patients in enough detail that you can make a comparison with patients in your clinical setting. The patients' characteristics and the way in which they are defined should be described explicitly. One factor rarely reported in prognostic studies that could strongly influence outcome is treatment. Therapeutic strategies often vary markedly among institutions and change over time as new treatments become available or old treatments regain popularity. To the extent that interventions are therapeutic or detrimental, overall patient outcome could improve or become worse.

Was Follow-up Sufficiently Long?

Because the presence of illness often long precedes the development of an outcome, investigators must follow patients long enough to detect the outcomes of interest. For example, recurrence of cancer in some women with early breast cancer can occur many years after initial diagnosis and treatment.[10] A prognostic study may provide an unbiased assessment of outcome over a short period if it meets the validity criteria in Table 7-1, but it may be of little use if a patient is interested in prognosis over a long period.

Can I Use the Results in the Management of Patients in My Clinical Setting?

Knowing the expected clinical course of a patient's condition can help to guide nursing actions. Nurses will be able to answer the questions of patients or family members about the course of the condition and provide either reassurance or counseling, as appropriate. Knowing that a patient is at risk of developing problems such as hearing difficulties or pressure sores, nurses can educate patients about signs and symptoms to look for, monitor patients for these problems, or refer patients for ongoing monitoring and assessment. Knowing that certain patients, such as adolescents, may be at high risk of engaging in behaviors such as smoking or risky sexual activity, nurses can recommend to decision makers in clinical settings that prevention programs be designed, implemented, and evaluated.

CLINICAL RESOLUTION

Our review of the validity criteria suggests that the investigators obtained an unbiased assessment of the risk of disability after meningitis in their cohort study.[1] The 10-month-old infant introduced at the beginning of this chapter resembles those in the cohort study who acquired the infection postneonatally, did not have preexisting conditions, were not premature or of low birth weight, and were infected with *Neisseria meningitidis*. The follow-up period in the study allows us to provide estimates for children 5 years of age.

The study by Bedford and colleagues provides important information about the risk of moderate or severe disability at 5 years of age in children who had meningitis in infancy. However, it fails to provide an adjusted analysis that accounts for the combined influences of age at infection, organism of infection, gestational age, and birth weight, all of which influence the risk of disability. You are therefore faced with the common situation of having to extrapolate from less than ideal data to estimate the patient's prognosis. You can quickly surmise that this child is likely to be at a lower risk than some of the children in the study because she was not infected as a neonate, was infected with *Neisseria meningitidis*, and was a term baby of normal birth weight.

The percentage of children who had meningitis and who developed moderate or severe disability and were of normal birth weight was 9.9%, and the rate for term babies was also 9.9%. Of those children infected with *Neisseria meningitidis*, 9.5% developed moderate or severe disability. You estimate that this child has a 10% risk of developing moderate or severe disability compared with 1.5% in children who have not had meningitis. This is an absolute difference of 8.5%. You tell the parents that there is about a 1 in 12 chance (inverse of the absolute difference) that their baby will develop moderate to severe disabilities that she would not otherwise have had. You encourage the parents to have regular monitoring of the child's development over the next 5 years and to have her hearing and vision checked even if she does not appear to have symptoms.

REFERENCES

1. Bedford H, de Louvois J, Halket S, Peckham C, Hurley R, Harvey D. Meningitis in infancy in England and Wales: follow up at age 5 years. *BMJ*. 2001;323:533-536.
2. Berlowitz DR, Ash AS, Brandeis GH, Brand HK, Halpern JL, Moskowitz MA. Rating long-term care facilities on pressure ulcer development: importance of case-mix adjustment. *Ann Intern Med*. 1996;124: 557-563.
3. Ellenberg JH, Nelson KB. Sample selection and the natural history of disease: studies of febrile seizures. *JAMA*. 1980;243:1337-1340.
4. Kriel RL, Krach LE, Jones-Saete C. Outcome of children with prolonged unconsciousness and vegetative states. *Pediatr Neurol*. 1993;9:362-368.
5. Pincus T, Brooks RH, Callahan LF. Prediction of long-term mortality in patients with rheumatoid arthritis according to simple questionnaire and joint count measures. *Ann Intern Med*. 1994;120:26-34.
6. Dawber TR, Kannell WB, Lyell LP. An approach to longitudinal studies in a community: the Framingham study. *Ann NY Acad Sci*. 1963;107:539.
7. Sims AC. Importance of high tracing-rate in long-term medical follow up studies. *Lancet*. 1973;2:433.
8. Walsh JS, Welch G, Larson EB. Survival of outpatients with Alzheimer-type dementia. *Ann Intern Med*. 1990;113:429-434.
9. Wood LA, Coupland RW, North SA, Palmer MC. Outcome of advanced stage low grade follicular lymphomas in a population-based retrospective cohort. *Cancer*. 1999;85:1361-1368.
10. Early Breast Cancer Trialists' Collaborative Group. Systemic treatment of early breast cancer by hormonal, cytotoxic, or immune therapy: 133 randomised trials involving 31,000 recurrences and 24,000 deaths among 75,000 women. *Lancet*. 1992;339:1-15.

8

Qualitative Research

Cynthia Russell, David Gregory, Jenny Ploeg, Alba DiCenso,
and Gordon Guyatt

The following Editorial Board members also made substantive contributions to this chapter: Marlene Cohen, Mark Newman, and Ania Willman.

We gratefully acknowledge the work of Mita Giacomini and Deborah Cook on the original chapter that appears in the Users' Guides to the Medical Literature, *edited by Guyatt and Rennie.*

In This Chapter

Finding the Evidence

Are the Results Valid?
  Was the Research Question Clear and Adequately Substantiated?
  Was the Design Appropriate for the Research Question?
  Was the Sampling Appropriate for the Research Question and Design?
  Were Data Collected and Managed Systematically?
  Were Data Analyzed Appropriately?

What Are the Results?
  Was the Description of Results Thorough?

How Can I Apply the Results to Patient Care?
  What Meaning and Relevance Does the Study Have for My Patient Care?
  Does the Study Help Me Understand the Context of My Patient Care?
  Does the Study Enhance My Knowledge About My Patient Care?

How Do Older Adults With Early-Stage Dementia Learn to Live With Their Memory Loss?

You are a primary care nurse practitioner who is seeing an elderly couple. The 75-year-old man is in for his flu shot, and his 70-year-old wife has recently been diagnosed with Alzheimer's disease. He is quite worried about his wife's recent diagnosis. His wife is also concerned and talks openly about her memory loss. She explains that she has always prided herself on her excellent memory but now finds herself not being able to remember things and having to ask her husband for help in answering questions. Her husband reports that he has noticed a big change in her memory. She repeats herself often and becomes frustrated when she cannot remember. During your visit with them, the woman turns to her husband for help in answering questions such as "What year did I have that fall?" She worries about becoming a burden to her husband. Her husband remarks that they have no choice but to learn to live with this. As they leave, you ask yourself: "How does one learn to live with memory loss?"

FINDING THE EVIDENCE

In your office, you access the Web site for the journal, *Evidence-Based Nursing,* which allows you to search for methodologically filtered studies that have appeared in the literature. You search *www.evidencebasednursing.com* with the word "dementia" and find 27 items. Most do not appear relevant. You then limit your search to the words "early dementia" and find one item, a *grounded theory* study that explores the process of learning to live with early-stage dementia.[1] You review the abstract and commentary and decide that because the study appears to address the question you are interested in answering, you will order the full text article from the library.[2]

Quantitative and qualitative modes of inquiry are complementary paths to building knowledge in a discipline. *Quantitative designs* are used for such studies as evaluating the effectiveness and safety of nursing interventions, the accuracy and precision of nursing assessment measures or diagnostic tests, the power of prognostic markers, the strength of causal relationships, and the cost-effectiveness of nursing interventions. *Qualitative designs* are well-suited for understanding the illness experience. Nurses may engage in research-based treatment of a patient's health problem but find that the patient's condition does not improve. The ways in which patients manage their lives, health problems, and dying are based on the meanings they accord to their illnesses and life circumstances. Quantitative research does not address questions of meaning and individual interpretations in the same manner that qualitative research does. Such questions are appropriately addressed using qualitative research methods.

Qualitative and quantitative research methods make different contributions to knowledge. Each method may be used *solely* in an ongoing program of research; for example, researchers use either qualitative or quantitative methods to explore phenomena of interest more completely. They may also be used *sequentially,* with a qualitative study following a quantitative study or vice versa, and in this additive fashion, the two methods contribute to knowledge about a phenomenon. In sequential use, the results of studies are used to inform subsequent studies, or they can be used sequentially within a single study. For example, Friedemann and Smith[3] tested a screening tool for family effectiveness by asking 30 participants to complete the questionnaire, explain their thought process for their responses to each question, and participate in semistructured interviews about their perceptions of family stability and growth patterns. Qualitative and quantitative methods can be used *simultaneously* in research studies. Russell and colleagues[4] combined ethnographic and epidemiologic methods to arrive at a comprehensive, holistic description of the health of a community and its residents. Finally, some researchers build their programs of research on a *mixture* of qualitative and quantitative methods, engaging in a back-and-forth interplay between the methods in an attempt to enlarge and expand the understanding of the phenomenon of interest. A program of research that illustrates these connections is that of Beck,[5] who used qualitative and quantitative approaches to explore maternal-child health issues.

Many authors have proposed criteria for appraising qualitative research.[6-18] There are some who question the appraisal process because of the lack of consensus among qualitative researchers on quality criteria.[12,13,15,17] We encourage readers interested in these debates to review these references. Despite this controversy, and recognizing that criteria will continue to evolve, we provide a set of guides to help nurses identify methodologically sound qualitative research that can inform their practice.

Our standard approach to using an article from the health care literature is readily applicable (Table 8-1). We ask the following questions: Are the results of this study valid? What are the results? How do the results apply to patient care?

ARE THE RESULTS VALID?

Qualitative researchers do not speak about validity in the same terms as quantitative researchers. In keeping with the worldviews and paradigms from which qualitative research arises, *validity,* or the extent to which the research reflects the best standards of

Table 8-1 Users' Guides for an Article Reporting Qualitative Research in Health Care

Are the Results Valid?
- Was the research question clear and adequately substantiated?
- Was the design appropriate for the research question?
- Was the sampling appropriate for the research question and design?
- Were data collected and managed systematically?
- Were data analyzed appropriately?

What Are the Results?
- Was the description of results thorough?

How Can I Apply the Results to Patient Care?
- What meaning and relevance does the study have for my patient care?
- Does the study help me understand the context of my patient care?
- Does the study enhance my knowledge about my patient care?

qualitative science, is described in terms of rigor, credibility, trustworthiness, and believability. Numerous articles and books focus on validity issues for qualitative research.[19-26] There are several qualitative research designs, and each has somewhat different conventions for appropriate conduct. This chapter is intended to provide a general approach to the critical appraisal of qualitative research; however, as with various quantitative research designs, the criteria for assessing rigor and validity vary somewhat depending on the specific study design.

Was the Research Question Clear and Adequately Substantiated?

Before proceeding with a full-fledged review of the study, readers should look for the precise question the study sought to answer and consider its relevance to their own clinical question. In addition, readers should review the article for clear documentation describing what is known about the phenomenon of interest.

Was the Design Appropriate for the Research Question?

Some sources list 40 or more unique approaches to qualitative research methods.[27] We describe three common approaches in published health care research including ethnography, grounded theory, and phenomenology. Other approaches that you may encounter include case studies, narrative research, and historical research. Patton[24] and Munhall[23] offer a description of several different qualitative research approaches. The goal of traditional *ethnography* is to learn about culture from the people who actually live in that culture.[28] Culture is present in societies, communities, organizations, spatial locations, or social worlds.[29] Kleinmen[30] suggested the need for clinical, or focused, ethnographies, in which the lives of patients and clinicians intersect. Although they are in keeping with the general intent of traditional ethnography, clinical ethnographies are more narrowly delimited and focus on health and illness experiences. Data collection approaches include participant observation, in-depth interviews, and fieldwork. We refer readers elsewhere for further information about ethnographic approaches.[28,29,31]

An ethnographic approach was used to answer the following research question: "What are the experiences of African-American youths who have at least one family member afflicted with human immunodeficiency virus (HIV) infection or acquired immunodeficiency syndrome and who deliberately seek exposure to HIV?"[32] Stories of six young people were developed through an extensive 4-year period of in-depth fieldwork that included telephone and in-person interviews and participant observation. The stories powerfully illustrate how the culture in which the youths had to survive was so alienating that they deliberately sought exposure to HIV. The ethnographic approach was uniquely suited to bring attention to the important influence of marginalization, insensitive social policies, and demanding caretaking responsibilities on the lives of these youths.

The purpose of a *grounded theory* approach to qualitative research is to discover the social-psychological processes inherent in a phenomenon.[33] Glaser and Strauss developed the grounded theory approach in the 1960s, and it is based on the theoretical perspective of *symbolic interactionism*.[34,35] One of the premises of symbolic interactionism is that we, as human beings, assign meaning to the people and objects with which we interact, and this assigned meaning is influenced by and influences our subsequent interactions. Distinct features of grounded theory include theoretical sampling and the constant comparative method. *Theoretical sampling* refers to sampling decisions made throughout the entire research process in which data sources (which could be individuals or documents or settings) are selected based on emerging study findings. The *constant comparative method* refers to the researcher's ongoing incorporation of the products of data analysis (e.g., incidents, categories, and constructs) in subsequent decisions about theoretical sampling. The ultimate goal of a grounded theory study is to develop a theory that is grounded in the data of the study and accounts for behavioral variation. Both observation and interviews are commonly used for data collection. We refer readers to classic references that describe grounded theory research in detail.[33-36]

Grounded theory was used to answer the following research question: "What is the process of reimaging after an alteration in body appearance or function?"[37] The theoretical sample consisted of 28 participants who had experienced body image disruptions, such as significant weight change, amputation or paralysis of body parts, or scars from burns, surgery, or trauma. Participants were interviewed 3, 6, 12, and 18 months after the physical alteration. The constant comparative method of concurrent data collection and analysis was used to develop a three-phase theory of the process of reimaging: (1) body image disruption, (2) wishing for restoration, and (3) reimaging the self. The grounded theory approach was ideally suited to discovering the social-psychological process of reimaging.

The aim of a *phenomenologic* approach to qualitative research is to gain a deeper understanding of the nature or meaning of the everyday "lived" experiences of people.[38] The origins of phenomenology are in philosophy, particularly the works of Husserl, Heidegger, and Merleau-Ponty. Because the primary sources of data are the perspectives and life worlds of the persons studied, in-depth interviews are the most common means of data collection. We refer readers elsewhere for details about phenomenologic research.[38,39]

Phenomenology was used to answer the following research question: "What is the lived experience of adults who are integrating a hearing loss into their lives?"[40] The *convenience sample* consisted of 32 adults with mild to profound degrees of hearing loss. Data were collected through semistructured, audiotaped interviews with participants. Analysis involved identification of core and major themes in the data and validation of the findings with selected participants. The core theme of "dancing with" eloquently captured the participants' perceptions of moving, gracefully or awkwardly, with the changes required by hearing loss, never sure of the next steps. The major themes of dancing with—loss and fear, fluctuating feelings, courage amid change, and an altered life perspective—provide a rich description of the participants' perceptions of what it was like to live with hearing loss. The phenomenologic approach was key to uncovering participants' meanings of the complex and dynamic process of integrating hearing loss into their lives.

Qualitative approaches arise from specific disciplines and are influenced by particular theoretical perspectives within those disciplines. A critical analysis of a research study considers the "fit" of the research question with the qualitative method used in the study.[41] Although the specific criteria for proper application of each methodological approach vary somewhat, similarities among the approaches are sufficient to discuss them as a whole.

Was the Sampling Appropriate for the Research Question and Design?

The emergent nature of qualitative research that results from the interaction between data collection and data analysis requires that investigators not prespecify a sample for data collection in strict terms, lest important data sources be overlooked. Whereas in quantitative studies, the ideal sampling standard is random sampling, most qualitative studies use *purposeful sampling*, a conscious selection of a small number of data sources meeting particular criteria. The logic and power of purposeful sampling lie in selecting information-rich cases (participants or settings) for in-depth study to illuminate the questions of interest.[24] This type of sampling usually aims to address a range of potentially relevant social phenomena and perspectives from an appropriate array of data sources. Selection criteria often evolve over the course of analysis, and investigators return repeatedly to the data to explore new cases or new perspectives.

Readers of qualitative studies should look for sound reasoning describing and justifying the selection strategies for data sources. Patton[24] offers a succinct, clear, and comprehensive discussion of the various sampling strategies used in qualitative research. Convenience sampling is one of the most commonly used, but one of the least appropriate, sampling strategies. Participants are primarily selected in terms of ease of access to the researcher and, secondarily, for their knowledge of the relevant subject matter. Purposive nonprobability sampling strategies include the following:

1. *Judgmental sampling,* in which theory or knowledge points the researcher to select specific cases: maximum variation sampling, to document range or diversity; extreme or deviant case sampling, in which one selects cases that are unusual or special in some way; typical or representative case sampling, to describe and illustrate what is typical and common in terms of the phenomenon of interest; critical sampling, to make a point dramatically; and criterion sampling, in which all cases that meet some predetermined criteria of importance are studied (this sampling strategy is commonly used in quality assurance).
2. *Opportunistic sampling,* in which availability of participants guides on-the-spot sampling decisions.
3. *Snowball, network,* or *chain sampling,* in which people nominate others for participation.
4. *Theory-based operational construct sampling,* in which incidents, time periods, people, or other data sources are sampled on the basis of their potential manifestation or representation of important theoretical constructs. Participant observation studies typically make use of opportunistic sampling strategies, whereas grounded theory studies make use of theory-based operational construct sampling.

Sample size is a critical question for all research studies. A study with a sample size that is too small may have such unique and particular findings that its qualitative transferability or quantitative generalizability is called into question. Qualitatively, however, even studies with small samples may help to identify theoretically provocative ideas that merit further exploration. Studies with sample sizes that are too large can be equally problematic. Sample size influences the trade-off between breadth and depth. Studies with smaller samples can explore a broader range of participants' experiences more fully, whereas studies with larger samples typically focus on a narrower range of experiences. Qualitative researchers judge the adequacy of the sample by how comprehensively and completely the research questions were answered. Readers of qualitative studies should review the researcher's documentation of sample size and selection throughout the course of the research.

Were Data Collected and Managed Systematically?

Qualitative researchers commonly use one or more of three basic strategies for collecting data (Figure 8-1). One strategy, *field observation*, involves witnessing events and recording them as they occur. Another strategy, *interviews*, involves questioning participants

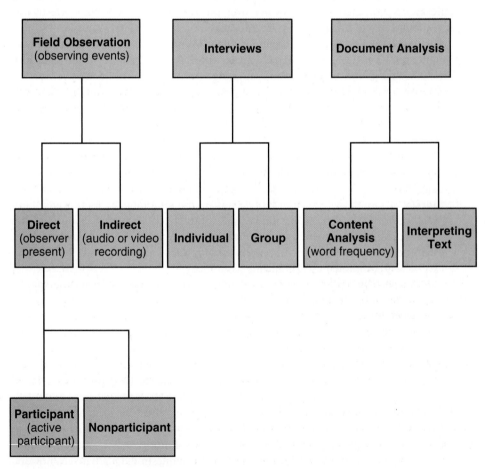

Figure 8-1. Sources of information in qualitative research.

directly about their experience. A third strategy, *document analysis*, involves reviewing written material. Readers should consider which data collection strategies researchers have used and whether those used would be expected to offer the most complete and accurate understanding of the phenomenon of interest.

Field Observation

The purpose of field observation is to observe the unfolding of social phenomena directly and prospectively. Researchers using field observations may enact different roles, ranging from full participation in a setting to that of a true observer. Researchers affect the social setting that they are observing, but these effects may be mitigated by the number of other people in that setting. For example, a researcher in a crowded waiting room may go unnoticed and hence will be able to observe the natural unfolding of events. By contrast, in a clinic examining room a researcher may be conspicuous and may significantly change the social interactions being observed. Field observations are most often recorded using written or audiotaped field notes, but some researchers use video cameras to record activities in the field.

Participant observation can open up settings that would normally be closed to a certain vantage point and can thus allow researchers to approximate the experience of informants. As a participant, the researcher sees things, cognitively, that may not otherwise be seen, leading to opportunities to understand the research topic in a different way. Participation in a setting increases the prospect that the researcher will feel the moral propriety and obligations of the setting. When researchers participate, they are witnessing a scene unfold in a manner that would not be possible given a controlled and contrived setting. Finally, participation helps researchers to see more clearly how people get things done. The causal question of "why?" so often preoccupies researchers that the practical, technical, and tacit question of "how?" is forgotten. Participation promotes a focus on the *how*, the skills necessary to be an actor in the setting, the *dynamic processes* in settings that affect the ongoing flow of activity and changes over time.

Interviews

Another data collection strategy commonly used in qualitative research is the interview. Standardized questionnaires are usually inappropriate for qualitative research because they presuppose too much of what respondents may say and do not allow respondents to relate experiences in their own terms. These problems limit opportunities to gain insight into personal and social phenomena. In addition, they can impose the researchers' preconceived notions on the data.

Qualitative interviews range from structured and controlled to unstructured and informal. The determination of an appropriate type of interview depends on the research interest, the circumstances of the setting or people to be studied, and the practical limitations of the researcher. Similarly, the types of questions used in interviews range from nondirective to probing and even confrontational. The use of a given type of question also depends on the specific purpose of the study. In grounded theory studies, for example, questions during the initial interviews are generally broad as the researcher attempts to elicit information about the dimensions of the phenomenon of interest. During later interviews, however, the researcher typically narrows the focus of questions and tests the developing theory with interviewees.

The most popular types of interviews are semistructured in-depth individual interviews and focus groups. The selection of a particular type of interview depends on the topic. Individual interviews tend to be more useful than focus group interviews for evoking personal experiences and perspectives, particularly on sensitive topics. Focus group interviews tend to be more useful than individual interviews for capturing interpersonal dynamics. They can be appropriate for discussing emotionally sensitive topics if participants feel empowered while speaking in the presence of peers; however, the public forum of a focus group can also inhibit candid disclosure.[42-45]

Interviews are often audiotaped and may be conducted on a one-time basis, repeated over time, face to face, over the telephone, or by computer. Various strategies enhance interviews, including setting the climate, listening analytically, probing thoughtfully, motivating the interviewee, and directing the interview.

Critical readers should look for the rationale for choosing a particular interview approach and should assess its appropriateness for the topics addressed. Using more than one type of interview may be helpful in capturing a wide range of information.

Document Analysis

Finally, documents such as medical charts, journals, correspondence, and other material artifacts can provide qualitative data.[46] These are especially useful in policy, historic, or organizational studies of health care. There are different approaches to the analysis of documents. One involves counting specific content elements (e.g., frequencies of particular words), whereas another involves interpreting text as one would interpret any other form of communication (e.g., seeking nuances of meaning and considering context). The former approach, especially if used alone, rarely provides adequate information for a qualitative, interpretive analysis.

Regardless of the choice of data collection strategy, the approach to data collection must be comprehensive to avoid focusing on particular, potentially misleading aspects of the data. Several aspects of a qualitative report indicate how extensively the investigators collected data: the number of observations, interviews, or documents; the duration of the observations; the duration of the study period; the diversity of units of analysis and data collection techniques; the number of investigators involved in collecting and analyzing data; and the degree of investigators' involvement in data collection and analysis.[47-50] Taping and transcribing interviews (or other dialogue) are often desirable but not necessary for all qualitative studies.

Were Data Analyzed Appropriately?

Qualitative researchers often begin with a general exploratory question and preliminary concepts. They then collect relevant data, observe patterns in the data, organize these into a conceptual framework, and resume data collection to explore and challenge their developing conceptualizations. This cycle may be repeated several times. The iterations among data collection and data interpretation continue until the analysis is well developed and further observations yield redundant, minimal, or no new information to challenge or elaborate the conceptual framework or in-depth descriptions of the phenomenon (a point often referred to as *saturation*[51] or *informational redundancy*[52]). This analysis-stopping criterion is so basic to qualitative analysis that authors seldom declare that they have reached this point; they assume readers will understand.

In the course of analysis, key findings may also be corroborated using multiple sources of information, a process called data *triangulation*. Triangulation is a metaphor and does not mean literally that three or more sources are required. The appropriate number of sources will depend on the importance of the findings, their implications for theory, and the investigators' confidence in their validity. Because no two qualitative data sources will generate exactly the same interpretation, much of the art of qualitative interpretation involves exploring why and how different information sources yield slightly different results.[53]

Readers may encounter several useful triangulation techniques for validating qualitative data and their interpretation in analysis.[54,55] *Investigator triangulation* requires more than one investigator to collect and analyze the data, such that the findings emerge through consensus among investigators. This is typically accomplished by an investigative team. Inclusion of team members from different disciplines helps to prevent the personal or disciplinary biases of a single researcher from excessively influencing the findings. *Theory triangulation*[56] is a process whereby emergent findings are examined in relation to existing social science theories.[54] Authors usually report how their qualitative findings relate to prevailing social theories, although some qualitative researchers suggest that such theories should not be used to guide research design or analysis.

Some researchers seek clarification and further explanation of their developing analytic framework from study participants, a step known as *member checking*. Most commonly, researchers specify that member checking is done to inquire whether participants' viewpoints were faithfully interpreted, determine whether there are gross errors of fact, and ascertain whether the account makes sense to participants with different perspectives.

Some qualitative research reports describe the use of qualitative analysis software packages.[57-59] Readers should not equate the use of computers with analytic rigor. Such software is merely a data management tool offering efficient methods for storing, organizing, and retrieving qualitative data. These programs do not perform analysis. The investigators themselves conduct the analysis as they create the key words, categories, and logical relationships used to organize and interpret the electronic data. The soundness of qualitative study findings depends on these investigator judgments, which cannot, as yet, be programmed into software packages.

We indicated earlier that qualitative data collection must be comprehensive, that is, of adequate breadth and depth to yield a meaningful description. The closely related criterion for judging whether the data were analyzed appropriately is whether this comprehensiveness was determined in part by the research findings, with the aims of challenging, elaborating, and corroborating the findings. This is most apparent when researchers state that they alternated between data collection and analysis, collected data with the purpose of elucidating the analysis in progress, collected data until analytic saturation or redundancy was reached, or triangulated findings using any of the methods mentioned.

Using the Guide

The purpose of the study by Werezak and Stewart[2] was to explore and conceptualize the process of learning to live with memory loss in older adults with early-stage dementia. The authors explained that research in this area is not usually based on self-reports of persons with dementia. To update readers on what was known about this topic, they described two preliminary models that conceptualized the experience of persons with dementia, beginning with initial memory loss and ending with terminal disability. Werezak and Stewart[2] explained that although these two models explicate the entire process of dementia from diagnosis to death, their aim was to develop a model that focused exclusively on the early stage of dementia.

The authors appropriately used a grounded theory method to explore how older adults learned to live with memory loss and the behavioral variations in this process. Their question was not appropriate for a phenomenologic study, given that they were not interested in the meaning of living with memory loss; nor was their question appropriate for a traditional ethnographic study, because they were not interested in the culture of persons living with early-stage dementia.

The sample consisted of three men and three women who were diagnosed with early-stage dementia and ranged in age from 61 to 79 years. All participants lived at home with their spouses. The authors described their theoretical sampling as including five participants with Alzheimer's disease and one with vascular dementia and noted that participants were selected on the basis of meeting inclusion criteria and ability to provide data relevant to the development of emerging conceptual categories. The authors did not provide a clear trajectory of how study participants were accrued and selected in relation to the progression of the study. It is not uncommon for authors to describe theoretical sampling in broad terms, given space limitations in journal articles.

The researchers recruited participants from various agencies. Agency personnel distributed letters to potential participants and provided contact information for the study. One of the researchers then contacted potential participants who indicated an interest in the study and arranged a meeting to give them further information. Given the researchers' interest in persons living with early-stage dementia, it was appropriate and necessary to involve community agencies in identifying potential participants, because these persons likely would not have been receiving special care for their dementia. Recruitment from specialized dementia-care providers or other dementia-related agencies would not have offered the researchers access to a sample of persons with early-stage dementia.

The authors ensured that participants had early-stage dementia by using a three-stage screening process. First, community agency personnel provided a clinical assessment of early-stage dementia, which served as a basis for initial interviews. At the conclusion of the first interview, researchers administered two screening instruments to confirm the stage of dementia and cognitive decline of each participant. Two potential participants were excluded at this point because their Modified Mini-Mental State Examination scores fell below the cut-off point considered by the researchers as indicative of early-stage dementia. Third, participants' health care providers were contacted by mail for confirmation of a diagnosis of dementia. It is important that researchers clearly articulate the steps involved in selecting participants who meet the criteria for study inclusion as did Werezak and Stewart.[2] This approach increases one's confidence that the study's results will be applicable to the intended group.

Continued

Werezak and Stewart used semistructured interviews and interviewed each participant twice. Proxies (e.g., family members) could be present during the interviews, but they were informed that the researchers were interested in the perspectives of the person with dementia. Data from the first round of interviews were coded and analyzed, yielding a preliminary theory. The second interviews occurred 1 to 3 months later, to verify and clarify the emerging theory. The researchers noted that the interview process evolved during this second round of interviews, and it became more unstructured and open-ended as the investigators sought clarification about issues that had emerged during the first round of interviews. Research using a grounded theory method typically involves either multiple interviews with participants to clarify and extend the boundaries of the developing theory or the inclusion of purposefully selected additional participants who offer insights into the researchers' conceptualizations.

Interviews were audiotaped, transcribed, and analyzed using the constant comparison method of analysis that is foundational to grounded theory. The researchers used NVivo, a qualitative, computer data management program to facilitate coding of the data. They specifically described using open, axial, and selective coding, reflecting their use of coding procedures specific to grounded theory.

WHAT ARE THE RESULTS?

Was the Description of Results Thorough?

Qualitative researchers are challenged to make sense of massive amounts of data and transform their understanding to a written mode to make this evident to readers. The written report is often a barrier to research utilization because of its lack of clarity and relevance except to a limited audience.[60] Sandelowski[60] described the challenges facing authors as they make decisions in balancing description (the facts of the cases observed) with analysis (the breakdown and recombining of data) and interpretation (the new meanings created from this process).

Holliday[26] offered a comprehensive discussion about the appropriate role of "cautious detachment" in qualitative research. The "truths" of qualitative research are relative to the research setting, and it is important that authors not overstep the interpretive boundaries of their studies in making it seem as though all their questions have been answered with certainty and without raising additional questions. A comparison of the findings and discussion sections of a study is helpful for judging the local context of the study and whether authors are truthful to their data.

Werezak and Stewart[2] described five core categories or stages that evolved over time and formed the basis for "the continuous process of adjusting to early-stage dementia" (p. 72), the theory that emerged from their data. The five categories were antecedents,

Continued

anticipation, appearance, assimilation, and acceptance. Different levels of aware-ness connected the stages. The researchers described these five categories in detail and offered quotes from participants to illustrate their findings. First, *antecedents* were subprocesses that made it difficult to obtain a diagnosis of dementia. Most participants were initially unaware of their memory problems, largely because of the insidious onset of symptoms, which they attributed to benign forgetfulness or work stress. When discussing the onset of memory loss, many participants recalled their previous memory quality, identified family members with and without dementia, and often described confounding health problems that made it difficult for them to identify which disease process was causing their memory loss. Second, in the *anticipation* stage, participants anticipated obtaining a diagnosis and described common reactions of shock and horror. They then began consid-ering future losses. They anticipated losing the ability to care for themselves and worried about "becoming a burden." Participants felt anxious about telling others about their memory loss and wondered how people would respond. Third, in the *appearance* stage, participants slowly became aware that family members, friends, and co-workers were noticing their memory loss. They recounted hurtful situations in which others were insensitive or indifferent to their disease-related experiences. Participants described seeing themselves as the same person despite their memory impairments. Fourth, *assimilation* referred to the cyclic and contin-uous process of fitting dementia into one's life. Participants described assimilating the disease into their inner world (e.g., feelings and thoughts about the disease and physiologic changes) and their outer world (e.g., lifestyle changes related to memory loss and interacting with supportive and unsupportive significant others). Positive-mediating experiences, such as feeling supported by others and retaining abilities that gave life meaning and purpose, facilitated the transition from inner to outer worlds. In response to negative-mediating experiences, such as disease progression and inability to function in social or work situations, par-ticipants withdrew into their inner worlds. Finally, in the *acceptance* stage, all par-ticipants described achieving a degree of acceptance of their dementia that allowed them to focus on enjoying the remainder of their lives. Factors facilitat-ing such acceptance included others' acceptance of the disease, using humor, hope, and altruism.

Werezak and Stewart[2] discussed the study's theoretical, clinical, and research impli-cations and used phrases such as "one of the factors participants saw" (p 80) and "many of the participants in the current study" (p 81) to situate their discussion of other literature on dementia with their unique sample of participants. In a review of the limitations of their study, the investigators identified the homogeneity of their sample (all well-educated, married, financially secure, and retired from work outside the home), the selection of participants (all volunteers), the prior attendance at support groups by two thirds of the sample, and their use of negative case analysis as areas that could influence the transferability of the findings. In addition, the authors noted the tentativeness of their findings and encouraged others to avoid overgeneralization of the study's findings.

HOW CAN I APPLY THE RESULTS TO PATIENT CARE?

What Meaning and Relevance Does the Study Have for My Patient Care?

Thorne[8] pointed out that critiquing qualitative research in health sciences disciplines demands not merely a focus on traditional appraisal criteria, but also an examination of the more complex question of what meaning can be made of the findings. The moral question of how research results might be used in ways not intended and not benefiting health science disciplines and patients is important, given that "health science disciplines exist because of a social mandate that entails a moral obligation toward benefiting individuals and the collective" (p 119).[8] Thorne describes five criteria for appraising the disciplinary relevance and usefulness of a study:

1. Moral defensibility: are there convincing claims about why this knowledge is needed?
2. Disciplinary relevance: is the knowledge appropriate to the development of the discipline?
3. Pragmatic obligation: does the study produce usable knowledge?
4. Contextual awareness: is the study situated in a historical context and within a disciplinary perspective?
5. Probable truth: is there evidence of ambiguity and creation of meaning?

In relation to the five appraisal criteria, Werezak and Stewart[2] clearly illustrated the limited attention that has been paid to the perspective of persons with early-stage dementia (moral defensibility). The disciplinary relevance is described in terms of the small body of literature that suggests that the views of persons with dementia may be different from those of their caregivers and, thus, the understanding of this disease obtained solely from caregivers may be incomplete or inaccurate. Werezak and Stewart[2] discussed the clinical implications of their study, thereby attending to the pragmatic obligation of qualitative research. They offered a nursing perspective of the proposed framework that helps readers to see the immediate relevance and long-term applicability of the findings (contextual awareness). Finally, the probable truth criterion was noted in their clear description of the factors that might influence the transferability of the study's findings.

Does the Study Help Me Understand the Context of My Patient Care?

The context in which the research is conducted influences the results of all research, but it is particularly important in qualitative research. In qualitative research, readers determine the potential applicability of a study's findings to their contexts. Inadequate reporting of the social and historical contexts of a study makes it difficult for readers to determine whether a study's findings can be "transferred" with any legitimacy to their situation.

Werezak and Stewart[2] provided an adequate description of the context and setting. They clearly acknowledged the factors that could influence the transferability of their findings, including the homogeneous sample, the fact that participants volunteered for the study, and participants' attendance at support groups.

Does the Study Enhance My Knowledge About My Patient Care?

One criterion for the generalizability of a qualitative study is whether it provides a useful map for readers to understand and navigate in similar social settings. Werezak and Stewart[2] described a theoretical framework of the process of learning to live with early-stage dementia. The small, homogeneous sample of financially secure, married, community-residing older adults with Alzheimer's disease or vascular dementia who lived in Canada was selected based on the ability to provide data relevant to the development of the emerging grounded theory. Readers would need to consider the similarity of their own patients and settings to those in this study.

CLINICAL RESOLUTION

Reflecting on the study by Werezak and Stewart,[2] you think back to the couple you saw earlier this week. The woman is similar to the study participants in terms of age, education and marital, socioeconomic, and employment status. You recall the emotional strain they both showed as they spoke about their reactions to the diagnosis of Alzheimer's disease and concerns about what lay ahead for them. Their escalating anxiety and uncertainty were consistent with the anticipation stage that Werezak and Stewart[2] described. You begin to consider how you could help them. You decide to arrange a home visit, thinking that visiting them in their own home may minimize further emotional distress and provide opportunities for more detailed assessment. Before you make the visit, you plan to investigate whether there is a community support group for the woman, who may appreciate the opportunity to talk with other people with dementia. You also plan to talk with her husband to determine his needs for information and support.

REFERENCES

1. Hall S. Learning to live with early-stage dementia involved a continuous process of adjustment that comprised 5 stages [abstract]. *Evid Based Nurs.* 2003;6:64. Taken from: *Can J Nurs Res.* 2002;34:67-85.
2. Werezak L, Stewart N. Learning to live with early dementia. *Can J Nurs Res.* 2002;34:67-85.
3. Friedemann ML, Smith AA. A triangulation approach to testing a family instrument. *West J Nurs Res.* 1997;19:364-378.
4. Russell CK, Gregory DM, Wotton D, Mordoch E, Counts MM. ACTION: application and extension of the GENESIS community analysis model. *Public Health Nurs.* 1996;13:187-194.
5. Beck CT. Developing a research program using qualitative and quantitative approaches. *Nurs Outlook.* 1997;45:265-269.
6. Giacomini MK, Cook DJ. Users' guides to the medical literature: XXIII. Qualitative research in health care A. Are the results of the study valid? Evidence-Based Medicine Working Group. *JAMA.* 2000;284:357-362.
7. Giacomini MK, Cook DJ. Users guides to the medical literature: XXIII. Qualitative research in health care B. What are the results and how do they help me care for my patients? Evidence-Based Medicine Working Group. *JAMA.* 2000;284:478-482.
8. Thorne S. The art (and science) of critiquing qualitative research. In: Morse JM, ed. *Completing a Qualitative Project: Details and Dialogue.* Thousand Oaks, CA: Sage Publications; 1997:117-132.
9. Hoddinott P, Pill R. A review of recently published qualitative research in general practice: more methodological questions than answers? *Fam Pract.* 1997;14:313-319.

10. Mays N, Pope C. Qualitative research in health care: assessing quality in qualitative research. *BMJ.* 2000;320:50-52.

11. Mays N, Pope C. Rigour and qualitative research. *BMJ.* 1995;311:109-112.

12. Sandelowski M, Barosso J. Reading qualitative studies. *Int J Qualitative Methods* [serial online]. 2002;1:Article 5. Available at http://www.ualberta.ca/~ijqm/. Accessed July 7, 2002.

13. Morse JM, Barrett M, Mayan M, Olson K, Spiers J. Verification strategies for establishing reliability and validity in qualitative research. *Int J Qualitative Methods* [serial online]. 2002;1:Article 2. Available at http://www.ualberta.ca/~ijqm/. Accessed July 7, 2002.

14. Knafl KA, Howard MJ. Interpreting and reporting qualitative research. *Res Nurs Health.* 1984;7:17-24.

15. Barbour RS. Checklists for improving rigour in qualitative research: a case of the tail wagging the dog? *BMJ.* 2001;322:1115-1117.

16. Forchuk C, Roberts J. How to critique qualitative research articles. *Can J Nurs Res.* 1993;25:47-55.

17. Chapple A, Rogers A. Explicit guidelines for qualitative research: a step in the right direction, a defence of the "soft" option, or a form of sociological imperialism? *Fam Pract.* 1998;15:556-561.

18. Elder NC, Miller WL. Reading and evaluating qualitative research studies. *J Fam Pract.* 1995;41:279-285.

19. Streubert Speziale HJ, Rinaldi Carpenter D. *Qualitative Nursing Research: Advancing the Humanistic Perspective.* Philadelphia, PA: Lippincott Williams & Wilkins; 2002.

20. Denzin NK, Lincoln YS, eds. *Handbook of Qualitative Research.* 2nd ed. Thousand Oaks, CA: Sage Publications; 2000.

21. Grbich C. *Qualitative Research in Health: An Introduction.* St. Leonards, Australia: Allen & Unwin Publishers; 1999.

22. Lincoln YS, Guba E. *Naturalistic Inquiry.* Beverly Hills, CA: Sage Publications; 1985.

23. Munhall PL. *Nursing Research: A Qualitative Perspective.* 3rd ed. Boston, MA: Jones & Bartlett Publishers; 2001.

24. Patton MQ. *Qualitative Research and Evaluation Methods.* 3rd ed. Newbury Park, CA: Sage Publications; 2002.

25. Taylor SJ, Bogdan R. *Introduction to Qualitative Research Methods: A Guidebook and Resource.* 3rd ed. New York: John Wiley & Sons; 1998.

26. Holliday A. *Doing and Writing Qualitative Research.* Thousand Oaks, CA: Sage Publications; 2002.

27. Tesch R. *Qualitative Research: Analysis Types and Software Tools.* Bristol, PA: Falmer Press; 1990.

28. Atkinson P, Coffey A, Delamont S, Lofland J, Lofland L, eds. *Handbook of Ethnography.* London, UK: Sage Publications; 2001.

29. Bernard HR, ed. *Handbook of Methods in Cultural Anthropology.* Walnut Creek, CA: AltaMira Press; 1998.

30. Kleinman A. Local worlds of suffering: an interpersonal focus for ethnographies of illness experience. *Qual Health Res.* 1992;2:127-134.

31. LeCompte MD, Schensul JJ. *Ethnographers' Toolkit.* Walnut Creek, CA: AltaMira Press; 1999.

32. Tourigny SC. Some new dying trick: African American youths "choosing" HIV/AIDS. *Qual Health Res.* 1998;8:149-167.

33. Strauss A, Corbin J. *Basics of Qualitative Research: Grounded Theory Procedures and Techniques.* Newbury Park, CA: Sage Publications; 1990.

34. Glaser BG, Strauss AL. *Discovery of Grounded Theory: Strategies for Qualitative Research.* Chicago, IL: Aldine; 1967.

35. Chenitz WC, Swanson JM. *From Practice to Grounded Theory: Qualitative Research in Nursing.* Menlo Park, CA: Addison-Wesley; 1986.

36. Glaser BG. *Theoretical Sensitivity: Advances in the Methodology of Grounded Theory.* Mill Valley, CA: Sociology Press; 1978.

37. Norris J, Kunes-Connell M, Spelic SS. A grounded theory of reimaging. *ANS Adv Nurs Sci.* 1998;20:1-12.

38. Van Manen M. *Researching Lived Experience: Human Science for an Action Sensitive Pedagogy.* London, Ont, Canada: Althouse Press; 1990.

39. Cohen MZ, Kahn DL, Steeves RH. *Hermeneutic Phenomenological Research: A Practical Guide for Nurse Researchers.* Thousand Oaks, CA: Sage Publications; 2000.

40. Herth K. Integrating hearing loss into one's life. *Qual Health Res.* 1998;8:207-223.

41. Crotty M. *The Foundations of Social Research: Meaning and Perspective in the Research Process.* St. Leonards, Australia: Allen & Unwin Publishers, 1998.

42. Kitzinger J. Qualitative research: introducing focus groups. *BMJ.* 1995;311:299-302.

43. Steward DW, Shamdasani PN. Group dynamics and focus group research. In: *Focus Groups: Theory and Practice.* London, UK: Sage Publications; 1990:33-50.

44. Krueger RA. *Focus Groups: A Practical Guide for Applied Research.* 2nd ed. Thousand Oaks, CA: Sage Publications; 1994.

45. Kidd PS, Parshall MB. Getting the focus and the group: enhancing analytical rigor in focus group research. *Qual Health Res.* 2000; 293-308.

46. Hodder I. The interpretation of documents and material culture. In: Denzin N, Lincoln Y, eds. *Handbook of Qualitative Research.* London, UK: Sage Publications; 1994:393-402.

47. Kirk J, Miller ML. *Reliability and Validity in Qualitative Research.* London, UK: Sage Publications; 1986.

48. Schatzman L, Strauss AL. Strategy for recording. In: *Field Research: Strategies for a Natural Sociology.* Englewood Cliffs, NJ: Prentice-Hall; 1973:94-107.

49. Lincoln YS, Guba EG. Implementing the naturalistic inquiry. In: *Naturalistic Inquiry.* London, UK: Sage Publications; 1985:250-288.

50. Patton MQ. Fieldwork strategies and observation methods. In: *Qualitative Research and Evaluation Methods.* 3rd ed. London, UK: Sage Publications; 2002:199-276.

51. Glaser B, Strauss AL. The constant comparative methods of qualitative analysis. In: *Discovery of Grounded Theory.* New York, NY: Aldine de Gruyter; 1967:101-116.

52. Lincoln YS, Guba EG. Designing a naturalistic inquiry. In: *Naturalistic Inquiry.* London, UK: Sage Publications; 1985:221-249.

53. Stake R. Triangulation. In: *The Art of Case Study Research.* London, UK: Sage Publications; 1995:107-120.

54. Lincoln YS, Guba EG. Establishing trustworthiness. In: *Naturalistic Inquiry.* London, UK: Sage Publications; 1985:289-331.

55. Patton MQ. Enhancing the quality and credibility of qualitative analysis. In: *Qualitative Research and Evaluation Methods.* 3rd ed. London, UK: Sage Publications; 2002:460-506.

56. Denzin NK. *Sociological Methods.* New York, NY: McGraw-Hill; 1978.

57. Russell CK, Gregory DM. Issues for consideration when choosing a qualitative data management system. *J Adv Nurs.* 1993;18:1806-1816.

58. Richards L, Richards T. Computing in qualitative analysis: a healthy development? *Qualitative Health Res.* 1991;1:234-262.

59. Weitzman EA. Software and qualitative research. In: Denzin NK, Lincoln YS, eds. *Handbook of Qualitative Research.* 2nd ed. London, UK: Sage Publications; 2000; 803-820.

60. Sandelowski M. Writing a good read: strategies for re-presenting qualitative data. *Res Nurs Health.* 1998;21:375-382.

9

Summarizing the Evidence Through Systematic Reviews

Donna Ciliska, Alba DiCenso, and Gordon Guyatt

The following Editorial Board members also made substantive contributions to this chapter: Carole Estabrooks, Sarah Hayward, Andrew Jull, Susan Marks, and Janet Pinelli.

We gratefully acknowledge the work of Andrew Oxman, Deborah Cook, and Victor Montori on the original chapter that appears in the Users' Guides to the Medical Literature, *edited by Guyatt and Rennie.*

In This Chapter

Finding the Evidence

What is a Systematic Review?

Are the Results Valid?
Did the Review Explicitly Address a Sensible Clinical Question?
Was the Search for Relevant Studies Detailed and Exhaustive?
Were the Primary Studies of High Methodological Quality?
Were Assessments of Studies Reproducible?

What Are the Results?
Were the Results Similar From Study to Study?
What Were the Overall Results of the Review?
How Precise Were the Results?

How Can I Apply the Results to Patient Care?
How Can I Best Interpret the Results to Apply Them to Patient Care?
Were All Patient-Important Outcomes Considered?
Are the Benefits Worth the Costs and Potential Risks?

CLINICAL SCENARIO

Should Women With Stress Incontinence Be Taught Pelvic-Floor Muscle Exercises?

You are a nurse working in a primary care clinic. Several times per week you meet women who have symptoms of stress urinary incontinence. You think there may be some benefit in teaching pelvic-floor exercises to help alleviate these symptoms, but some of your colleagues disagree. The clinic has no policy on the topic. During a clinical staff meeting, you ask whether anyone is interested in developing a clinic policy on interventions for stress urinary incontinence. Two colleagues offer to help you. At the first meeting, you decide to begin by looking for a recent systematic review. You know that systematic reviews are a good place to start because they summarize existing relevant research.

FINDING THE EVIDENCE

Having recently read an article showing that Cochrane reviews are higher in quality than systematic reviews published in journals,[1] you begin by looking in the *Cochrane Library.* You enter the terms "incontinence" and "muscle training," locate a relevant review by Hay-Smith and colleagues in the Cochrane Database of Systematic Reviews, and find that the latest update was in November 2000.[2]

WHAT IS A SYSTEMATIC REVIEW?

Basing clinical decisions on a single research study can be a mistake. Individual studies may have inadequate sample sizes to detect patient-important differences[3] between comparison groups (leading to false-negative results); the results of apparently similar studies may vary because of chance; and subtle differences in the design of studies and the participants may lead to different or even discrepant findings. Whenever possible, nurses should base their clinical decisions on a recent, high-quality systematic review. A *systematic review* is a rigorous summary of all the research evidence that relates to a specific question, be it a question about harm, diagnosis, prognosis, or the effectiveness of health care interventions.

How does a systematic review differ from a traditional literature review? Traditional literature reviews, commonly found in journals and textbooks, typically provide an overview of a disease or condition. Such overviews may provide a discussion of one or more aspects of a particular health issue, including causation, diagnosis, prognosis, and nursing management, and may address various clinical, background, and theoretical questions. For example, a review article or a chapter from a textbook on asthma may include sections on causation, assessment, and prognosis and may examine many different options for the prevention and management of asthma. Typically, authors of traditional reviews make little or no attempt to be systematic in the formulation of questions, the search for relevant evidence, or the summary of the evidence. Nursing students and practicing nurses looking for background information often find these reviews useful for obtaining a broad picture of a clinical condition or area of inquiry (see Chapter 2, Finding the Evidence). Unfortunately, authors of traditional reviews often make conflicting practice recommendations, and their advice frequently lags behind or is inconsistent with the best available evidence.[4] One important reason for this phenomenon is the use of unsystematic approaches to collect and summarize evidence. Indeed, a study by Oxman and Guyatt showed that self-rated expertise was inversely related to the methodological rigor of a review; that is, as the author's rating of his or her own expertise increased, the rigor of the review methods decreased.[5]

Systematic reviews differ from unsystematic reviews in that they attempt to overcome possible biases at all stages by following a rigorous methodology. Investigators must make several decisions when preparing a systematic review: formulating the question; identifying, selecting, and critically appraising relevant studies; abstracting and synthesizing (either quantitatively or nonquantitatively) relevant study findings; and drawing conclusions. Table 9-1 outlines the general process for conducting a systematic review. In the first step, the question is formulated through the specification of the population, intervention or exposure, and outcomes of interest (see Chapter 2, Finding the Evidence). Once the question is formulated, the next step is to specify the minimum methodological standards that studies must meet to be included in the review. Next, any restrictions for study inclusion are specified. These restrictions include language (e.g., studies reported in English only), time frame (e.g., studies conducted since 1980), and publication status (e.g., only published studies). For example, a systematic review of sex education may specify the population as adolescents, the intervention as sex education, the outcome as avoidance of adolescent pregnancy, the minimum methodological standard as randomized controlled trials (RCTs), the language as studies reported in any language, the time frame as studies published since 1970, and the publication status as published and unpublished studies. These selection criteria inform the search strategy.

The next step involves a comprehensive search of multiple sources to identify all relevant studies. This process usually yields large numbers of potentially relevant titles and abstracts. Through application of the selection criteria to the titles and abstracts of study reports, the review team identifies a smaller number of relevant articles for retrieval. The selection criteria are then applied to the complete study reports. After the selection process is completed, the team evaluates each relevant study for methodological quality and abstracts the data. Finally, data from all relevant studies are summarized either quantitatively or nonquantitatively. The most rigorous approach to statistically combining the results of more than one study is called *meta-analysis*. This strategy effectively increases the sample size and produces a more precise estimate of effect than can be obtained from any of the individual studies included in the review.

The analysis includes an examination of differences among individual study findings (heterogeneity), an attempt to explain these differences, and an assessment of precision (using confidence intervals). If studies are too different from one another with respect to population, nature of the intervention or exposure, or outcomes, the review team can systematically summarize (but not meta-analyze) the study findings in a nonquantitative or narrative review.

To date, most systematic reviews have summarized quantitative studies. Recently, review teams have summarized qualitative studies in the form of systematic reviews, often called *meta-syntheses*.[6] For example, Clemmens conducted a meta-synthesis of 25 qualitative studies on the phenomenon of adolescent motherhood and found five overarching metaphors: (1) the reality of motherhood brings hardship; (2) living in the two worlds of adolescence and motherhood; (3) motherhood as positively transforming; (4) baby as stabilizing influence; and (5) supportive context as turning point for the future.[7]

Table 9-1 The Process of Conducting a Systematic Review

Formulate the Question

- Specify:
    Population
    Intervention or exposure
    Outcome
    Methodology
- Specify inclusion and exclusion criteria.
- Determine restrictions: time frame, unpublished data, language.

Conduct Literature Search

- Decide on information sources: bibliographical databases, handsearching of key journals, reference lists of retrieved articles, experts, personal files, funding agencies, pharmaceutical companies, registries.
- Identify titles and abstracts.

Apply Inclusion and Exclusion Criteria

- Apply inclusion and exclusion criteria to titles and abstracts.
- Obtain full study reports for eligible titles and abstracts.
- Apply inclusion and exclusion criteria to full study reports.
- Select final eligible studies.

Abstract Data

- Assess methodological quality of studies (validity assessment).
- Abstract data from each study about participants, exposure or intervention, study design.
- Abstract results.

Conduct Analysis

- Explore heterogeneity.
- Determine method for summarizing results.
- Combine results (if appropriate).

A high-quality systematic review provides a comprehensive summary of research-based knowledge on a topic, taking into account the validity of the primary studies; however, not all systematic reviews are high quality, and appraisal of their validity before applying their results to clinical practice is essential. As in other chapters of this book, we use the framework of assessing the validity of the methods, interpreting the results, and applying the results to patients (Table 9-2).

ARE THE RESULTS VALID?

Did the Review Explicitly Address a Sensible Clinical Question?

In Chapter 2, Finding the Evidence, we describe the importance of formulating an answerable question by specifying the population, the intervention or exposure, and the outcomes of interest. When reading a systematic review, the first step is to determine the question the review is addressing. Have the authors of the review specified a question that describes the population, the exposure or intervention, and the outcomes? If they have, the next step is to determine whether the question is a sensible one. Readers need to ask themselves whether they would expect the same effect across the range of patients, interventions or exposures, and outcomes included in the review.

Consider a systematic review designed to summarize all studies that evaluated any public health nursing intervention for clients of any age to determine if the interventions reduced subsequent use of health services. We would reject such a systematic review because it is too broad. Some interventions might be effective in certain age groups or populations, whereas others might not be effective and may be harmful. Combining the results of these studies would yield a meaningless estimate of effect that would not be applicable to any of the interventions or clients.

Table **9-2**   Users' Guides for a Review Article

Are the Results Valid?

- Did the review explicitly address a sensible clinical question?
- Was the search for relevant studies detailed and exhaustive?
- Were the primary studies of high methodological quality?
- Were assessments of studies reproducible?

What Are the Results?

- Were the results similar from study to study?
- What were the overall results of the review?
- How precise were the results?

How Can I Apply the Results to Patient Care?

- How can I best interpret the results to apply them to patient care?
- Were all patient-important outcomes considered?
- Are the benefits worth the costs and potential risks?

On the other hand, if a review is focused on a narrow group of study participants (e.g., 14-year-old girls), intervention (e.g., a didactic sex education program), outcome (e.g., improvement in knowledge about contraception), or studies (e.g., those only in the English language), it will limit the generalizability of the findings. What makes a systematic review too broad or too narrow? Clinicians need to ask themselves whether factors such as underlying biology or behavioral responses are such that they would expect the same effect of an intervention across the range of patients. They should ask parallel questions about the other components of the study question. For example, do they expect more or less the same effect across the range of interventions and outcomes? In summary, readers must determine whether it is plausible that an intervention will have a similar effect across the range of patients, interventions, and outcomes specified in the systematic review.

Was the Search for Relevant Studies Detailed and Exhaustive?

Authors of systematic reviews should outline selection criteria (also known as inclusion and exclusion criteria) based on a specified range of patients, exposures or interventions, outcomes, and methodological considerations similar to those described for reports of primary studies in other parts of this book (Table 9-3). They should conduct a thorough search for studies that meet these inclusion criteria. Their search should include the use of bibliographical databases such as CINAHL, ERIC, PsycINFO, MEDLINE, EMBASE/Excerpta Medica, the Cochrane Central Register of Controlled

Table 9-3 Guides for Selecting Articles That Are Most Likely to Provide Valid Results

Health Care Intervention
- Were patients randomized?
- Was follow-up complete?

Harm
- Were groups shown to be similar in all known determinants of outcome, or were analyses adjusted for differences?
- Was follow-up sufficiently complete?

Diagnosis
- Was the diagnostic test evaluated in a spectrum of patients with a low to high probability of having the target disorder?
- Was there a blind comparison with an independent reference (gold) standard applied similarly to all patients?

Prognosis
- Was the sample of patients representative?
- Were the patients sufficiently homogeneous with respect to prognostic risk?
- Was follow-up sufficiently complete?

Trials (containing more than 400,000 controlled trials), and databases of current research.[8] They should handsearch key journals in the field, check the reference lists of the articles they retrieve, and contact experts in the area. It may also be important to examine recently published abstracts from scientific meetings and to access less frequently used databases, such as databases of doctoral theses (e.g., Dissertation Abstracts Online) and of ongoing trials held by relevant manufacturing companies. Unless the authors describe what they did to locate relevant studies, it is difficult to determine the likelihood that they missed relevant studies.

The review team should contact experts in the area of interest for two reasons. The first is to identify published studies that they may have missed (including studies that are in press and those that have not yet been indexed or referenced). The second is to identify unpublished studies to avoid publication bias. *Publication bias* occurs when the publication of research depends on the direction of the study results and whether they are statistically significant. Studies in which a new intervention is not found to be effective often are not published. Because of this, systematic reviews that fail to include unpublished studies may overestimate the true effect of an intervention[9-13] (see Chapter 23, Publication Bias).

Were the Primary Studies of High Methodological Quality?

Even if a systematic review includes only RCTs, it is important to know whether the studies were of good quality because peer review does not guarantee the validity of published research (see Chapter 4, Health Care Interventions).[14] For the same reasons that the guides for reviewing individual research studies begin by asking whether the results are valid, it is essential to consider the validity of the primary studies included in systematic reviews.

Differences in study methods may explain important differences in results.[15-17] For example, less rigorous studies tend to overestimate the effectiveness of therapeutic and preventive interventions.[18] Even if the results of different studies are consistent, determining their validity remains important. Consistent results are less compelling if they come from methodologically weak rather than strong studies. A systematic review of adolescent pregnancy prevention identified 13 RCTs and 17 observational studies.[19] When estimates of the effect of the interventions were computed for both types of studies, the summary odds ratios for the observational studies showed a significant intervention benefit, whereas the RCTs found no benefit for any outcome in either boys or girls.

There is no single correct way to assess the quality of studies, although in the context of a systematic review, the focus should be on the consistent use of criteria to evaluate study methods. Quality rating scales are sometimes used; however, summing quality ratings into an overall score can be problematic. Rather than using a summary score, the review team can assess relevant methodological aspects individually and explore their influence on the effect size.[20,21] Some investigators use long checklists to evaluate methodological quality, whereas others focus on three or four key criteria. If there are many studies to consider, the authors of the review may decide to apply a quality rating threshold for inclusion of studies in the review. When considering whether to trust the results of a review, check to see whether the authors used criteria similar to those we have presented in other sections of this book (see Chapter 4, Health Care Interventions; Chapter 5, Harm; Chapter 6, Diagnosis; and Chapter 7, Prognosis). Authors of systematic reviews should apply these criteria when selecting studies for inclusion and assessing the validity of the included studies (see Tables 9-1, 9-3).

Were Assessments of Studies Reproducible?

As we have seen, authors of systematic reviews must decide which studies to include, how valid they are, and which data to abstract. These decisions require judgment by the reviewers and are subject to mistakes (i.e., random errors) and bias (i.e., systematic errors). Having two or more people participate in each decision guards against errors; if there is good agreement beyond chance between reviewers and if they incorporate a strategy for dealing with discrepancies, readers can have more confidence in the results of the systematic review (see Chapter 30, Measuring Agreement Beyond Chance).

Using the Guide

Hay-Smith and colleagues specified their question as follows: what are the effects of pelvic-floor muscle training in the management of female urinary (stress, mixed, urge) incontinence?[2] They described the participants as adult women with stress, mixed, or urge urinary incontinence diagnosed on the basis of symptoms or urodynamic evaluation. They excluded women with nocturnal enuresis or urinary incontinence associated with factors outside the urinary tract, such as neurological disorders or cognitive impairment. They described the intervention as a pelvic-floor muscle training program designed to ameliorate symptoms of existing urine leakage and excluded studies that evaluated programs for primary prevention of urinary incontinence. Pelvic-floor muscle training was defined as a program of repeated voluntary pelvic-floor muscle contractions taught by a health care professional. They specified the following outcome measures: women's observations (e.g., symptom scores, perception of cure/improvement, satisfaction with outcome); quantification of symptoms (e.g., number of leakage episodes, pad tests); clinicians' measures (e.g., measures of pelvic-floor muscle activity, such as perineometry and palpation); quality of life (e.g., general and specific quality of life measures and psychosocial measures); socioeconomics (e.g., direct and indirect costs of interventions, resource implications, formal economic analysis); and other (e.g., adverse events, compliance, incontinence at long-term follow-up). Their methodological inclusion criteria limited the review to RCTs, excluding quasi-randomized and other nonrandomized controlled clinical trials. Their selection criteria also specified no restrictions on language of publication or publication status (i.e., published or unpublished). In summary, the authors addressed a sensible clinical question and formulated appropriate selection criteria.

The authors searched the Cochrane Incontinence Group Trials Register, the Cochrane Rehabilitation and Related Therapies Field database, MEDLINE, EMBASE/Excerpta Medica, the Dutch National Institute of Allied Health Professions database, and the Physiotherapy Index. In addition, they searched the proceedings of the International Continence Society, handsearched selected physical therapy journals, contacted experts in the field, and checked reference lists of relevant articles. Given this comprehensive search, it is unlikely that the authors missed relevant RCTs.

Of the 43 trials that met the selection criteria, 31 RCTs included only women with stress incontinence, and 12 included women with a range of symptoms or urodynamic diagnoses. Only seven trials had adequate allocation concealment, and nine trials used outcome assessors who were blinded to group allocation. Thirteen trials reported no losses to follow-up, seven trials had loss to follow-up rates less than 10%, and the remaining trials had loss to follow-up rates of 12% to 41%. Only five trials clearly reported some or all of their analyses on the basis of intention to treat. In an *intention-to-treat analysis,* outcomes are analyzed based on the group to which patients were randomized regardless of whether they actually received the planned intervention. (see Chapter 15, The Principle of Intention to Treat).

Two of the review's authors independently decided whether potentially eligible trials met inclusion criteria, assessed trials for methodological quality, and extracted data. Disagreements were resolved through discussion.

The methods of the systematic review were strong. However, the methodological quality of the primary studies included in the review was variable. Many studies failed to conceal allocation, blind outcome assessors to group allocation, and minimize loss to follow-up.

WHAT ARE THE RESULTS?

Were the Results Similar From Study to Study?

The decision about whether the results of individual studies should be combined statistically in a *meta-analysis* rests on the degree of similarity among the results of the individual studies. In other words, were results similar across studies? The authors of a review should present the results in a way that allows clinicians to check the similarity in findings across studies. The more results differ from study to study, the more one should question the decision to combine the results of studies.

If there appear to be differences among study results, readers need to ask whether these are true differences or whether they are due to chance. There are two ways to determine whether the differences among the results of individual studies are greater than one would expect by chance. First, readers can make an initial assessment by examining the extent to which the confidence intervals of the individual studies overlap. The greater the overlap is, the more comfortable one can be with combining results. Widely separated confidence intervals flag the presence of important variability in results that requires explanation (see Chapter 24, Evaluating Differences in Study Results).

Second, authors of reviews can conduct statistical analyses called *tests of heterogeneity* to assess the degree of difference among study findings. These tests (often chi-square tests) determine the extent to which differences between the results of individual studies are greater than one would expect if all studies were measuring the same underlying effect and the observed differences were only due to chance. The more significant the test of heterogeneity (e.g., $P < 0.05$), the less likely that the observed differences were due to chance alone (see Chapter 28, Hypothesis Testing). Unfortunately, higher P values ($P = 0.1$, or even 0.3) do not necessarily rule out important heterogeneity. The reason is that the test of heterogeneity is not very powerful when the number of studies and their sample sizes are both small. Hence, large differences in the apparent magnitude of effects among studies (i.e., the point estimates) dictate caution in interpreting the overall findings, even in the presence of a nonsignificant test of heterogeneity. Conversely, if the differences in results across studies are not clinically important, then heterogeneity is of little concern, even if it is statistically significant (see Chapter 24, Evaluating Differences in Study Results).

Authors of reviews should try to explain between-study differences in findings. Possible explanations include differences among patients (e.g., pelvic-floor muscle training may be more effective in women who are younger rather than older or in those with stress rather than urge incontinence), interventions (e.g., pelvic-floor muscle training alone or combined with behavioral interventions), outcome measurements (self-reported "improvement" versus "cure"), timing of measurement (e.g., different effects if the outcome is measured at 30 days rather than at 1 year after pelvic-floor muscle training), or study methods (e.g., smaller effects in trials with blinded outcome assessors or those with more complete follow-up). Although appropriate and necessary, this search for explanations of heterogeneity in study results may be misleading (see Chapter 16, When to Believe a Subgroup Analysis). Furthermore, how can readers deal with the residual heterogeneity in study results that remains unexplained? We deal with this issue in our discussion of the applicability of the results of systematic reviews.

What Were the Overall Results of the Review?

In clinical studies, investigators collect data from individual patients. Because of the limited capacity of the human mind to handle large amounts of information, investigators use statistical methods to summarize and analyze data. In systematic reviews, investigators collect data from individual studies. Investigators must also summarize these data, and increasingly, they rely on quantitative methods to do so.

Simply comparing the number of positive studies with the number of negative studies is not an adequate way to summarize the results. With this sort of "vote counting," large and small studies are given equal weight, and (unlikely as it may seem) one investigator may interpret a study result as positive, whereas another may interpret the same study result as negative.[22] For example, a clinically important effect that is not statistically significant could be interpreted as positive in light of clinical importance and negative in light of statistical significance. There is a tendency to overlook small, but important, effects if studies with statistically nonsignificant (but potentially clinically important) results are counted as negative.[23] Moreover, readers cannot tell anything about the magnitude of an effect from a vote count even if studies are appropriately classified using additional categories for study results with positive or negative trends.

Typically, meta-analysts weight studies according to their size, such that larger studies receive more weight. Thus, the overall results represent a weighted average of the results of the individual studies. Occasionally, studies are also given more or less weight depending on their quality, or poorer-quality studies are given a weight of zero (excluded) in the primary analysis or in a secondary analysis that tests the extent to which different assumptions lead to different results (*a sensitivity analysis*).

Different statistical approaches can be used in meta-analysis.[24] *Fixed-effects models* are usually used when no significant heterogeneity exists among studies. The goal of this model is to provide the best estimate of the treatment effect in the studies that are part of the analysis.[25] The error term for a fixed-effects model comes only from within-study variation (study variance), and the model ignores between-study variation or heterogeneity. The goal of the *random-effects model* is to provide the best estimate of treatment effect in a hypothetical set of all possible studies of the relevant question, and assumes the available studies are a random sample of those studies. The calculation of the summary statistic (e.g., relative risk or odds ratio) in the random-effects model incorporates both within-study and between-study variation[26] (see Chapter 25, Fixed-Effects and Random-Effects Models).

Readers should look at the overall results of a systematic review in the same way they look at the results of primary studies. In a systematic review of the effects of a health care intervention, they should look for the summary relative risk and relative risk reduction or the summary odds ratio (see Chapter 27, Measures of Association). In systematic reviews of a diagnostic test, readers should look for summary estimates of likelihood ratios (see Chapter 6, Diagnosis).

Figure 9-1 is a graphical display summarizing the results of a meta-analysis of studies evaluating the efficacy of probiotics for prevention of antibiotic-associated diarrhea.[27] It is useful to learn how to interpret these figures as they can convey a large amount of information at a glance. First, focus on the far left column. Looking down, readers will see a row for each of the nine studies included in this comparison, referenced by the name of the first author. The dark square that corresponds to each row represents the odds ratio for that study, and the horizontal line extending from both sides of the square represents the 95% confidence interval around that odds ratio. The larger is the square, the larger is the study sample size. The vertical solid line represents an odds ratio of 1.0 indicating no difference between the treatment and control groups in the proportion of patients with antibiotic-associated diarrhea. When the square representing the odds ratio for an individual study appears to the left of the vertical line, it favors treatment, indicating that there were fewer patients with antibiotic-associated diarrhea in the probiotics group (e.g., first study by Surawicz[28]). When the square representing the odds ratio for an individual study appears to the right of the vertical line, it favors the control, indicating that there were fewer patients with antibiotic-associated diarrhea in the control group (e.g., third study by Lewis[29]). When the confidence interval around the odds ratio crosses over the solid vertical line representing an odds ratio of 1.0, it signifies that the findings of that study were not significant (e.g., third study by Lewis[29]). When the confidence interval does not cross over the vertical line, it signifies that the findings of that study were significant (e.g., first study by Surawicz[28]). The width of the confidence interval line reflects the size of the study. The larger is the study, the shorter is the line (representing a more narrow confidence interval).

Readers can get an overall sense of the heterogeneity of the study results simply by looking at how the lines are scattered. Ideally, all estimates of the odds ratio will be on the same side of the solid vertical line, and all confidence intervals will overlap. In Figure 9-1, one of the odds ratios appears on the right side of the solid vertical line (study by Lewis), and although all of the confidence intervals overlap, two appear to the left of the solid

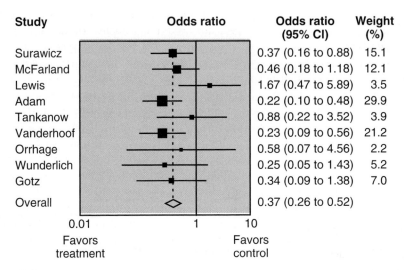

Figure 9-1. Meta-analysis of probiotics vs control in preventing antibiotic-associated diarrhea. *(Modified and reproduced with permission of the BMJ Publishing Group from D'Souza AL, Rajkumar C, Cooke J, Bulpitt CJ. Probiotics in prevention of antibiotic associated diarrhoea: meta-analysis. BMJ. 2002;324:1361-1366.)*

vertical line (studies by Adam and Vanderhoof) and barely overlap with the confidence interval around the odds ratio on the right of the line (study by Lewis). The authors of the review performed a test of heterogeneity (sometimes called a test of homogeneity), which was not significant ($P = 0.2$), indicating that one cannot reject the hypothesis that the true underlying odds ratio was the same across studies, and the observed differences between study findings could be due to chance.[27] Because this test was not significant, the authors decided to combine the data using a fixed-effects method. Despite the nonsignificant test for heterogeneity (which may have resulted from the small number of studies in the analysis) and given the barely overlapping confidence intervals, readers would want to scrutinize this systematic review for possible variations in the patient population, intervention, outcomes, and study methods that might explain differences in individual study findings.

Continuing toward the right of the figure, the odds ratios and 95% confidence intervals are provided for each study, and the weight given to each study in the analysis is specified as a percent, with larger studies given more weight. At the bottom of the figure is the overall summary statistic depicted as a diamond encompassing the 95% confidence interval. The edges of the diamond do not cross or touch the vertical line, which indicates a statistically significant difference in favor of probiotics.

As noted earlier, when outcomes are dichotomous (e.g., alive or dead, diarrhea or no diarrhea), meta-analyses generally report relative risks or odds ratios as the summary statistic. When the outcomes are continuous (e.g., blood pressure, blood glucose, or weight), the calculation is a mean difference or mean effect size. When mean difference or other continuous measures are reported, the vertical line of no difference represents 0 rather than 1.

Sometimes, the outcome measures used in different studies are similar but not identical. For example, different trials may measure health-related quality of life using different instruments. If the patients and the interventions are reasonably similar, estimating the average effect of the intervention on quality of life still may be worthwhile. One way of doing this is to summarize the results of each study as an effect size.[30] The *effect size* is the difference in outcomes between the intervention and control groups divided by the standard deviation. The effect size summarizes the results of each study in terms of the number of standard deviations of difference between the intervention group and the control group. Investigators can then calculate a weighted average of effect sizes from studies that measured a given outcome in different ways.

Readers may find it difficult to interpret the importance of an effect size for patients. For example, is a weighted average effect of one half of a standard deviation clinically trivial or large? Once again, one should look for a presentation of the results that conveys their practical importance (e.g., by translating the summary effect size back into natural units).[31] For instance, clinicians may be familiar with the importance of differences in walk test scores in patients with chronic lung disease. Investigators can convert the effect size of an intervention on certain measures of functional status (e.g., the walk test and stair climbing) back into differences in walk test scores.[32]

How Precise Were the Results?

Just as with single studies, the true effect in a meta-analysis can never be known. Confidence intervals around the point estimate tell us about the neighborhood within which the true effect likely lies. The confidence interval around the summary statistic is almost always more narrow than the confidence intervals around the point estimates of any of the individual studies because the analysis in effect creates one study with a large sample size and therefore, a more precise estimate of effect.

In Figure 9-1, the overall summary odds ratio is 0.37 and the 95% confidence interval is 0.26 to 0.52. Put into words, this means that the risk of developing antibiotic-associated diarrhea is reduced by 37% in patients who take probiotics. The confidence interval indicates that there is a 95% chance that the true risk reduction lies somewhere between 26% and 52%. Given this positive finding, the lower boundary of the confidence interval helps inform decision making. If clinicians consider reducing the risk of developing antibiotic-associated diarrhea by as little as 26%, the minimum plausible effect, to be a worthwhile benefit (i.e., clinically important), they are likely to be comfortable recommending the use of probiotics (see Chapter 29, Confidence Intervals).

USING THE GUIDE

In the review by Hay-Smith et al,[2] seven of 43 trials compared pelvic-floor muscle training with no treatment. Three trials included women with genuine stress incontinence only; one trial included women with a urodynamic diagnosis of genuine stress or mixed incontinence, and three trials included women with symptoms of urine leakage. Two trials of women with genuine stress incontinence or mixed incontinence measured self-reported cure. In the pelvic-floor muscle training group, 16.7% of women self-reported cure compared with 1.9% in the no-treatment group. Results were consistent across studies. Meta-analysis was conducted using a fixed-effects model and resulted in a summary relative

Continued

risk (RR) of 7.3 and a 95% confidence interval (CI) of 2.0 to 26.5. The wide confidence interval reflects a lack of precision resulting from the inclusion of a small number of small trials.

Combined data from three trials demonstrated a significant reduction in leakage episodes over 24 hours for women who received pelvic-floor muscle training compared with no treatment (weighted mean difference −1.3; 95% CI −1.6 to −0.9); however, statistically significant heterogeneity was observed ($P = .0059$), which the authors attributed to variations in study quality and provision of an intervention to the control group.

The authors did not combine data on the pad test, clinicians' measures, and quality of life. A variety of pad tests in three trials consistently found a greater reduction in leakage in women who had pelvic-floor muscle training. Of the three trials in which clinicians measured pelvic-floor muscle activity, two trials reported greater improvement in the pelvic-floor muscle measures after training. Only one trial examined quality of life and found that women in the pelvic-floor muscle activity group had significant improvements on a Social Activity Index ($P < 0.01$) compared with the no-treatment group. None of the trials included an economic analysis. Two trials reported adverse events associated with pelvic-floor muscle training (e.g., pain with contractions), and these were reversible.

Combined data from three trials showed that women who received "intensive" pelvic-floor muscle training were more likely to report cure than those who received "standard" pelvic-floor muscle training (38% vs 25%; summary RR, 1.47; 95% CI 1.17 to 1.84). There was no significant heterogeneity across trials.

The authors concluded that although larger, higher-quality studies are needed, some evidence supports a recommendation to offer pelvic-floor muscle training as a first-line conservative treatment for women with stress or mixed incontinence.

HOW CAN I APPLY THE RESULTS TO PATIENT CARE?

How Can I Best Interpret the Results to Apply Them to Patient Care?

Even if the true underlying effect is identical in each of several studies, chance will ensure that the observed results differ (see Chapter 26, Bias and Random Error). As a result, systematic reviews risk capitalizing on the play of chance. Perhaps studies of older patients, by chance, had smaller treatment effects. Reviewers may erroneously conclude that a treatment is less effective in elderly patients. The greater the number of subgroup analyses conducted, the greater is the risk of a chance finding.

Clinicians can apply certain criteria to distinguish between subgroup analyses that are credible and those that are not (see Chapter 16, When to Believe a Subgroup Analysis). A hypothesized difference in subgroups is more credible if (1) conclusions are based on within-study rather than between-study comparisons; (2) a large difference in treatment effect exists across subgroups; (3) there is a highly statistically significant difference in treatment effect (e.g., the lower the P value when comparing different effect sizes in subgroups, the more credible the difference); (4) a hypothesis was made before the study began and was one of only a few hypotheses tested; (5) consistency was found across studies; and (6) indirect evidence supported the difference (e.g., biologic plausibility). If these criteria are not met, the results of a subgroup analysis are less likely to be trustworthy, and it may be more appropriate to assume that the overall effect across all patients and all interventions, rather than the subgroup effect, applies to the patient at hand and to the treatment under consideration.

What if subgroup analyses fail to provide an adequate explanation for unexplained heterogeneity in study results? Although several reasonable alternatives exist, including ignoring the combined results, we suggest that clinicians consider a summary measure from all of the best available studies for the most accurate estimate of the effect of the intervention.[33-35]

Were All Patient-Important Outcomes Considered?

Although it is a good idea to look for focused systematic reviews because they are more likely to provide valid results, this does not mean that clinicians should ignore outcomes that are not included in a review. For example, the potential benefits of hormone replacement therapy may include a reduced risk of fractures and colorectal cancer, and potential disadvantages may include an increased risk of breast cancer and stroke. Focused reviews are more likely to provide valid results of the effects of hormone replacement therapy on each of these four outcomes, but a clinical decision requires consideration of all of them.

Systematic reviews frequently do not report the adverse effects of treatment. One reason is that individual studies often measure adverse effects in different ways or not at all, thus making it difficult to summarize the results. Costs are an additional outcome that are often absent from systematic reviews.

Are the Benefits Worth the Costs and Potential Risks?

Finally, either explicitly or implicitly, clinicians and patients must weigh the expected benefits against the costs and potential risks of an intervention. Although this is most obvious when deciding whether to implement a health care intervention, providing patients with information about causes of disease or prognosis also can have both benefits and risks. For example, informing city dwellers about the health risks of air pollution exposures may lead them to reduce the risk of exposure, with potential benefits; however, it may also cause anxiety or make peoples' lives less convenient. Informing an asymptomatic woman with newly detected cancer about her prognosis may help her to plan better, but it may also label her, cause anxiety, or increase the period during which she is "sick."

A valid systematic review provides the best possible basis for quantifying the expected outcomes, but these outcomes still must be considered in the context of a patient's values and concerns about the expected outcomes of a decision. Ultimately, trading off benefits and risks will involve value judgments, and in clinical decision making, these values should come from the patient (see Chapter 34, Incorporating Patient Values).

Clinical Resolution

The group arrives at several conclusions. First, although the methodological quality of the systematic review is strong, many of the trials included in the review were small and had methodological shortcomings, which limit the conclusions that could be

Continued

drawn. Second, compared with no treatment, pelvic-floor muscle training appeared to increase the likelihood of self-reported cure in women with stress or mixed incontinence. In absolute terms, seven women would need to be given pelvic-floor muscle training to have a single additional self-reported cure [1/absolute risk reduction = 100%/(16.7% − 1.9%) or 1/(0.167 − 0.019)] (see Chapter 32, Number Needed To Treat). Third, evidence suggested that more intensive pelvic-floor muscle training was better than standard pelvic-floor muscle training. Fourth, side effects of pelvic-floor muscle training were uncommon and reversible. Fifth, most of the trials studied the effect of training in younger, premenopausal women.

The group concluded that many areas of uncertainty remain: whether pelvic-floor muscle training is effective in older women; whether training is effective over a long term; whether training is better or worse than other treatments, such as electrical stimulation or behavioral training; and whether training is more effective if combined with treatments such as vaginal cones or intravaginal resistance.

Despite these uncertainties, and given the uncommon risk of side effects and the increased self-reported cure rates, the group decides to offer pelvic-floor muscle training for premenopausal women with stress or mixed incontinence. However, before doing this, they plan to review the individual trials that contributed to the meta-analyses to learn more about the specific components of pelvic-floor muscle training in each study, such as how it was taught, types (quick or hold) and number of contractions, and length of training.

REFERENCES

1. Jadad AR, Cook DJ, Jones A, et al. Methodology and reports of systematic reviews and meta-analyses: a comparison of Cochrane reviews with articles published in paper-based journals. *JAMA*. 1998;280:278-280.
2. Hay-Smith EJ, Bo K, Berghmans LC, et al. Pelvic floor muscle training for urinary incontinence in women. *Cochrane Database of Syst Rev.* 2001;(1):CD001407.
3. Guyatt GH, Montori VM, Devereaux PJ, Schunemann HJ, Bhandari M. Patients at the center: in our practice, and in our use of language [editorial]. *ACP Journal Club. 2004;140:A11.*
4. Antman EM, Lau J, Kupelnick B, Mosteller F, Chalmers TC. A comparison of results of meta-analyses of randomized control trials and recommendations of clinical experts: treatments for myocardial infarction. *JAMA.* 1992;268:240-248.
5. Oxman AD, Guyatt GH. The science of reviewing research. *Ann NY Acad Sci.* 1993;703:125-133; discussion 133-134.
6. Paterson BL, Thorne SE, Canam C, et al. *Meta-study of Qualitative Health Research: A Practical Guide to Meta-analysis and Meta-synthesis.* Thousand Oaks, CA: Sage Publications; 2001.
7. Clemmens D. Adolescent motherhood: a meta-synthesis of qualitative studies. *MCN Am J Matern Child Nurs.* 2003;28:93-99.
8. The *meta*Register of Controlled Trials (*m*RCT). Current controlled trials. Available at: *http://www.controlled-trials.com/.* Accessed November 21, 2002.
9. Dickersin K, Min Y, Meinert CL. Factors influencing publication of research results. JAMA. 1992;267:374-378.
10. Dickersin K. How important is publication bias? A synthesis of available data. *AIDS Educ Prev.* 1997;9(suppl 1):15-21.
11. Stern JM, Simes RJ. Publication bias: evidence of delayed publication in a cohort study of clinical research projects. *BMJ.* 1997;315:640-645.
12. Ioannidis JP. Effect of the statistical significance of results on the time to completion and publication of randomized efficacy trials. *JAMA.* 1998;279:281-286.

13. Egger M, Smith G. Bias in location and selection of studies. *BMJ*. 1998;316:61-66.
14. Williamson JW, Goldschmidt PG, Colton T. The quality of medical literature: analysis of validation assessments. In: Bailar JC, Mosteller F, eds. *Medical Uses of Statistics*. 2nd ed. Waltham, MA: NEJM Books; 1992:370-391.
15. Horwitz RI. Complexity and contradiction in clinical trial research. *Am J Med*. 1987;82:498-510.
16. Detsky AS, Naylor CD, O'Rourke K, McGeer AJ, L'Abbe KA. Incorporating variations in the quality of individual randomized trials into meta-analysis. *J Clin Epidemiol*. 1992;45:255-265.
17. Moher D, Pham B, Jones A, et al. Does quality of reports of randomised trials affect estimates of intervention efficacy reported in meta-analyses? *Lancet*. 1998;352:609-613.
18. Kunz R, Oxman AD. The unpredictability paradox: review of empirical comparisons of randomised and non-randomised clinical trials. *BMJ*. 1998;317:1185-1190.
19. Guyatt GH, DiCenso A, Farewell V, Willan A, Griffith L. Randomized trials versus observational studies in adolescent pregnancy prevention. *J Clin Epidemiol*. 2000;53:167-174.
20. Moher D, Jadad AR, Nichol G, Penman M, Tugwell P, Walsh S. Assessing the quality of randomized controlled trials: an annotated bibliography of scales and checklists. *Control Clin Trials*. 1995;16:62-73.
21. Juni P, Witschi A, Bloch R, Egger M. The hazards of scoring the quality of clinical trials for meta-analysis. *JAMA*. 1999;282:1054-1060.
22. Glass GV, McGaw B, Smith ML. *Meta-analysis in Social Research*. Beverly Hills, CA: Sage Publications; 1981:18-20.
23. Cooper HM, Rosenthal R. Statistical versus traditional procedures for summarizing research findings. *Psychol Bull*. 1980;87:442-449.
24. Fleiss JL. The statistical basis of meta-analysis. *Stat Methods Med Res*. 1993;2:121-145.
25. Lau J, Ioannidis JP, Schmid CH. Summing up evidence: one answer is not always enough. *Lancet*. 1998;351:123-127.
26. DerSimonian R, Laird N. Meta-analysis in clinical trials. *Control Clin Trials*. 1986;7:177-188.
27. D'Souza AL, Rajkumar C, Cooke J, Bulpitt CJ. Probiotics in prevention of antibiotic associated diarrhoea: meta-analysis. *BMJ*. 2002;324:1361-1366.
28. Surawicz CM, Elmer GW, Speelman P, McFarland LV, Chinn J, Van Belle G. Prevention of antibiotic associated diarrhoea by *Saccharomyce boulardii*. *Gastroenterology*. 1989;96:981-988.
29. Lewis SJ, Potts LF, Barry RE. The lack of therapeutic effect of *S boulardii* in the prevention of antibiotic related diarrhoea in elderly patients. *J Infect*. 1998;36:171-174.
30. Rosenthal R. *Meta-analytic Procedures for Social Research*. 2nd ed. Newbury Park, CA: Sage Publications; 1991.
31. Smith K, Cook D, Guyatt GH, Madhavan J, Oxman AD. Respiratory muscle training in chronic airflow limitation: a meta-analysis. *Am Rev Respir Dis*. 1992;145:533-539.
32. Lacasse Y, Wong E, Guyatt GH, King D, Cook DJ, Goldstein RS. Meta-analysis of respiratory rehabilitation in chronic obstructive pulmonary disease. *Lancet*. 1996;348:1115-1119.
33. Peto R. Why do we need systematic overviews of randomized trials? *Stat Med*. 1987;6:233-244.
34. Oxman AD, Guyatt GH. A consumer's guide to subgroup analyses. *Ann Intern Med*. 1992;116:78-84.
35. Yusuf S, Wittes J, Probstfield J, Tyroler HA. Analysis and interpretation of treatment effects in subgroups of patients in randomized clinical trials. *JAMA*. 1991;266:93-98.

10

Moving From Evidence to Action Using Clinical Practice Guidelines

Alba DiCenso, Donna Ciliska, Maureen Dobbins, and Gordon Guyatt

The following Editorial Board members also made substantive contributions to this chapter: Nancy Edwards, Linda Johnston, Dorothy McCaughan, Mark Newman, and Ania Willman.

We gratefully acknowledge the work of Robert Hayward, Scott Richardson, Lee Green, Mark Wilson, Jack Sinclair, Deborah Cook, Paul Glasziou, Alan Detsky, and Eric Bass on the original chapter that appears in the Users' Guides to the Medical Literature, *edited by Guyatt and Rennie.*

In This Chapter

Finding the Evidence

Are the Results Valid?
Were All Relevant Patient Groups, Management Options, and Possible Outcomes Considered?
Was an Explicit and Sensible Process Used to Identify, Select, and Combine Evidence?
Was There an Appropriate Specification of Values or Preferences Associated With Outcomes?
Is the Guideline Likely to Account for Important Recent Developments?
Has the Guideline Been Subjected to Peer Review and Testing?

What Are the Results?
Were Practical, Clinically Important Recommendations Made?
Did the Authors Indicate the Strength of Their Recommendations?

How Can I Apply the Results to Patient Care?
Is the Primary Objective of the Guideline Consistent With My Objective?
Are the Recommendations Applicable to My Patient Care?

Implementation of Clinical Practice Guidelines

CLINICAL SCENARIO

Preventing Falls in the Elderly: Can a Clinical Practice Guideline Help?

You are a nurse manager in the local health department in a community where many seniors live. You have recently been assigned to a new program that focuses on healthy aging in the community. You have a team of enthusiastic public health nurses who have many years of experience in working with the elderly. You have been meeting with these nurses regularly to review the existing services they provide and to identify unmet health care needs in this population. The nurses are concerned about the number of falls that occur among elderly clients and share their frustration about whether they are doing enough to prevent falls. Your team agrees that prevention of falls in this population is a high priority. Various interventions are suggested at the meeting, such as in-home assessment of risk of falls, exercise programs for the general elderly population, and targeted exercise and balance interventions. The team is unsure about how to proceed. One of the nurses notes that a number of nursing organizations have recently become involved in the development of best practice guidelines and wonders whether a guideline exists on prevention of falls in the elderly. You volunteer to find out.

FINDING THE EVIDENCE

You bring up your Web browser and go to your favorite search engine, *Google.com*. You enter the term "practice guidelines," and the first item on the results list is "National Guideline Clearinghouse" at *http://www.guideline.gov/*. This looks promising because the server is sponsored by the Agency for Healthcare Research and Quality (AHRQ), a US government agency formerly known as the Agency for Health Care Policy and Research (AHCPR), which, you recall, created a series of guidelines using formal evidence-based guidelines methodology.[1]

After linking to the Clearinghouse, you enter the terms "falls," "prevention," and "elderly" in the search box, which yields 16 guidelines. The fourth one on the list seems promising: "Guidelines for the prevention of falls in people over 65." The guideline is summarized on the Clearinghouse site and has been published in the peer-reviewed literature.[2] You click on "Complete Summary" and print the text that appears. You also note that the guideline summary is linked to the full text of the article in *BMJ*, so you link there and print the entire article. You look forward to reading the material, although with some concern, because you are aware that some guidelines are poorly constructed.[3,4]

In this chapter, we focus on evaluating and implementing clinical practice guidelines. *Practice guidelines*, or "systematically developed statements to assist practitioner and patient decisions about appropriate health care for specific clinical circumstances,"[5] represent an attempt to distill a large body of health care knowledge into a convenient, readily usable format.[6-10] Like systematic reviews, practice guidelines gather, appraise, and combine evidence. Guidelines, however, go beyond systematic reviews in attempting to address all the issues relevant to a clinical decision and all the values that could sway a clinical recommendation. Guidelines refine clinical questions and balance trade-offs between benefits and risks. Guidelines make explicit recommendations, often on behalf of health organizations, with a definite intent to influence what clinicians do.

Guideline development can include up to eight steps (Figure 10-1).[9] In step 1, guideline developers select a topic and frame a well-developed decision-making question. In step 2, they search appropriate databases for existing guidelines that address the clinical problem; if they locate a suitable guideline, they update it with a literature review; if they do not find a suitable guideline, they conduct an explicit and systematic search

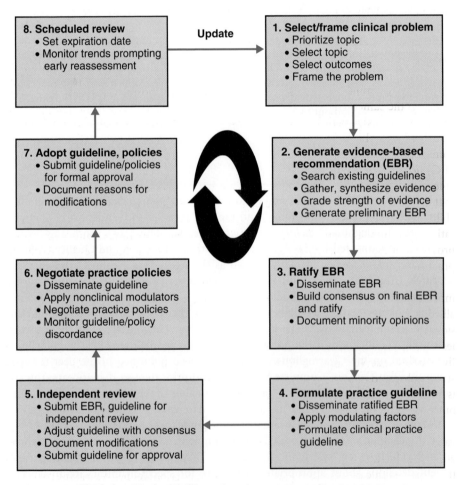

Figure 10-1. The practice guidelines development cycle. *(Modified and reproduced with permission of the American Society of Clinical Oncology from Browman GP, Levine MN, Mohide EA, et al. The practice guidelines development cycle: a conceptual tool for practice guidelines development and implementation. J. Clin Oncol. 1995;13:502-512.)*

of the original literature to create a guideline. In this case, priority is given to locating high-quality systematic reviews. In step 3, the guideline developers document the consensus process they used to ratify the evidence-based recommendations. During step 4, the guideline is formulated with consideration of clinical modulating factors (e.g., reconciling desirability to maintain conventional practice with strength of guideline evidence for an alternative practice). Step 5 involves an independent review of the guideline and its recommendations. Steps 6 to 8 focus on the implementation of the guideline in a specific clinical setting and involve (1) consideration of clinical, practical, and administrative constraints that need to be addressed to implement the guideline; (2) formal adoption of the guideline by the sponsoring organization; and (3) scheduling of guideline reviews and updates. Occasionally, one may need to reframe the clinical problem, which feeds back into step 1.[9]

Practice guideline methodology relies on the consensus of a group of decision makers—ideally experts, front-line clinicians, and patients—who carefully consider the evidence and decide on its implications. The guideline developers mandate may be to develop recommendations for a country, region, city, hospital, or clinic. Guidelines based on the same evidence may differ depending on the country (e.g., Philippines or the United States), whether the region is urban or rural, whether the institution is a large teaching hospital or a small community hospital, and whether the clinic serves a poor community or an affluent one. For this reason, however, some people (e.g., the editors of *Clinical Evidence;* see Chapter 2, Finding the Evidence) believe that we should not provide recommendations, but rather provide only summaries of evidence. They believe that differences in baseline risks, in preferences of individual patients and, in local availability of interventions will always mean that the evidence must be individually interpreted rather than applied universally. For this reason, *Clinical Evidence* limits itself to the provision of the evidence that readers can use for developing locally applicable clinical practice guidelines.

Thomas and colleagues conducted a systematic review to evaluate the effects of introducing clinical practice guidelines in nursing, midwifery, and other professions allied to medicine.[11] They found 18 studies in which nurses were the targeted professional group and one study aimed solely at dieticians. The behaviors targeted in the studies included management of hypertension, low back pain, and hyperlipidemia. Three of five studies observed improvements in at least some processes of care, and six of eight studies observed improvements in outcomes of care. The reviewers concluded that there is some evidence that guideline-driven care is effective in changing the process and outcome of care provided by nurses.

Practice guidelines can be methodologically strong or weak and thus may yield either valid or invalid recommendations. Numerous instruments for appraising clinical practice guidelines exist.[12] In Table 10-1, we outline our standard approach for using an article from the health care literature that describes a practice guideline. We ask the following questions: (1) Are the results valid? (2) What are the results? and (3) How do the results apply to patient care?

Figure 10-2 presents the steps involved in developing a recommendation, along with the formal strategies for doing so. The first step in clinical decision making is to define

Table **10-1** Users' Guides for an Article Describing Clinical Practice
Guidelines

Are the Results Valid?

- Were all relevant patient groups, management options, and possible outcomes considered?
- Was an explicit and sensible process used to identify, select, and combine evidence?
- Was there an appropriate specification of values or preferences associated with outcomes?
- Is the guideline likely to account for important recent developments?
- Has the guideline been subjected to peer review and testing?

What Are the Results?

- Were practical, clinically important recommendations made?
- Did the authors indicate the strength of their recommendations?

How Can I Apply the Results to Patient Care?

- Is the primary objective of the guideline consistent with my objective?
- Are the recommendations applicable to my patient care?

---

the decision. This involves specifying alternative courses of action and possible outcomes. Often, treatments are designed to prevent or ameliorate outcomes such as pain, pressure ulcers, or urinary incontinence. As usual, we refer to the outcomes that interventions are designed to prevent or ameliorate as *target outcomes*. Interventions are associated with adverse outcomes such as side effects and inconvenience. In addition, new interventions may markedly increase or decrease costs. Ideally, the definition of the decision will be comprehensive. All reasonable alternatives will be considered, and all possible beneficial and adverse outcomes will be identified. In elderly patients at risk for falls, such as those patients described in the opening scenario, options may include doing nothing, recommending exercise programs or balance training, providing home assessments, or recommending hip protectors. Outcomes may include falls and fractures, increased muscle strength, improved balance, the inconvenience associated with the interventions, and costs to the patient, the health care system, and society.

Decision makers must then evaluate the links between the identified options and outcomes. What will the alternative management strategies yield in terms of benefits and harm?[13,14] How are potential benefits and risks likely to vary in different groups of patients?[14,15] Once these questions are answered, making treatment recommendations involves value judgments about the relative desirability or undesirability of possible outcomes. We will use the term *preferences* synonymously with *values* or *value judgments* in referring to the process of trading off positive and negative consequences of alternative management strategies.

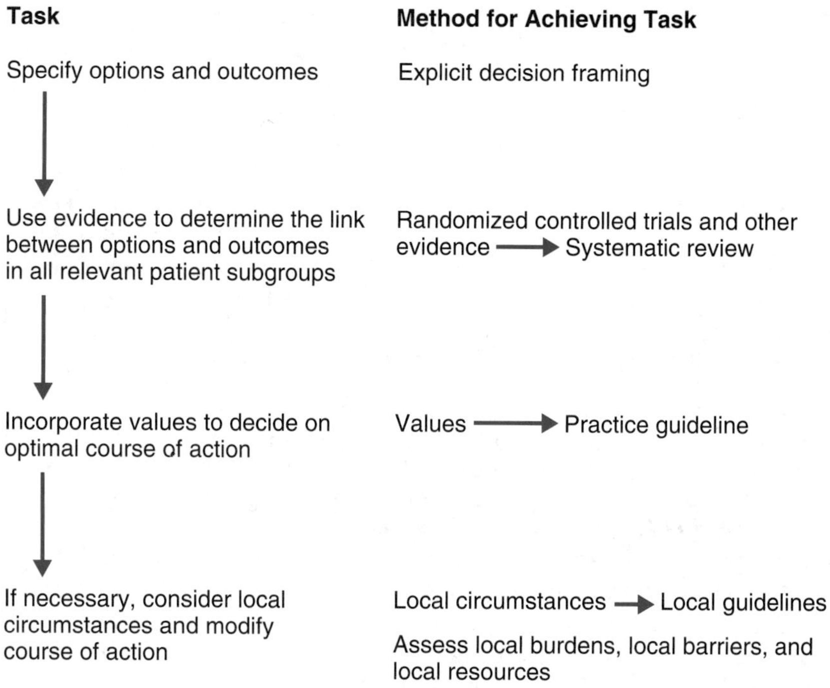

Task	Method for Achieving Task
Specify options and outcomes	Explicit decision framing

↓

| Use evidence to determine the link between options and outcomes in all relevant patient subgroups | Randomized controlled trials and other evidence ⟶ Systematic review |

↓

| Incorporate values to decide on optimal course of action | Values ⟶ Practice guideline |

↓

| If necessary, consider local circumstances and modify course of action | Local circumstances ⟶ Local guidelines
Assess local burdens, local barriers, and local resources |

Figure 10-2. A schematic view of the process of developing a health care recommendation.

ARE THE RESULTS VALID?

Were All Relevant Patient Groups, Management Options, and Possible Outcomes Considered?

Guidelines pertain to decisions, and decisions involve particular groups of patients, choices for those patients, and the consequences of the choices. Regardless of whether guideline developers are formulating guidelines that apply to prevention, treatment, diagnosis, or rehabilitation, they should specify all relevant patient groups, the interventions of interest, and sensible alternative practices. Treatment recommendations often vary for different subgroups of patients. In particular, those at lower risk for *target outcomes* are less likely to benefit from the intervention than those who are at higher risk (see Chapter 33, Applying Results to Individual Patients).

Guideline developers must consider not only all relevant patient groups and management options, but also all important outcomes that could be influenced by the management options. Evidence concerning the effects on morbidity, mortality, and quality of life are all relevant to patients, and efficient use of resources dictates attention to costs. Costs can be considered from the perspectives of patients, insurers, the health care system, or society (see Chapter 18, Economic Evaluation). To illustrate, a clinical practice guideline that makes recommendations regarding pain management must specify the patient groups to whom the recommendations apply (e.g., children, adults, or both; those with acute or chronic pain, or both), the interventions of interest (e.g., inclusion of nontraditional pain control measures), and the outcomes (e.g., pain control, quality of life, and health care costs).

Was an Explicit and Sensible Process Used to Identify, Select, and Combine Evidence?

After the options and outcomes have been specified, the next task for guideline developers is to estimate the likelihood that each outcome will occur. In effect, guideline developers have a series of specific questions. For prevention of falls in the elderly, the initial question is, what is the effect of alternative approaches on the incidence of falls and fractures, quality of life, and health care costs? Guideline recommendations must consolidate and combine all the relevant evidence in an appropriate manner. In carrying out this task, guideline developers must avoid bias that will distort the results. Ideally, they should have access to, or conduct, a systematic review of the evidence bearing on each question. Chapter 9, Summarizing the Evidence Through Systematic Reviews, provides guidelines for assessing the likelihood that collection and summarization of evidence will be free of bias.

Unsystematic approaches to identification and collection of evidence may result in underestimation or, more commonly, overestimation of treatment effects, and side effects may be exaggerated or ignored. Even if the evidence has been identified and collected in a systematic fashion, unsystematic methods of summarizing the collected evidence can result in similar risks of bias. Unsystematic approaches may lead to recommendations advocating harmful interventions or a failure to encourage effective treatment.

Systematic reviews deal with this problem by explicitly stating inclusion and exclusion criteria for evidence to be considered, conducting a comprehensive search for the evidence, and summarizing the results according to explicit rules that include examining how effects may vary in different patient subgroups (see Chapter 9, Summarizing the Evidence Through Systematic Reviews). When a systematic review pools data across studies to provide a quantitative estimate of overall treatment effect, we call it a *meta-analysis*. Systematic reviews provide strong evidence when the quality of primary study designs is good and sample sizes are large; they provide weaker evidence when study designs are poor and sample sizes are small. Because many of the steps in a systematic review involve judgment (e.g., specifying inclusion and exclusion criteria, applying these criteria to potentially eligible studies, evaluating the methodological quality of primary studies, and selecting an approach to data analysis), systematic reviews are not immune to bias. Nevertheless, in their rigorous approach to identifying and summarizing data, systematic reviews reduce the likelihood of bias in estimating causal links between management options and patient outcomes.

The highest-quality treatment guidelines define admissible evidence, report how it was selected and combined, make key data available for the reader's review, and report randomized trials that link interventions with outcomes. However, such randomized trials may be unavailable, and the authors of systematic reviews may reasonably abandon their project if there are no high-quality studies to summarize. Persons who produce guidelines do not have this luxury. For important but ethically, technically, or economically difficult questions, strong scientific evidence may never become available. Because guideline developers must deal with the best (often inadequate) evidence available, they may have to consider various studies (published and unpublished) as well as reports of expert and consumer experience. This means that the strength of the evidence in support of the recommendations can vary widely. Thus, even recommendations that are grounded in rigorous collection and summarization of evidence may yield weak recommendations if the quality of the evidence is poor. Although guideline developers must formulate recommendations, they should be candid about the quality of evidence on which those recommendations are based.

A quality-of-evidence scale can be used to rate different categories of evidence (e.g., research studies or expert opinion) and methods for producing it (e.g., blinded or non-blinded outcome assessment). By applying a systematic approach to the appraisal and classification of evidence, the strength of the evidence in support of the recommendations can be reported.

Was There an Appropriate Specification of Values or Preferences Associated With Outcomes?

Linking treatment options with outcomes is largely a question of fact and a matter of science. In contrast, assigning preferences to outcomes is a matter of values. Clinicians should look for information about who was involved in assigning values to outcomes or who, by influencing recommendations, was implicitly involved in assigning values. Expert panels and consensus groups are often used to develop the guideline recommendations. You should review the names and affiliations of the "expert" panel members and bear in mind that panels dominated by members of specialty groups may be subject to intellectual, territorial, and even financial biases. Panels that include a balance of experts in research methodology, practitioners, and public representatives are more likely to have considered diverse views in their deliberations than panels restricted to content experts.

Even with broad representation, the actual process of deliberation can influence recommendations. Therefore, clinicians should look for a report of methods used to synthesize preferences from multiple sources. Informal and unstructured processes may be vulnerable to undue influence by individual panel members, particularly that of the panel chair. Explicit strategies for describing and dealing with dissent among judges, or frank reports of the degree of consensus, strengthen the credibility of the recommendations.

Knowing the extent to which patient preferences were considered is particularly important. Many guideline reports, by their silence on the matter of patient preferences, assume that guideline developers adequately represent patients' interests. Although these preferences are reported rarely, it also would be valuable to know which principles, such as patient autonomy (a patient's control over decisions about her health), nonmaleficence (avoiding harm), or distributive justice (the fair distribution of health care resources), were given priority in guiding decisions about the value of alternative interventions. Excellent guidelines will state whether the guideline is intended to optimize values for individual patients, reimbursement agencies, or society as a whole. Ideally, guidelines will state the underlying value judgments on which they are based.

Is the Guideline Likely to Account for Important Recent Developments?

Guidelines often concern controversial health problems about which new knowledge is actively sought in ongoing studies. Because of the time required to assemble and review evidence and to achieve consensus about recommendations, the guideline may be out of date by the time you see it. For example, in light of the recent studies that have shown a negative association between hormone replacement therapy and coronary heart disease,[16,17]guidelines about the use of hormone replacement therapy in post-menopausal women are under revision. You should look for two important dates: the publication date of the most recent evidence considered and the date on which the final recommendations were made. Some authorities also identify important studies in progress and new information that could change the guideline. Ideally, these considerations may be used to qualify guidelines as temporary or provisional, to specify dates for expiration or review, or to identify key research priorities. Usually, however, you must scan the bibliography to obtain an impression of how current a particular guideline may be.

Has the Guideline Been Subjected to Peer Review and Testing?

People may interpret evidence differently and their values may differ, and guidelines are subject to both sorts of differences. Your confidence in the validity of a guideline increases if external reviewers have judged the conclusions to be reasonable and if clinicians have found the guidelines to be applicable to practice. If the guidelines differ from those developed by others, you should look for an explanation. Conversely, if the guidelines meet the first four validity criteria (Table 10-1) and the underlying evidence is strong, rejection by, clinicians or peer reviewers may have more to do with their biases than with any limitation of the guidelines.

If the underlying evidence is weak, clinicians' confidence in the validity of the guideline will be limited, regardless of the degree of consensus or peer review. The weaker the underlying evidence, the greater is the argument for actually testing the guideline to determine whether its application improves patient outcomes. The question for any such test would be, Are patient outcomes better, or are outcomes equivalent at decreased cost, when clinicians operate on the basis of the practice guidelines?

Weingarten and colleagues[18] conducted such an investigation to examine the impact of implementation of a practice guideline recommending that low-risk patients admitted to coronary care units receive early discharge. On alternate months over a 1-year period, clinicians either received or did not receive a reminder of the guideline recommendations. During the months in which the intervention was in effect, mean hospital stay was approximately 1 day shorter, and the average cost of stay was about $1000 less. Mortality and health status at 1 month were similar in the two groups. The investigators concluded that the guideline reminder reduced the length of hospital stays and associated costs without adversely affecting measured patient outcomes. Although the authors used alternate-month allocation, which makes the study weaker than a true randomized trial, a study of this type helps to validate the predicted consequences of guideline implementation for defined outcomes.

Using the Guide

The authors of the guidelines for the prevention of falls in people older than 65 years[2] specified the patient group, management options, and outcomes. The patient group consisted of people aged 65 years or older who were living in the community or in residential care; management options included all interventions designed to minimize or prevent exposure to risk factors for falling or fracture that had been evaluated in randomized controlled trials, except drug or dietary treatments for prevention of fractures; and outcomes included the number of people who had fallen or the number of falls or fractures. The authors did not explicitly consider the effects of the interventions on muscle strength, balance, costs, or quality of life. The effect of the intervention on quality of life, for example, would be important to know because elderly people might not be willing to participate in the intervention if it negatively influenced quality of life.

The authors used an explicit and sensible process to identify and select evidence. They updated two previous systematic reviews to identify any new evidence. They searched MEDLINE for all randomized controlled trials and systematic reviews by using the terms "falls," "accidental falls," "fracture," "elderly," "aged," "older," and "senior." They followed up relevant references in articles and contacted researchers for information about other trial evidence and about studies from journals not catalogued by the National Library of Medicine. The guideline development group assigned a methodology quality score to trials according to the criteria used for the related Cochrane review with the addition of sample size. Evidence statements were graded according to the quality score and sample size. The grade of evidence was based on three categories: A, consistent findings in multiple randomized controlled trials or a meta-analysis; B, single randomized controlled trial or weak inconsistent findings in multiple randomized controlled trials; and C, limited scientific evidence, cohort studies, flawed randomized controlled trials, or panel consensus.

With respect to considering the relative value of different outcomes, members of the development group included two general practitioners, a social worker, a falls prevention researcher, a district nurse, a physician specializing in care of the elderly, a community nurse manager, and a guidelines facilitator. The authors noted that the absence of a physical therapist or exercise specialist in the development group was partly mitigated by their inclusion on the review panel. There did not appear to be a lay representative of the elderly population on the panel. There was little discussion about how patient preferences were considered (e.g., willingness to attend exercise sessions), although the authors did mention that compliance with wearing hip protectors was a problem for patients.

The guideline developers considered the importance of recent developments. They explicitly stated that they had updated two previous reviews to include any new evidence up to March, 1998. The guideline was published in an October 2000 issue of the *BMJ;* however, the authors stated that because the prevention of falls in older people is an active research area, they recommended that their guidelines be revised by March, 2001.

The authors identified an external review panel, which comprised a public health nurse for the elderly, a physician specializing in care of the elderly, a general practitioner, falls researchers, and an exercise physiologist, to review the guideline. To test the

Continued

---

acceptability of the recommendations to potential users and their feasibility in different care settings, the authors piloted them in two general practices, a residential home, and a general hospital, after which changes were made to the presentation of the recommendations. Unfortunately, no detailed results of the pilot tests were provided.

In summary, this guideline meets the criteria for validity in the inclusion of all falls prevention interventions other than drug or dietary treatments, focus on relevant outcomes, explicit and rigorous search for high-quality evidence, use of a sensible quality-of-evidence scale, multidisciplinary membership of the guideline development panel and the review panel, and piloting of the guideline. It could have been strengthened by participation of a lay representative of the elderly population on the guideline development panel, explicit consideration of issues related to patient preferences and values, and a more detailed reporting of the results of the pilot testing.

WHAT ARE THE RESULTS?

Once you are confident that the clinical practice guideline addresses your clinical question and is based on a rigorous up-to-date assessment of the relevant evidence, you can review the recommendations to determine how useful they will be in your patient care.

Were Practical, Clinically Important Recommendations Made?

To be useful, recommendations should give practical, unambiguous advice about a specific health problem. For guidelines about managing health conditions, you should determine whether the intent is to prevent, screen for, diagnose, treat, or palliate the disorder. For guidelines about the appropriate uses of health interventions, the recommendations should include a definition of the intervention and its optimal role in patient management.

To be clinically important, a practice guideline should convince you that the benefits of following the recommendations are worth the expected harms and costs. You should consider both the relative and absolute changes in outcomes. A 25% reduction in the relative risk of death from a disease is more compelling if it involves a reduction in the proportion of deaths from 40 of 100 to 30 of 100 (an absolute risk reduction of 10 in 100) than if it involves a reduction from 4 of 100 to 3 of 100 (an absolute risk reduction of 1 in 100).[19]

Did the Authors Indicate the Strength of Their Recommendations?

Multiple considerations should inform the strength or grade of recommendations: the quality of the sources contributing to the systematic review or reviews that bring together the relevant evidence, the magnitude and consistency of the intervention effects in different studies, the magnitude of adverse effects, the burden to patients and the health care system, the costs, and the relative value placed on different outcomes. Thus, recommendations may vary from those that rely on evidence from a systematic review of randomized controlled trials that shows large intervention effects on important patient outcomes with minimal side effects, inconvenience, and costs (yielding a strong recommendation) to those that rely on evidence from observational studies showing a small magnitude of intervention effects with appreciable side effects and costs (yielding a weak recommendation).

Grades of Recommendation

The strength of recommendations in practice guidelines can be formally graded. The Canadian Task Force on the Periodic Health Examination proposed the first formal taxonomy of levels of evidence[20,21] focusing on individual studies. Since then, numerous hierarchies for ranking levels of evidence and grades of recommendation have been developed. In Chapter 35, Interpreting Levels of Evidence and Grades of Health Care Recommendations, we review and describe these hierarchies and outline the most recent system currently under development by the Grades of Recommendation Assessment, Development and Evaluation (GRADE) Working Group.

For the purposes of this chapter, we describe an existing framework that has been modified to reflect the fact that practice guidelines should ideally be based on systematic reviews that bring together evidence from the best available individual studies (Table 10-2). The letter grades in Table 10-2 (A, B, C+, and C) reflect a hierarchy of methodological strength that ranges from systematic reviews of randomized trials with consistent results to systematic reviews of observational studies with inconsistent results. Systematic reviews of randomized trials yield the strongest evidence (grade A). Because inferences about the health effects of interventions are weakened when there are unexplained major differences in effects in different studies, guidelines based on systematic reviews of randomized trials are stronger when the results of individual studies are similar (grade A), and guidelines are weaker when major differences between studies (i.e., *heterogeneity*) exist (grade B). Recommendations from observational studies yield weaker evidence (grade C). If the evidence linking interventions and outcomes comes from systematic reviews of original studies, clinicians can apply the criteria for a valid systematic review and the schema in Table 10-2 to decide on the strength of evidence supporting specific recommendations.

The numbers 1 and 2 under Grade of Recommendations in Table 10-2 reflect the balance between the benefits and risks of an intervention. If the benefits clearly outweigh the risks (or vice versa), and virtually all patients would make the same choice, the recommendation is designated as grade 1. When the balance is less certain, and different patients may make different choices, the recommendation is designated as grade 2. Numerous factors may contribute to the uncertainty in the balance between benefits and risks, including variation in patient values and a wide range of confidence intervals around estimates of benefit and risk (see Chapter 35, Interpreting Levels of Evidence and Grades of Health Care Recommendations).

If recommendations are developed based on systematic reviews of observational studies or if the estimate of the magnitude of the intervention effect is imprecise, clinicians can conclude that the recommendations are relatively weak. Investigators can deal with this weakness in recommendations by testing the effect of the guideline on patient outcomes in real-world clinical situations.

Guidelines on hormone replacement therapy demonstrate the limitations of recommendations based on weak evidence. To date, these guidelines have been based largely on observational studies (which would be characterized as 2C in the schema presented in Table 10-2) and have suggested that hormone replacement therapy reduces coronary

Table 10-2 An Approach to Grading Treatment Recommendations Based on Systematic Reviews of the Relevant Evidence

Grade of Recommendation	Balance Between Benefits and Risks	Methodological Strength of Supporting Evidence in Systematic Reviews	Implications
1A	Clear	RCTs without important limitations	Strong recommendation; can apply to most patients in most circumstances without reservation
1B	Clear	RCTs with important limitations (inconsistent results, methodological flaws*)	Strong recommendations; likely to apply to most patients in most circumstances
1 C+	Clear	No RCTs directly addressing the question, but results from closely related RCTs can be unequivocally extrapolated, or evidence from observational studies may be overwhelming	Strong recommendation; can apply to most patients in most circumstances
1C	Clear	Observational studies	Intermediate-strength recommendation; may change when stronger evidence is available
2A	Unclear	RCTs without important limitations	Intermediate-strength recommendation; best action may differ depending on circumstances or patient or societal values
2B	Unclear	RCTs with important limitations (inconsistent results, methodological flaws*)	Weak recommendation; alternative approaches likely to be better for some patients under some circumstances
2C	Unclear	Observational studies	Very weak recommendation; other alternatives may be equally reasonable

*These situations include RCTs with both lack of blinding and subjective outcomes in which the risk of bias in measurement of outcomes is high, and RCTs with large losses to follow-up. Because grade B and C studies are flawed, it is likely that most recommendations in these classes will be level 2. The following considerations will bear on whether the recommendation is grade 1 or 2: the magnitude and precision of the treatment effect, patient risk of the target event being prevented, the nature of the benefit and the magnitude of the risk associated with treatment, variability in patient preferences, variability in regional resource availability and health care delivery practices, and cost considerations. Inevitably, weighing these considerations involves subjective judgment.
RCT, Randomized controlled trial.

Table **10-3**   A Hierarchy of Rigor in Making Treatment
Recommendations

Level of Rigor	Systematic Summary of Evidence	Consideration of Relevant Options and Outcomes	Explicit Statement of Values	Sample Methodologies
High	Yes	Yes	Yes	Practice guideline*
Intermediate	Yes	Yes or no	No	Systematic review*
Low	No	Yes or no	No	Traditional review; article reporting primary research

*Sample methodologies may not reflect the level of rigor shown. Exceptions may occur in either direction. For example, if the author of a practice guideline neither systematically collects nor summarizes information and if neither societal nor patient values are explicitly considered, resulting recommendations will be low in rigor. Conversely, if the author of a systematic review does consider all relevant options and at least qualitatively considers values, resulting recommendations will approach high rigor.

events. A recent randomized controlled trial, however, found that women who received estrogen plus progestin had a greater incidence of total cardiovascular disease than did women who received placebo.[16] Clearly, clinicians should be cautious in their implementation of grade C recommendations.

Table 10-3 presents a schema for classifying the methodological quality of treatment recommendations and emphasizes three key components: a systematic summary of the evidence, consideration of all relevant options and outcomes, and an explicit or quantitative consideration of societal or patient preferences. For example, if a practice guideline is based on a systematic summary of evidence, considers all relevant options and outcomes, and explicitly considers values, the rigor of recommendations will be high. When any of these three components are missing, the rigor of the recommendations will be reduced.

USING THE GUIDE

The authors made a series of practical recommendations related to each of the interventions designed to minimize or prevent exposure to risk factors for falling or fracture in people aged 65 years or older. However, it is difficult to evaluate the clinical importance of the recommendations because no information was provided about the relative or absolute changes in outcomes. Recommendations were graded, incorporating the strength of evidence with the additional considerations of applicability to, and feasibility within, health and social care in the United Kingdom. Grading of recommendations ranged from one to three stars. A one-star recommendation was directly based on grade C evidence (limited scientific evidence, cohort studies, flawed randomized controlled trials, or panel consensus) or was extrapolated from grade A or B evidence; a two-star recommendation was directly based on grade B evidence (single randomized controlled trial or weak inconsistent findings in multiple randomized

Continued

controlled trials) or extrapolated from grade A evidence; a three-star recommendation was directly based on grade A evidence (consistent findings in multiple randomized controlled trials or a meta-analysis).

The recommendations were based on 21 trials. The authors summarized the evidence for each intervention (exercise alone, multifaceted interventions, community-based assessment, and residential setting–based interventions) and provided separate evidence statements for the unselected population and a selected group that included women who were older than 80 years of age, followed by separate recommendations for each of these groups. The authors provided two three-star recommendations:

1. With the possible exception of training in balance (t'ai chi), exercise programs for prevention of falls in unselected older people living in the community should not be established.
2. Programs for prevention of falls should be multifaceted.

They also provided seven two-star recommendations:

1. Individually tailored exercise programs administered by qualified professionals targeted at persons older than 80 years of age should be established.
2. T'ai chi classes with individual instruction should be offered to unselected older people living in the community.
3. Multifaceted programs should prioritize correction of postural hypotension, rationalization of drug use, and interventions to improve balance, transfers, and gait.
4. A structured, interdisciplinary medical and occupational therapy program should be established for older people who have presented to emergency departments for a fall.
5. Nonselective exercise programs for prevention of falls should not be implemented in residential settings.
6. Residents in residential settings who have had at least one fall should be offered a risk assessment program, with referral to their primary physician for specific preventive measures if necessary.
7. All residents of nursing homes should be offered hip protectors.

HOW CAN I APPLY THE RESULTS TO PATIENT CARE?

Is the Primary Objective of the Guideline Consistent With My Objective?

In determining whether to apply the recommendations of a clinical practice guideline to your patients, ask yourself (1) is the purpose of the guideline consistent with the question I am asking? and (2) is the guideline intended for use by clinicians in my type of setting? For example, guidelines that have been developed for use in a primary care setting may not be relevant to other types of settings.

Are the Recommendations Applicable to My Patient Care?

Having established that the clinical practice guideline is valid, you must consider the extent to which the recommendations may apply to the people in your community or the patients in your care. For instance, if the patients in your setting have different prevalences of disease or risk factors, the recommendations may not apply. The flexibility of the recommendations may be indicated by patient or practice characteristics that require individualizing recommendations or that justify departures from the recommendations.

You should consider whether information must be obtained from and provided to patients and how to elicit patient preferences. It is important to consider whether the values assigned (implicitly or explicitly) to outcomes could differ enough from the preferences of patients in your setting to change a decision about whether to adopt a recommendation.

CLINICAL RESOLUTION

You bring a copy of the article by Feder and colleagues[2] to the next team meeting with the public health nurses in the healthy aging program. You note that the guideline developers clearly specified the patient population, interventions, and outcomes to which their recommendations would pertain. They used a comprehensive strategy to locate all relevant evidence on which to base their recommendations, and they rated the quality of the evidence using an established scale. The guideline development panel included representation from numerous relevant disciplines. The authors were careful to ensure that the guidelines were current by updating two previous reviews and specifying a date after which the guidelines should be revised. They asked an external panel to review the guidelines and pilot tested them in numerous settings. You note that the guideline development process could have been strengthened by the following:

- Assessment of the effects of drug and dietary treatments on falls
- Inclusion of additional outcomes such as muscle strength, balance, quality of life, and costs
- Inclusion of a lay representative of the elderly population on the development panel
- Explicit consideration of patient preferences and values
- Presentation of data on relative and absolute changes in outcomes
- Provision of more details about the results of pilot testing.

You add that the authors explained in their conclusion that none of the trials included an economic evaluation and that exercise was not well defined in the trials and could include several different elements, such as muscle strengthening and balance training.

You then review the recommendations with the team and pay special attention to the grading of the recommendations. To ensure that you have the most up-to-date information, you have also brought along a copy of the Cochrane review on interventions for preventing falls in elderly people (latest update July 2003).[22] There are several similarities between the recommendations in the guidelines and the interventions shown to be beneficial in the systematic review. However, because the guideline developers did not examine the effects of drug and dietary treatments on falls, there is additional information in the Cochrane review that could inform the public health nurses' practice. The nurses decide that a small group will review the guideline recommendations in conjunction with the Cochrane review and return to the next team meeting with suggestions for changes in practice.

IMPLEMENTATION OF CLINICAL PRACTICE GUIDELINES

Implementing clinical practice guidelines is recognized as a significant process of change for an organization, particularly if current practice differs from guideline recommendations.[23-25] Systematic reviews suggest that clinical practice guidelines are most likely to be adopted in practice when dissemination and implementation strategies incorporate several features, such as involvement of end-user clinicians in guideline development, active involvement of learners in the educational intervention, and integration of the guideline into the process of care (e.g., restructuring of medical records).[26] A multifaceted dissemination and implementation strategy is more likely to increase the probability of uptake in practice than is reliance on a single intervention.[26-29] DiCenso and colleagues[30] developed a toolkit for implementation of clinical practice guidelines, which is available on the Internet *(www.rnao.org)*. The toolkit is based on a conceptual model that depicts five essential components of guideline implementation:

1. Selection of a high-quality, up-to-date, evidence-based guideline
2. Identification and engagement of key stakeholders who can influence implementation success
3. Assessment of environmental readiness for guideline implementation
4. Use of multiple proven implementation strategies (e.g., interactive education sessions and reminder systems; see Chapter 11, Changing Nursing Practice in an Organization)
5. Evaluation of guideline implementation.

To ensure successful guideline implementation, an organization must be willing to provide the necessary human, physical, and financial resources. Because this toolkit was developed only recently, its effectiveness and utility in facilitating guideline implementation requires validation by empirical research.

REFERENCES

1. Eddy DM. *A Manual for Assessing Health Practices and Designing Practice Policies: The Explicit Approach.* Philadelphia: American College of Physicians, 1992.
2. Feder G, Cryer C, Donovan S, Carter Y. Guidelines for the prevention of falls in people over 65. *BMJ.* 2000;321:1007-1011.
3. Shaneyfelt TM, Mayo-Smith MF, Rothwangl J. Are guidelines following guidelines? The methodological quality of clinical practice guidelines in the peer-reviewed medical literature. *JAMA.* 1999;281:1900-1905.
4. Grilli R, Magrini N, Penna A, Mura G, Liberati A. Practice guidelines developed by specialty societies: the need for a critical appraisal. *Lancet.* 2000;355:103-106.
5. Field MJ, Lohr KN, eds. *Clinical Practice Guidelines: Directions for a New Program.* Washington, DC: National Academy Press, 1990.
6. Hayward RS, Laupacis A. Initiating, conducting and maintaining guidelines development programs. *Can Med Assoc J.* 1993;148:507-512.
7. Grimshaw J, Eccles M, Russell I. Developing clinically valid practice guidelines. *J Eval Clin Pract.* 1995;1:37-48.
8. Field MJ, Lohr KN, eds. *Guidelines for Clinical Practice: From Development to Use.* Washington, DC: National Academy Press, 1992.
9. Browman GP, Levine MN, Mohide EA, et al. The practice guidelines development cycle: a conceptual tool for practice guidelines development and implementation. *J Clin Oncol.* 1995;13:502-512.
10. Grinspun D, Virani T, Bajnok I. Nursing best practice guidelines: the RNAO project. *Hosp Q.* 2002;5:56-60.

11. Thomas L, Cullum N, McColl E, Rousseau N, Soutter J, Steen N. Guidelines in professions allied to medicine. *Cochrane Database Syst Rev.* 2000;(2):CD000349.

12. Graham ID, Calder LA, Hebert PC, Carter AO, Tetroe JM. A comparison of clinical practice guideline appraisal instruments. *Int J Technol Assess Health Care.* 2000;16:1024-1038.

13. Glasziou PP, Irwig LM. An evidence based approach to individualising treatment. *BMJ.* 1995;311:1356-1358.

14. Sinclair JC, Cook RJ, Guyatt GH, Pauker SG, Cook DJ. When should an effective treatment be used? Derivation of the threshold number needed to treat and the minimum event rate for treatment. *J Clin Epidemiol.* 2001;54:253-262.

15. Smith GD, Egger M. Who benefits from medical interventions? *BMJ.* 1994;308:72-74.

16. Rossouw JE, Anderson GL, Prentice RL, et al. Risks and benefits of estrogen plus progestin in healthy post-menopausal women: principal results from the Women's Health Initiative randomized controlled trial. *JAMA.* 2002;288:321-333.

17. Grady D, Herrington D, Bittner V, et al. Cardiovascular disease outcomes during 6.8 years of hormone therapy: Heart and Estrogen/progestin Replacement Study follow-up (HERS II). *JAMA.* 2002;288:49-57.

18. Weingarten SR, Reidinger MS, Conner L, et al. Practice guidelines and reminders to reduce duration of hospital stay for patients with chest pain. *Ann Intern Med.* 1994;120:257-263.

19. Laupacis A, Naylor CD, Sackett DL. How should the results of clinical trials be presented to clinicians? *ACP J Club.* 1992;116:A12-A14.

20. Canadian Task Force on the Periodic Health Examination. The periodic health examination. *Can Med Assoc J.* 1979;121:1193-1254.

21. Woolf SH, Battista RN, Anderson GM, Logan AG, Wang E. Assessing the clinical effectiveness of preventive maneuvers: analytic principles and systematic methods in reviewing evidence and developing clinical practice recommendations. *J Clin Epidemiol.* 1990;43:891-905.

22. Gillespie LD, Gillespie WJ, Robertson MC, Lamb SE, Cumming RG, Rowe BH. Interventions for preventing falls in elderly people. *Cochrane Database Syst Rev.* 2003;(4):CD000340.

23. Grol R. Successes and failures in the implementation of evidence-based guidelines for clinical practice. *Med Care.* 2001;39:1146-1154.

24. Moulding NT, Silagy CA, Weller DP. A framework for effective management of change in clinical practice: dissemination and implementation of clinical practice guidelines. *Qual Health Care.* 1999;8:177-183.

25. Solberg LI, Brekke ML, Fazio CJ, et al. Lessons from experienced guideline implementers: attend to many factors and use multiple strategies. *Jt Comm J Qual Improv.* 2000;26:171-188.

26. Davies J, Freemantle N, Grimshaw J, et al. Implementing clinical practice guidelines: can guidelines be used to improve clinical practice? *Eff Health Care.* 1994;8:1-12.

27. Grimshaw JM, Russell IT. Effect of clinical guidelines on medical practice: a systematic review of rigorous evaluations. *Lancet.* 1993;342:1317-1322.

28. Oxman AD, Thomson MA, Davis DA, et al. No magic bullets: a systematic review of 102 trials of interventions to improve professional practice. *Can Med Assoc J.* 1995;153:1423-1431.

29. Bero LA, Grilli R, Grimshaw JM, Harvey E, Oxman AD, Thomson MA. Closing the gap between research and practice: an overview of systematic reviews of interventions to promote the implementation of research findings. *BMJ.* 1998;317:465-468.

30. DiCenso A, Virani T, Bajnok I, et al. A toolkit to facilitate the implementation of clinical practice guidelines in healthcare settings. *Hosp Q.* 2002;5:55-60.

11

Changing Nursing Practice in an Organization

Maureen Dobbins, Donna Ciliska, Carole Estabrooks, and Sarah Hayward

The following Editorial Board members also made substantive contributions to this chapter: Linda Johnston, Cathy Kessenich, Dorothy McCaughan, Mark Newman, and Ania Willman.

In This Chapter

Framework for Adopting an Evidence-Based Innovation in an Organization
    Knowledge
    Persuasion
    Decision
    Implementation
    Confirmation

CLINICAL SCENARIO

Promoting Control of Asthma: How to Change Clinical Practice in an Organization

You are a clinical educator in an asthma clinic in a large community hospital. You recently attended the annual conference of the Registered Nurses Association of Ontario (RNAO) and learned that the association is developing, pilot testing, evaluating, and disseminating *best practice guidelines* for nurses.[1] One of the recently completed practice guidelines is related to asthma control. You learn that the RNAO is seeking organizations to pilot test the implementation of this guideline. You review the guideline and find considerable variation between current practice in your clinic and the guideline recommendations. You decide to talk with your immediate supervisor about submitting a proposal to the RNAO to implement the *Adult Asthma Care Guidelines for Nurses*[2] in your clinic. Although your supervisor is generally supportive, she asks you first to do a bit of homework to answer three questions: (1) Do other asthma control guidelines exist, and, if so, why implement this one? (2) Is the methodology used to create this guideline sufficiently rigorous, and are the recommendations based on high-quality evidence? and (3) What is the best process for implementing practice change in an organization? Prepared for a challenge, you go off to find the answers to these questions.

The completion and publication of high-quality research do not ensure its translation into practice. In fact, there can be a substantial time lag of 8 to 15 years between the generation of technical information and its use in practice[3] or in policy development.[4]

In the case of nursing practice, this situation is further complicated by the fact that most nurses work in organizations such as hospitals, public health departments, or long-term care settings and must adhere to the policies and procedures stipulated by the setting. Thus, even if a nurse learns about a new evidence-based strategy, he or she must often wait until administrators of the organization choose to adopt the strategy before a change in practice can occur. In the case of pressure sore prevention, for example, nurses have the decision-making autonomy to make some changes in their practice, such as ensuring frequent position changes and massaging areas of weight bearing.[5] However, other interventions, such as the purchase of high-specification foam mattresses,[5] require approval of senior administrators. In this chapter, we describe a framework to facilitate the adoption of an evidence-based practice in an organization. To illustrate the framework, we have created a hypothetical scenario and have drawn partially from the RNAO's experience in the pilot implementation and evaluation of the *Adult Asthma Care Guidelines for Nurses.*[2]

FRAMEWORK FOR ADOPTING AN EVIDENCE-BASED INNOVATION IN AN ORGANIZATION

Several frameworks describe the process of transferring research findings to practice,[6-10] some of which are specific to nursing.[11-20] Although the frameworks vary in terminology and structure, they include similar innovation adoption processes and identify similar explanatory variables. In this chapter, we use the framework by Dobbins and colleagues[7] to illustrate the steps involved in changing practice in a group, unit, ward, or organization. The framework is based on the Diffusion of Innovations theory,[21] which includes five stages: knowledge, persuasion, decision, implementation, and confirmation (Figure 11-1). Innovations in health care may be preventive, curative, rehabilitative, or palliative, and they may encompass instruments, equipment, drugs, procedures, services, and programs used in the delivery of health care.[22]

During the knowledge phase, we identify the relevant evidence about a new health care intervention and appraise the quality of the evidence. Having determined that the evidence is of high quality, we move to the persuasion stage of the framework to consider how characteristics of the innovation, organization, environment, and individual influence decisions to adopt the innovation. During the decision stage, we consider the research evidence along with other relevant information, such as health care resources, organizational culture, patient preferences, clinical circumstances, and clinical expertise, and we make a decision to adopt or not to adopt the innovation. If we choose to adopt it, we move on to the implementation stage, during which we may use multiple strategies to spread the word about the innovation to those responsible for its implementation. In the final stage, confirmation, we evaluate whether the innovation was successfully adopted into practice. Depending on the results of the evaluation, we affirm our decisions or revisit them in light of new information. Confirmation therefore creates an iterative loop in the process and leads back to the knowledge stage. Having provided an overview of the framework, we offer a series of guides to help readers move systematically through the process of changing nursing practice in an organization.

Knowledge

Did the Search for the Evidence Identify the Most Highly Synthesized Current Information?

The innovation adoption process begins with the identification of a clinical or health care system problem that leads to a search of the research literature for a potential solution. As we describe in Chapter 2, Finding the Evidence, information seekers should begin by looking at the most current and highest level resource available for the problem.[23] At the top of the resource hierarchy are *systems,* which include practice guidelines, clinical pathways, or evidence-based textbook summaries that integrate evidence-based information about specific clinical problems and provide regular updates. When no evidence-based information system exists for a clinical problem, then *synopses of syntheses (systematic reviews)* are the next best source. These synopses encapsulate the key methodological details and findings of a systematic review and often include a commentary with recommendations for application of the findings to practice. Moving down the hierarchy, *syntheses* provide clinicians with a systematic review of all evidence addressing a focused clinical question. Toward the bottom of the hierarchy are *synopses of single studies,* followed by preprocessed *single studies* that have been selected because they are both highly relevant and have study designs that minimize bias and thus permit a high strength of inference.

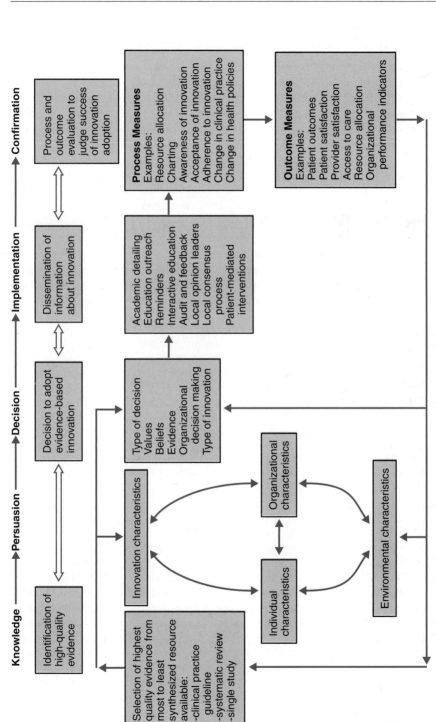

Figure 11–1. Framework for adopting an evidence-based innovation in an organization.

Were the Results of the Research Valid and Applicable to Patients in My Setting?

Once the evidence is found, we use the corresponding guides to evaluate the validity of the results and the applicability to patients in our setting. For *clinical practice guidelines*, we apply the guides described in Chapter 10, Moving from Evidence to Action Using Clinical Practice Guidelines; for systematic reviews, we apply the guides described in Chapter 9, Summarizing the Evidence Through Systematic Reviews; and for single studies evaluating health care interventions, we apply the guides described in Chapter 4, Health Care Interventions. If we conclude, based on the relevant guides, that the results are valid and applicable to our patients, we move on to the persuasion stage of the framework.

USING THE GUIDE

You consider whether the RNAO *Adult Asthma Care Guidelines for Nurses*[2] represent the most highly synthesized current information available and include valid recommendations applicable to patients in your setting. Your first instinct is to go to the National Guideline Clearinghouse (*www.guideline.gov*), a major source of clinical practice guidelines of relevance to nursing (see Chapter 2, Finding the Evidence, and Chapter 10, Moving from Evidence to Action Using Clinical Practice Guidelines). However, you note that the RNAO guideline developers conducted an extremely comprehensive search of MEDLINE, EMBASE/Excerpta Medica, CINAHL, the Cochrane Library, and 42 Web sites for existing asthma guidelines, and one of the Web sites was the National Guideline Clearinghouse. The developers decided to formulate the guideline on the basis of seven existing guidelines that met the following criteria: published in English, developed in 1995 or later, focused solely on asthma, based on evidence, and assigned high scores in rigor based on the Appraisal Instrument for Clinical Guidelines.[24,25] You conclude that although many other asthma care guidelines exist, this one is likely to be the most current, while at the same time taking into account the content of existing well-developed guidelines.

You next determine whether the methodology used to create this guideline is sufficiently rigorous and whether the recommendations are based on high-quality evidence (see Chapter 10, Moving from Evidence to Action Using Clinical Practice Guidelines for guides to appraise clinical practice guidelines). You note that the panel began by extracting recommendations and content from the seven guidelines and identified key areas for nursing intervention recommendations. The panel reviewed systematic reviews and primary research studies to formulate recommendations and categorized them by *level of evidence,* with level 1 based on "randomized controlled trials (or meta-analyses of such trials) of adequate size to ensure a low risk of incorporating false-positive or false-negative results."[2] The developers used an explicit and sensible process to identify, select, and combine evidence. They sent the guidelines to external stakeholders for peer review and made minor revisions as a result of this feedback. You determine that the RNAO *Adult Asthma Care Guidelines for Nurses* represent highly synthesized current information and were carefully and rigorously developed.

There are three recommendations in the guidelines supported by level 1 evidence, and you would like to begin by proposing the implementation of one of these three. The recommendation you have chosen to implement states that "every client with asthma should have an individualized asthma action plan for guided self-management based on evaluation of symptoms with or without peak flow measurement developed in partnership with a health care professional."[2] An action plan is "an individualized written plan developed for the purpose of client self-management of asthma."[26] The plan guides self-monitoring of asthma based on the level of asthma control and directs patient management according to that level (e.g., seeking medical attention and/or adjusting medication). It is developed in partnership between individual patients and asthma care providers. Often, asthma action plans use a traffic light analogy, having green, yellow, and red zones. The green zone represents stable asthma control; the yellow zone represents signs of worsening asthma and the need to adjust medications and/or seek medical assistance; and the red zone represents asthma that is out of control and severe enough to warrant urgent medical attention (Figure 11-2 is an example of an action plan).

According to the RNAO guideline, it is the role of the nurse to facilitate the attainment and effective use of an individualized action plan developed in partnership with the physician and the rest of the asthma care team. A Cochrane review [26] concluded that self-management programs for adults with asthma that involved self-monitoring, either by peak flow or symptoms, combined with a written action plan and regular medical review, resulted in reduced health services use, fewer days lost from work, and fewer episodes of nocturnal asthma. Your hospital does not currently use individualized action plans.

The third question posed by your supervisor focused on the best process for implementing practice change in an organization. You contact a nursing faculty colleague and you learn from her that certain frameworks facilitate the transfer of research findings to practice. You review these frameworks, find substantial consistency among them, and decide to use one developed by Dobbins and colleagues.[7]

You are now ready to meet with your supervisor to answer her questions. She is sufficiently impressed with the information you provide and agrees to support your decision to submit a proposal to the RNAO to pilot test the implementation of the *Adult Asthma Care Guidelines for Nurses*, initially beginning with one recommendation. You submit the proposal and are successful. Your next step is to identify characteristics that could influence the decision to adopt the recommendation in your clinic.

Persuasion

What Characteristics of the Innovation, Organization, Environment, and Individual Are Likely to Influence the Adoption of the New Practice?

During the persuasion stage, decision makers and practitioners form attitudes about the innovation and consider the consequences of adopting or not adopting it.[27] Characteristics of the innovation, organization, environment, and individual play key roles in influencing innovation adoption behaviors. To date, most of the research examining the relationship between these characteristics and innovation adoption has used a design that examines the relationship between two or more variables at one point in time. The weakness of this design is that, depending on the nature of the characteristic, it is sometimes impossible to tell which came first. Did the characteristic influence innovation adoption or did the innovation adoption influence the characteristic? Longitudinal designs in which information about the characteristic is gathered before adoption of the innovation establish a temporal relationship and are therefore preferable.

Individuals have the ability to shape their organizations and environments just as organizations and environments shape individual behavior.[28,29] This relationship was highlighted many decades ago when Hassinger[30] suggested that even if individuals are exposed to an innovation, this exposure will have little effect unless the innovation is perceived as relevant and consistent with the individual's attitudes and the perceived attitudes of others in the organization. Rogers[21] noted that information about the consequences of adoption is usually sought from like-minded peers who have previously

	LEVEL	STATUS	ACTION
All Clear • No symptoms of an asthma episode • Able to do usual activities • Usual medications control asthma	1	Doing well	**Take:** Medicine Dose Max # times/day _____ _____ _____ _____ _____ _____ _____ _____ _____
Caution • Increased asthma symptoms (including wakening at night due to asthma) • Usual activities somewhat limited • Increased need for asthma medications	2	Increase in symptoms	**Add:** Medicine Dose Max # times/day _____ _____ _____ _____ _____ _____ Return to Level 1 when symptoms improve.
Medical Alert • Increased symptoms longer than 24 hrs • Very short of breath • Usual activities severely limited • Asthma medications have not reduced symptoms	3	No improvement after___hrs OR Even more symptoms	**Add:** Medicine Dose _____ _____ _____ _____ And call your provider.
	Danger signs	• Difficulty walking and talking due to shortness of breath • Lips or fingernails are blue ⇒ **Go to the hospital now** ⇒ **Or call 911 now**	

Figure 11–2,A. An asthma action plan (symptom monitoring). *(Modified and reproduced with permission of the Kaiser Permanente Center for Health Research, Portland, OR.)*

	LEVEL	STATUS	ACTION

Green Zone: All Clear
My best peak flow:_____
 	
Peak flow ____ to ____
(100% to 80% of my best
peak flow)
• No symptoms of an
  asthma episode
• Able to do usual activities
• Usual medications control
  asthma
	1	Doing well	**Take:**
			Medicine Dose Max #
			                                times/day
			_____ _____ _____
			_____ _____ _____
			_____ _____ _____

Yellow Zone: Caution
Peak flow ____ to ____
(80% to 50% of my best
peak flow)
• Increased asthma symptoms
  (including wakening at night
  due to asthma)
• Usual activities somewhat
  limited
• Increased need for asthma
  medications
	2	Increase in
		symptoms
			Add:
			Medicine Dose Max #
			                                times/day
			_____ _____ _____
			
			Return to Level 1 when
			symptoms improve.

Red Zone: Medical Alert
Peak flow less than_____
(50% of my best peak flow)
• Increased symptoms longer
  than 24 hrs
• Very short of breath
• Usual activities severely
  limited
• Asthma medications have
  not reduced symptoms
	3	No
		improvement
		after___hrs
		OR
		even more
		symptoms
			Add:
			Medicine Dose
			
			_____ _____
			_____ _____
			
			And call your provider.

	Danger signs	• Difficulty walking and talking due to shortness of breath • Lips or fingernails are blue ⇒ **Go to the hospital now** ⇒ **Or call 911 now**	

Figure 11–2,B. An asthma action plan (peak flow monitoring).

adopted the innovation. If colleagues are positive about adopting an innovation, motivation to adopt it increases. We now examine how characteristics of the innovation, organization, environment, and individual influence change in practice.

Innovation Characteristics. Rogers[21] suggested that five specific attributes of an innovation are associated with higher diffusion rates: advantage, compatibility, complexity, trialability, and observability. Innovations that are perceived to provide more relative advantage and are more compatible, less complex, easier to assess by trial, and easier to observe are more readily adopted. Table 11-1 defines and summarizes the impact of these five innovation characteristics on innovation adoption.

Researchers have shown that (1) previous practice provides a familiar standard against which an innovation can be interpreted and compared *(compatibility)*;[21] (2) potential adopters prefer to read research studies that are written plainly, have minimal statistical data explained in uncomplicated language, and are presented in an attractive way *(complexity)*;[31,32] (3) organizations imitate other organizations that are proximate either geographically or in their communication networks and will adopt innovations when other organizations have adopted them *(trialability)*;[33-36] and (4) the greater is the degree of *observability*, the greater is the rate of adoption.[37]

Organizational Characteristics. Organizational context has a major influence on decision makers' and practitioners' behaviors in response to innovation.[14,22,32,38] This influence was first identified in 1971 in a study conducted on a national sample of hospitals in the United States. Veney and colleagues[39] found that organizational variables accounted for 41% of the observed variation in innovation adoption among health care professionals compared with 5% of the observed variation explained by characteristics of the chief administrator of the hospital. Since that time, numerous studies have been published describing and assessing the impact of organizational characteristics on innovation adoption. Table 11-2 defines and summarizes organizational characteristics found to influence innovation adoption.

Organizations that have high functional differentiation, a culture that values the use of research evidence in practice, effective communication systems, decentralized decision making, managerial support for change, and adequate resources are more likely to adopt innovations. Innovation promoters can assess these characteristics within their organization to identify naturally occurring facilitators and barriers to evidence-based practice and can use that knowledge to optimize the impact of those characteristics that facilitate innovation and minimize those that pose barriers.

Environmental Characteristics. There is increasing emphasis on the importance of environmental factors in the adoption of research evidence in policy and practice. Environmental characteristics that influence adoption of innovations among health services organizations include reporting relationships, urbanization, network embeddedness, and regulations and legislation. Table 11-3 defines and summarizes environmental characteristics found to be significantly associated with innovation adoption.

Organizations that have positive reporting relationships between senior administrators and the governing board, those that are located in affluent urban centers where peer pressure and competition are present, and those that are viewed as prestigious are more likely to adopt innovations. Persons responsible for promoting a change in practice can conduct an environmental scan to identify and address potential barriers and to identify factors that will promote the use of evidence in practice.

Table **11-1** Characteristics of the Innovation That Influence Its Adoption

Characteristic[21]	Definition	Effect on Adoption
Relative advantage	Degree to which an innovation is perceived as better than the idea it supersedes; measured in economic terms, social prestige, satisfaction, and savings in time and effort	Positive association between relative advantage and innovation adoption[21]
Compatibility	Degree to which an innovation is perceived as being consistent with the existing values, needs, and past experiences of potential adopters	Positive association between high compatibility and innovation adoption[21]
Complexity	Degree to which an innovation is perceived as difficult to understand and use	Negative association between the complexity of the innovation and adoption[31, 32]
Trialability	Extent to which the innovation can be implemented on a small scale to determine its advantages or disadvantages	Positive association between increased trialability and innovation adoption[33-36]
Observability	Evaluation of the consequences of adopting the innovation; measured using organizational performance indicators (i.e., decreased costs, improved efficiency), patient outcomes (i.e., decreased mortality or morbidity, increased quality of life, patient satisfaction) or health systems outcomes (i.e., resource allocation, expenditures)	Positive association between increased observability and innovation adoption[37]

Table **11-2** Characteristics of the Organization That Influence Adoption of an Innovation

Characteristic[40]	Definition	Effect on Adoption
Structure		
Organizational size	Full-time equivalent staff	Direction of association varies across organizations[40, 41]
Functional differentiation	Number of divisions	Positive association between number of divisions and innovation adoption[40, 42]
Administrative intensity	Manager-to-staff ratio	Direction of association varies across organizations[40]
Complexity	Number of services	Positive association between number of services and innovation adoption[38, 40-44]
Workplace Culture		
Values	Value organization places on use of research evidence	Positive association between value organization places on research use and innovation adoption[38, 45-47]
Communication Systems		
Internal and external communication channels	Mechanisms that promote the flow of information into and within an organization	Positive association between increased flow of information into and within an organization and innovation adoption[38, 40, 42]
Leadership Support		
Decision making	Centralized or decentralized	Negative association between centralized decision making and innovation adoption[38, 42]
Managerial attitude toward change	Support given by managers toward changes based on evidence	Positive association between managerial attitude and innovation adoption[40]
Resources	Resources available to facilitate the implementation of the innovation	Positive association between increased availability of resources and innovation adoption[40]

Table 11-3 Characteristics of the Environment That Influence Adoption of an Innovation

Characteristic	Definition	Effect on Adoption
Reporting Relationships		
Senior administrators and the board of their agency (e.g., hospital board)	Quality of the relationship between senior administrators and the board	Positive association between quality of relationship and innovation adoption[41]
Urbanization		
Urban or rural	Location of organization in an urban or rural area	Positive association between urban location and innovation adoption[42]
City or regional resources	Amount of financial resources of the city or region in which the organization is situated	Positive association between financial resources of the city or region and innovation adoption[48]
Network Embeddedness		
Decision making autonomy of organization	Degree to which the organization must negotiate decisions with other organizations in the city or region	Direction of association varies across studies[49]
Peer pressure	Extent of pressure exerted by peers to adopt innovation	Positive association between adoption behavior of peers at the organization level and innovation adoption[33,41]
Competition	Level of competition for resources and patients existing in the city or region	Positive association between level of competition between organizations and innovation adoption[43]
Prestige	Level of prestige assigned to the organization in comparison to other organizations	Positive association between level of prestige an organization has in a city or region and innovation adoption[41]
Regulation and Legislation		
Local, state or provincial, federal	Impact of regulations and legislation on innovation adoption	Direction of association varies across studies and type of innovation[48]

Individual Characteristics. Estabrooks and colleagues[50] completed a systematic review in which they examined six categories of potential individual determinants of research use: beliefs and attitudes, involvement in research activities, information seeking, professional characteristics, education, and other socioeconomic factors. These investigators found that methodological problems surfaced in all the studies, and, except for attitude to research, there was little to suggest that any potential individual determinant influences research use.

However, certain individual characteristics have been identified as barriers to use of research evidence in practice and provide a useful guide for evidence-based promoters in identifying characteristics of nurses that will hinder evidence-based practice. For example, many health care practitioners and decision makers perceive research findings as irrelevant to their practice or decision-making needs.[12,45,51-55] Other barriers include limited decision-making authority to change patient care procedures, insufficient time to implement new ideas, insufficient time to review literature, and lack of critical appraisal skills.[45,51,55-61] Early identification of individual-level barriers allows incorporation of strategies to overcome these barriers into the implementation plan.

A clinical nurse educator may determine that some nurses have negative attitudes toward the relevance of research to practice and do not perceive themselves as having the decision-making authority to change practice. In this instance, the nurse educator could include activities in the implementation plan to help nurses understand the specific relevance of the innovation to their practice and to highlight those practice decisions they have the authority to make.

Readiness for adoption of an innovation will depend on how the innovation itself, the organization, the environment, and the individual members of the organization score on the characteristics described earlier. Based on this assessment, we can create a list of the facilitators and barriers that may influence adoption of the innovation. Careful analysis of the list of barriers determines whether to proceed with implementing an innovation and what must be done in the setting before or during the implementation phase.

USING THE GUIDE

You assess the characteristics of the innovation, organization, environment, and individual to identify factors that will either facilitate or hinder the implementation process. Your assessment reveals the following:

Innovation Characteristics

In discussion with your team, you determine that the implementation of individualized action plans represents a more effective management strategy than what currently exists in the asthma clinic (relative advantage) and that the move toward enhanced asthma control among adult patients is compatible with the goals and objectives of the clinic as well as the hospital as a whole (compatibility). Although the initial work to implement the recommendation is complex and requires considerable discussion and negotiation (complexity), it will be possible to try out the action plans on a small scale before full implementation (trialability). Finally, you determine several indicators of success, some of which can be evaluated in the short term, to demonstrate the effectiveness of the implementation plan (observability). You realize, however, that new data collection mechanisms will need to be developed to evaluate some of these measures.

Organizational Characteristics

You identify the following characteristics in your organization that should facilitate implementation of the guideline recommendation. Your organization is a large, acute care, community hospital with many divisions (high functional differentiation) and provides a wide variety of services (high complexity). The culture of your organization, at least at the senior management level, is one that values and recognizes the need for the use of evidence in practice (workplace culture), and your direct supervisor strongly supports the implementation of the *Adult Asthma Care Guidelines for Nurses* (managerial support for change). Without funding from the RNAO to pilot test the implementation of the asthma guidelines, there would be inadequate resources within the organization's budget to implement these guidelines (resources). You recognize that your organization has two characteristics that could act as barriers to implementing the guidelines. Decisions in your organization historically tend to be more centralized than decentralized, and communication systems are inadequate to promote the flow of information effectively within the organization. You realize you will need to address these issues early in the implementation process.

Environmental Characteristics

You identify certain characteristics that should facilitate the implementation process. You know that a positive relationship exists between senior administrators and the chief executive officer and the hospital board (reporting relationship). You are also situated in a large urban center (urbanization). Finally, you are regarded as an organization of high prestige by the community (prestige). You identify, however, two characteristics that could act as barriers to the implementation process: peer pressure and competition. Given that you are the largest hospital in the area and the only one to provide asthma services to adults in the region, there is little pressure exerted from peers to change practice, nor is there competition from other services. You take note of these two issues, but you realize that these factors are out of your control and decide to focus your attention on highlighting those environmental characteristics that could facilitate the implementation process.

Individual Characteristics

You complete your assessment by considering characteristics of the individual members of your organization. You are particularly interested in identifying characteristics that are likely to hinder the implementation process. You identify two factors that will need to be addressed early in the implementation process. Nurses perceive their decision-making authority to change practice as being very low, and they have little time to implement new ideas, particularly if it requires additional activities on their part.

Having completed your assessment of the innovation, organization, environment, and individuals, and having identified many more facilitators than barriers, you feel more positive about the task ahead and begin to plan the next steps of the implementation process. You are careful to consider characteristics that will help to facilitate the process and begin to brainstorm around actions that can be taken to overcome, or at least minimize, the effects of the identified barriers. You are now ready to engage the necessary stakeholders in the organization.

Decision

Who Are the Key Stakeholders Who Should Be Involved in the Decision to Adopt the Innovation?

The early identification and support of stakeholders who influence whether and how an innovation is implemented are central to changing nursing practice.[19] *Stakeholders* are individuals, groups, or organizations that can directly or indirectly affect the decision to adopt the innovation and its implementation. Stakeholders can include staff nurses, the chief nursing officer, advanced practice nurses, physicians, other members of the health care team, and senior management from other sectors, for example, accounting, quality improvement, pharmacy, and nutrition. A *stakeholder analysis* assesses the values, interests, and beliefs of key persons who may have an impact on the proposed change, assesses their level of support, and identifies possible ways to engage their interests.[62] Through this process, champions of the practice change are identified. It is important to reassess stakeholder values, beliefs, and interests routinely throughout the implementation process.[19]

A study by Davies and colleagues[63] emphasized the importance of stakeholder influence on promoting the use of high-quality evidence for women in labor. The investigators evaluated the effect of a tailored intervention to promote continuous labor support by nurses and to decrease the use of electronic fetal monitoring for low-risk women. Results of this intervention study, as determined by chart audits and randomly selected observations of nursing practice, were mixed. At the hospitals where practice changes occurred, there was good stakeholder involvement in the implementation of the specific recommendation, whether it was labor support or electronic fetal monitoring.

What Factors Need to Be Considered to Make an Evidence-Based Decision?

During the decision stage, administrators and other key stakeholders in the organization engage in decision-making activities to decide whether to adopt the innovation. The decision-making process consists of a series of actions and choices through which an organization evaluates a new idea.[21] This process is shaped by the values, interests, and beliefs of the individual decision makers. For example, persons tend to expose themselves to ideas that are in accordance with their interests, needs, and attitudes, and they consciously or unconsciously avoid messages that conflict with their predispositions.[21] An evidence-based decision-making process considers not only the research findings, but also the values and beliefs of the organization, the health care resources, and, depending on the nature of the intervention, the clinical expertise of the staff. The decision makers may choose to adopt a specific research finding in whole or in part or in a modified way; they may choose not to adopt it; or they may choose to use the research evidence to justify their current practice.

USING THE GUIDE

You realize that adoption of the guideline recommendation will require considerable discussion and negotiation among the key stakeholders including physicians, respiratory specialists, and nurses. You also realize that support from senior administrators and department heads will be necessary for the organization to accept the new role of nurses as coordinators of patient care. As coordinators of patient care, nurses will ensure that all treatment plans are agreed to and signed off by the necessary health disciplines within the asthma care team.

As a result of developing the proposal for RNAO, many of the necessary stakeholders are already aware of the guideline implementation project. You also know that some of the key stakeholders, for example the director of the asthma clinic, the director of nursing, and the emergency department director, are in favor of implementing individualized action plans. However, you are aware that front-line staff, particularly nurses in the asthma clinic and emergency department, as well as physicians and respiratory specialists, have resisted changes to practice in the past.

This provides an opportune time to assist the organization in moving away from centralized decision making toward a decentralized process. Your initial strategies purposefully include activities that will facilitate decentralized decision making. For example, you begin by scheduling a meeting with the asthma clinic director, the director of nursing, and the emergency department director. During the meeting, you outline the scope of the implementation project, identify other key stakeholders, and devise a plan to facilitate the participation of all key stakeholders in the planning and implementation phases of the project.

With the endorsement of the directors, you write a letter inviting all stakeholders to the official launch of the guideline project, at which time you will ask for representatives from each stakeholder group to work collaboratively in developing a template for individualized action plans. You negotiate with the three directors that they will each take a leadership role during the launch event in presenting the project, expressing their commitment to the project, and garnering support from the necessary stakeholders. To facilitate support from the necessary stakeholder groups, the directors agree to speak personally with practitioners who are well respected by their peers and to ensure their participation in the planning and implementation phases of the project. The hope is that these practitioners will act as champions of the new practice recommendation. After weeks of planning and the development of promotional material, an official launch event is held.

You recall from your environmental scan that some barriers to the successful implementation of the recommendation were identified in your organization. Your early activity of holding a planning meeting with the three key directors and obtaining their support in bringing front-line staff into the decision-making process will facilitate a shift from centralized to decentralized decision making, for this decision at least. Feedback about previous attempts to change clinical practice in the organization indicates that there was an inadequate flow of information within the organization, often causing some front-line staff members to feel isolated and excluded from the process. You plan to address this barrier by developing a protocol for the communication of information between departments and among team members.

You also realize that the success of implementing the recommendation will be contingent on the nurses' belief that they have the decision-making authority to implement the recommendation, as well as the physicians' acceptance of this authority.

Continued

To address this issue, you ensure that well-respected members of the nursing and medical departments are included in the planning process so that each member will feed back decisions from the group to their respective disciplines. You also plan to include discussions on this topic in all the educational sessions you hold. Finally, you realize that there will be significant resistance to implementing the recommendation if it requires additional time on the part of nurses. You are sure to include in the promotional materials and discussions during the launch, research findings showing that although implementation of this recommendation initially requires additional time, it has resulted in better asthma control in patients and consequently, fewer return visits for uncontrolled episodes of asthma.[26]

After the launch, you organize several meetings with the stakeholder groups to develop and gain consensus for new practice patterns in your hospital that will support individualized asthma action plans. Progress, albeit slow and difficult at times, has been made. Key factors in successfully moving the process forward are the continued involvement and support of the three directors. It was decided early on that at least one director would always be in attendance at scheduled meetings.

To determine whether patients are currently managing their asthma well, you conduct a chart audit on a random sample of adult patients with asthma who have attended the clinic over the past year. You determine that many patients are not managing their asthma at an optimal level, require additional visits to the clinic and the emergency department, and report missing several days of work or school. You compare these data to state or provincial data and determine that your hospital has a higher number of return visits and days missed from work or school than do patients with asthma who attend other institutions.

After reviewing the data, and with considerable discussion and negotiation, the group decides to implement individualized action plans. You provide examples of individualized asthma action plans used in hospitals that are similar to yours and use these to guide the development of an individualized action plan template that satisfies each stakeholder group. You also work with the group to identify changes in practice that will be required by clinicians to implement the action plan successfully. You prepare new policies and procedures to reflect these changes. With support from this working group as well as from senior management, you are now ready to begin implementing strategies to help clinicians change their practice and begin using individualized action plans for patients with asthma.

Implementation

If the decision to adopt the innovation is made, the organization engages in activities to facilitate its integration into clinical practice or policy decisions. Implementation activities may begin with strategies that first translate the research evidence into a small number of relevant and usable key messages.[64]

What Strategies Will Promote Behavioral Change and Implementation of Research Findings Among My Colleagues?

Researchers have evaluated the effectiveness of strategies designed to change provider behavior; however, most of this research has focused on medical practice, and therefore the results must be interpreted cautiously in terms of nursing practice. Table 11-4 summarizes interventions that have been evaluated most rigorously and their respective impact on behavioral change.[65–72]

Convincing evidence exists that the more interactive strategies such as *academic detailing* (also known as educational outreach visits),[67] *interactive workshops,*[66] *reminder systems,*[71] *audit and feedback,*[69] and *opinion leaders,*[68] have a greater impact on physician practice.[73] Given their moderate effect size, low cost, and feasibility, reminders should be strongly encouraged.[71] *Academic detailing* produces modest effects but may not be feasible from a cost perspective or for changing nursing practice in a large hospital, given its one-to-one nature.[73] Passive dissemination of information such as continuing nursing education and workshops is generally ineffective in changing practice.[66,70]

USING THE GUIDE

You plan specific implementation strategies to highlight the introduction and use of individualized action plans:

1. To enhance communication in your large organization, you prepare regular columns for the hospital newsletter, beginning with a description of action plans and followed by regular updates on progress with implementation of the action plan.

2. To help identify and heighten awareness about the action plan, you use a logo (a stoplight) to "brand" memos, posters, and printed material related to the action plan.

3. To teach the nurses about action plans, you:
   - Develop and tailor education sessions for nurses in different clinical areas, specifically, those in the emergency department, inpatient units, and the asthma clinic.
   - Develop patient pathways and documentation tools to allow nurses to target their assessment and teaching to the patients' needs.
   - Prepare preworkshop packages to allow nurses to familiarize themselves with some of the content before they attend the education workshop; this reduces the amount of content to cover in the workshop, allows for more active involvement by participants in the workshop, and serves as review material after the workshop.
   - Develop 2-hour workshops for nurses in each of the different clinical areas (emergency department, inpatient units, asthma clinic).
   - Identify nurses who are well respected in the various clinical settings and train them first, using the train-the-trainer approach; after the training, ask these nurses to wear the stoplight logo on their nametag so they can be identified as having completed the training and serve as resources for others.
   - Recognizing how little time nurses have during the workday, arrange for nurses to be paid to come in on their day off for the workshop.
   - Provide opportunities for nurses to share their concerns about the introduction and use of asthma action plans and to participate actively in the discussion.
   - Provide free coffee and donuts, and, at the end of the session, give nurses certificates acknowledging their attendance at the workshop.

Continued

- Once the initial education is completed, book time on the nursing units to conduct 15-minute review in-service sessions; use games and activities to help nurses review skills with medication devices, drug categories, and use of a patient teaching booklet.
- Work with nurse educators to build asthma patient education into the orientation of new nurses.

4. To remind staff about the organization's support for the action plan, unit leaders speak to staff members and indicate their strong support for its adoption.

5. To maintain visibility of the action plan, you hang posters at strategic spots in the hospital.

Throughout the implementation, you are accessible and proactive in supporting nurses. Your strategy is implemented over several months. At times, nurses express concern about the new practice and are somewhat resistant to the changes. However, over time, attitudes toward the change in practice become more positive. Having completed the implementation phase of the project, you now focus your attention on evaluating the impact of introducing individualized action plans in your hospital.

Confirmation

After information about the new practice has been disseminated to clinicians and efforts have been undertaken to facilitate its implementation, it is time to evaluate whether a change in practice has occurred and whether it has had its intended impact. The results of the evaluation provide feedback to the implementation process and the initial decision to adopt the innovation. Initially, the data will be used to determine whether the innovation is actually being implemented in the way in which it was intended. If changes in practice are suboptimal, the data will provide rationale for conducting additional dissemination strategies and possibly using different strategies. If the data show that patient outcomes and/or organizational outcomes such as number of readmissions or length of stay remain unchanged despite changes in practitioner practice, then the decision to adopt the innovation could be revisited.

What Indicators Should I Measure to Evaluate the Success of Implementing the Evidence-Based Decision?

Although the outcome of the diffusion process has traditionally been measured as a dichotomous variable (adopt or not adopt), researchers have determined that adoption is not an "all or nothing" process.[74,75] Innovation adoption should be measured along a continuum from no adoption to full adoption. During this stage, evaluation of the success of the implementation process should be based on structure, process, and intermediary outcome indicators. *Structure evaluation* assesses whether the physical and human resources required to implement the new practice are available and in place (e.g., numbers and qualifications of staff members, supplies, and equipment).[19] *Process evaluation* examines whether and how the new practice is implemented; for example, if an educational

Table 11-4 Strategies to Promote Behavioral Change Among Health Professionals

Consistently Effective Strategies	Strategies With Mixed Effects	Strategies Having Little or No Effect
Academic Detailing or Education Outreach Visits	**Audit and Feedback**	**Educational Materials**
Use of a trained person who meets with professionals in their practice settings to provide information with the intent of changing practice	Any written or verbal summary of clinical performance of professionals (e.g., based on review of charting or one-to-one observation of clinical practice) over a specified period; the summary may also include recommendations for clinical action.	Distribution of published or printed recommendations for clinical care, including clinical practice guidelines, audiovisual materials, and electronic publications
Shown to be most effective with changing physician prescribing practices[67,72]	Shown to be most effective in changing physician prescribing practices[69,72,73]	May result in change in knowledge, but does not translate into changes in professional practice among nurses[65,72]
Reminders	**Local Opinion Leaders**	**Didactic Educational Meetings, Conferences, or Workshops**
Any intervention, manual or computerized, that prompts professionals to perform a clinical action	Use of respected academic and clinical professionals nominated by their colleagues as educationally influential	Lectures Not effective in changing nursing practice[66,70,72]
Shown to be effective in changing both physician and nursing practice[71,72]	Shown to be effective in changing physician prescribing practices; limited evidence of effect on changing nursing practice[68,72]	
Multifaceted Interventions	**Local Consensus Process**	
A combination that includes two or more of: audit and feedback, reminders, local	Inclusion of participating professionals in discussion to ensure that they agreed that the	

Continued

Table 11-4 Strategies to Promote Behavioral Change Among Health Professionals—cont'd

Consistently Effective Strategies	Strategies With Mixed Effects	Strategies Having Little or No Effect
consensus processes, patient-mediated interventions	chosen clinical problem is important and the approach to managing the problem is appropriate	
Shown to be effective in multiple settings among different health care professionals in changing practice[65,70–72]	Shown to be effective in changing nursing and physician practice[72]	
Interactive Education Meetings or Workshops	**Patient-Mediated Interventions**	
Participation of professionals in workshops that include interaction and discussion	Any intervention aimed at changing the performance of professionals where specific information was sought from, or given to, patients	
Shown to be effective in changing practice in health care professionals in multiple settings[66]	Shown to have no effect on prescribing practices or provision of preventive services, but positive results in changing physician behavior related to clinical practice guidelines when combined with academic detailing[69]	

program to introduce staff nurses to a new practice is delivered effectively, it is likely that there will be an improvement in knowledge and attitudes about the practice after attendance at the educational session.[19] Other examples include changes in policies and clinical practice, changes in professional behavior, and changes in patient behavior.

What Organizational, Patient, or Health Systems Outcome Indicators Should I Measure to Evaluate the Success of the Change in Nursing Practice?

In the final stage of the framework, the organization seeks reinforcement for the decision. The innovation characteristic of observability takes on an important role during this stage because it provides direct feedback to the decision makers about the impact of their decision.[21] Data are collected about relevant outcome indicators to determine whether the change in nursing practice had its intended effect. Commonly measured outcomes include patient outcomes and compliance with practice and policy recommendations.[73] Important outcomes rarely evaluated include the impact of the innovation on health care resource allocation and expenditures and on organizational performance indicators.[73] Table 11-5 summarizes structure, process, and outcome indicators that can be used to evaluate success in implementing practice guidelines.

USING THE GUIDE

Before implementing the individualized asthma action plans, you develop an evaluation scheme. You determine that you will need to assess factors related to structure (what you need to have), process (how you go about it), and outcomes (what happens) before, during, and after implementing the change in practice. Although data are currently collected on most of these variables, some have not previously been assessed in your organization. You develop strategies to facilitate the collection of data on these additional variables. As much as possible, you develop a data collection system that does not increase work for nurses. The four data collection periods you decide on are: before the implementation, 3 months into the implementation, at the completion of the implementation, and 1 year after the implementation. You realize that this represents additional work for you but understand that you will need data at all these points to determine whether the implementation strategies are effective and to identify issues that may arise at different stages of the implementation process. To assist you in your thinking, you develop an evaluation framework (Table 11-6).

You discuss the evaluation plan with your immediate supervisor. She supports the four data collection points. You schedule a meeting with her and with the directors of nursing and the emergency departments to discuss the baseline findings. You also schedule a meeting with them to discuss the findings 3 months into the implementation of the individualized action plans. During this meeting, you assess how the implementation process is going and determine whether new approaches are required. You discuss realistic expectations for observing changes in patient outcomes, such as nocturnal symptoms, days missed from work or school, clinic and emergency department visits, and hospital admissions. You determine that, in addition to measuring patient outcomes at the end of the implementation phase, it will be necessary to collect patient outcome data 1 year after implementation because it will take time for asthma control to become established. You will then use these data to report back to key stakeholders on the long-term outcomes of implementing individualized action plans. Along with the key stakeholders, you will assess whether the move to individualized action plans for promoting asthma control is having the desired effect. If the answer is yes, then the decision to adopt this innovation will be maintained. If the answer is no, then the organization will revisit the decision and potentially change or alter the initial decision. The final component of the evaluation framework you develop is a proposed budget and timeline for collecting and analyzing the data.

Table 11-5 Indicators to Evaluate the Implementation of a Practice Guideline

Category	Structure (What You Need to Have)	Process (How You Go About It)	Outcome (What Happens)
Organization or Unit	Organizational stability Culture and support for change Quality assurance mechanisms Policy and procedures Nursing care delivery system Physical facilities Equipment	Development or modification of policies and procedures Charting	Achievement of targets for patient outcome improvement Achievement of condition-specific goals
Provider	Number and qualifications of staff Ratio of staff to patients or clients Roles and responsibilities Multidisciplinary collaboration Educational program	Awareness of and attitude to practice guideline Knowledge and skill level	Attendance at educational program Adherence to practice guideline Number and completeness of assessments done Number and range of appropriate treatments Provider satisfaction

Patient, Client, or Family	Patient or client characteristics (demographics, level of risk) Patient-centered approach Involvement in decisions	Patient awareness of and attitude to practice guideline Family, community acceptance Patient, family knowledge	Physical, psychological, social, patient, or client outcomes Family health Satisfaction with care Access to care
Financial Costs	Costs of additional staff and physical resources required New equipment	Costs of implementation strategies Staff education Patient or client education	Incremental costs of innovation, including product and drug costs Revenue or growth of service Length of stay Number of diagnostic tests, interventions Visits to emergency department, readmission rates

Modified and reproduced with permission of the Registered Nurses Association of Ontario (RNAO). Toolkit: Implementation of Clinical Practice Guidelines. Toronto: RNAO; 2002.

Table **11-6** Evaluating the Implementation of Individualized Action Plans for Adult Patients With Asthma

Category	Structure (What You Need to Have)	Process (How You Go About It)	Outcome (What Happens)
Organization or Unit	Management support for individualized action plans	Development or modification of policies and procedures to facilitate appropriate referrals	Achievement of targets for patient outcome improvement: reduced number of hospital readmissions, unscheduled clinic visits, and emergency department visits.
	Quality assurance mechanisms	Asthma action plans completed for each patient, and completion documented in the patients' charts	Achievement of condition-specific goals: less frequent and shorter episodes of uncontrolled asthma
	Promote education		
	Seek patient opinion		
	Feedback to nurses		
	Policy or procedures that reflect change in practice		
	Nursing role as coordinator of patient care		
	Availability of patient education resources (sample action plans, referral information)		
Provider	Roles, responsibilities, multidisciplinary collaboration	Self-assessed knowledge of asthma action plans	Attendance at educational training
	Educational program	Self-reported awareness of referral sources for people with asthma	Documentation of completion and review of individualized action plans for self-management of asthma symptoms
	Dedicated staff to implement strategies to facilitate change in practice	Self-reported positive attitude toward usefulness of asthma plans	Appropriate follow-up when action plan indicates that asthma
		High level of knowledge	

	and skill related to interventions to implement when action plan indicates poorly controlled asthma	is poorly controlled or uncontrolled (e.g., provision of patient education, referral of patient to appropriate services) Nurse satisfaction
Patient, Client, or Family	Patient or client characteristics (demographics, level of risk) Patient-centered approach Involvement in decisions	Patient awareness of and attitude to individualized action plans Patient or family knowledge of asthma control Written information on asthma Individualized action plan on discharge Adherence to individualized action plan	Proportion of clients with asthma plans Proportion of clients with acceptable asthma control Experience of daytime symptoms Experience of nighttime and/or awakening symptoms Absence from school or work Satisfaction with care Quality of life
Financial Costs	Costs of implementation strategies Staff education Patient or client education		Length of hospital stay Number of diagnostic tests, interventions Visits to emergency department, readmissions

Modified and reproduced with permission of the Registered Nurses Association of Ontario (RNAO) from Edwards N, Davies B, Dobbins M, Griffin P, Ploeg J, Skelly J. RNAO Evaluation Team, Nursing Best Practice Guidelines Project, Cycle 3; 2003.

Changing practice in an organization is a multistage, time- and resource-intensive process. The framework described in this chapter illustrates that the process of the adoption of research evidence is iterative and influenced by a variety of complex factors. This framework may guide evidence-based promoters in health care organizations in their research transfer activities, and it may help decision makers to use scarce resources most effectively with respect to research transfer.

REFERENCES

1. Grinspun D, Virani T, Bajnok I. Nursing best practice guidelines: the RNAO project. *Hosp Q.* 2002;5: 56-60.
2. Registered Nurses Association of Ontario. *Adult Asthma Care Guidelines for Nurses: Promoting Control of Asthma.* Toronto: Registered Nurses Association of Ontario; 2003.
3. Utterback JM. Innovation in industry and the diffusion of technology. *Science.* 1974;183:620-626.
4. Power EJ, Tunis SR, Wagner JL. Technology assessment and public health. *Annu Rev Public Health.* 1994;15:561-579.
5. Registered Nurses Association of Ontario. *Assessment and Management of Stage I to IV Pressure Ulcers.* Toronto: Registered Nurses Association of Ontario; 2002. Available at: http://www.rnao.org/bestprac-tices/completed_guidelines/BPG_Guide_C2_pressure_ulcer.asp. Accessed November 6, 2003.
6. Champagne F. The use of scientific evidence and knowledge by managers. Third Conference on the Scientific Basis of Health Care, Toronto; 1999.
7. Dobbins M, Ciliska D, DiCenso A. Dissemination and use of research evidence for policy and practice: a framework for developing, implementing and evaluating strategies. *Online J Knowledge Synthesis Nurs.* 2002;9:Document 7.
8. Landry R, Amara N, Laamary M. Utilization of social science research knowledge in Canada. *Res Policy.* 2001;30:333-349.
9. Lavis JN. Towards a new research transfer strategy for the Institute for Work and Health. Toronto: Institute for Work and Health; 1999.
10. Grol R, Grimshaw J. Evidence-based implementation of evidence-based medicine. *Jt Comm J Qual Improv.* 1999;25:503-513.
11. Horsley JA, Crane J, Crabtree MK. *Using Research to Improve Nursing Practice: A Guide.* New York: Grune & Stratton; 1983.
12. Titler MG, Kleiber C, Steelman V, et al. Infusing research into practice to promote quality care. *Nurs Res.* 1994;43:307-313.
13. Stetler CB. Refinement of the Stetler/Marram model for application of research findings to practice. *Nurs Outlook.* 1994;40:15-25.
14. Kitson A, Ahmed LB, Harvey G, Seers K, Thompson DR. From research to practice: one organizational model for promoting research-based practice. *J Adv Nurs.* 1996;23:430-440.
15. Kitson A. Towards evidence-based quality improvement: perspectives from nursing practice. *Int J Qual Health Care.* 2000;12:459-464.
16. Kitson A, Harvey G, McCormack B. Enabling the implementation of evidence based practice: a conceptual framework. *Qual Health Care.* 1998;7:149-158.
17. Estabrooks CA. Mapping the research utilization field in nursing. *Can J Nurs Res.* 1999;31:53-72.
18. Logan J, Graham IK. Towards a comprehensive interdisciplinary model of health care research use. *Sci Commun.* 1998;20:227-246.
19. Registered Nurses Association of Ontario. *Toolkit: Implementation of Clinical Practice Guidelines.* Toronto: Registered Nurses Association of Ontario; 2002. Available at: http://www.rnao.org/bestpractices/com-pleted_guidelines/BPG_Guide_C1_Toolkit.asp. Accessed November 6, 2003.
20. DiCenso A, Virani T, Bajnok I, et al. A toolkit to facilitate the implementation of clinical practice guidelines in healthcare settings. *Hosp Q.* 2002;5:55-60.
21. Rogers EM. *Diffusion of Innovations.* 4th ed. New York: Free Press; 1995.
22. Battista RN. Innovation and diffusion of health-related technologies: a conceptual framework. *Int J Technol Assess Health Care.* 1989:5;227-248.

23. Haynes RB. Of studies, summaries, synopses, and systems: the "4S" evolution of services for finding current best evidence. *Evidence-Based Mental Health.* 2001;4:37-39.
24. Cluzeau F, Littlejohns P, Grimshaw J, Feder G, Moran S. Development and application of generic methodology to assess the quality of clinical guidelines. *Int J Qual Health Care.* 1999;11:21-28.
25. AGREE Collaboration. Appraisal of guidelines for research and evaluation (AGREE) instrument. Available at: www.agreecollaboration.org. Accessed November 6, 2003.
26. Gibson PG, Powell H, Coughlan J, et al. Self-management education and regular practitioner review for adults with asthma. *Cochrane Database Syst Rev.* 2003;1:CD001117.
27. Warner KE. A "desperation-reaction" model of medical diffusion. *Health Serv Res.* 1975;10:369-383.
28. Orlandi MA. Health promotion technology transfer: organizational perspectives. *Can J Public Health.* 1996;87:S28-S33.
29. Granovetter M. Economic action and social structure: the problem of embeddedness. *Am J Sociol.* 1985;91;481-510.
30. Hassinger E. Stages in the adoption process. *Rural Sociol.* 1959;24:52-53.
31. Meah S, Luker KA, Cullum NA. An exploration of midwives' attitudes to research and perceived barriers to research utilisation. *Midwifery.* 1996;12:73-84.
32. McCaughan D, Thompson C, Cullum N, Sheldon TA, Thompson DR. Acute care nurses' perceptions of barriers to using research information in clinical decision-making. *J Adv Nurs.* 2002;39:46-60.
33. Abrahamson E. Managerial fads and fashions: the diffusion and rejection of innovations. *Acad Manage Rev.* 1991;16:586-612.
34. Abrahamson E, Rosenkoff E. Institutional and competitive bandwagons: using mathematical modeling as a tool to explore innovation diffusion. *Acad Manage Rev.* 1991;16:586-612.
35. Brown LA. *Innovation Diffusion: A New Perspective.* New York: Methuen; 1981.
36. Burt R. Social contagion and innovation: cohesion versus structural equivalence. *Am J Sociol.* 1987;92:1287-1335.
37. Teisberg EO. McCaw Cellular Communications, Inc. in 1990. *Harvard Business Rev.* 1992;53:127-133.
38. Kaluzny AD. Innovation in health services: theoretical framework and review of research. *Health Serv Res.* 1974;9:101-120.
39. Veney JE, Kaluzny AD, Gentry JT, Sprague JB, Duncan DP. Implementation of health programs in hospitals. *Health Serv Res.* 1971;6:350-362.
40. Damanpour F. Organizational innovation: a meta-analysis of effects of determinants and moderators. *Acad Manage J.* 1991;34:555-590.
41. Burns LR, Wholey DR. Adoption and abandonment of matrix management programs: effects of organizational characteristics and interorganizatonal networks. *Acad Manage J.* 1993;36:106-138.
42. Kimberly JR, Evanisko MJ. Organizational innovation: the influence of individual, organizational, and contextual factors on hospital adoption of technological and administrative innovations. *Acad Manage J.* 1981;24:689-713.
43. Kaluzny AD, Veney JE, Gentry JT. Innovation of health services: a comparative study of hospitals and health departments. *Milbank Mem Fund Q Health Soc.* 1974;52:51-82.
44. Hage J, Dewar R. The prediction of organizational performance: the case of program innovation. *Admin Sci Q.* 1973;18:279-285.
45. Funk SG, Champagne MT, Wiese RA, Tornquist EM. Barriers to using research findings in practice: the clinician's perspective. *Appl Nurs Res.* 1991;4:90-95.
46. Dobbins M, Cockerill R, Barnsley J. Factors affecting the utilization of systematic reviews: a study of public health decision makers. *Int J Technol Assess Health Care.* 2001;17:203-214.
47. Royle JA, Blythe J, DiCenso A, Baumann A, Fitzgerald D. Do nurses have the information resources and skills for research utilization? *Can J Nurs Admin.* 1997;10:9-30.
48. Meyer AD, Goes JB. Organizational assimilation of innovation: a multilevel contextual analysis. *Acad Manage J.* 1998;31:897-923.
49. Scott WR. Innovation in medical care organizations: a synthetic review. *Med Care Rev.* 1990;47:165-192.
50. Estabrooks CA, Floyd JA, Scott-Findlay S, O'Leary KA, Gushta M. Individual determinants of research utilization: a systematic review. *J Adv Nurs.* 2003;43:506-520.
51. Funk SG, Tornquist EM, Champagne MT. Barriers and facilitators of research utilization: an integrative review. *Nurs Clin North Am.* 1995;30:395-407.

52. Bero LA, Jadad AR. How consumers and policymakers can use systematic reviews for decision making. *Ann Intern Med*. 1997;127:37-42.

53. Greenwood J. Nursing research: a position paper. *J Adv Nurs*. 1984;9:77-82.

54. Miller JR, Messenger SR. Obstacles to applying nursing research findings. *Am J Nurs*. 1978;78:632-634.

55. Walczak JR, McGuire DB, Haisfield ME, Beezley A. A survey of research-related activities and perceived barriers to research utilization among professional oncology nurses. *Oncol Nurs Forum*. 1994;21:710-715.

56. Hicks C. A study of nurses' attitudes towards research: a factor analytic approach. *J Adv Nurs*. 1996;23:373-379.

57. Lacey EA. Research utilization in nursing practice: a pilot study. *J Adv Nurs*. 1994;19:987-995.

58. McSherry R. What do registered nurses and midwives feel and know about research? *J Adv Nurs*. 1997;25:985-998.

59. Pettengill MM, Gillies DA, Clark CC. Factors encouraging and discouraging the use of nursing research findings. *Image J Nurs Sch*. 1994;26:143-147.

60. Tisdale NE, Williams-Barnard CL, Moore PA. Attitudes, activities, and involvement in nursing research among psychiatric nurses in a public-sector facility. *Issues Ment Health Nurs*. 1997;18:365-375.

61. Sellick K, McKinley S, Botti M, Kingsland S, Behan J. Victorian hospital nurses' research attitudes and activity. *Aust J Adv Nurs*. 1996;13:5-14.

62. Varvasovszky Z, Brugha R. A stakeholder analysis. *Health Policy Plan*. 2000;15:338-345.

63. Davies B, Hodnett E, Hannah M, O'Brien-Pallas L, Pringle D, Wells G. Fetal health surveillance: a community wide approach versus a tailored intervention for the implementation of clinical practice guidelines. *Can Med Assoc J*. 2002;167:469-474.

64. Rogers EM. The innovation-decision process. In: *Diffusion of Innovations*. 3rd ed. London: Collier Macmillan; 1983:163-209.

65. Thomson MA. Closing the gap between nursing research and practice. *Evid Based Nurs*. 1998;1:7-8.

66. Thomson O'Brien MA, Freemantle N, Oxman AD, Wolf F, Davis DA, Herrin J. Continuing education meetings and workshops: effects on professional practice and health care outcomes. *Cochrane Database Syst Rev*. 2001;2:CD003030.

67. Thomson O'Brien MA, Oxman AD, Davis DA, Haynes RB, Freemantle N, Harvey EL. Educational outreach visits: effects on professional practice and health care outcomes. *Cochrane Database Syst Rev*. 2000;2:CD000409.

68. Thomson O'Brien MA, Oxman AD, Haynes RB, Davis DA, Freemantle N, Harvey EL. Local opinion leaders: effects on professional practice and health care outcomes. *Cochrane Database Syst Rev*. 2000;2:CD000125.

69. Jamtvedt G, Young JM, Kristoffersen DT, Thomson O'Brien MA, Oxman AD. Audit and feedback: effects on professional practice and health care outcomes. *Cochrane Database Syst Rev*. 2003;3:CD000259.

70. Bero LA, Grilli R, Grimshaw JM, Harvey E, Oxman AD, Thomson MA. Closing the gap between research and practice: an overview of systematic reviews of interventions to promote the implementation of research findings. *BMJ*. 1998;317:465-468.

71. Grimshaw JM, Shirran L, Thomas R, et al. Changing provider behavior: an overview of systematic reviews of interventions. *Med Care*. 2001;39(8 Suppl 2):II2-II45.

72. NHS Centre for Reviews and Dissemination. Getting evidence into practice. *Effective Health Care*. 1999;5:1-16. Available at: http://www.york.ac.uk/inst/crd/ehc51.pdf. Accessed November 6, 2003.

73. Dobbins M, Ciliska D, DiCenso A. *Dissemination and Use of Research Evidence for Policy and Practice: A Framework for Developing, Implementing and Evaluating Strategies*. Ottawa, Canada: Canadian Nurses Association; 1998. Available at: http://www.cna-nurses.ca/pages/resources/dumac.html. Accessed November 6, 2003.

74. Calsyn RJ, Tornatzky LG, Dittmar S. Incomplete adoption of an innovation: the case of goal attainment scaling. *Evaluation*. 1977;4;128-130.

75. Larsen JK, Agarwalla-Rogers R. Re-invention of innovative ideas: Modified? Adopted? None of the above. *Evaluation*. 1977;4:136-140.

Beyond the Basics: Using and Teaching the Principles of Evidence-Based Nursing

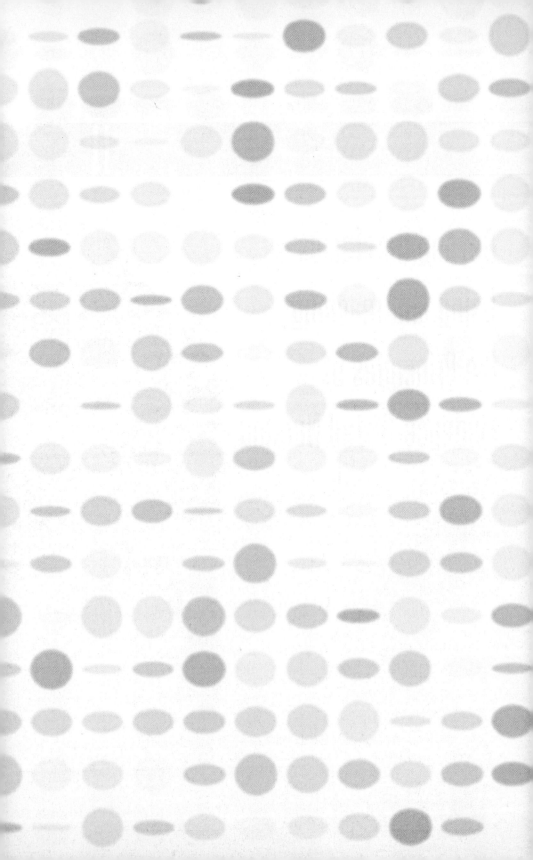

Health Care Interventions

Chapter **12**   Quality of Life

Chapter **13**   Surrogate Outcomes

Chapter **14**   Surprising Results of
Randomized Controlled Trials

Chapter **15**   The Principle of Intention
to Treat

Chapter **16**   When to Believe a Subgroup
Analysis

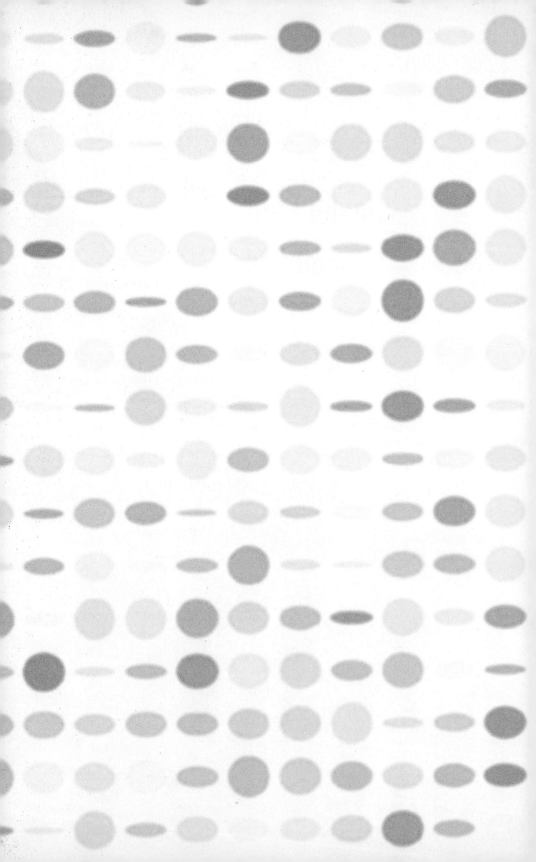

Quality of Life

12

Donna Ciliska, Alba DiCenso, and Gordon Guyatt

*We gratefully acknowledge the work of David Naylor, Elizabeth Juniper,
Daren Heyland, Roman Jaeschke, and Deborah Cook on the original chapter that
appears in the* Users' Guides to the Medical Literature, *edited by Guyatt and Rennie.*

In This Chapter

When is it Important to Consider Health-Related Quality of Life?

Are the Results Valid?
  Did the Investigators Measure Aspects of Patients' Lives That Patients
    Consider Important?
  Did the Health-Related Quality of Life Instruments Work in the Intended Way?
  Were Important Aspects of Health-Related Quality of Life Omitted?
  If There Were Trade-offs Between Quality of Life and Quantity of Life, or if an
    Economic Evaluation Was Performed, Were the Most Appropriate Measures
    Used?

What Are the Results?
  How Can We Interpret the Magnitude of Effect on Health-Related Quality
    of Life?

How Can I Apply the Results to Patient Care?
  Will the Information From the Study Help Patients to Make Informed Decisions
    About Their Health Care?
  Did the Study Design Simulate Clinical Practice?

CLINICAL SCENARIO

Coping Skills Training for Youth With Diabetes: Does It Improve Quality of Life?

You are a nurse working in a pediatric diabetes clinic. You are concerned about the number of adolescents in your clinic with high glycosylated hemoglobin levels despite intensive diabetes management. In particular, you are currently seeing a 16-year-old boy who has poor metabolic control despite frequent insulin adjustment. He has had diabetes for 2 years, and his most recent glycosylated hemoglobin value was 9.0%. During your last clinic visit with this young man, he talked about how managing his diabetes interferes excessively with his life. The need for vigilance about food choices, blood glucose testing, and insulin dosages makes him feel different from his friends. Sometimes he chooses not to join in social activities rather than be singled out, and at other times, he simply chooses to ignore the diet restrictions or does not bother testing his blood glucose levels.

You are impressed by both the methodology and results of a recent randomized controlled trial showing that adolescents in an intensive diabetes management program benefited from coping skills training.[1] The goal of the training program was to help youth to cope with their lives in the context of diabetes management; skills included social problem solving, cognitive behavior modification, and conflict resolution. After reviewing the study with your colleagues, your team decides to offer this training program at your clinic. You suggest to the patient that he consider participating in this new program. Not surprisingly, when you explain that he will need to attend six weekly 1-hour sessions and monthly follow-ups, the patient is hesitant. "How will it make my life any better?" he asks.

When we offer health care to patients, we strive to increase longevity, prevent future morbidity, and help them feel better. Feeling better includes avoiding discomfort (e.g., pain, nausea, breathlessness), disability (loss of function), and distress (emotional suffering).[2] At times, however, an intervention designed to improve certain patient outcomes may have a negative effect on how patients feel or the extent to which they are able to enjoy life. Increasingly, we are recognizing the importance of measuring the effect of an intervention on a patient's quality of life as well as on traditional outcomes such as survival, tumor size reduction, and physiologic or laboratory measures.

Both qualitative and quantitative research studies have contributed to the investigation of *quality of life*. Investigators have used qualitative approaches to consider the effects of deinstitutionalization on quality of life in people with long-term mental illness,[3] as well as to understand how adults with disabilities describe their quality of life in relation to physical and social environments.[4] Qualitative designs have contributed to the development of quality-of-life measurement tools for various conditions, including peripheral arterial disease.[5] Chapter 8, Qualitative Research, provides criteria for evaluating qualitative studies. This chapter focuses on quantitative measurement of quality of life.

Because clinicians are most interested in aspects of quality of life that directly relate to health rather than such issues as financial solvency or the quality of the environment, we frequently refer to measurements of how people are feeling as *health-related quality of life* (HRQL).[6] Investigators measure HRQL using questionnaires that typically include questions about how patients are feeling or what they are experiencing, and response options in the form of "yes/no" answers, seven-point (or any other number) Likert-type scales, or visual analogue scales. Investigators aggregate responses to the questions into domains or dimensions (e.g., physical or emotional function) that yield an overall score. In this chapter, we use HRQL to refer to the health aspects of life that people generally value, and we accept patients' statements of what they value without precise determination of ranking of items or domains.[7-9]

Clinicians are accustomed to asking patients how they feel, yet they are often unfamiliar with methods of measuring how patients feel. At the same time, clinicians read articles that recommend implementing or avoiding a health care intervention on the basis of its impact on patient well-being. This chapter is designed for clinicians who want to know if a given health care intervention will make the patient feel better. As in other chapters of this book, we use the framework for assessing the validity of the methods, interpreting the results, and applying the results to patients (Table 12-1). We preface our discussion with a commentary on when one should and should not consider HRQL measurement.

WHEN IS IT IMPORTANT TO CONSIDER HEALTH-RELATED QUALITY OF LIFE?

Until about 1980, few, if any, intervention studies included measurements of HRQL. When should readers be concerned if investigators have not paid adequate attention to how patients feel? Patients generally agree that, under most circumstances, prolonging their lives is a sufficient reason to accept a course of treatment. Some years ago, investigators showed that 24-hour oxygen administration in patients with severe chronic

Table 12-1   Users' Guides for an Article About Health-Related
                  Quality of Life

Are the Results Valid?

Primary guides

- Did the investigators measure aspects of patients' lives that patients consider important?
- Did the health-related quality of life instruments work in the intended way?

Secondary guides

- Were important aspects of health-related quality of life omitted?
- If there were trade-offs between quality and quantity of life, or if an economic evaluation was performed, were the most appropriate measures used?

What Are the Results?

How can we interpret the magnitude of effect on health-related quality of life?

How Can I Apply the Results to Patient Care?

- Will the information from the study help patients to make informed decisions about their health care?
- Did the study design simulate clinical practice?

airflow limitation reduced mortality.[10] The omission of HRQL data from the original article ultimately was not important. Because the intervention prolongs life, our enthusiasm for continuous oxygen administration is not diminished by a subsequent report suggesting that more intensive oxygen therapy had little or no impact on HRQL.[11] Similarly, although feeling better is important to patients with heart failure, when interventions either extend[12] or shorten[13] the life span, we usually do not need an HRQL assessment to inform our clinical decisions.

There are exceptions to this rule. Although many life-prolonging treatments have a negligible impact on or actually improve HRQL, this is not always the case. If treatment leads to deterioration in HRQL, patients may be concerned that small gains in life expectancy come at too high a cost. This concern is vividly illustrated by patient decisions regarding whether to accept toxic cancer chemotherapy that will provide marginal gains in longevity. In the extreme, an intervention such as mechanical ventilation may prolong the life of a patient in a vegetative state, but the patient's family may wonder whether their loved one would be better off dead.

When the goal of an intervention is to improve how people feel (rather than to prolong their lives) and physiologic correlates of patients' experience are lacking, measurement of HRQL is imperative. For example, we would pay little attention to studies of distraction strategies for pain relief that failed to measure patients' pain.

Difficult decisions arise when the relation between physiologic or laboratory measures and HRQL outcomes is uncertain. Practitioners have relied on substitute end points because they assumed a strong link between physiologic measurements and patients' well-being. As we argue elsewhere (see Chapter 13, Surrogate Outcomes), substitute end points such as bone density for fractures, cholesterol level for coronary artery disease deaths, and laboratory exercise capacity for ability to undertake day-to-day activities, have often proved misleading. Changes in conventional measures of health status show only weak to moderate correlations with changes in HRQL,[14,15] and they fail to detect patient-important changes in HRQL.[16] Randomized trials that measure both physiologic end points and HRQL may show effects on one but not the other. For example, trials of patients with chronic lung disease have shown treatment effects on peak flow rates without improvement in HRQL.[17,18] We therefore advocate caution when relying on surrogate outcomes.

Using the Guide

The investigators reported the results of a randomized trial of coping skills training in 77 patients, 12 to 20 years of age, who had type 1 diabetes mellitus and were receiving intensive diabetes management.[1] At 1-year follow-up, participants who received coping skills training had lower glycosylated hemoglobin levels than those who received intensive diabetes management alone (7.5% vs 8.5%, $P = 0.001$).

Is additional information about HRQL necessary to interpret the results of this study? A patient's decision to attend the coping skills training depends on the balance between the benefits and inconvenience; the patient's question about whether his life will be better will also be relevant to his decision. Without information about the effect of coping skills training on HRQL, the patient cannot make a fully informed choice.

ARE THE RESULTS VALID?

Did the Investigators Measure Aspects of Patients' Lives That Patients Consider Important?

We have described how investigators often substitute their own end points—ones that make intuitive sense to them — for those that patients value. Readers can recognize these situations by asking themselves the following question: If the end points measured by the investigators were the only thing that changed, would patients be willing to receive the intervention? In addition to changes in clinical or physiologic variables, patients would want to feel better or live longer. For instance, if a treatment for osteoporosis increased bone density without preventing back pain, loss of height, or fractures, patients would not be interested in risking the side effects—or incurring the costs and inconvenience—of treatment.

How can nurses be secure that investigators have measured aspects of life that patients value? Investigators may show that the outcomes they have measured are important to patients by asking them directly. For example, in a study examining HRQL in patients with chronic airflow limitation, investigators used a literature review and interviews with health care workers and patients to identify 123 items reflecting possible ways that chronic airflow limitation could affect patients' HRQL.[19] They then asked 100 patients to identify the items that were problems for them and to indicate the importance of those items. The most important problem areas for patients were dyspnea during day-to-day activities and chronic fatigue. An additional problem area was emotional function, which included feelings of frustration and impatience.

If authors do not present direct evidence that outcome measures are important to patients, they may cite previous relevant research. For example, a randomized trial of respiratory rehabilitation in patients with chronic lung disease used an HRQL measure based on the responses of patients in the study described above.[20]   Ideally, the report would include a sufficiently detailed summary of how the measure was developed to avoid the need to return to the original study report.

Alternatively, investigators may describe the content of their outcome measures in detail. An adequate description of the content of a questionnaire allows readers to use their own experience to decide whether the outcomes are important to patients. For example, a randomized trial of surgery versus watchful waiting for benign prostatic hyperplasia "assessed the degree to which urinary difficulties bothered the patients or interfered with their activities of daily living, sexual function, social activities, and general well-being."[21] Few would doubt the importance of these items and, because patients in primary care often are untroubled by minor symptoms of benign prostatic hyperplasia, the importance of including them as outcomes.

Using the Guide

In the study of coping skills training for adolescents with type 1 diabetes, participants completed the Diabetes Quality of Life for Youth Measure, which comprises three intercorrelated scales: a 17-item Diabetes Life Satisfaction scale, a 23-item Disease Impact scale, and an 11-item Disease-Related Worries scale. This instrument is an adaptation of a diabetes quality of life measure for adults.[22] The article describing the

Continued

USING THE GUIDE—CONT'D

coping skills training study provided a brief description of the instrument. Review of the article that described the development of the instrument[22] revealed that clinicians who specialized in pediatric diabetes care reviewed the adult version, identified items that were not applicable to children and adolescents, and identified additional items related to school life and peers. The investigators who adapted the instrument did not ask adolescents to identify areas that were problems for them; however, they did field test the instrument in a sample of youths, and this testing resulted in rewording of questions to improve readability.

Did the Health-Related Quality of Life Instruments Work in the Intended Way?

Measuring how people feel is not easy. Investigators must demonstrate that their instruments allow strong inferences about the effect of an intervention on HRQL. We now review how an HRQL instrument should perform (i.e., its measurement properties) if it is to be useful.

Signal and Noise

Investigators use HRQL instruments in two distinct ways: to help clinicians distinguish between people who have better or worse levels of HRQL at a particular point, or to measure whether people feel better or worse over time.[23] Consider a trial of people at risk for pressure ulcers, which shows that a pressure-relieving mattress successfully prevents pressure ulcers in patients with scores of 12 or less on the Braden Scale for Predicting Pressure Sore Risk. We could use the Braden score for two purposes. First, we could use it to discriminate between patients who do and do not need to use pressure-relieving mattresses.[24] Second, we could monitor whether pressure-relieving mattresses reduce patients' risk of pressure ulcers over time and in so doing monitor changes in the Braden score.

If, when we are trying to discriminate among people at a single point, everyone has the same score, we will not be able to tell who is doing better and who is doing worse. The key differences we are trying to detect—the *signal*—come from differences in scores among patients. The larger those differences are, the better we will be able to discriminate. At the same time, if patients' scores on repeated measurement fluctuate wildly—we call this fluctuation the *noise*—we will not be able to say much about their relative well-being.[25] The greater is the noise, which comes from variability within patients, the more difficulty we will have in detecting the signal. For instance, consider an instrument in which scores range from 20 to 100. If we measure stable patients once and again 2 weeks later, and if each patient's scores on the two occasions are within five points of one another, we may feel satisfied with the instrument's reproducibility. However, if all patients score between 55 and 60 on the two repetitions, we will be unable to comment on which patients have less HRQL impairment and which have more (the instrument's ability to discriminate between patients).

The technical term usually used to describe the ratio of variability between patients (the signal) to the total variability (the signal plus the noise) is *reliability.* If patients' scores change little over time but are very different from patient to patient, reliability will be high.

If the change in score within patients is high in relation to differences among patients, reliability will be low. The mathematical expression of reliability is the variance (or variability) among patients divided by the variance among patients plus the variance within patients.

By contrast, instruments used to evaluate change over time must be able to detect important changes in the way patients feel, even if those changes are small. Thus, the signal comes from the difference in scores in patients whose status has improved or deteriorated, and the noise comes from the variability in scores in patients whose status has not changed. The term we use for the ability to detect change (the ratio of signal to noise over time) is *responsiveness*.

An unresponsive instrument can result in false-negative results, in which the intervention improves how patients feel, yet the instrument fails to detect the improvement. This problem may be particularly applicable to questionnaires that cover all relevant areas of HRQL, but cover each area superficially.

In studies that show no difference in HRQL when patients receive a new versus a conventional intervention, nurses should look for evidence that the instrument was able to detect small or medium-sized effects in previous investigations. In the absence of such evidence, instrument unresponsiveness becomes a plausible reason for the failure to detect differences in HRQL. For example, researchers who conducted a randomized trial of a diabetes education program reported no changes in two measures of well-being and attributed the results to, among other factors, lack of integration of the program with standard therapy.[26] However, participants in the educational program showed improvements in knowledge and self-care and decreased feelings of dependence on physicians when compared with a control group. Given these changes, the lack of difference in well-being between groups may be explained by inadequate responsiveness of the two well-being measures.

Using the Guide

The study that describes the development of the Diabetes Quality of Life for Youth Measure reported estimates of reliability (Cronbach alpha) ranging from 0.82 to 0.85 for the three scales.[22] This measure proved to be responsive in the coping skills trial as it detected statistically significant differences between intervention and control groups over time.

Validity

Validity has to do with whether an instrument measures what it is intended to measure. The absence of a reference, gold, or criterion standard for HRQL creates a challenge for anyone hoping to measure how patients feel. We can be more confident that an instrument is doing its job if the items appear to measure what is intended (the instrument's *face validity*), although face validity alone is of limited help.

Empirical evidence that an instrument measures the domains of interest allows stronger inferences. To provide such evidence, investigators have borrowed validation strategies from psychologists, who have long struggled with determining whether questionnaires assessing intelligence, attitudes, and emotional function really do measure what is intended. Investigators who are interested in underlying attitudes may find apparent differences between persons that actually reflect variability in the tendency to provide socially acceptable answers, rather than differences in attitudes. For example, if investigators find apparent effects of rehabilitation on HRQL, in reality they may be merely detecting differences in satisfaction with care. If this were true, the instrument would be detecting a signal, but it would be the wrong signal.

Establishing validity therefore involves examining the logical relationships that should exist between assessment measures. For example, we would expect that patients with lower treadmill exercise capacity generally would have more dyspnea in daily life than would patients with higher exercise capacity. We would also expect substantial correlations between a new measure of emotional function and existing emotional function questionnaires. When we are interested in evaluating change over time, we examine correlations of change scores. For example, patients who deteriorate in their treadmill exercise capacity should, in general, show increases in dyspnea, whereas those whose exercise capacity improves should experience less dyspnea. Similarly, a new emotional function measure should show improvement in patients who improve on existing measures of emotional function. The technical term for this process is testing an instrument's *construct validity*.

Readers should look for evidence of the validity of HRQL measures used in clinical studies. Reports of randomized trials using HRQL measures seldom include evidence of the validity of the instruments they use, but clinicians can be reassured by statements (backed by citations) that the questionnaires have been validated previously. In the absence of evident face validity or empirical evidence of validity, readers are entitled to be skeptical about a study's measurement of HRQL.

USING THE GUIDE

In the study that described the development of the Diabetes Quality of Life for Youth Measure,[22] the investigators reported that the three scales did not correlate with metabolic control as measured by glycosylated hemoglobin values, but they did correlate with self-rated health status ($r = 0.54$). Although practitioners may have a tendency to equate good metabolic control with quality of life, these data suggest that self-perceived quality of life has a different meaning to adolescents with type 1 diabetes.

Were Important Aspects of Health-Related Quality of Life Omitted?

Although investigators may have addressed HRQL issues, they may not have done so comprehensively. The importance of exhaustive measurement may depend on the particular context. Imagine a hierarchy that begins with symptoms, moves on to the functional consequences of symptoms, and ends with more complex elements such as emotional function. If, as a clinician, you believe that your patient's sole interest is in whether an intervention relieves the primary symptoms and most important functional limitations, you will be satisfied with a limited range of assessment. Randomized trials of patients with migraine[27,28] and postherpetic neuralgia[29] primarily measured pain; studies of patients with rheumatoid arthritis[30,31] and back pain[32] measured pain and physical function, but not emotional or social function.

Although such omissions are unimportant to some patients, they may be critical to others (see Chapter 34, Incorporating Patient Values). We encourage you to consider the broader impact of disease on patients' lives. Disease-specific measures that explore the full range of patients' problems and experiences remind us of domains we might otherwise forget. We can trust these measures to be comprehensive if the developers have conducted a detailed survey of patients who have the illness or condition.

If you are interested in going beyond the specific illness and comparing the impact of interventions on HRQL across diseases or conditions, you will require a more comprehensive assessment. None of the measures, whether they are disease specific, system or organ specific, function specific (e.g., sleep or sexual function), or problem specific (e.g., pain), are adequate for comparisons across conditions. Such comparisons require generic measures that cover all relevant areas of HRQL and are designed for administration to people with any kind of underlying health problem (or no problem at all). One type of generic measure, a *health profile*, yields scores for all domains of HRQL (e.g., mobility, self-care, and physical, emotional, and social function). Numerous well-established health profiles exist, including the Sickness Impact Profile[33] and the short forms of the instruments used in the Medical Outcomes Study,[34,35] with notable advantages such as simplicity, self-administration, and the ability to put changes in specific functions in the context of overall HRQL. Inevitably, however, such instruments cover each area superficially. This feature may limit their responsiveness. Indeed, several randomized trials have found that generic instruments were less powerful in detecting treatment effects than were specific instruments.[7,14,36-40] Ironically, generic instruments also may not be sufficiently comprehensive; in certain cases, they may completely omit patients' primary symptoms.

USING THE GUIDE

Disease-specific measures may comprehensively sample all aspects of HRQL relevant to a specific illness and may also be responsive. The Diabetes Quality of Life for Youth Scales measure all important disease-specific areas of HRQL, including life satisfaction, impact of diabetes, and worries specific to diabetes. The investigators could have administered a generic instrument to tap into non–diabetes-related aspects of HRQL, but they likely would have failed to measure diabetes-specific issues in sufficient detail.

If There Were Trade-offs Between Quality of Life and Quantity of Life, or if an Economic Evaluation Was Performed, Were the Most Appropriate Measures Used?

Although health profiles provide information about broad domains of HRQL and therefore permit comparisons across conditions, they are ill-suited for health care policy decisions that involve integrating costs. Such decisions require choices about resource allocation across diseases, conditions, or health problems, and they inevitably mandate cost considerations (see Chapter 18, Economic Evaluation). Choosing among health care programs requires standardized comparisons of very different interventions (e.g., rehabilitation programs or health education) for very different conditions (e.g., heart disease, diabetes, or asthma). Inevitably, they involve putting a value on health states; they may thus require sophisticated weighting for patient preferences and may necessitate relating health states to anchors of death and full health. Such measures may aid policy makers in making the right decisions about how public money is allocated.

Most HRQL questionnaires describe the resultant health states of programs and interventions in a way that is sufficient to inform clinicians and patients, but they do not quantify how much individual patients or members of a society value specific health states or services. Additional economic measures of a different dimension are needed to ascertain the value of the health state. Studies that measure both descriptive aspects of HRQL (using generic health indices) and the valuation of that health state in the same patient show poor correlation between how patients describe health states and how they value them.[41] Measures that provide a single number that summarizes HRQL are preference weighted or value weighted; these have the preferences or values anchored to death and full health and are called *utility measures*. Typically, utility measures use a scale from zero (death) to 1.0 (full health) to summarize HRQL. Because they weight the duration of life according to its quality, their output is often called *quality-adjusted life-years (QALYs)* or *disability-adjusted life-years (DALYs)*. Thus, utilities are holistic measures that ask patients to express, in a single value, their strengths of preferences for particular health states (see Chapter 18, Economic Evaluation).

An instrument called the *standard gamble* provides one way of determining the utility a patient attaches to a health state. One may ask a patient to picture himself or herself at age 60 years in good health, except for severe osteoarthritis of the right hip, which results in severe pain with movement and marked functional limitation. The patient chooses between two options (Figure 12-1). In one option (the *lower arm* of Figure 12-1), the patient will live in the current state of health, limited by pain and disability, for 20 years and then will die. In the other hypothetical option (the *upper arm* of Figure 12-1), the patient will either return to full health and live for 20 years and then die, or he or she will die immediately. One may start by setting the probability of full health in the gamble arm (*x* in Figure 12-1) at 95% and the probability of immediate death (*y* in Figure 12-1) at 5%. If the patient chooses the gamble, one progressively lowers *x* and increases *y* until the patient becomes indifferent. If the patient becomes indifferent at a probability of full health of 90%, he or

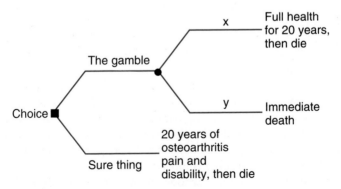

Figure 12–1. The standard gamble.

she is indicating that the utility attached to living with the pain and limitation of hip osteoarthritis is 0.90 (with full health having a utility of 1.0). If he or she becomes indifferent when *x* is 60%, this means that the utility associated with living with hip osteoarthritis is 0.60. The standard gamble is only one of numerous ways to measure patient utilities.

In a classic article, Boyle and colleagues[42] used a utility measure to calculate that treating critically ill infants weighing 1000 to 1499 g at birth cost $3200 per QALY gained, whereas treating infants with birth weights of 500 to 999 g cost $22,400 per QALY gained (in 1978 Canadian dollars). Estimates of the cost per QALY for treating patients undergoing renal dialysis have ranged from approximately US$30,000 to $50,000.[43,44] Different weighting schemes yield different results and may therefore be considered arbitrary. However, increasingly simple utility measures are now available, have provided interesting results in clinical trials, and may facilitate integrating cost into policy decisions. Nevertheless, the use, measurement, and interpretation of utility measures remain controversial (see Chapter 18, Economic Evaluation).[45]

> ### Using the Guide
>
> The investigators in the coping skills training trial[1] did not use a health profile or a utility measure, which limited the data for comparisons across disease states and prevented a formal economic analysis.

WHAT ARE THE RESULTS?

How Can We Interpret the Magnitude of Effect on Health-Related Quality of Life?

Understanding the results of a trial measuring HRQL involves special challenges. Patients with acute back pain who were prescribed bed rest had mean scores on the Oswestry Back-Disability Index, a measure of disease-specific functional status, that were 3.9 points worse than those of control patients.[32] Patients with severe rheumatoid arthritis who were allocated to treatment with cyclosporine had a mean disability score that was 0.28 units better than that of control patients.[30] Are these differences trivial, are they small but important, are they of moderate magnitude, or do they reflect large and extremely important differences in efficacy among interventions?

These examples show that the interpretability of most HRQL measures is not self-evident. When trying to interpret HRQL results, we must consider that different patients will place different values on the same change in function or capacity. This explains why, in some lines of research (particularly health economics), investigators set aside HRQL measures with multiple domains in favor of holistic measures (utilities) that rely on each individual patient's preferences (e.g., the standard gamble). Although we can try to set "minimal important differences," it is likely that for some patients even smaller differences will be important or, conversely, that much larger differences will be required before a given change in HRQL will be seen as worthwhile.

The result is a series of trade-offs that are often assessed informally in the interaction between health care workers and patients. For example, patient A may be desperate for small improvements in a particular domain of HRQL and willing to participate in time-intensive, inconvenient education sessions to achieve that improvement. Patient B may have a very different view. Eliciting these preferences is an integral part of practicing evidence-based health care effectively and sensitively (see Chapter 1, Introduction to Evidence-Based Nursing, and Chapter 34, Incorporating Patient Values).

However, when reading the literature, clinicians still must arrive at some estimate of how well a given intervention performs with regard to effecting improvements in HRQL. Numerous methods are available for understanding the magnitude of HRQL effects. Investigators may relate changes in HRQL questionnaire scores to well-known functional measures (e.g., the New York Heart Association functional classification), clinical diagnosis (e.g., the change in score needed to move people into or out of the diagnostic category of depression), or the impact of major life events.[46] They may relate changes in HRQL scores to patients' global ratings of the magnitude of change they have experienced[47] or the extent to which they rate themselves as feeling better or worse than other patients.[48] Regardless of strategy, if investigators do not provide an indication of how to interpret changes in HRQL scores, the findings will be of limited use to clinicians.

These strategies lead to estimates of change in HRQL measures that, for individual patients or groups of patients, constitute trivial, small, medium, and large differences. For example, we may establish that 3.9 points on the Oswestry Back-Disability Index or 0.28 units on a rheumatoid arthritis disability index signifies, on average, small but important changes for individual patients. This still leaves a problem for interpretation of results from clinical trials. For instance, if the mean change on the Oswestry Back-Disability Index is only 2.0, does this mean that we can dismiss the difference as unimportant to patients?

Investigators have gained insight into this issue by examining the distribution of change in HRQL in individual patients and by calculating the proportion of patients who achieved small, medium, and large gains from interventions and the associated numbers needed to treat (NNTs).[49]

USING THE GUIDE

The investigators of the trial of coping skills training in adolescents with type 1 diabetes reported that the intervention improved quality of life over a 1-year period ($P = 0.005$).[1] This statement alone does not allow clinicians to interpret the magnitude of difference in HRQL.

Contact with the primary author of the study revealed the following: mean differences in change between treatment and control groups of 6.0 on the Diabetes Life Satisfaction Scale (where 23 is the poorest quality of life and 115 is excellent quality of life); a difference in change on the Disease Impact Scale of 6.1 (where 17 is the best quality of life and 85 the worst); and a difference in change on the Disease-Related Worries Scale of 2.0 (where 11 represents the best quality of life and 55 the poorest). All differences favored the intervention group (M. Grey [Margaret.Grey@yale.edu], e-mail, January 8, 2003).

These numbers are still of limited help. They would be considerably more useful if we knew the change in score that constitutes a small but important difference (the minimal important difference). Unfortunately, this information is not available.

Using the Guide—cont'd

We can nevertheless gain some insight into the size of the effect by converting the differences into standard deviation units; that is, we can look at the magnitude of the effects in terms of the standard deviation. For instance, for the Life Satisfaction Scale, the mean difference in change between the two groups was 6.0, and the largest standard deviation observed in the treatment and control groups was approximately 15. Thus, the effect size is 6/15 or 0.4. Making similar calculations (that is, dividing the mean difference in changes between the two groups by the standard deviation), the effect sizes on the three domains vary from about 0.3 to 0.6.

These effect sizes remain, however, difficult to interpret. To facilitate interpretation, one can set a threshold for a small but important improvement in quality of life. Then, one can calculate the proportion of patients in each group who achieved this particular improvement. The difference in proportions then forms the basis for calculating the number of patients one would need to treat (NNT) to produce a small but important difference in quality of life (see Chapter 4, Health Care Interventions and Chapter 27, Measures of Association).[50]

Rather conveniently, there is a more or less constant relationship between the effect size and the proportion improved, irrespective of the choice of the threshold of the minimal important difference. Table 12-2 describes that relationship between the effect size (first row), the proportion improved by the intervention (second row), and the NNT (third row). You can see from the table that effect sizes ranging from 0.3 to 0.6 correspond to NNTs of nine to five.

In other words, the number of adolescents who would need to participate in the program for a single person to achieve a small but important improvement in quality of life is in the range of five to nine (third row of Table 12-2). Another way to express this is that an individual patient's likelihood of achieving important improvement as a result of the intervention is in the range of 11% to 20% (second row of Table 12-2).

HOW CAN I APPLY THE RESULTS TO PATIENT CARE?

Will the Information From the Study Help Patients to Make Informed Decisions About Their Health Care?

People with the same chronic disease often vary markedly in the problems they experience. Even if the problems are the same, the magnitude of the impact of these problems on their lives may differ. Assessment of HRQL helps in the care of an individual patient only if that patient's problems are similar to those of patients in the trial.

Table **12-2**   Calculation of NNTs From Effect Sizes

Effect size	0.1	0.2	0.3	0.4	0.5	0.6	0.7	0.8	0.9	1.0
Proportion improved by intervention	0.05	0.08	0.11	0.14	0.20	0.20	0.25	0.25	0.33	0.33
NNT*	20	13	9	7	5	5	4	4	3	3

NNT, *Number needed to treat.*
NNT = 1/proportion improved by intervention.

Knowing whether the HRQL results of a study are relevant for patients requires understanding of the illness experience of those patients. Even the most common problems of a chronic disease do not affect all patients who are comparably afflicted. For example, 92% of patients with inflammatory bowel disease complain of frequent bowel movements, and 82% complain of abdominal cramps.[51] With respect to emotional function, 78% feel frustrated, and 76% feel depressed. These percentages come from a study that recruited patients from a secondary care setting;[51] the proportion of patients with these problems would likely have been smaller if investigators had sampled from primary care settings. Furthermore, the patients who experienced these difficulties varied in the extent to which they believed the problems to be important.

USING THE GUIDE

Thinking back to our opening clinical scenario, before answering the question about how coping skills training would affect the adolescent's life, the nurse would need to be aware of the problems the adolescent was currently experiencing, the importance he attached to these problems, and the value he would attach to having the problems improved (see Chapter 34, Incorporating Patient Values).

Ideally, one would measure the impact of the intervention on the individual patient. However, this is often not feasible. When nurses use data collected from other patients to inform the patient under consideration, HRQL instruments that focus on specific aspects of patients' function and symptoms may be of more use than global measures or measures that tell us simply about patients' satisfaction or well-being. For instance, people with chronic lung disease may find it more informative to know that other patients who received the intervention became less dyspneic and fatigued in daily activity, rather than simply that they judged their quality of life to be improved. HRQL measures are most useful when results facilitate their practical use by you and the patients in your care.

Did the Study Design Simulate Clinical Practice?

Interventions may affect quality of life by reducing disease symptoms and consequences and by creating new problems (e.g., side effects). In fact, negative effects may make the cure worse than the disease. Investigators conducting trials are usually blind to treatment allocation, and they try to keep patients in study interventions for as long as possible. Patients may therefore persist despite considerable detrimental effects; ultimately, this may be reflected in their HRQL measure.

This is not how we normally practice. If patients experience significant negative effects, we discontinue the intervention. Thus, the design of clinical trials may create an artificial situation, with misleading estimates of the impact of an intervention on HRQL. This issue is of particular concern for patients receiving treatment with medications such as antihypertensive agents, in which much of the impairment in HRQL may result from the treatment, rather than from the medical condition.

USING THE GUIDE

The trial of coping skills training in adolescents with type 1 diabetes is likely to have simulated clinical practice well. Managing the physical, emotional, and social demands of type 1 diabetes is challenging enough that if coping skills training is beneficial, patients are likely to continue with the intervention despite the time and travel requirements. If the adolescent is experiencing problems similar to those of the trial patients and if those problems are important to him, he will likely achieve benefits comparable to that of patients in the trial.

CLINICAL RESOLUTION

In light of the available information, you inform the adolescent patient that, on average, adolescents who participated in the coping skills program felt more satisfied with life and were less worried. The magnitude of the effect, however, was not large. The young man would have about a 1 in 5 chance of gaining important benefits from the program. The patient decides to reflect on what you have told him for the next week and return at that time with his decision.

We encourage nurses to consider the impact of interventions on patients' HRQL and to look for information about this impact in clinical trials. Responsive, valid, and interpretable instruments measuring experiences of importance to most patients should increasingly help guide our clinical decisions.

REFERENCES

1. Grey M, Boland EA, Davidson M, Li J, Tambolane WV. Coping skills training for youth with diabetes mellitus has long-lasting effects on metabolic control and quality of life. *J Pediatr*. 2000;137:107-113.
2. Fletcher RH, Fletcher SW, Wagner EH. *Clinical Epidemiology: The Essentials*. 3rd ed. Baltimore: Williams & Wilkins; 1996:4-6.
3. Newton L, Rosen A, Tennant C, et al. Deinstitutionalization for long-term mental illness: an ethnographic study. *Aust NZ J Psychiatry*. 2000;34:484-490.
4. Albrecht GL, Devlieger PJ. The disability paradox: high quality of life against all odds. *Soc Sci Med*. 1999;48:977-988.
5. Treat-Jacobson D, Halverson SL, Ratchford A, Regensteiner JG, Lindquist R, Hirsch AT. A patient-derived perspective of health-related quality of life with peripheral arterial disease. *J Nurs Scholarship*. 2002;34:55-60.
6. Guyatt GH, Feeny DH, Patrick DL. Measuring health-related quality of life. *Ann Intern Med*. 1993;118:622-629.
7. Gill TM, Feinstein AR. A critical appraisal of the quality of quality-of-life measurements. *JAMA*. 1994;272:619-626.
8. Wilson IB, Cleary PD. Linking clinical variables with health-related quality of life: a conceptual model of patient outcomes. *JAMA*. 1995;273:59-65.
9. Guyatt GH, Cook DJ. Health status, quality of life, and the individual. *JAMA*. 1994;272:630-631.
10. Nocturnal Oxygen Therapy Trial Group. Continuous or nocturnal oxygen therapy in hypoxemic chronic obstructive lung disease: a clinical trial. *Ann Intern Med*. 1980;93:391-398.
11. Heaton RK, Grant I, McSweeny AJ, Adams KM, Petty TL. Psychologic effects of continuous and nocturnal oxygen therapy in hypoxemic chronic obstructive pulmonary disease. *Arch Intern Med*. 1983;143:1941-1947.

12. Mulrow CD, Mulrow JP, Linn WD, Aguilar C, Ramirez G. Relative efficacy of vasodilator therapy in chronic congestive heart failure: implications of randomized trials. *JAMA*. 1988;259:3422-3426.

13. Packer M, Carver JR, Rodeheffer RJ, et al, for the PROMISE Study Research Group. Effect of oral milrinone on mortality in severe chronic heart failure. *N Engl J Med*. 1991;325:1468-1475.

14. Juniper EF, Svensson K, O'Byrne PM, et al. Asthma quality of life during 1 year of treatment with budesonide with or without formoterol. *Eur Respir J*. 1999;14:1038-1043.

15. Juniper EF, Norman GR, Cox FM, Roberts JN. Comparison of the standard gamble, rating scale, AQLQ and SF-36 for measuring quality of life in asthma. *Eur Respir J*. 2001;18:38-44.

16. Juniper EF, Price DB, Stampone P, Creemers JP, Mol SJ, Fireman P. Clinically important improvements in asthma-specific quality of life, but no difference in conventional clinical indexes in patients changed from conventional beclomethasone dipropionate to approximately half the dose of extrafine beclomethasone dipropionate. *Chest*. 2002;121:1824-1832.

17. COMBIVENT Inhalation Solution Study Group. Routine nebulized ipratropium and albuterol together are better than either alone in COPD. *Chest*. 1997;112:1514-1521.

18. Jaeschke R, Guyatt GH, Willan A, et al. Effect of increasing doses of beta agonists on spirometric parameters, exercise capacity, and quality of life in patients with chronic airflow limitation. *Thorax*. 1994;49:479-484.

19. Guyatt GH, Berman LB, Townsend M, Pugsley SO, Chambers LW. A measure of quality of life for clinical trials in chronic lung disease. *Thorax*. 1987;42:773-778.

20. Goldstein RS, Gort EH, Stubbing D, Avendano MA, Guyatt GH. Randomised controlled trial of respiratory rehabilitation. *Lancet*. 1994;344:1394-1397.

21. Wasson JH, Reda DJ, Bruskewitz RC, Elinson J, Keller AM, Henderson WG, for the Veterans Affairs Cooperative Study Group on Transurethral Resection of the Prostate. A comparison of transurethral surgery with watchful waiting for moderate symptoms of benign prostatic hyperplasia. *N Engl J Med*. 1995;332:75-79.

22. Ingersoll GM, Marrero DG. A modified quality-of-life measure for youths: psychometric properties. *Diabetes Educ*. 1991;17:114-118.

23. Kirshner B, Guyatt GH. A methodological framework for assessing health indices. *J Chronic Dis*. 1985;38:27-36.

24. Bergstrom N, Demuth PJ, Braden BJ. A clinical trial of the Braden scale for predicting pressure sore risk. *Nurs Clin North Am*. 1987; 22:417-428.

25. Guyatt GH, Kirshner B, Jaeschke R. Measuring health status: what are the necessary measurement properties? *J Clin Epidemiol*. 1992;45:1341-1345.

26. de Weerdt I, Visser AP, Kok GJ, de Weerdt O, van der Veen EA. Randomized controlled multicentre evaluation of an education programme for insulin-treated diabetic patients: effects on metabolic control, quality of life, and costs of therapy. *Diabet Med*. 1991;8:338-345.

27. Salonen R, Ashford E, Dahlof C, et al, for the International Intranasal Sumatriptan Study Group. Intranasal sumatriptan for the acute treatment of migraine. *J Neurol*. 1994;241:463-469.

28. Mathew NT, Saper JR, Silberstein SD, et al. Migraine prophylaxis with divalproex. *Arch Neurol*. 1995;52:281-286.

29. Tyring S, Barbarash RA, Nahlik JE, et al, for the Collaborative Famciclovir Herpes Zoster Study Group. Famciclovir for the treatment of acute herpes zoster: effects on acute disease and postherpetic neuralgia: a randomized, double-blind, placebo-controlled trial. *Ann Intern Med*. 1995;123:89-96.

30. Tugwell P, Pincus T, Yocum D, et al, for the Methotrexate-Cyclosporine Combination Study Group. Combination therapy with cyclosporine and methotrexate in severe rheumatoid arthritis. *N Engl J Med*. 1995;333:137-141.

31. Kirwan JR, for the Arthritis and Rheumatism Council Low-Dose Glucocorticoid Study Group. The effect of glucocorticoids on joint destruction in rheumatoid arthritis. *N Engl J Med*. 1995;333:142-146.

32. Malmivaara A, Hakkinen U, Aro T, et al. The treatment of acute low back pain: bed rest, exercises, or ordinary activity? *N Engl J Med*. 1995;332:351-355.

33. Bergner M, Bobbitt RA, Carter WB, Gilson BS. The Sickness Impact Profile: development and final revision of a health status measure. *Med Care*. 1981;19:787-805.

34. Tarlov AR, Ware JE Jr, Greenfield S, Nelson EC, Perrin E, Zubkoff M. The Medical Outcomes Study: an application of methods for monitoring the results of medical care. *JAMA.* 1989;262:925-930.

35. Ware JE Jr, Kosinski M, Bayliss MS, McHorney CA, Rogers WH, Raczek A. Comparison of methods for the scoring and statistical analysis of SF-36 health profile and summary measures: summary of results from the Medical Outcomes Study. *Med Care.* 1995;33(suppl 4):AS264-AS279.

36. Tandon PK, Stander H, Schwarz RP Jr. Analysis of quality of life data from a randomized, placebo-controlled heart-failure trial. *J Clin Epidemiol.* 1989;42:955-962.

37. Smith D, Baker G, Davies G, Dewey M, Chadwick DW. Outcomes of add-on treatment with lamotrigine in partial epilepsy. *Epilepsia.* 1993;34:312-322.

38. Chang SW, Fine R, Siegel D, Chesney M, Black D, Hulley SB. The impact of diuretic therapy on reported sexual function. *Arch Intern Med.* 1991;151:2402-2408.

39. Tugwell P, Bombardier C, Buchanan WW, et al. Methotrexate in rheumatoid arthritis: impact on quality of life assessed by traditional standard-item and individualized patient preference health status questionnaires. *Arch Intern Med.* 1990;150:59-62.

40. Laupacis A, Wong C, Churchill D, for the Canadian Erythropoietin Study Group. The use of generic and specific quality-of-life measures in hemodialysis patients treated with erythropoietin. *Control Clin Trials.* 1991;12(suppl 4):168S-179S.

41. Bosch JL, Hunink MG. The relationship between descriptive and valuational quality-of-life measures in patients with intermittent claudication. *Med Decis Making.* 1996;16:217-225.

42. Boyle MH, Torrance GW, Sinclair JC, Horwood SP. Economic evaluation of neonatal intensive care of very-low-birth-weight infants. *N Engl J Med.* 1983;308:1330-1337.

43. Hornberger JC, Garber AM, Chernew ME. Is high-flux dialysis cost-effective? *Int J Technol Assess Health Care.* 1993;9:85-96.

44. Hornberger JC, for the Renal Physicians Association Working Committee on Clinical Guidelines. The hemodialysis prescription and cost effectiveness. *J Am Soc Nephrol.* 1993;4:1021-1027.

45. Naylor CD. Cost-effectiveness analysis: are the outputs worth the inputs? *ACP J Club.* 1996;124:A12-A14.

46. Testa MA, Anderson RB, Nackley JF, Hollenberg NK, for the Quality-of-Life Hypertension Study Group. Quality of life and antihypertensive therapy in men: a comparison of captopril with enalapril. *N Engl J Med.* 1993;328:907-913.

47. Juniper EF, Guyatt GH, Willan A, Griffith LE. Determining a minimal important change in a disease-specific quality of life questionnaire. *J Clin Epidemiol.* 1994;47:81-87.

48. Redelmeier DA, Guyatt GH, Goldstein RS. Assessing the minimal important difference in symptoms: a comparison of two techniques. *J Clin Epidemiol.* 1996;49:1215-1219.

49. Guyatt GH, Juniper EF, Walter SD, Griffith LE, Goldstein RS. Interpreting treatment effects in randomised trials. *BMJ.* 1998;316:690-693.

50. Norman GR, Gwadry Sridhar F, Guyatt GH, Walter SD. The relation of distribution- and anchor-based approaches in interpretation of changes in health-related quality of life. *Med Care.* 2001;39:1039-1047.

51. Mitchell A, Guyatt G, Singer J, et al. Quality of life in patients with inflammatory bowel disease. *J Clin Gastroenterol.* 1988;10:306-310.

13

Surrogate Outcomes

Alba DiCenso and Gordon Guyatt

The following Editorial Board members also made substantive contributions to this chapter: Andrew Jull, Cathy Kessenich, Andrea Nelson, and Mary van Soeren.

We gratefully acknowledge the work of Heiner Bucher, Deborah Cook, Anne Holbrook, and Finlay McAlister on the original chapter that appears in the Users' Guides to the Medical Literature, *edited by Guyatt and Rennie.*

In This Chapter

Finding the Evidence

Surrogate Outcomes

Are the Results Valid?
    Is There a Strong, Independent, Consistent Association Between the Surrogate End Point and the Clinical End Point?
    Have Randomized Trials of Other Interventions Shown That Improvement in the Surrogate End Point Has Consistently Led to Improvement in the Target Outcome?

What Are the Results?
    How Large, Precise, and Lasting Was the Intervention Effect?

How Can I Apply the Results to Patient Care?
    Are the Likely Intervention Benefits Worth the Potential Risks and Costs?

Should We Recommend Exercise for a Postmenopausal Woman to Prevent Osteoporotic Fractures on the Basis of Its Effect on Bone Density?

You are a primary health care nurse practitioner seeing a 52-year-old postmenopausal woman for a periodic health assessment. She has enjoyed good health all her life, is not taking any medications, works in an office, and leads a sedentary life. She tells you that her mother fell and fractured her hip at the age of 70. She has read that osteoporosis leads to fractures and wonders whether she is at risk. Her physical examination is normal. She has no history of back pain, no height loss, no back tenderness or pain with movement during the examination, and no evidence of kyphosis.

She dislikes exercise but would consider it to avoid fractures. Because this woman finds exercise distasteful, you believe that it is important to provide her with specific information about the relationship of exercise, osteoporosis, and fractures. You tell her that you would like to look up the most recent research related to her question and get back to her.

FINDING THE EVIDENCE

You are interested in both what experts recommend about the patient's question and whether there are any systematic reviews that summarize the evidence on which the experts are basing their recommendations. You access the Internet to look for both a clinical practice guideline and a systematic review on the topic. You connect to the Canadian clinical practice guidelines database, CMA Infobase (*http://mdm.ca/ cpgsnew/cpgs/index.asp*), and select the Basic Search option. You conduct a search by entering the keyword "exercise" and the MeSH term "osteoporosis." The most recent guideline is one produced by the Osteoporosis Society of Canada entitled "2002 Clinical Practice Guidelines for the Diagnosis and Management of Osteoporosis in Canada."[1] You then connect to the Cochrane Library and search the Cochrane Database of Systematic Reviews using the keywords "exercise AND osteoporosis AND post-menopausal." You find a systematic review entitled "Exercise for Preventing and Treating Osteoporosis in Postmenopausal Women."[2]

People do not want to develop osteoporosis because it increases their risk of fractures. Therefore, the ideal study of the influence of exercise on osteoporosis will evaluate its effect on fracture rates. However, the guideline[1] tells you that there are no randomized controlled trials that evaluate the effect of physical activity on fracture prevention. As it turns out, there is one such trial. Although the objective of the Cochrane systematic review was to examine the effectiveness of exercise therapy in preventing bone loss and fractures in postmenopausal women, only one of the 18 identified trials evaluated the effect of exercise on vertebral fractures; the others examined its effect on bone density.

Unfortunately, the one study that assessed changes in fracture rates[3] is too small (n = 97) to provide reliable estimates (the trend was for exercise to increase vertebral fracture rates after 2 years of follow-up, with an odds ratio of 3.42, but the 95% confidence interval [CI] was extremely wide: 0.57 to 20.53). The authors of the systematic review recommended that long-term studies of exercise be conducted to determine its effect on fracture rates. In the meantime, you wonder whether you can substitute the findings of studies of exercise effects on a *surrogate outcome*, bone density, for the unavailable data on the *patient-important outcome*, fractures.

SURROGATE OUTCOMES

Ideally, clinicians considering the effectiveness of an intervention should refer to methodologically strong clinical trials assessing patient-important outcomes such as health-related quality of life, prevention of bone fractures, smoking cessation, and prevention of adolescent pregnancy. Often, however, these trials require such large sample sizes or such lengthy patient follow-up, that researchers look for alternatives. Substituting surrogate end points for target events permits researchers to conduct smaller and shorter trials and thus offers an apparent solution to the dilemma.

A *surrogate end point* may be defined as an intermediate outcome used as a substitute for an end point that directly measures how a patient feels, functions, or survives.[4] Surrogate end points include physiologic variables (e.g., bone density as a surrogate end point for bone fractures, blood pressure as a surrogate end point for stroke, cholesterol as a surrogate end point for heart disease, and CD4 cell count as a surrogate end point for morbidity and mortality related to acquired immunodeficiency syndrome [AIDS]) or intermediate measures of behavior change (e.g., intention to quit smoking as a surrogate end point for smoking cessation and knowledge and attitudes about sexual behavior as surrogate end points for avoidance of adolescent pregnancy or sexually transmitted diseases).

The use of surrogate end points is indispensable for drug evaluation in *phase II trials* and early *phase III trials* geared to establish or verify a drug's promise of benefit. In many countries, companies can obtain drug approval by demonstrating a positive impact on surrogate end points. The use of surrogate end points for regulatory purposes reflects drug approval decisions that regulators must make in the presence of public health realities.

Reliance on surrogate end points may be beneficial or harmful. Use of surrogate end points may lead to the rapid and appropriate dissemination of new treatments. For example, the decision of the United States Food and Drug Administration to approve new antiretroviral drugs based on information from trials using surrogate end points recognized the enormous need for effective therapies for patients with human immunodeficiency virus (HIV) infection. Subsequently, several of these drugs proved effective in randomized trials focusing on patient-important outcomes.[5-8] Conversely, reliance on surrogate end points could influence clinicians to offer interventions that may have no effect or, at worst, a negative effect on patient-important outcomes. For example, although fluoride improves lumbar spine bone density, it has also shown a strong trend toward increasing nonvertebral fractures[9] (see Chapter 14, Surprising Results of Randomized Controlled Trials).

How can clinicians distinguish between these two situations? A surrogate outcome will be consistently reliable only if there is a causal connection between changes in the surrogate outcome and changes in the clinically important outcome. Thus, the surrogate outcome must be in the causal pathway of the disease process or behavior; and an intervention's entire effect on the clinical outcome of interest should be fully captured by a change in the surrogate. In this chapter, we build on previous discussions of how one can establish a causal relationship (see Chapter 5, Harm), and we present an approach to the critical appraisal of studies using surrogate end points and the application of their results to the management of individual patients.

As our discussion demonstrates, clinicians need to assess the results of more than one study to make decisions about the adequacy of specific surrogate outcomes. Evaluation may require a comprehensive review of observational studies of the relationship between the surrogate end point and the target end point, along with review of some or all of the randomized trials that have evaluated the effect of the intervention on both end points. Although most clinicians would hesitate to take the time to conduct such an investigation, our guidelines will allow them to evaluate experts' arguments for recommending interventions on the basis of their effects on *surrogate end points*.

ARE THE RESULTS VALID?

When we consider the validity of a surrogate end point, we must address two issues. First, to be consistently reliable, the surrogate must be in the causal pathway from the intervention to the outcome. Second, we must be confident that there are no important effects of the intervention on the outcome of interest that are not mediated through or captured by the surrogate outcome. Our guides for validity, as presented in Table 13-1, bear directly on these two issues.

Is There a Strong, Independent, Consistent Association Between the Surrogate End Point and the Clinical End Point?

To function as a valid substitute for a target outcome, a surrogate end point must be associated with that target outcome. In general, researchers choose surrogate end points because they have found a *correlation* between a *surrogate outcome* and a *target outcome* in observational studies, and their understanding of biologic and behavior characteristics gives them confidence in the plausibility that changes in the surrogate will invariably lead to changes in the target outcome. The stronger the association, the more likely is a causal link between the surrogate and target outcomes. The strength of an association is reflected in statistical measures such as the *relative risk* or *odds ratio* (see Chapter 27, Measures of Association). Many biologically plausible surrogate outcomes are associated only weakly with clinically important outcomes. For example, measures of respiratory function in patients with chronic lung disease and conventional exercise tests in patients with heart and lung disease are correlated only weakly with capacity to undertake activities of daily living.[10,11] When correlations are low, the surrogate is likely to be a poor substitute for the target outcome.

One's confidence in the validity of the association also depends on whether it is consistent across different studies and after adjustment for known confounding variables. For example, ecologic studies such as the Seven Countries Study[12] suggested a strong

Table 13-1 Users' Guides for an Article Reporting a Surrogate End Point

Are the Results Valid?

- Is there a strong, independent, consistent association between the surrogate end point and the clinical end point?
- Have randomized trials of other interventions shown that improvement in the surrogate end point has consistently led to improvement in the target outcome?

What Are the Results?

- How large, precise, and lasting was the intervention effect?

How Can I Apply the Results to Patient Care?

- Are the likely intervention benefits worth the potential risks and costs?

---

correlation between serum cholesterol levels and coronary heart disease mortality even after adjusting for other predictors such as age, smoking, and systolic blood pressure. When a surrogate is associated with an outcome after adjusting for multiple other potential *prognostic factors* (also known as determinants of outcome), the association is an *independent association* (see Chapter 31, Regression and Correlation). Subsequent cohort studies confirmed this association and suggested that long-term reductions in serum cholesterol of 0.6 mmol/L would lower the risk of coronary heart disease by approximately 30%.[13] Similarly, cohort studies have consistently shown that a single measurement of plasma viral load predicts the subsequent risk of AIDS or death in patients with HIV infection.[14–19] For example, in one study, the proportion of patients who progressed to AIDS after 5 years in the lowest through the highest quartiles of viral load was 8%, 26%, 49%, and 62%, respectively.[19] Moreover, this association retained its predictive power after adjustment for other potential predictors such as CD4 cell count.[14–18]

USING THE GUIDE
The studies in the systematic review of exercise and prevention of osteoporosis examined the effect of exercise on a surrogate outcome, bone density, rather than on the patient-important outcome, fractures. A systematic review of observational studies has shown that increased bone density does indeed have a relatively strong, consistent, independent association with fractures.[20] Thus, bone density meets the first criterion for an acceptable surrogate end point.

Meeting this first criterion is necessary, but not sufficient, to support reliance on a surrogate outcome. Before offering an intervention on the basis of its effects on a surrogate outcome, a consistent relationship must be demonstrated between the surrogate and target outcomes based on data from randomized trials; the effect of the intervention on the surrogate outcome must be large, precise, and lasting; and the benefit-to-risk trade-off must be clear.

Have Randomized Trials of Other Interventions Shown That Improvement in the Surrogate End Point Has Consistently Led to Improvement in the Target Outcome?

Given the possibility that an association may not be causal, pathophysiologic studies, ecologic studies, and cohort studies are insufficient to establish a definitive link between surrogate and clinically important outcomes. We can confidently rely on surrogate end points only when long-term randomized controlled trials have consistently shown that modification of the surrogate is associated with concomitant modifications in the target outcome. For example, although sex education increases knowledge about sexuality and birth control,[21] a systematic review of randomized trials found that it did not delay initiation of sexual intercourse, improve use of birth control, or reduce adolescent pregnancies.[22] Thus, an increase in knowledge does not necessarily translate into an improvement in sexual behavior and is therefore an invalid surrogate outcome for the clinically important outcome of pregnancy prevention.

Similarly, although ventricular ectopic beats are associated with adverse prognosis in patients with myocardial infarction,[23] and although class I antiarrhythmic agents effectively suppress ventricular arrhythmias,[24] these drugs actually increased mortality when they were evaluated in randomized trials.[25] In this case, reliance on the surrogate end point of suppression of nonlethal arrhythmias led to the deaths of tens of thousands of patients.[26] This experience led investigators evaluating other classes of antiarrythmic drugs to realize that reduction in nonlethal arrythmias provides insufficient evidence of benefit.

The treatment of heart failure provides another instructive example. Trials of angiotensin-converting enzyme (ACE) inhibitors in patients with heart failure demonstrated parallel increases in exercise capacity[27-30] and decreases in mortality.[31] These findings suggested that clinicians might be able to use exercise capacity as a valid surrogate outcome for mortality in studies of patients with heart failure. Both milrinone[32] and epoprostenol[33] improved exercise tolerance in patients with symptomatic heart failure. However, when these drugs were evaluated in randomized controlled trials, both showed an associated increase in cardiovascular mortality, which in one case was statistically significant[34] and in the second case led to early termination of the study.[35] Thus, exercise tolerance is inconsistent in predicting reduced mortality and is therefore an invalid surrogate outcome.

Other suggested surrogate end points in patients with heart failure have included ejection fraction, heart rate variability, and markers of autonomic function.[36] The dopaminergic agent ibopamine positively influences all three surrogate end points; yet, a randomized trial showed that the drug increased mortality in patients with heart failure.[37] In another example, the positive effect of growth hormone on certain surrogate outcomes, including nitrogen balance and facilitating weaning from mechanical ventilation, led to optimism about its likely effect on mortality in critically ill patients.[38,39] However, two randomized trials found large increases in mortality with growth hormone.[40]

We can contrast these examples with randomized trials that have consistently shown that modification of CD4 cell count is associated with changes in important outcomes. Numerous trials comparing different classes of antiretroviral therapies have demonstrated that patients randomized to more potent drug regimens had higher CD4 cell counts and were less likely to progress to AIDS or death.[8,41] Although there is no guarantee that the next trial using a different class of drugs will show the same pattern, these results strengthen our inference that if therapy for HIV infection increases CD4 cell count, a reduction in AIDS-related mortality will result.

These examples highlight the point made earlier: confidence in a surrogate outcome depends on the assumption that the surrogate captures the full relationship between the treatment and the outcome.[42,43] This assumption can be violated in two ways. First, treatment may have a beneficial mechanism of effect on the outcome independent of its effect on the surrogate outcome. For instance, although ACE inhibitors and calcium-channel blockers both appear to reduce blood pressure and stroke equally well, one explanation for the superior effect of ACE inhibitors over calcium antagonists on other patient-important outcomes in hypertension (e.g., myocardial infarction or congestive heart failure) is that ACE inhibitors may have biologic effects independent of blood pressure lowering that calcium antagonists do not share.[44,45]

Second, treatment may have a deleterious effect on the outcome independent of its effect on the surrogate outcome. For instance, clofibrate was shown to successfully lower cholesterol in a trial of the primary prevention of ischemic heart disease. If the investigators had not also examined the patient-important outcome of mortality, they would have missed the increase in all-cause mortality in the treatment group.[46]

USING THE GUIDE

Systematic reviews of alendronate[47] and risedronate[48] for prevention of osteoporotic fractures in postmenopausal women have shown parallel increases in bone density and reductions in the incidence of new vertebral fractures. This finding suggests that clinicians could rely on bone density to evaluate new interventions for prevention of osteoporosis and assume that increases in bone density would be accompanied by reductions in fractures.

However, a secondary prevention trial of postmenopausal women using sodium fluoride showed divergent results.[49] Although sodium fluoride increased bone density at the lumbar spine by 35% over a 5-year period, more vertebral and nonvertebral fractures occurred in the intervention group than in the placebo group (163 vertebral and 72 nonvertebral fractures occurred in 101 women receiving sodium fluoride, versus 136 vertebral and 24 nonvertebral fractures in 101 women receiving placebo). In another randomized trial, sodium fluoride again showed a large increase in bone density without any change in fracture rate.[50] Inferences on the basis of unchanged bone density may also be problematic. A study of calcium carbonate malate and vitamin D in elderly patients showed virtually no change in bone density, but researchers noted a reduction in fracture risk of approximately 50%.[51] Thus, increase in bone density as a surrogate end point has shown an inconsistent relationship with osteoporotic fractures.

Further exploration of the results of randomized trials of antiosteoporotic therapy has reinforced the message that bone density measurements capture only part of the

o   USING THE GUIDE—CONT'D

treatment effects. If change in bone density were the sole determinant of the effect of an intervention on fractures, one would expect a strong relationship between change in bone density and relative risk of fracture. The weaker the relationship is, the more likely it will be that other effects of treatment (e.g., effects on the bone architecture or matrix) affect fracture risk and the less clinicians can rely on changes in bone density as a surrogate for fracture reduction. More recent analyses have suggested that changes in bone density account for a small proportion of the variability in reduction in fracture risk.[52] Through regression models, investigators were able to predict substantial relative risk reductions in vertebral fractures even with no change in bone density. They concluded that bone density was unhelpful for predicting the impact of antiosteoporotic treatment on nonvertebral fractures.

Thus, increase in bone density as a surrogate end point has shown an inconsistent relationship with osteoporotic fractures. The discrepant results of these studies illustrate how cautious we must be when substituting surrogate outcomes for patient-important outcomes.

WHAT ARE THE RESULTS?

How Large, Precise, and Lasting Was the Intervention Effect?

When considering results, we are interested not only in whether an intervention alters a *surrogate end point*, but also in the magnitude, precision, and duration of the effect. If an intervention shows large reductions in the surrogate end point, the 95% confidence intervals around those reductions are narrow, and the effect persists over a sufficiently long time, our confidence that the target outcome will be favorably affected increases. We are less confident if effects are smaller, have wider confidence intervals, and a shorter follow-up.

USING THE GUIDE

The systematic review on exercise for preventing and treating osteoporosis in post-menopausal women included 18 randomized controlled trials.[2] Meta-analyses showed that a combined aerobics and weight-bearing program increases bone density of the spine (weighted mean difference [WMD], 1.79%; 95% CI, 0.58% to 3.01%), walking increases bone density of the hip (WMD, 0.92%; 95% CI, 0.21% to 1.64%), and aerobic exercise increases bone density of the wrist (WMD, 1.22%; 95% CI, 0.71% to 1.74%). These differences are relatively small compared with, for example, alendronate, which increases bone density of the lumbar spine, hip, and forearm by 7.48%, 4.24%, and 2.08%, respectively. [52]

HOW CAN I APPLY THE RESULTS TO PATIENT CARE?

The questions clinicians should ask when applying the results are the same ones we have suggested for any issue of treatment or prevention (see Chapter 4, Health Care Interventions). These questions have to do with whether the results can be applied to the care of patients in your setting, whether all important outcomes were considered, and whether the likely benefits are worth the risks of the intervention.

The first question—can the results be applied to my patient?—refers to the extent to which your patient is similar to those in the published studies under consideration and the extent to which the intervention, along with the associated technologies for monitoring and responding to complications, is available in your setting. The second question—were all important outcomes considered?—relates to the focus of this chapter, namely, was the primary outcome really of interest to patients? This question also draws attention to issues of adverse intervention effects. The third question—were the benefits worth the risks of the intervention?—presents particular challenges when investigators have used surrogate end points, and we discuss this in the next section.

Are the Likely Intervention Benefits Worth the Potential Risks and Costs?

When deciding whether to offer an intervention to patients, clinicians must be able to estimate the magnitude of the likely benefit. When available data are limited to the effect on a surrogate end point, estimating the extent to which an intervention will improve patient-important outcomes becomes a challenge.

One approach is to extrapolate from one or more randomized controlled trials that assess a related intervention in a similar patient population and provide data on both surrogate and target outcomes. For example, until recently, few long-term data existed on the efficacy of lovastatin, a cholesterol-lowering drug, for reducing patient-important outcomes in any population. However, one could extrapolate from short-term efficacy studies assessing the surrogate end point of cholesterol lowering. Thus, because treatment with 40 mg of lovastatin daily lowered low-density lipoprotein cholesterol levels similarly to treatment with 40 mg of pravastatin (31% reduction versus 34% reduction in the CURVES Study[53]), one could theorize that long-term benefits from lovastatin would be similar to those of pravastatin. Subsequently, the AFCAPS/TexCAPS Trial (a 5-year trial assessing the efficacy of lovastatin for primary prevention of ischemic heart disease)[54] confirmed that this agent had a benefit profile similar to that of pravastatin (as determined by the 5-year primary prevention WOSCOPS trial).[55] The relative risk reductions and 95% confidence intervals for myocardial infarction were 40% (17% to 57%) and 31% (17% to 43%), respectively.

This approach is likely to be seriously flawed when one extrapolates from trials of interventions that are very different from one another. Consider the consequences of trying to ascertain the effect of exercise on fractures on the basis of bone density results. Recognizing the limitations of the approach described earlier, we could examine the results of randomized controlled trials of alendronate, a drug for which we have data on bone density and fractures. A systematic review of alendronate trials[52] reported that taking 10 to 40 mg of alendronate for 2 to 4 years improved bone density at the lumbar spine (WMD, 7.48%; 95% CI, 6.12% to 8.85%), the hip (WMD, 4.24%; 95% CI, 3.45% to 5.02%), and the forearm (WMD, 2.08%; 95% CI, 1.53% to 2.63%). The weighted mean differences for the effect of exercise were smaller for the spine (WMD, 1.79%; 95% CI, 0.58% to 3.01%), hip (WMD, 0.92%; 95% CI, 0.21% to 1.64%), and wrist (WMD, 1.22%; 95% CI, 0.71% to 1.74%). The same systematic review of alendronate[52] reported a 49% reduction in relative risk of nonvertebral fracture. Because the improvement in bone density with exercise is about one fourth of the effect of alendronate, we would anticipate a considerably lower reduction in fracture risk with exercise.

CLINICAL RESOLUTION

Although there is some evidence of an association between bone density and vertebral and nonvertebral fractures, randomized controlled trials have failed to show a consistent association between increased bone density and reduced fracture rates across all osteoporosis interventions. After reviewing the guideline[1] and systematic review,[2] you are now prepared to talk with your patient about the relationship of exercise, osteoporosis, and fractures. You explain that although exercise has been shown to improve bone density, you cannot say with confidence that this translates into a reduction in risk of bone fractures.

When we use surrogate end points to make inferences about expected benefits, we make assumptions about the link between the surrogate end point and the target outcome. In this chapter, we outlined criteria to help you decide when these assumptions may be appropriate. Even if a surrogate end point meets all of these criteria, inferences about the benefit of an intervention may still prove to be misleading. Thus, recommendations based on the effects on surrogate outcomes can never be as strong as those based on patient-important outcomes.

These considerations emphasize that the only definitive solution to the surrogate outcome dilemma is to wait for the results of randomized trials assessing the effect of an intervention on outcomes of importance to patients. The large number of examples in which reliance on surrogate end points has led—or could have led—clinicians astray underscores the wisdom of this conservative approach (see Chapter 14, Surprising Results of Randomized Controlled Trials). Conversely, when a patient's risk of serious morbidity or mortality is high, a wait-and-see strategy may pose problems for many patients and their health care providers.

We encourage clinicians to critically question therapeutic interventions in which the only proof of efficacy is based on surrogate end point data. Clinicians may choose to recommend an intervention based on randomized controlled trials reporting only surrogate end points when (1) the surrogate end point meets all our validity criteria; (2) the effect of the intervention on the surrogate end point is large; (3) the patient's risk of the target outcome is high; (4) the patient places a high value on avoiding the target outcome; and (5) no satisfactory alternative interventions exist. In other situations, clinicians must carefully consider the known side effects and costs of treatment, along with the possibility of unanticipated adverse effects, before recommending an intervention on the basis of surrogate end point data.

REFERENCES

1. Brown JP, Josse RG, for the Scientific Advisory Council of the Osteoporosis Society of Canada. 2002 clinical practice guidelines for the diagnosis and management of osteoporosis in Canada. *Can Med Assoc J.* 2002;167(10 suppl):S1-S34.

2. Bonaiuti D, Shea B, Iovine R, et al. Exercise for preventing and treating osteoporosis in postmenopausal women. *Cochrane Database Syst Rev.* 2002;3:CD000333.

3. Ebrahim S, Thompson PW, Baskaran V, Evans K. Randomized placebo-controlled trial of brisk walking in the prevention of postmenopausal osteoporosis. *Age Aging.* 1997;26:253-260.

4. Temple RJ. A regulatory authority's opinion about surrogate endpoints. In: Nimmo WS, Tucker GT, eds. *Clinical Measurement in Drug Evaluation.* New York: John Wiley & Sons; 1995:3-22.

5. Hammer SM, Katzenstein DA, Hughes MD, et al, for the AIDS Clinical Trials Group Study 175 Study Team. A trial comparing nucleoside monotherapy with combination therapy in HIV-infected adults with CD4 cell counts from 200 to 500 per cubic millimeter. *N Engl J Med.* 1996;335:1081-1090.

6. Delta Coordinating Committee. Delta: a randomised double-blind controlled trial comparing combinations of zidovudine plus didanosine or zalcitabine with zidovudine alone in HIV-infected individuals. *Lancet.* 1996;348:283-291.

7. Saravolatz LD, Winslow DL, Collins G, et al, for the Investigators for the Terry Beirn Community Programs for Clinical Research on AIDS. Zidovudine alone or in combination with didanosine or zalcitabine in HIV-infected patients with the acquired immunodeficiency syndrome or fewer than 200 CD4 cells per cubic millimeter. *N Engl J Med.* 1996;335:1099-1106.

8. Hammer SM, Squires KE, Hughes MD, et al, for the AIDS Clinical Trials Group 320 Study Team. A controlled trial of two nucleoside analogues plus indinavir in persons with human immunodeficiency virus infection and CD4 cell counts of 200 per cubic millimeter or less. *N Engl J Med.* 1997;337:725-733.

9. Haguenauer D, Welch V, Shea B, Tugwell P, Adachi JD, Wells G. Fluoride for the treatment of postmenopausal osteoporotic fractures: a meta-analysis. *Osteoporos Int.* 2000;11:727-738.

10. Guyatt GH, Thompson PJ, Berman LB, et al. How should we measure function in patients with chronic heart and lung disease? *J Chronic Dis.* 1985;38:517-524.

11. Mahler DA, Weinberg DH, Wells CK, Feinstein AR. The measurement of dyspnea: contents, interobserver agreement, and physiologic correlates of two new clinical indexes. *Chest.* 1984;85:751-758.

12. Verschuren WM, Jacobs DR, Bloemberg BP, et al. Serum total cholesterol and long-term coronary heart disease mortality in different cultures: twenty-five-year follow-up of the Seven Countries Study. *JAMA.* 1995;274:131-136.

13. Law MR, Wald NJ, Thompson SG. By how much and how quickly does reduction in serum cholesterol concentration lower risk of ischaemic heart disease? *BMJ.* 1994;308:367-372.

14. Mellors JW, Rinaldo CR Jr, Gupta P, White RM, Todd JA, Kingsley LA. Prognosis in HIV-1 infection predicted by the quantity of virus in plasma. *Science.* 1996;272:1167-1170.

15. Mellors JW, Kingsley LA, Rinaldo CR Jr, et al. Quantitation of HIV-1 RNA in plasma predicts outcome after seroconversion. *Ann Intern Med.* 1995;122:573-579.

16. Ruiz L, Romeu J, Clotet B, et al. Quantitative HIV-1 RNA as a marker of clinical stability and survival in a cohort of 302 patients with a mean CD4 cell count of 300×10^6/l. *AIDS.* 1996;10:F39-F44.

17. O'Brien TR, Blattner WA, Waters D, et al. Serum HIV-1 RNA levels and time to development of AIDS in the Multicenter Hemophilia Cohort Study. *JAMA.* 1996;276:105-110.

18. Yerly S, Perneger TV, Hirschel B, et al, for the Swiss HIV Cohort Study. A critical assessment of the prognostic value of HIV-1 RNA levels and CD4[+] cell counts in HIV-infected patients. *Arch Intern Med.* 1998;158:247-252.

19. Ho DD. Viral counts count in HIV infection. *Science.* 1996;272:1124-1125.

20. Marshall D, Johnell O, Wedel H. Meta-analysis of how well measures of bone mineral density predict occurrence of osteoporotic fractures. *BMJ.* 1996;312:1254-1259.

21. Visser AP, van Bilsen P. Effectiveness of sex education provided to adolescents. *Patient Educ Couns.* 1994;23:147-160.

22. DiCenso A, Guyatt G, Willan A, Griffith L. Interventions to reduce unintended pregnancies among adolescents: systematic review of randomised controlled trials. *BMJ.* 2002;324:1426-1430.

23. Bigger JT Jr, Fleiss JL, Kleiger R, Miller JP, Rolnitzky LM. The relationships among ventricular arrhythmias, left ventricular dysfunction, and mortality in the 2 years after myocardial infarction. *Circulation.* 1984;69:250-258.

24. McAlister FA, Teo KK. Antiarrhythmic therapies for the prevention of sudden cardiac death. *Drugs.* 1997;54:235-252.

25. Echt DS, Liebson PR, Mitchell LB, et al, for the Cardiac Arrhythmia Suppression Trial. Mortality and morbidity in patients receiving encainide, flecainide, or placebo. *N Engl J Med.* 1991;324:781-788.

26. Moore TJ. *Deadly Medicine: Why Tens of Thousands of Heart Patients Died in America's Worst Drug Disaster.* New York: Simon & Schuster; 1995.

27. Drexler H, Banhardt U, Meinertz T, Wollschlager H, Lehmann M, Just H. Contrasting peripheral short-term and long-term effects of converting enzyme inhibition in patients with congestive heart failure: a double-blind, placebo-controlled trial. *Circulation.* 1989;79:491-502.

28. Lewis GR. Comparison of lisinopril versus placebo for congestive heart failure. *Am J Cardiol.* 1989;63:12D-16D.

29. Giles TD, Fisher MB, Rush JE. Lisinopril and captopril in the treatment of heart failure in older patients: comparison of a long- and short-acting angiotensin-converting enzyme inhibitor. *Am J Med.* 1988;85: 44-47.

30. Riegger GA. Effects of quinapril on exercise tolerance in patients with mild to moderate heart failure. *Eur Heart J.* 1991;12:705-711.

31. Garg R, Yusuf S. Overview of randomized trials of angiotensin-converting enzyme inhibitors on mortality and morbidity in patients with heart failure: Collaborative Group on ACE Inhibitor Trials. *JAMA.* 1995;273:1450-1456.

32. DiBianco R, Shabetai R, Kostuk W, Moran J, Schlant RC, Wright R. A comparison of oral milrinone, digoxin, and their combination in the treatment of patients with chronic heart failure. *N Engl J Med.* 1989;320:677-683.

33. Sueta CA, Gheorghiade M, Adams KF Jr, et al, for the Epoprostenol Multicenter Research Group. Safety and efficacy of epoprostenol in patients with severe congestive heart failure. *Am J Cardiol.* 1995;75: 34A-43A.

34. Packer M, Carver JR, Rodeheffer RJ, et al, for the PROMISE Study Research Group. Effect of oral milrinone on mortality in severe chronic heart failure. *N Engl J Med.* 1991;325:1468-1475.

35. Califf RM, Adams KF, McKenna WJ, et al. A randomized controlled trial of epoprostenol therapy for severe congestive heart failure: the Flolan International Randomized Survival Trial (FIRST). *Am Heart J.* 1997;134:44-54.

36. Yee KM, Struthers AD. Can drug effects on mortality in heart failure be predicted by any surrogate measure? *Eur Heart J.* 1997;18:1860-1864.

37. Hampton JR, van Veldhuisen DJ, Kleber FX, et al, for the Second Prospective Randomised Study of Ibopamine on Mortality and Efficacy (PRIME II) Investigators. Randomised study of effect of ibopamine on survival in patients with advanced severe heart failure. *Lancet.* 1997;349:971-977.

38. Jiang ZM, He GZ, Zhang SY, et al. Low-dose growth hormone and hypocaloric nutrition attenuate the protein-catabolic response after major operation. *Ann Surg.* 1989;210:513-524.

39. Knox JB, Wilmore DW, Demling RH, Sarraf P, Santos AA. Use of growth hormone for postoperative respiratory failure. *Am J Surg.* 1996;171:576-580.

40. Takala J, Ruokonen E, Webster NR, et al. Increased mortality associated with growth hormone treatment in critically ill adults. *N Engl J Med.* 1999;341:785-792.

41. Cameron DW, Heath-Chiozzi M, Danner S, et al, for the Advanced HIV Disease Ritonavir Study Group. Randomised placebo-controlled trial of ritonavir in advanced HIV-1 disease. *Lancet.* 1998;351:543-549.

42. Prentice RL. Surrogate endpoints in clinical trials: definition and operational criteria. *Stat Med.* 1989;8:431-440.

43. Fleming TR. Surrogate markers in AIDS and cancer trials. *Stat Med.* 1994;13:1423-1435.

44. Pahor M, Psaty BM, Alderman MH, et al. Health outcomes associated with calcium antagonists compared with other first-line antihypertensive therapies: a meta-analysis of randomised controlled trials. *Lancet.* 2000;356:1949-1954.

45. Neal B, MacMahon S, Chapman N. Effects of ACE inhibitors, calcium antagonists, and other blood-pressure-lowering drugs: results of prospectively designed overviews of randomised trials: Blood Pressure Lowering Treatment Trialists' Collaboration. *Lancet.* 2000;356:1955-1964.

46. Report of the Committee of Principal Investigators. W.H.O. cooperative trial on primary prevention of ischaemic heart disease using clofibrate to lower serum cholesterol: mortality follow-up. *Lancet.* 1980;2:379-385.

47. Cranney A, Wells G, Willan A, et al. Meta-analyses of therapies for postmenopausal osteoporosis. II. Meta-analysis of alendronate for the treatment of postmenopausal women. *Endocr Rev.* 2002;23:508-516.

48. Cranney A, Waldegger L, Zytaruk N, et al. Risedronate for the prevention and treatment of post-menopausal osteoporosis. *Cochrane Database Syst Rev.* 2003;(4):CD004523.

49. Riggs BL, Hodgson SF, O'Fallon WM, et al. Effect of fluoride treatment on the fracture rate in post-menopausal women with osteoporosis. *N Engl J Med.* 1990;322:802-809.

50. Meunier PJ, Sebert JL, Reginster JY, et al. Fluoride salts are no better at preventing new vertebral fractures than calcium-vitamin D in postmenopausal osteoporosis: the FAVO study. *Osteoporos Int.* 1998;8:4-12.

51. Dawson-Hughes B, Harris SS, Krall EA, Dallal GE. Effect of calcium and vitamin D supplementation on bone density in men and women 65 years of age or older. *N Engl J Med.* 1997;337:670-676.

52. Guyatt GH, Cranney A, Griffith L, et al. Summary of meta-analyses of therapies for postmenopausal osteoporosis and the relationship between bone density and fractures. *Endocrinol Metab Clin North Am.* 2002;31:659-679.

53. Jones P, Kafonek S, Laurora I, Hunninghake D. Comparative dose efficacy study of atorvastatin versus simvastatin, pravastatin, lovastatin, and fluvastatin in patients with hypercholesterolemia (the CURVES Study). *Am J Cardiol.* 1998;81:582-587.

54. Downs JR, Clearfield M, Weis S, et al, for the Air Force/Texas Coronary Atherosclerosis Prevention Study. Primary prevention of acute coronary events with lovastatin in men and women with average cholesterol levels: results of AFCAPS/TexCAPS. *JAMA.* 1998;279:1615-1622.

55. Shepherd J, Cobbe SM, Ford I, et al, for the West of Scotland Coronary Prevention Study Group. Prevention of coronary heart disease with pravastatin in men with hypercholesterolemia. *N Engl J Med.* 1995;333:1301-1307.

14

Surprising Results of Randomized Controlled Trials

Alba DiCenso and Gordon Guyatt

The following Editorial Board members also made substantive contributions to this chapter: Paola DiGiulio, Kate Flemming, Teresa Icart Isern, and Sharon Lock.

We gratefully acknowledge the work of Christina Lacchetti on the original chapter that appears in the Users' Guides to the Medical Literature, *edited by Guyatt and Rennie.*

In This Chapter

Surrogate End Points and Observational Studies Provide Weaker Evidence Than Do Randomized Controlled Trials of Patient-Important End Points

When Randomized Controlled Trial Results Have Contradicted Those of Studies of Surrogate End Points

When Randomized Controlled Trial Results Have Contradicted Those of Observational Studies of Patient-Important End Points

SURROGATE END POINTS AND OBSERVATIONAL STUDIES PROVIDE WEAKER EVIDENCE THAN DO RANDOMIZED CONTROLLED TRIALS OF PATIENT-IMPORTANT END POINTS

Ideally, evidence of the effectiveness of preventive, therapeutic, or diagnostic interventions will come from rigorous *randomized controlled trials* (RCTs) measuring effects on patient-relevant outcomes. Historically, however, clinicians have often relied on weaker evidence. Evidence may be weaker in two ways. First, the methodology may be pristine—as is the case in rigorous RCTs—but the participants may differ in important ways from those of interest, or the outcomes may not be important to patients. For instance, demonstrating that a particular pain management strategy reduces the severity of pain in adults with chronic illness is important, but it provides weak evidence for administration of that same intervention to young children postoperatively. Similarly, demonstrating the effect of a sex education intervention on adolescent knowledge and attitudes about birth control may be interesting, but trials examining the effect of the intervention on the initiation of sexual intercourse, use of birth control, and incidence of adolescent pregnancy are imperative before clinicians can confidently recommend such a program.

Second, evidence may be weak if investigators examine the apparent effect of a health care intervention on patient-important outcomes such as quality of life, pain, or satisfaction with care, but do so using observational study designs. In Chapter 5, Harm, we describe a number of observational study designs including *cohort studies* and *case-control studies*. Of these, investigators most frequently use cohort designs to address issues of treatment efficacy. In these cohort studies, patients' preferences, or the judgement of clinicians, determine whether study participants receive an experimental or control intervention.

Observational studies differ from RCTs, in which allocation of patients according to chance minimizes bias resulting from known and unknown prognostic differences between comparison groups. The power of randomization is that intervention and control groups are far more likely to be balanced with respect to both known and unknown determinants of outcome (e.g., age, underlying severity of illness, comorbid conditions). By balancing these factors, investigators can look specifically at the effect of the intervention on the outcome of interest. In an observational study, however, those who determine who will receive the intervention and who will not are often influenced, consciously or unconsciously, by known prognostic factors. Therefore, it is likely that prognostic factors will be unbalanced between groups, and the study will yield biased, and therefore misleading, results, which underestimate or overestimate the intervention's effect.

Our message is not to dismiss weaker forms of evidence; however, health care interventions should be evaluated using the strongest form of evidence possible. Observational studies may occasionally provide such compelling results that they mandate clinical use of an intervention. Often, they provide the best available evidence. We do emphasize, however, that when clinicians rely on weak evidence, they should acknowledge the risk of administering useless or even harmful interventions. Our concern arises from examples of conclusions based on observational studies that were subsequently refuted by RCTs (see Table 14-1, pp. 238-242).

When Randomized Controlled Trial Results Have Contradicted Those of Studies of Surrogate End Points

In this section, we illustrate how studies that use surrogate or substitute end points may not yield results that are consistent with studies that examine the same question but use patient-relevant outcomes. A *surrogate end point* may be defined as a measurement (e.g., laboratory or physiologic) used as a substitute for an end point that measures directly how a patient feels, functions, or survives. Examples of surrogate outcomes include the measurement of knowledge and attitudes instead of behavior, bone mineral density instead of bone fractures, blood pressure instead of stroke, and degree of atherosclerosis on coronary angiography instead of myocardial infarction or coronary death. The use of surrogate end points often allows investigators to conduct studies with fewer patients or shorter follow-up periods. For example, measuring change in knowledge and attitudes of adolescents toward birth control immediately after a sex education class would require a much shorter follow-up period than determining the number of girls who become pregnant, which would require months or years of follow-up (see Chapter 13, Surrogate Outcomes, for more details). The following examples compare the results of studies of similar interventions that used surrogate outcomes and patient-relevant outcomes.

Two RCTs compared the effect of active compression-decompression (ACD) cardiopulmonary resuscitation (CPR) with standard CPR for patients in cardiac arrest.[1,2] In the first trial,[1] patients in cardiac arrest were randomized to receive 2 minutes of either ACD CPR or standard CPR, followed by 2 minutes of the alternate technique. Rather than looking at survival, the investigators examined surrogate outcomes consisting of mean end-tidal carbon dioxide concentrations, systolic arterial pressure, velocity time integral, and diastolic filling time. For all four outcomes, ACD CPR resulted in highly statistically significant improvements, and the investigators concluded that ACD CPR improved cardiopulmonary circulation.

In the second trial,[2] investigators compared the same interventions but examined survival as an outcome. They found no significant difference between the groups for survival at 1 hour or survival until hospital discharge. The investigators concluded that ACD CPR did not improve survival in patients with cardiac arrest.

The second example focuses on the evaluation of sex education programs for adolescents. Over the years, investigators have conducted numerous studies to determine whether sexuality and birth control education programs for adolescents improve knowledge and attitudes about these topics. These studies were based on the assumption that improvement in knowledge and attitudes would translate into responsible sexual behavior. However, literature reviews have shown otherwise. Although a review of numerous observational studies and one RCT concluded that sex education increased knowledge about sexuality and birth control and shifted attitudes toward a more liberal and tolerant view of sexuality,[3] a more recent systematic review of RCTs evaluating sex education programs found that they did not delay initiation of sexual intercourse, improve use of birth control, or reduce adolescent pregnancies.[4]

These examples illustrate how studies that report surrogate or substitute outcomes could influence clinicians to offer interventions that may have no effect or, at worst,

Table 14-1 Comparison of Same End Points From Observational Studies and Randomized Controlled Trials*

Question	Evidence From Observational Studies	Evidence From RCTs
What is the effect of sodium fluoride on vertebral fractures?	In a before/after study using quantitative computed tomography to measure TVBD in the lumbar spine of 18 women with osteoporosis, mean TVBD was significantly greater in the intervention group than for an age-matched group of untreated women with osteoporosis ($P < 0.001$). Only 1 of the 18 fluoride-treated women with osteoporosis continued to have spinal fractures during therapy, accounting for 4 fractures per 872 patient-years of observation, a value that is significantly lower than the published incidence of 76 fractures per 91 patient-years for untreated patients with osteoporosis ($P < 0.001$).[9]	An RCT allocated 202 women with osteoporosis to either sodium fluoride or placebo, in addition to daily supplements of calcium. Compared with the placebo group, the treatment group had an increase in median bone mineral density of 35% in the lumbar spine ($P < 0.0001$), 12% in the femoral neck ($P < 0.0001$), and 10% in the femoral trochanter ($P < 0.0001$). However although the number of new vertebral fractures was similar in the two groups (163 and 136, respectively; $P = 0.32$), 3 times as many fluoride-treated women had nonvertebral fractures as did women given placebo (72 and 24, respectively; 95% CI, 1.8 to 5.6, $P < 0.01$).[10]
Does hormone replacement therapy (estrogen or estrogen plus progestin) alter the risk of CHD events in postmenopausal women with established coronary disease?	A meta-analysis of 16 cohort studies with internal controls and 3 cross-sectional angiography studies (including studies of women with established CHD) demonstrated an RR of 0.50 (95% CI, 0.43 to 0.56) for CHD among estrogen users. Investigators concluded that "…the preponderance of the evidence strongly suggests women taking postmenopausal estrogen therapy are at a decreased risk for CHD."[11]	A randomized controlled secondary prevention trial did not find a reduction in the overall rate of CHD events in postmenopausal women with established CHD (relative hazard [RH] of non-fatal MI or CHD mortality, 0.99; 95% CI, 0.80 to 1.22). Investigators concluded that "based on the finding of no overall cardiovascular benefit and a pattern of early increase in risk of CHD events, we do not recommend starting this treatment for the purpose of secondary prevention of CHD."[12]

Does hormone replacement therapy (estrogen plus progestin) reduce the risk of CHD events in healthy postmenopausal women?

In an observational study of 70,533 postmenopausal women, the risk for major coronary events was lower among current users of hormone therapy, including short-term users, compared with never-users (RR, 0.61; 95% CI, 0.52 to 0.71). Investigators concluded "postmenopausal hormone use that appears to decrease risk for major coronary events in women without previous heart disease."[13]

The Women's Health Intitiative Investigators randomly allocated 16,608 healthy postmenopausal women to estrogen plus progestin or placebo. The trial was stopped after a mean of 5.2 years of follow-up because of early increases in breast cancer. At the time the study was stopped, estimated hazard ratios were as follows: CHD (hazard ratio, 1.29; 95% CI, 1.02 to 1.63); stroke (hazard ratio, 1.41; 95% CI,1.07 to 1.85); pulmonary embolism (hazard ratio, 2.13; 95% CI, 1.39 to 3.25); for total cardiovascular disease (arterial and venous disease) (hazard ratio, 1.22; 95% CI, 1.09 to 1.36). Investigators concluded that " … the results indicate that this regimen should not be initiated or continued for primary prevention of CHD."[14]

Does a diet low in fat and high in fiber alter the risk of colorectal adenomas?

A cohort study prospectively examined the risk of colorectal adenoma in 7284 male health professionals according to quintiles of nutrient intake and found that dietary fiber was inversely associated with the risk of adenoma ($P < 0.0001$); RR for men in the highest versus the lowest quintile was 0.36 (95% CI, 0.22 to 0.60). Furthermore, for men on a high-saturated fat, low-fiber diet, the RR was 3.7 (95% CI, 1.5 to 8.8) compared with those on a low-saturated fat, high-fiber diet.

Investigators randomly allocated 2079 participants, who had had 1 or more histologically confirmed colorectal adenomas removed within 6 months, to 1 of 2 groups: an intervention group (given intensive counseling and assigned to follow a low-fat, high-fiber diet) and a control group (given a standard brochure on healthy eating and assigned to follow their usual diet). Results showed that 39.7% of participants in the intervention group and 39.5% in the control group had at least 1 recurrent adenoma (RR,1.00; 95% CI,

Continued

Table 14-1 Comparison of Same End Points from Observational Studies and Randomized Controlled Trials*—cont'd

Question	Evidence From Observational Studies	Evidence From RCTs
	Investigators concluded that "... a diet high in saturated fat and low in fiber increases the risk of colorectal adenoma."[15]	0.90 to 1.12). Moreover, among participants with recurrent adenomas, the mean number of such lesions was 1.85 ± 0.08 and 1.84 ± 0.07 in the intervention and control groups, respectively ($P = 0.93$). Investigators concluded that "adopting a diet that is low in fat and high in fiber, fruits, and vegetables does not influence the risk of recurrence of colorectal adenomas."[16]
Does supplementation with beta-carotene alter the risk of major coronary events?	Analysis of a cohort from the Lipid Research Clinics Coronary Primary Prevention Trial and Follow-up Study (LRC-CPPT) found that, after adjustment for known CHD risk factors including smoking, serum carotenoids were inversely related to CHD events. Men in the highest quartile of serum carotenoids had an adjusted RR of 0.64 (95% CI, 0.44 to 0.92) for CHD compared with the lowest quartile. For men who never smoked, this RR was 0.28 (95% CI, 0.11 to 0.73). Investigators concluded that those "... with higher serum carotenoid levels had a decreased risk of incident CHD."[17]	An RCT randomized 22,071 male physicians to beta-carotene or placebo. They found no statistically significant effect of beta-carotene on the number of myocardial infarctions (RR, 0.96; 95% CI, 0.84 to 1.09), strokes (RR, 0.96; 95% CI, 0.83 to 1.11), deaths from cardiovascular causes (RR, 1.09; 95% CI, 0.93 to 1.27), or deaths from all causes (RR, 1.02; 95% CI, 0.93 to 1.11). Investigators concluded that "beta-carotene produced neither benefit nor harm in terms of the incidence of ... cardiovascular disease."[18]

| Does dietary supplementation with vitamin E alter the risk of major coronary events? | A cohort of 5133 Finnish men and women showed an inverse association between dietary vitamin E intake and coronary mortality in both men and women, with relative risks of 0.68 (*P* for trend = 0.01) and 0.35 (*P* for trend < 0.01), respectively, between the highest and lowest tertiles of intake. Investigators concluded that "... antioxidant vitamins protect against coronary heart disease." [19] | An RCT of 2545 women and 6996 men at high risk of cardiovascular events randomized to vitamin E or placebo found no significant differences in the number of deaths from cardiovascular causes (RR, 1.05; 95% CI, 0.90 to 1.22), myocardial infarction (RR, 1.02; 95% CI, 0.90 to 1.15), or stroke (RR, 1.17; 95% CI, 0.95 to 1.42). Investigators concluded that "...in patients at high risk for cardiovascular events, treatment with vitamin E had no apparent effect on cardiovascular outcomes." [20] |
| Does treatment with growth hormone alter mortality risk in critically ill patients? | A before/after study of 53 patients who had failed standard ventilator weaning protocols and were subsequently treated with human growth hormone found that 81% of previously unweanable patients were eventually weaned from mechanical ventilation, with an overall survival of 76%. Researchers concluded that "... this study presents clinical evidence supporting the safety and efficacy of human growth hormone in promoting respiratory independence in a selected group of surgical intensive care unit patients." [21] | Two multicenter RCTs assessed patients in intensive care units who received either human growth hormone or placebo until discharge from intensive care or for a maximum of 21 days. Results showed that the in-hospital mortality rate was higher in patients who received human growth hormone than in those who did not (*P* < 0.001 for both studies). The RR of death for patients receiving human growth hormone was 1.9 (95% CI, 1.3 to 2.9) in one study and 2.4 (95% CI, 1.6 to 3.5) in the other. Among the survivors, the length of stay in the intensive care unit and in the hospital and the duration of mechanical ventilation were prolonged |

Continued

Table 14-1 Comparison of Same End Points From Observational Studies and Randomized Controlled Trials*—cont'd

Question	Evidence From Observational Studies	Evidence From RCTs
		in the human growth hormone group. Researchers concluded that "in patients with prolonged critical illness, high doses of growth hormone are associated with increased morbidity and mortality."[22]
Do educational and community interventions modify the risk of adolescent pregnancy?	A meta-analysis of observational studies demonstrated a statistically significant delay in initiation of intercourse (OR, 0.64; 95% CI, 0.44 to 0.93) and a reduction in pregnancy (OR, 0.74; 95% CI, 0.56 to 0.98) in girls in studies of adolescent pregnancy prevention educational or community interventions.[23]	A meta-analysis of randomized trials provided no support for the effect of adolescent pregnancy prevention educational or community interventions in girls for initiation of intercourse (OR, 1.09; 95% CI, 0.90 to 1.32) or pregnancy (OR, 1.08; 95% CI, 0.91 to 1.27).[23]

*Note: Data are expressed as reported in the original literature.
CHD, Coronary heart disease; CI, confidence interval; OR, odds ratio; RR, relative risk; TVBD, trabecular vertebral body density.

a negative effect on patient-relevant outcomes. Beware of such studies, and instead look for studies that report patient-relevant outcomes before you offer interventions to patients.

When Randomized Controlled Trial Results Have Contradicted Those of Observational Studies of Patient-Important End Points

Observational studies tend to show larger intervention effects than do randomized trials,[5-7] although systematic underestimation of intervention effects also may occur.[8] Kunz and Oxman[8] conducted a systematic review to summarize empirical studies of the relation between randomization and estimates of effect. They found that the deviation of the estimates of effect for observational studies compared with randomized trials ranged from an underestimation of effect of 76% to an overestimation of 160%. Reasons for the discrepancies between estimates of effect derived from RCTs and observational studies likely relate to an imbalance in prognostic factors between study groups. For example, if patients with a poor prognosis were more likely to be in the control group in observational studies, this would result in larger estimates of treatment effect in the observational studies. Conversely, if patients with a poor prognosis were more likely to be in the treatment group in observational studies, this would result in larger estimates of effect in RCTs. Table 14-1 provides examples of observational studies and RCTs that focused on the same patient-important end points. In many cases, the observational study results would lead clinicians to offer useless or even harmful interventions to patients.

CONCLUSION

Although an observational study may accurately predict the results of an RCT, this is not always the case. The problem is that one never knows in advance whether the particular instance is one in which the observational study findings reflect the truth or whether they are misleading. Confident clinical action must generally await the results of RCTs.

REFERENCES

1. Cohen TJ, Tucker KJ, Lurie KG, et al. Active compression-decompression: a new method of cardiopulmonary resuscitation. Cardiopulmonary Resuscitation Working Group. *JAMA*. 1992;267:2916-2923.
2. Stiell IG, Hebert PC, Wells GA, et al. The Ontario trial of active compression-decompression cardiopulmonary resuscitation for in-hospital and prehospital cardiac arrest. *JAMA*. 1996;275:1417-1423.
3. Visser AP, van Bilsen P. Effectiveness of sex education provided to adolescents. *Patient Educ Couns*. 1994;23:147-160.
4. DiCenso A, Guyatt G, Willan A, Griffith L. Interventions to reduce unintended pregnancies among adolescents: systematic review of randomised controlled trials. *BMJ*. 2002;324:1426-1430.
5. Sacks HS, Chalmers TC, Smith H Jr. Sensitivity and specificity of clinical trials: randomized v historical controls. *Arch Intern Med*. 1983;143:753-755.
6. Chalmers TC, Celano P, Sacks HS, Smith H Jr. Bias in treatment assignment in controlled clinical trials. *N Engl J Med*. 1983;309:1358-1361.
7. Colditz GA, Miller JN, Mosteller F. How study design affects outcomes in comparisons of therapy. I. Medical. *Stat Med*. 1989;8:441-454.

8. Kunz R, Oxman AD. The unpredictability paradox: review of empirical comparisons of randomised and non-randomised clinical trials. *BMJ*. 1998;317:1185-1190.

9. Farley SM, Libanati CR, Odvina CV, et al. Efficacy of long-term fluoride and calcium therapy in correcting the deficit of spinal bone density in osteoporosis. *J Clin Epidemiol*. 1989;42:1067-1074.

10. Riggs BL, Hodgson SF, O'Fallon WM, et al. Effect of fluoride treatment on the fracture rate in post-menopausal women with osteoporosis. *N Engl J Med*. 1990;322:802-809.

11. Stampfer MJ, Colditz GA. Estrogen replacement therapy and coronary heart disease: a quantitative assessment of the epidemiologic evidence. *Prev Med*. 1991;20:47-63.

12. Hulley S, Grady D, Bush T, et al. Randomized trial of estrogen plus progestin for secondary prevention of coronary heart disease in postmenopausal women: Heart and Estrogen/progestin Replacement Study (HERS) Research Group. *JAMA*. 1998;280:605-613.

13. Grodstein F, Manson JE, Colditz GA, Willett WC, Speizer FE, Stampfer MJ. A prospective, observational study of postmenopausal hormone therapy and primary prevention of cardiovascular disease. *Ann Intern Med*. 2000;133:933-941.

14. Writing Group for the Women's Health Initiative Investigators. Risks and benefits of estrogen plus progestin in healthy postmenopausal women: principal results from the Women's Health Initiative randomized controlled trial. *JAMA*. 2002;288:321-333.

15. Giovannucci E, Stampfer MJ, Colditz G, Rimm EB, Willett WC. Relationship of diet to risk of colorectal adenoma in men. *J Natl Cancer Inst*. 1992;84:91-98.

16. Schatzkin A, Lanza E, Corle D, et al. Lack of effect of a low-fat, high-fiber diet on the recurrence of colorectal adenomas: Polyp Prevention Trial Study Group. *N Engl J Med*. 2000;342:1149-1155.

17. Morris DL, Kritchevsky SB, Davis CE. Serum carotenoids and coronary heart disease: The Lipid Research Clinics Coronary Primary Prevention Trial and Follow-up Study. *JAMA*. 1994;272:1439-1441.

18. Hennekens CH, Buring JE, Manson JE, et al. Lack of effect of long-term supplementation with beta carotene on the incidence of malignant neoplasms and cardiovascular disease. *N Engl J Med*. 1996;334:1145-1149.

19. Knekt P, Reunanen A, Jarvinen R, Seppanen R, Heliovaara M, Aromaa A. Antioxidant vitamin intake and coronary mortality in a longitudinal population study. *Am J Epidemiol*. 1994;139:1180-1189.

20. Yusuf S, Dagenais G, Pogue J, Bosch J, Sleight P. Vitamin E supplementation and cardiovascular events in high-risk patients: The Heart Outcomes Prevention Evaluation Study Investigators. *N Engl J Med*. 2000;342:154-160.

21. Knox JB, Wilmore DW, Demling RH, Sarraf P, Santos AA. Use of growth hormone for postoperative respiratory failure. *Am J Surg*. 1996;171:576-580.

22. Takala J, Ruokonen E, Webster NR, et al. Increased mortality associated with growth hormone treatment in critically ill adults. *N Engl J Med*. 1999;341:785-792.

23. Guyatt GH, DiCenso A, Farewell V, Willan A, Griffith L. Randomized trials versus observational studies in adolescent pregnancy prevention. *J Clin Epidemiol*. 2000;53:167-174.

15

The Principle of Intention to Treat

Alba DiCenso and Gordon Guyatt

The following Editorial Board members also made substantive contributions to this chapter: Cathy Kessenich and Andrea Nelson.

We gratefully acknowledge the work of P.J. Devereaux on the original chapter that appears in the Users' Guides to the Medical Literature, *edited by Guyatt and Rennie.*

In This Chapter

How Should Randomized Trials Deal With Intervention Group Patients Who Do Not Receive the Intervention?
  A Hypothetical Randomized Controlled Trial in Which Patients Experience the Target Event Before Receiving the Intervention
  A Hypothetical Randomized Controlled Trial in Which Patients Do Not Adhere to the Intervention

Misleading Use of Intention-to-Treat Terminology

HOW SHOULD RANDOMIZED TRIALS DEAL WITH INTERVENTION GROUP PATIENTS WHO DO NOT RECEIVE THE INTERVENTION?

One does not need randomized controlled trials (RCTs) to determine the effect of a smoking cessation program in persons who do not adhere to it. Intuitively, it follows that, in an RCT, one should compare persons in the experimental group who adhered to the intervention with those in the control group. As it turns out, however, doing so is a mistake. We need to know the outcomes of all participants in a trial, including those in the experimental group who do not adhere to the intervention, and we need to include data about outcomes for these nonadherent persons in the analysis to arrive at an unbiased estimate of the intervention effect.

One argument for incorporating all study participants in the final analysis, including those who did not adhere to the intervention, has to do with the effect of the intervention on members of the community. If one is interested in knowing the effect of a smoking cessation program on a given population, one must include all members of that population. When participants do not adhere to an intervention, particularly if adverse effects caused nonadherence, reservations will arise about the effect of the intervention on a community. This chapter focuses on reasons that it is important to incorporate all study participants in the final analysis, whether they receive the intervention or not.

A Hypothetical Randomized Controlled Trial in Which Patients Experience the Target Event Before Receiving the Intervention

There are occasions when patients are randomized to an intervention, and between the time of randomization and the initiation of the intervention, these patients experience the target event that the intervention is designed to prevent. Picture an RCT of women at risk for postpartum depression. The trial compares an experimental program of weekly home visits by a nurse with provision of usual care in a primary care practice. Assume that, although the investigators do not know it, the underlying true effect of the nurse home visiting program is zero, and women in the home visit group do neither better nor worse than those in the primary care group.

Of 100 women randomized at hospital discharge to nurse home visits, 10 are readmitted with postpartum depression in the first week after discharge before they receive a home visit. Of the 90 women who receive home visits, 10 experience postpartum depression in the subsequent 3 months (Figure 15-1). What will happen to the women in the control group? Because randomization creates groups with the same fate or destiny and because we have already established that the home visit intervention has no effect on outcome, we predict that 10 women in the control group will be readmitted with postpartum depression in the first week after discharge and another 10 will experience postpartum depression in the subsequent 3 months.

The *intention-to-treat principle* dictates that we count all events in all randomized patients, regardless of whether they receive the intended intervention. When we apply the intention-to-treat principle in our study of nurse home visits for prevention of postpartum depression, we find 20 events in each group and, therefore, no evidence of a positive

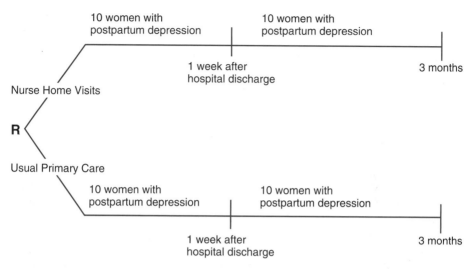

Figure 15-1. Results of a hypothetical trial of nurse home visits for women at risk of postpartum depression. *R,* Patients randomized to nurse home visits or usual primary care.

intervention effect. However, if we use the logic that we should not count events in women in the nurse home visit group who did not receive home visits, the event rate in the intervention group would be 11% (10/90) compared with 20% in the control group—a relative risk reduction of almost 50%. These data show how analyses restricted to patients who received their assigned intervention (sometimes referred to as per-protocol, as-treated, efficacy, or explanatory analyses) can provide a misleading estimate of the effect of an intervention.

A Hypothetical Randomized Controlled Trial in Which Patients Do Not Adhere to the Intervention

There are other occasions when patients are randomized to receive an intervention and choose not to adhere to it. Imagine an RCT of hip protectors to prevent fractures in elderly persons with a history of falling, in which 20 of 100 patients in the intervention group are nonadherent (Figure 15-2). Under what circumstances would a comparison between the control group and the 80 patients who wore hip protectors yield an unbiased result? An unbiased result would be possible only if the underlying prognosis in the 80 adherent patients were identical to that of the 20 nonadherent patients. If the 20 nonadherent patients were destined to do better than the other members of their group, the per-protocol analysis would provide a misleading underestimate of the true

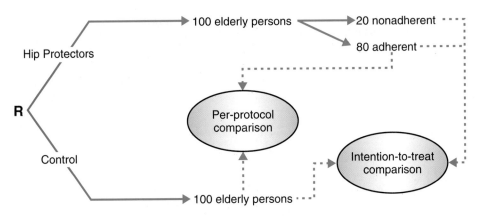

Figure 15-2. A schematic view of per-protocol and intention-to-treat comparisons. *R,* Randomization.

intervention effect. If, as is more often the case, nonadherent patients were more likely to have an adverse outcome (i.e., fracture), their omission would lead to a spurious overestimate of the benefit of the intervention.

To make our demonstration more vivid, we can illustrate with additional hypothetical data. Let us assume that the intervention (i.e., use of hip protectors) is ineffective and that the true underlying event rate of fractures in both the intervention and control groups is 20% (Figure 15-3). Let us assume that the event rate (fractures) among the 20 nonadherent participants is much higher (60%). Under these circumstances, nonadherent participants will experience 12 of the 20 events destined to occur in the intervention group. If one compares only the adherent patients (event rate of 8 out of 80, or 10%) with the control group (event rate of 20 out of 100, or 20%), one will mistakenly conclude that the intervention cuts the event rate in half.

These hypothetical examples illustrate common situations that occur in RCTs. In the first situation, patients in the intervention group experience the target event after randomization but before receiving the intervention, and in the second, patients in the intervention group do not adhere to the intervention. The intention-to-treat principle applies regardless of the intervention (e.g., support intervention, medication, or behavioral intervention) and regardless of the outcome (e.g., mortality, morbidity, or a behavioral outcome such as smoking cessation). Removing patients after randomization always risks introducing bias by creating noncomparable groups.

We have dealt with the situation of nonadherence in the intervention group. The situation may be equally problematic if patients in the control group do not adhere to the control intervention and instead receive the experimental intervention. Let us say, for instance, that hip protectors substantially reduce the risk of fractures in elderly people with a history of falling, but that 50% of participants in the no-hip protector group (control group) begin using hip protectors shortly after randomization. The intention-to-treat analysis will show an apparent intervention effect that is half of what investigators

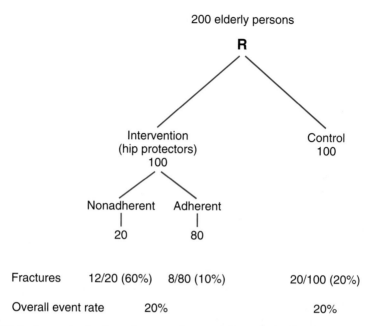

Figure 15-3. Impact of missed events in nonadherent individuals in the intervention group. *R,* Randomization.

would have observed if none of the control group participants had used hip protectors. The apparent relative risk reduction with hip protectors will be even less if the control group participants who used hip protectors were those at highest risk of adverse events.

MISLEADING USE OF INTENTION-TO-TREAT TERMINOLOGY

We have been careful to talk about the intention-to-treat principle rather than the commonly used term intention-to-treat analysis. The reason is that there is considerable ambiguity in the term *intention-to-treat analysis,* and its use can be very misleading. For instance, picture a trial in which 20% of intervention group patients and 20% of control group patients discontinue their assigned intervention (e.g., nurse home visits in the case of intervention group patients and usual primary care in the case of control group patients), and investigators elect to terminate their follow-up at that point. At the end of the trial, the investigators count events in all patients who completed follow-up and correctly assign the events to the groups to which they were allocated. Technically, the investigators could say that they had conducted an intention-to-treat analysis in that they counted all events of which they were aware against the group to which patients were allocated. Of course, this intention-to-treat analysis has in no way avoided the possible bias introduced by omission of outcome events in patients who discontinued the intervention.

One could argue whether investigators should include patients lost to follow-up in the denominator when calculating the proportion of patients who experienced target outcomes. The danger of including these patients is that if the investigators do not clearly state the proportion lost to follow-up (as is often the case), readers may believe that the study succeeded in following-up all patients. Whether the denominators include all patients or only those followed-up ultimately makes little difference, because large loss to follow-up opens a study to major bias. These observations highlight the close conceptual link between biases introduced in an as-treated analysis and those that arise through loss to follow-up.

The problem of misleading statements concerning intention-to-treat analysis in reports of RCTs is far from theoretical. Hollis and Campbell[1] surveyed all RCTs published in *BMJ*, *The Lancet*, *JAMA*, and the *New England Journal of Medicine* in 1997. They found that 119 (48%) of the trials used the term "intention-to-treat analysis." Of these 119 trials, 12 explicitly violated the principle of intention-to-treat by excluding patients who did not begin the treatment to which they were allocated. Investigators can justify such a policy if the reasons for not starting cannot have been affected by allocation. For instance, exclusion of patients who are blinded to the intervention and decide that they do not want to participate shortly after randomization and before starting the intervention is unlikely to bias study results. Although the approach is potentially justifiable, investigators who use it will mislead if they describe their study as conducting an intention-to-treat analysis.

In another three instances, the investigators' decision to exclude patients from analyses unequivocally violated intention-to-treat principles.[1] In many of the other trials, the reason for loss to follow-up may have been nonadherence with the intervention to which patients were allocated. The report by Hollis and Campbell[1] tells us that clinicians must look at the details of what actually happened in the methods sections of an article, and often in the results section as well, rather than accepting statements that the investigators undertook an intention-to-treat analysis.

REFERENCE

1. Hollis S, Campbell F. What is meant by intention to treat analysis? Survey of published randomised controlled trials. *BMJ*. 1999;319:670-674.

16

When to Believe a Subgroup Analysis

Donna Ciliska and Gordon Guyatt

We gratefully acknowledge the work of Andrew Oxman on the original chapter that appears in the Users' Guides to the Medical Literature, *edited by Guyatt and Rennie.*

In This Chapter

Why Do Investigators Conduct Subgroup Analyses?

Measures of Effect and Subgroup Analyses

Guidelines for Interpreting Subgroup Analyses
  Were Subgroup Differences Based on Comparisons Within, Rather Than Between, Studies?
  Did the Hypothesis Precede, Rather Than Follow, the Analysis?
  Was the Subgroup Effect One of a Small Number of Hypothesized Effects Tested?
  Was the Magnitude of the Effect Large?
  Was the Effect Statistically Significant?
  Was the Effect Consistent Across Studies?
  Does Indirect Evidence Support the Hypothesized Subgroup Effect?

In evaluations of health care interventions, and especially when an intervention does not appear to be efficacious for the average patient, investigators may conduct separate analyses for subgroups of patients, such as those at different stages of their illness, those with different comorbid conditions, those with different ages, and the like. Often these subgroup analyses were not planned ahead of time, and the data are simply dredged to see what might turn up. Investigators sometimes overinterpret these data-dependent analyses as demonstrating that the intervention really has a different effect in a subgroup of patients. For example, men, or patients who are sicker or older may be held up as benefiting substantially more or less than other subgroups of patients in the trial.

Readers should be skeptical about subgroup analyses. An intervention is likely to benefit a subgroup more or less than other patients only if the difference in the effects of the intervention in the subgroups is large and very unlikely to occur by chance. Even when these conditions apply, results may be misleading if investigators did not specify their hypotheses related to subgroup analyses before the study began, if they had a large number of hypotheses, or if other studies fail to replicate the finding. The more subgroup analyses investigators conduct, the greater is the risk of a spurious, or misleading, conclusion.

In a survey of 45 clinical trials reported in three leading health care journals, Pocock and colleagues found that 51% of the reports had at least one subgroup analysis that compared the response of different patient subgroups to the interventions.[1] In this chapter, we present guidelines for interpreting the results of *subgroup analyses*.

Although this chapter focuses on randomized controlled trials and meta-analyses of randomized controlled trials (systematic reviews), the same principles apply to other research designs. However, we begin with the assumption that the underlying design of the study of interest is sound. For trials evaluating health care interventions, sound design involves elements of randomization, blinding where possible, and completeness of follow-up (see Chapter 4, Health Care Interventions). If the study designs are not sound, the overall conclusions will be suspect, as will conclusions based on subgroup analyses.

WHY DO INVESTIGATORS CONDUCT SUBGROUP ANALYSES?

A statistically significant *subgroup analysis* suggests that there may be an important difference in *treatment effect* between subgroups in the intervention and control groups. This difference may be across types of patients (e.g., older or younger; sicker or less sick patients) or across interventions (e.g., low-intensity or high-intensity interventions). Although they are not usually as important, differences may also occur across measurements of outcome (e.g., thresholds for occurrence of stroke with important functional disability or early or late measurement of intervention effects). When an effect is real, we say there is an interaction between type of patient, intervention, or outcome and the magnitude of the intervention effect. When the magnitude of the difference between subgroups is both real and sufficiently large, it may influence patient management. For example, we may learn that a certain intervention is effective in men but not in women, and, therefore, will offer it only to men.

Determining which subgroup analyses should be done, and which should be believed, remains controversial. Critics of subgroup analysis decry fishing expeditions and data-dredging exercises,[2-5] which result in false inferences about subgroup effects. Advocates of subgroup analysis are concerned about the risks of missing important differences in effect,[6,7] particularly with cavalier pooling of results,[8] which can result in meaningless conclusions about "average" effects[9] or failure to detect important intervention effects as a result of overly heterogeneous study populations.[10]

Although the debate between these two camps can lead to some useful insights, clinicians need practical advice for when to believe an analysis that shows an apparent difference in intervention effects across subgroups. In considering this issue, we need to consider the different possible measures of effect and how the choice of measure of effect can influence inferences about subgroup differences.

MEASURES OF EFFECT AND SUBGROUP ANALYSES

Consider a 40-year-old woman who has an elevated serum cholesterol level, with a ratio of total cholesterol to high-density lipoprotein of 6. She does not smoke, have diabetes or a family history of heart disease, and her blood pressure is 110/70 mm Hg. Her risk of cardiovascular death in the next decade is 2% or less. Contrast this woman with a 70-year-old man who has an identical serum cholesterol level and ratio of total cholesterol to high-density lipoprotein, but who smokes, has diabetes and a positive family history of heart disease, and his blood pressure is 140/85 mm Hg. His risk of cardiovascular death in the next decade is 30% or more.

These two individual patients represent extremes of high- and low-risk subgroups of candidates for lipid-lowering therapy. If one considers the absolute risk reduction that these patients may achieve by taking a statin for the next decade, a subgroup effect will be almost certain. The greatest absolute benefit the younger woman could expect would be a risk reduction of about 1% (from 2% to 1%), whereas the older man could have a risk reduction of 10% or more (from 30% to 20%). We would thus conclude that an interaction exists between risk level and the magnitude of intervention effect (i.e., the largest effects are seen in the higher-risk group).

Conversely, the relative risk reduction (approximately 30% in meta-analyses of statin drugs[11]) may well be similar in high-risk and low-risk patients. Indeed, meta-analyses of randomized trials of statins suggest that relative risk reductions vary little across high-risk and low-risk groups. In general, when considering many different interventions, *relative risk reductions* tend to be similar across risk groups, whereas *absolute risk reductions* show greater variability (see Chapter 27, Measures of Association). In our discussion of subgroup analyses, we refer to relative risk reductions unless otherwise stated.

It is implausible that the underlying true intervention effect would be identical in any two subgroups. We are concerned about important differences that would result in a change in an intervention decision. We cannot offer a rule for the point at which differences in relative risk reductions become important because it will depend on a patient's baseline risk, prevention of the adverse outcome, and the side effects of treatment.

We suggest, however, that differences in relative risk reduction of less than 10% (e.g., from 20% to 10%) are seldom important.

In formulating guides for whether to believe a subgroup analysis, we build on criteria suggested by other authors.[12–15] Table 16-1 summarizes the approach that we will describe in detail. Because we believe that more serious errors tend to be committed when investigators present spurious subgroup analyses as real, we focus on the dangers of misleading analyses that suggest different intervention effects across subgroups. We do, however, acknowledge that when sample sizes are small and the power of analyses is limited, false-negative subgroup analyses also occur.

GUIDELINES FOR INTERPRETING SUBGROUP ANALYSES

Were Subgroup Differences Based on Comparisons Within, Rather Than Between, Studies?

To this point, this chapter has focused on subgroup analyses within the same study. This guideline emphasizes the importance of distinguishing within-study differences from between-study differences. Making inferences about different effect sizes in different groups on the basis of *between-study* differences is highly risky when compared with inferences based on *within-study* differences. For example, one would be reluctant to conclude that music therapy for preoperative stress results in a different level of relaxation than does an imagery exercise on the basis of two studies: one comparing music therapy with usual care and one comparing imagery with usual care. Drawing inferences about these two interventions from two different usual-care controlled studies would be making an indirect comparison of their effect. A direct comparison would involve a single study in which patients are randomized to music therapy, imagery, or usual care. If such a direct comparison in a single high-quality study demonstrated clinically important and statistically significant differences in the magnitude of effect between the two active interventions, the inference would be quite strong.

A meta-analysis examining the effectiveness of prophylaxis for gastrointestinal bleeding in critically ill patients[16] found that histamine-2-receptor (H_2) antagonists and antacids, each compared with placebo, had comparable effects in reducing overt bleeding (odds

Table **16-1**   Guidelines for Deciding Whether Apparent Differences in Subgroup Response Are Real

- Were subgroup differences based on comparisons within, rather than between, studies?
- Did the hypothesis precede, rather than follow, the analysis?
- Was the subgroup effect one of a small number of hypothesized effects tested?
- Was the magnitude of the effect large?
- Was the effect statistically significant?
- Was the effect consistent across studies?
- Does indirect evidence support the hypothesized subgroup effect?

ratios of 0.58 and 0.66, respectively). By contrast, direct comparison from studies in which patients were randomized to H_2 antagonists or antacids found a statistically significantly greater reduction in bleeding with H_2 antagonists (odds ratio, 0.56).

The reason that inference on the basis of between-study differences is potentially so misleading is that the apparent differentiating factor between studies will always be only one of many differences. For instance, aside from differences in the specific interventions used, the results could be explained by differences between studies in populations (e.g., varying risks of adverse outcomes), varying degrees of cointervention, or varying criteria for defining the outcome. This would not be the case when basing inferences on within-study differences because within the same study, factors such as the baseline characteristics of the population, control of cointervention, and outcome criteria are the same across comparison groups. In within-study subgroup analyses, there are only two possible explanations for the difference in effect across subgroups: either it is true or it is a chance phenomenon. Because chance so often leads clinicians astray, readers require other evidence for deciding when to believe a subgroup analysis, even for within-trial comparisons.

Did the Hypothesis Precede, Rather Than Follow, the Analysis?

Embedded within any large data set are certain apparent, but misleading, interactions. As a result, the credibility of any apparent interaction that arises out of post hoc exploration of a data set is questionable. By post hoc, we mean that rather than identifying questions or hypotheses before the data are collected, questions or hypotheses are generated and explored after the data are collected and some preliminary analyses are done. Post hoc comparisons differ from planned comparisons in which questions or hypotheses are specified before any analyses are conducted.

Through a post hoc analysis of sex differences, investigators in the first large trial of aspirin in patients with transient ischemic attacks stumbled across the finding that aspirin prevented stroke in men with cerebrovascular disease, but not in women.[17] For a considerable period, this finding led many clinicians to withhold aspirin from women with cerebrovascular disease. Subsequent studies and a meta-analysis summarizing these studies[18] refuted the finding.

Determining whether a hypothesis preceded analysis of a data set can be difficult. At one extreme, unexpected results could clearly be responsible for generating a new hypothesis in which the results are discovered by a post hoc analysis. At the other extreme, a subgroup analysis could clearly be planned—a priori (or in advance)—in a study protocol to test a hypothesis suggested by prior research. Between these two extremes is a range of possibilities, and the extent to which a hypothesis was generated before, during, or after data collection and analysis is often not clear. Nevertheless, if a hypothesis was previously, clearly, and unequivocally suggested by a different data set, one has moved from a hypothesis-generating framework to a hypothesis-testing framework.

Was the Subgroup Effect One of a Small Number of Hypothesized Effects Tested?

Post hoc hypotheses based on subgroup analyses often arise from exploration of a data set in which many such hypotheses are considered. The greater the number of hypotheses tested, the greater the number of interactions one will discover by chance. Even if investigators have clearly specified their hypotheses in advance, the strength of inference associated with the apparent confirmation of any single hypothesis will decrease if it is one of a large number that have been tested.

Clinicians and investigators tend to underestimate the impact of chance on the results of experiments. In an imaginative investigation entitled "The Miracle of DICE Therapy for Acute Stroke," Counsell and colleagues directed participants of a statistics class to roll different-colored dice numerous times to simulate 44 clinical trials of fictitious therapies.[19] Participants received the dice in pairs and were told that one die in each pair was an ordinary die representing control patients, whereas the other die was loaded to roll either more or fewer sixes than the control die. Rolling a six represented a patient's death, and all other numbers represented survival. Some pairs of dice were red, some white, and some green, each color representing a different medication used in administering "DICE therapy." The investigators simulated trials that differed in size (various numbers of rolls of paired dice), methodological rigor (high or low quality), peer review (yes or no), and publication status (published or unpublished). Subgroup analysis suggested that red DICE therapy had a nonsignificant trend toward excess mortality. When the inferior red drug was excluded, along with methodologically inferior and unpublished trials and data from inexperienced centers, DICE therapy offered an impressive 39% relative risk reduction for mortality in acute stroke.

The participants, however, had been deliberately misled: the dice were not loaded. The effects observed, which closely mimicked the patterns reported in actual health care literature, resulted entirely from chance. The impressive, statistically significant effect of "properly administered" DICE therapy resulted entirely from selective subgroup analyses and exclusions.

The DICE therapy demonstration suggests that clinicians should exercise great caution in interpreting apparent subgroup effects when investigators have conducted many such analyses on a data set. For instance, in a regression analysis concerning predictors of the effect of digoxin on heart failure patients in sinus rhythm, Lee and colleagues tested 16 variables and found that the presence of a third heart sound was an important predictor of digoxin response.[20] Clinicians should be skeptical of this finding because of the relatively large number of variables tested. The skepticism would increase if the investigators had examined each variable separately, rather than in a regression analysis that considered all 16 variables simultaneously (see Chapter 31, Regression and Correlation). Readers of studies with subgroup analysis cannot always be sure about the number of possible interactions that the investigators tested. If the investigators choose to withhold this information and report only those interactions that were significant, readers are likely to be misled.

Was the Magnitude of the Effect Large?

As a rule, the larger the difference between the effect in a particular subgroup and the overall effect, the more plausible it is that the difference is real. At the same time, as the difference in effect size between the anomalous subgroup and the remaining patients becomes larger, the clinical importance of the difference increases. When sample sizes are small, however, large differences in apparent effect will occur simply by chance. If you concluded that an interaction was real just because it was large, you would be wrong more often than you would be right.

For example, a meta-analysis of 24 randomized trials compared the effect of sucralfate with H_2 receptor antagonists and/or antacids on the incidence of nosocomial pneumonia in critically ill patients.[21] The pooled estimate showed a relative risk of 0.86 (95% confidence interval, 0.75 to 0.97), a finding suggesting a possible reduction of pneumonia with sucralfate.[21] The results of the individual studies varied, however, from a relative risk of 0.33 (a 67% reduction of pneumonia with sucralfate) to 1.84 (an 84% increase in pneumonia). These differences occurred even though the results were entirely consistent with a single underlying magnitude of intervention effect for all of these studies; that is, results of individual studies did not differ significantly from one another (heterogeneity P value, 0.33) (see Chapter 9, Summarizing the Evidence Through Systematic Reviews; see also Chapter 24, Evaluating Differences in Study Results). However, given that individual studies found contradictory results (some finding a reduction and some an increase in pneumonia), focusing on the results of the individual studies, and on possible subgroup effects, could easily have led the investigators to make erroneous inferences about subgroup effects, capitalizing on the play of chance.

Was the Effect Statistically Significant?

A key question that investigators must address when examining apparent subgroup differences is this: If the true underlying effect were the same in all patients, how likely is it that the observed differences between subgroups would have occurred by chance? (See Chapter 28, Hypothesis Testing.) For instance, in the GUSTO trial that found a 1% absolute reduction in mortality in patients with acute myocardial infarction treated with tissue-type plasminogen activator (tPA) rather than streptokinase, the mortality difference was 1.2% in the United States and 0.7% elsewhere.[22] Observers noted that patients in the United States underwent invasive revascularization with percutaneous transluminal angioplasty or coronary artery bypass surgery more frequently. These investigators therefore wondered whether the benefits of tPA could be greater in the context of this more aggressive approach; that is, was there a subgroup effect such that the effect of tPA was greater in the context of greater use of angioplasty and surgery?

How would one go about determining whether the difference in the magnitude of the apparent effects in the United States and elsewhere was a real phenomenon or an artifact of the play of chance? The wrong way would be to test whether the effect was significant in the United States and then separately test whether the effect was significant in other countries. Figure 16-1 illustrates just how misleading such an analysis could be.

Figure 16-1 depicts intervention effects in two hypothetical subgroups and a pooled estimate combining the subgroups. The vertical line represents a relative risk of 1.0, indicating neither a beneficial nor a harmful intervention effect. The underlying truth, reflected in the results, is that the intervention effect (represented by the solid squares) is identical in the two subgroups. If one looks only at subgroup 2, the effect is statistically significant (reflected in the confidence interval, which does not overlap the vertical line

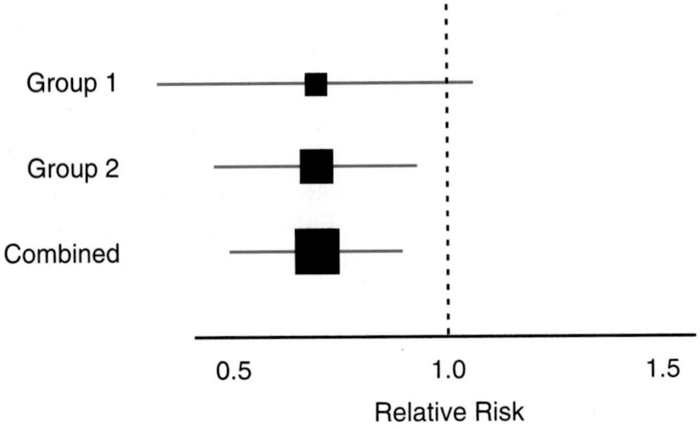

Figure 16-1. Two subgroups with an underlying identical treatment effect.

representing a relative risk of 1.0). In subgroup 1, because of a smaller sample size, the effect does not reach statistical significance (reflected in the confidence interval, which overlaps the vertical line representing a relative risk of 1.0). It would clearly be a mistake to conclude that the intervention works in subgroup 2, but not in subgroup 1.

How should one handle this situation? Rather than asking separately, is the intervention effective in subgroup 1? or, is it effective in subgroup 2?, one should ask, is the effect different in subgroup 1 compared with subgroup 2? According to Figure 16-1, the answer to that question is a resounding no. Putting the correct question into the formal framework of hypothesis testing, one would ask, if there was no difference between the true underlying intervention effects in the two subgroups, how often would one observe differences in apparent effects as large as or larger than those observed? (See Chapter 28, Hypothesis Testing). Returning to the example of the trial of thrombolytic therapy, the question would be as follows: If there was no true underlying gradient of effect, how often would investigators find differences as large as or larger than the difference between 1.2% and 0.7%? The *P* value for this test was 0.3. In other words, if there really was no difference in mortality between tPA and streptokinase in the United States and other countries, differences as large as or larger than those observed among subgroups in the United States and other countries would occur by chance 30% of the time. Thus, the data provide little support for the hypothesis that the effect of tPA differs across these settings.

Contrast this with a meta-analysis examining the effect of alendronate on nonvertebral fractures.[23] The investigators used regression methods to discover that a model that pooled all doses of alendronate was less powerful than a model that separated doses of less than 10 mg and 10 mg or more in explaining differences in results across studies ($P = 0.002$). The investigators therefore gained confidence that the apparently larger effect of doses of greater than 10 mg (relative risk reduction, 0.49) than that of lower doses (relative risk reduction, 0.13) was a real, rather than chance, phenomenon.

Investigators can use various statistical techniques to explore whether chance can explain apparent subgroup differences.[9,12,24–26] Readers should look for the results of a statistical test that addresses the possibility that the apparent difference in the magnitude of effect between subgroups is a chance finding.

We add two notes of caution. First, if investigators have examined large numbers of subgroup hypotheses, they run the risk of generating low P values in some of their analyses simply by chance. For example, a study of platelet-activating factor receptor antagonist (PAFra) in 262 patients with sepsis showed a weak, nonsignificant trend in favor of active therapy.[27] Subgroup analysis of 110 patients with gram-negative bacterial infection showed a large, statistically significant advantage for the use of PAFra. A subsequent larger study of 444 patients with gram-negative bacterial infection showed a small, nonsignificant trend in favor of PAFra almost identical to that of the previous trial analysis, which included all randomized patients.[28] The disappointed investigators may have been less surprised at the result of the second trial had they fully appreciated the limitations of their first subgroup analysis: the possible differential effect of PAFra in gram-negative bacterial infection was one of 15 subgroup hypotheses tested.[29]

Second, if a hypothesis about an interaction has arisen out of exploration of a data set, one could argue for excluding that study from a meta-analysis in which the hypothesis is tested. Certainly, if the hypothesis is confirmed in a meta-analysis that excludes data from the study that originally suggested the interaction, the inference rests on stronger ground. If the statistical significance of the interaction disappears or is substantially weakened when data from the original study are excluded, the strength of inference is reduced. For example, if a post hoc analysis found that aspirin did not reduce the risk of stroke in women, the inference would be strengthened if it was also found in a meta-analysis of other studies (excluding this original study).

Was the Effect Consistent Across Studies?

A hypothesis concerning differential response in a subgroup of patients may be generated by examination of data from a single study. The interaction becomes more credible if it is also found in other studies. The extent to which a rigorous systematic review of the relevant literature finds an interaction to be consistently present is probably the best single index of its credibility.

The hypothesis about a third heart sound (an abnormal sound that suggests ventricular "stiffness" or noncompliance during filling) as a predictor of response to digoxin in patients with heart failure who are in sinus rhythm was tested in a second randomized crossover trial.[30] The presence of a third heart sound proved to be a weaker predictor than in the initial study, although its association with response to digoxin did reach conventional levels of statistical significance. However, other factors that, like a third heart sound, reflect greater severity of heart failure also were associated with response to digoxin. Thus, the second study provided support for a more general hypothesis—that response is related to severity of heart failure.

Other studies that examined the efficacy of digoxin in patients with heart failure who were in sinus rhythm have been summarized in a meta-analysis.[31] Unfortunately, none of these studies conducted subgroup analyses addressing the issue of differential response according to severity of heart failure. If these analyses had been done in the other available studies, the hypothesis would likely have been confirmed or refuted with substantially greater confidence. As it is, we are inclined to view the conclusion as tentative (i.e., the strength of inference is only moderate).

Does Indirect Evidence Support the Hypothesized Subgroup Effect?

We are generally more inclined to believe a hypothesized interaction if indirect evidence (e.g., from animal studies or analogous situations in human biology) makes the interaction more plausible. In other words, to the extent that a hypothesis is consistent with our current understanding of the biologic mechanisms of disease, we are more likely to believe it. Such understanding comes from three types of indirect evidence: studies of different populations (including animal studies), observations of interactions for similar interventions, and results of studies of other related outcomes, particularly intermediary outcomes.

The extent to which indirect evidence strengthens an inference about a hypothesized interaction varies substantially. In general, the strongest type of indirect evidence is based on intermediary outcomes, such as evidence of differences in immune response that supports a conclusion that the clinical effectiveness of a vaccine differs depending on age.[32] Conversely, the weakest type of indirect evidence generally comes from related interventions, such as evidence of a similar interaction with other vaccines.

The human mind is sufficiently fertile that there is no shortage of biologically plausible explanations, or indirect evidence, to support almost any observation. An ironic example of biologic evidence that supported a possible interaction comes from an early trial, described previously, suggesting that aspirin reduced stroke in men but not in women.[17] This finding stimulated animal research, which provided a biologic basis for the interaction.[33] Ultimately, however, it turned out that aspirin was as effective in women as in men for stroke reduction.

CONCLUSION

Criteria suggested for determining whether to believe hypotheses about causation have proved helpful in understanding controversial causal claims.[2,34] The criteria suggested here should be useful in deciding when to believe an analysis that suggests a differential response to an intervention in a definable subgroup of patients or with a particular intervention intensity. At one extreme are relatively small, marginally significant interactions based on between-study differences or generated by post hoc exploration of a single data set. At the other extreme are large, important interactions, originally suggested by both indirect and direct evidence, and independently tested in a new trial or in a meta-analysis in which the possibility that the interaction resulted from chance is very low. The former should be viewed with great skepticism; the latter can form the basis of clinical decision making. The strength of inference can range from one end of this spectrum to the other. When criteria are partially satisfied, further information from new primary studies or meta-analyses will often be desirable to strengthen the inference (one way or the other) to the point at which it can be confidently applied as clinical policy.

Decisions about how much effort to put into accumulating more evidence and what clinical action to take will depend on the potential benefits, risks, and costs. Decision thresholds for undertaking further research and taking clinical action vary greatly. For interventions with large potential benefits and small risks and costs, we are generally willing to accept lower standards of evidence than for interventions with smaller potential benefits or larger risks or costs.

Decisions about whether to base clinical practice on the average estimate of effect from an overall analysis (one that is more robust) or on a subgroup analysis (one that more closely reflects the specific clinical situation at hand) hinges on the criteria described earlier. It is tempting to take one extreme or the other; that is, always to base decisions on the overall estimate of effect or always to base decisions on the most applicable subgroup analysis. However, a thoughtful approach based on these criteria is more likely to result in the most benefit and the least harm for patients.

REFERENCES

1. Pocock SJ, Hughes MD, Lee RJ. Statistical problems in the reporting of clinical trials: a survey of three medical journals. *N Engl J Med.* 1987;317:426-432.
2. Fletcher RH, Fletcher SW, Wagner EH. *Clinical Epidemiology: The Essentials.* 2nd ed. Baltimore: Williams & Wilkins; 1988:185-186.
3. Feinstein AR. *Clinical Epidemiology: The Architecture of Clinical Research.* Philadelphia: WB Saunders; 1985:306-307, 516-517.
4. Senn S, Harrell F. On wisdom after the event. *J Clin Epidemiol.* 1997;50:749-751.
5. Altman DG. Within trial variation: a false trail? *J Clin Epidemiol.* 1998;51:301-303.
6. Horwitz RI, Singer BH, Makuch RW, Viscoli CM. On reaching the tunnel at the end of the light. *J Clin Epidemiol.* 1997;50:753-755.
7. Feinstein AR. The problem of cogent subgroups: a clinicostatistical tragedy. *J Clin Epidemiol.* 1998;51: 297-299.
8. Goldman L, Feinstein AR. Anticoagulants and myocardial infarction: the problems of pooling, drowning, and floating. *Ann Intern Med.* 1979;90:92-94.
9. Furberg CD, Morgan TM. Lessons from overviews of cardiovascular trials. *Stat Med.* 1987;6:295-306.
10. Horwitz RI. Complexity and contradiction in clinical trial research. *Am J Med.* 1987;82:498-510.
11. Bucher HC, Griffith LE, Guyatt GH. Systematic review on the risk and benefit of different cholesterol-lowering interventions. *Arterioscler Thromb Vasc Biol.* 1999;19:187-195.
12. Buyse ME. Analysis of clinical trial outcomes: some comments on subgroup analyses. *Control Clin Trials.* 1989;10(suppl 4):187S-194S.
13. Bulpitt CJ. Subgroup analysis. *Lancet.* 1988;2:31-34.
14. Byar DP. Assessing apparent treatment: covariate interactions in randomized clinical trials. *Stat Med.* 1985;4:255-263.
15. Shuster J, van Eys J. Interaction between prognostic factors and treatment. *Control Clin Trials.* 1983;4: 209-214.
16. Cook DJ, Witt LG, Cook RJ, Guyatt GH. Stress ulcer prophylaxis in the critically ill: a meta-analysis. *Am J Med.* 1991;91:519-527.
17. The Canadian Cooperative Study Group. A randomized trial of aspirin and sulfinpyrazone in threatened stroke. *N Engl J Med.* 1978;299:53-59.
18. Antiplatelet Trialists' Collaboration. Secondary prevention of vascular disease by prolonged antiplatelet treatment. *Br Med J Clin Res Ed.* 1988;296:320-331.
19. Counsell CE, Clarke MJ, Slattery J, Sandercock PA. The miracle of DICE therapy for acute stroke: fact or fictional product of subgroup analysis? *BMJ.* 1994;309:1677-1681.
20. Lee DC, Johnson RA, Bingham JB, et al. Heart failure in outpatients: a randomized trial of digoxin versus placebo. *N Engl J Med.* 1982;306:699-705.
21. Cook DJ, Reeve BK, Guyatt GH, et al. Stress ulcer prophylaxis in critically ill patients: resolving discordant meta-analyses. *JAMA.* 1996;275:308-314.

22. GUSTO investigators. An international randomized trial comparing four thrombolytic strategies for acute myocardial infarction. *N Engl J Med.* 1993;329:673-682.
23. Cranney A, Guyatt G, Willan A, Griffith L, Krolicki N, Welch V, et al. A meta-analysis of alendronate for the treatment of osteoporosis in postmenopausal women. *Osteoporos Int.* 2001;12:140-151.
24. Schneider B. Analysis of clinical trial outcomes: alternative approaches to subgroup analysis. *Control Clin Trials.* 1989;10(suppl 4):176S-186S.
25. Breslow NE, Day NE. *Statistical Methods in Cancer Research.* Vol 1. *The Analysis of Case-Control Studies.* Lyon, France: International Agency for Research on Cancer; 1980:122-159, 192-246.
26. Beach ML, Meier P. Choosing covariates in the analysis of clinical trials. *Control Clin Trials.* 1989;10(suppl 4):161S-175S.
27. Dhainaut JF, Tenaillon A, Le Tulzo Y, et al, for the BN 52021 Sepsis Study Group. Platelet-activating factor receptor antagonist BN 52021 in the treatment of severe sepsis: a randomized, double-blind, placebo-controlled, multicenter clinical trial. *Crit Care Med.* 1994;22:1720-1728.
28. Dhainaut JF, Tenaillon A, Hemmer M, et al, for the BN 52021 Sepsis Investigator Group. Confirmatory platelet-activating factor receptor antagonist trial in patients with severe gram-negative bacterial sepsis: a phase III, randomized, double-blind, placebo-controlled, multicenter trial. *Crit Care Med.* 1998;26: 1963-1971.
29. Natanson C, Esposito CJ, Banks SM. The sirens' songs of confirmatory sepsis trials: selection bias and sampling error. *Crit Care Med.* 1998;26:1927-1931.
30. Guyatt GH, Sullivan MJ, Fallen EL, et al. A controlled trial of digoxin in congestive heart failure. *Am J Cardiol.* 1988;61:371-375.
31. Jaeschke R, Oxman AD, Guyatt GH. To what extent do congestive heart failure patients in sinus rhythm benefit from digoxin therapy? A systematic overview and meta-analysis. *Am J Med.* 1990;88:279-286.
32. Stieb DM, Frayha HH, Oxman AD, Shannon HS, Hutchison BG, Crombie FS. Effectiveness of *Haemophilus influenzae* type b vaccines. *Can Med Assoc J.* 1990;142:719-733.
33. Kelton JG, Hirsh J, Carter CJ, Buchanan MR. Sex differences in the antithrombotic effects of aspirin. *Blood.* 1978;52:1073-1076.
34. Hill AB. *Principles of Medical Statistics.* 9th ed. New York: Oxford University Press; 1971:312-320.

II

Health Services Research

Chapter **17**   Health Services Interventions

Chapter **18**   Economic Evaluation

Chapter **19**   Computer Decision Support Systems

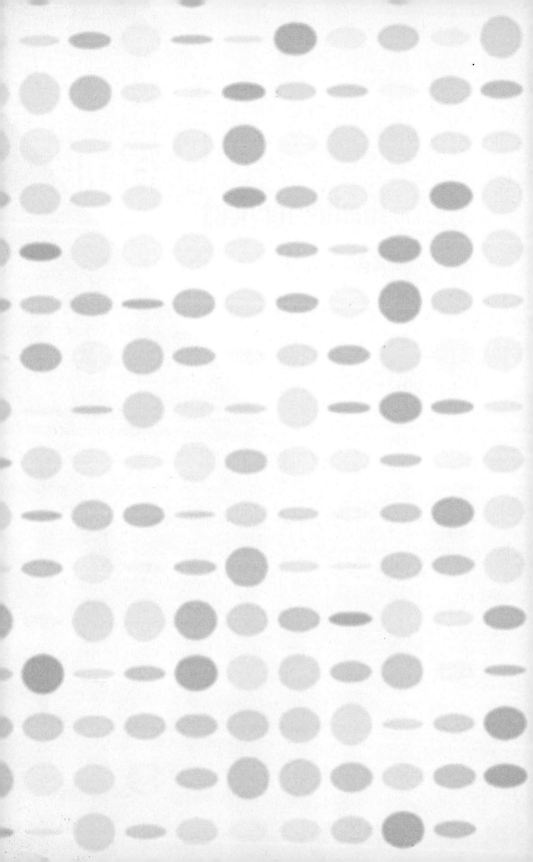

17

Health Services Interventions

Alba DiCenso, Brian Hutchison, Jeremy Grimshaw, Nancy Edwards,
and Gordon Guyatt

*The following Editorial Board members also made substantive contributions
to this chapter: Phyllis Brenner, Marie Driever, and Jenny Ploeg.*

In This Chapter

What Is Health Services Research?

Research Designs for Evaluating Health Services Interventions
Randomized Controlled Trials
Observational Designs
Mixed Methods
Systematic Reviews

Are the Results Valid?
Were Study Participants Randomized? If Yes, Was Randomization Concealed,
and Were Study Participants Analyzed in the Groups to Which They Were
Randomized?
Were Groups Shown to Be Similar in All Known Determinants of Outcome, or
Were Analyses Adjusted for Differences?
Were Valid Determinant, Process, and Outcome Measures Used?
Was Assessment of Exposure/Outcome Uniform and Unbiased?
Was Ascertainment of Exposure/Outcome Sufficiently Complete?
Were Analyses Adjusted for Unit of Assignment, if Cluster Assignment Was
Used?
Were Rival Plausible Explanations Considered for Results of Nonrandomized
Studies?

What Are the Results?
How Large Was the Intervention Effect?
How Precise Was the Estimate of the Intervention Effect?

How Can I Apply the Results to Health Services Decision Making?
Were the Study Setting and Context Similar to Mine?
Were All Important Processes and Outcomes Considered?

Can a Quality Improvement Program Improve Quality of Care and Mental Health Outcomes of Depressed Patients in Primary Care?

You are the administrative director of a primary care clinic in a managed care organization. You recently attended a conference where you learned that depression is the third most common reason for consultation in primary care. You are surprised to learn that despite its frequency and the availability of effective treatments, many patients who present with depression in managed primary care settings are not properly diagnosed, and of those who are diagnosed, many are not treated appropriately. The clinicians in your primary care clinic include internists, family physicians, and nurse practitioners. You meet with them to discuss this issue and find that they too are concerned about the number of patients they are seeing with depression, the limited amount of time they have to fully explore a patient's related life circumstances, the large number of patients who fail to respond completely to antidepressant medications or psychotherapy, and nonattendance at follow-up appointments by some patients.

You refer back to the handouts the conference presenter provided and find her summary of a recent systematic review on interventions to improve management of depression in primary care.[1] She has rated the review as high quality because the authors (1) performed an exhaustive search for relevant studies by searching (without language restriction) several medical, psychological, and health services databases, reviewing reference lists from all included studies, and contacting experts in the field; (2) specified appropriate inclusion criteria for study designs (randomized controlled trials, nonrandomized controlled clinical trials, controlled before-and-after studies, and interrupted time-series studies), the intervention (organizational or educational interventions targeted at primary health care professionals and patients), and outcomes of interest (management and outcomes of depression, quality of care, and costs); and (3) ensured that assessment of individual studies was reproducible by having two reviewers independently extract and check data on study setting, design, methodological quality, type of intervention, outcomes, follow-up, and results.

They found 36 studies that met the inclusion criteria, including 29 randomized controlled trials and nonrandomized controlled clinical trials, five controlled before-and-after studies, and two interrupted time-series studies. Because there were substantial differences in study designs, interventions, and outcomes, the authors conducted a narrative synthesis rather than combining the results quantitatively through a meta-analysis. You decide to retrieve a copy of the review to learn more about which interventions improved the management of depression.

The authors of the systematic review found that simply providing a clinical practice guideline or an educational program for clinicians was generally ineffective. Studies that showed a positive impact on the management and outcomes of depression used complex interventions consisting of two or more strategies, some of which involved changes in delivery systems, such as specialist clinics and nurse case management. The systematic review included a summary of effective and ineffective strategies. You review the summary of effective strategies, one of which is a quality improvement (QI) program, and wonder whether the program might be suitable for implementation in your clinic. You retrieve two papers that report the 1- and 2-year follow-up results of a large randomized trial that evaluated the QI program.[2,3]

These articles report a trial in which investigators randomized 46 primary care clinics in six managed care organizations in the United States to usual care or one of two similar QI programs: one with enhanced resources for supporting medication management (QI-Meds) and the other with enhanced resources for providing psychotherapy (QI-Therapy). For usual care, medical directors of each clinic were mailed the Agency for Healthcare Research and Quality depression practice guidelines, with copies of quick reference guides for each clinician. The QI component of each intervention (QI-Meds and QI-Therapy) consisted of the following: (1) 2-day training of an expert team (a primary care clinician, a nursing supervisor, a psychiatrist for QI-Meds, and a psychologist for QI-Therapy) in assessing and treating depression, educating primary care clinicians, and conducting quality assurance meetings; (2) training of clinic nurses to educate patients using a patient brochure and videotape, and to assess depressive symptoms and functioning; (3) training of intervention clinicians using a manual on detection, assessment, and treatment of depression; monthly or bimonthly lectures using teaching slides based on the manual; pocket reminder cards; and academic detailing; and (4) monthly quality assurance meetings to review intervention progress and clinical care of patients.

In addition to these common components, the QI-Meds program included nurse case managers and trained psychiatrists who supervised the case managers. Nurses used protocols to assess patient symptoms and discuss treatment adherence and side effects. The psychiatrists reviewed nurse reports and identified patients with poor treatment response at 6 to 8 weeks for possible specialty consultation. The QI-Therapy program included designated trained therapists who offered up to 12 sessions of individual or group cognitive behavioral therapy.

Within each managed care organization, the investigators grouped primary care clinics into sets of three, matching on mix of primary care and specialist clinicians, patient sociodemographics and ethnic mix, and type of relationship with behavioral health services. A clinic could be a single clinic, a cluster of small clinics, or a clinical care team within a large clinic. Within matched sets, they randomized clinics to usual care (443 patients), the QI-Meds program (424 patients), or the QI-Therapy program (489 patients). Outcomes were assessed every 6 months for 2 years and included quality of care, mental health outcomes, and employment.

This chapter focuses on the critical appraisal of studies that evaluate health services interventions. Such studies fall within the broad domain of health services research. We will begin by defining *health services research*, contrasting it with clinical research, and will then describe research designs used to evaluate health services interventions. We will outline criteria for assessing the validity, results, and applicability of studies that evaluate health services interventions. Examples of health services interventions include new models of care such as community mental health teams[4] and hospital-at-home services,[5] new care providers such as primary health care nurse practitioners,[6] and strategies to increase the use of health care interventions such as immunization.[7]

Health services research uses numerous research designs. However, this chapter focuses specifically on research designs that are most appropriate to evaluate health services interventions. Qualitative designs, although not generally used to evaluate the effectiveness of health services interventions, are used to address other important health services research questions (e.g., What are the perceived support needs of family caregivers of persons living with chronic disease and receiving home-care services, and what types of telephone services would meet these needs?).[8] Qualitative methods are also used alongside evaluative methods to provide insights into contextual factors that may influence the implementation, utilization, or effectiveness of a health services intervention (see Chapter 8, Qualitative Research). Having shown that a health services intervention is safe and effective, investigators will often be asked by policy and other decision makers about the cost-effectiveness or economic efficiency of the intervention. Therefore, economic evaluation plays a major role in health services research (see Chapter 18, Economic Evaluation, for a detailed description).

WHAT IS HEALTH SERVICES RESEARCH?

During recent decades, there has been increased interest in the financing, funding, organization, and delivery of health care. Concerns about costs, along with dramatic regional and international differences in practice patterns among clinicians and institutions, have focused the attention of administrators and policy makers on the interplay among the structure, processes, and outcomes of health services.

Academy Health, an interdisciplinary organization representing health services researchers and policy makers, defines *health services research* as "the multidisciplinary field of scientific investigation that studies how social, financing systems, organizational structures and processes, health technologies, and personal behaviors affect access to health care, the quality and cost of health care, and ultimately health and well-being. Its research domains are individuals, families, organizations, institutions, communities, and populations."[9] "The main goals of health services research are to identify the most effective ways to organize, manage, finance, and deliver high quality care; reduce medical errors; and improve patient safety."[9]

Health services research focuses on health services or health care delivery systems. Unlike clinical research, which has traditionally focused on the treatment and care of individual patients, health services research adopts a population or systems perspective. Health services research can aid in addressing care delivery problems in nursing through studies of the effectiveness of alternative care models (e.g., home visits versus outpatient visits to monitor the health status of seniors with congestive heart failure) and the mix of interdisciplinary health care professionals in care delivery.[10] Questions considered by health services research include the following: How should services be funded and delivered? Who should receive health services? How well are services being delivered? and, How effective are health services interventions?[11]

From the previous description, it is clear that health services research addresses a broad range of questions. This chapter focuses on only one type of question in this broad field—the effectiveness of health services interventions. These are studies that address questions such as, do nurse practitioners provide care equivalent to doctors in a primary care setting? In this question, the health services intervention is the nurse practitioner. In contrast, a clinical question of relevance to nurse practitioners might be, should a 3-day or 7-day course of antibiotics be given to children with otitis media? The key difference is that the evaluation of nurse practitioners informs us about how to deliver health services, whereas an evaluation of antibiotics informs us about a health care intervention or clinical treatment.

The dissemination of findings from *health services research* is directed at those who plan, manage, and fund the delivery of health services (e.g., policy makers who provide funding for health care, administrators who allocate funds for health services delivery in an organization or jurisdiction, and managers who design and implement service delivery models). In contrast, dissemination of findings from *clinical research* is directed primarily at clinicians who provide day-to-day patient care. Even more than in clinical research, context is a key component of health services research. Health services researchers must describe the context of their studies and often measure contextual variables and consider them in their analyses. This topic is discussed in more detail later in this chapter.

RESEARCH DESIGNS FOR EVALUATING HEALTH SERVICES INTERVENTIONS

Health services interventions (e.g., a change in the way a service is financed, funded, delivered, or organized) are challenging to evaluate because of their complexity.[12] Context plays a key role in studies of health services organization and delivery. Programs that appear similar may have different effects because of variations in contextual factors, such as location of setting (urban versus rural), size of setting, management characteristics, organizational culture, political climate, and organizational resources. Some researchers see context as a confounder or interference between an intervention and its intended outcome. Others see context as an integral part of the intervention that can itself be the primary focus of the research.[12]

Because randomized controlled trials seek to isolate an intervention in order to evaluate it, they can fail to consider the context within which a new intervention is introduced. For this reason, their use in health services research is sometimes criticized. Consideration of the study context contributes to the understanding and interpretation of study findings.[12] Tension often exists in health services research between research designs such as randomized controlled trials that minimize threats to *internal validity* by eliminating or controlling for contextual variability and designs that allow for an examination of the interplay among context, implementation of the intervention, and outcomes, and have a high degree of *external validity* (generalizability).

In this chapter, we focus on the most appropriate designs for evaluating the way health services are organized and delivered: randomized controlled trials; observational studies, including controlled before-and-after studies, interrupted time-series studies, cohort studies, and case-control studies; mixed methods studies; and systematic reviews. In our view, randomized controlled trials should be used whenever possible.

Observational studies are appropriate when there are practical, ethical, or logistic barriers to randomization. Such instances occur when an intervention operates at a level of the health care system that precludes randomization (e.g., if the intervention is a government decision to introduce, regulate, and fund midwifery care, patient choice rather than randomization will dictate who receives midwifery care and how comparison groups can be formed for evaluation of this service). When a policy decision has been made and the researcher has no control over the delivery of the intervention (e.g., the introduction of mobile speed cameras in reducing road traffic–related injuries), observational studies are also appropriate.

Randomized Controlled Trials

Randomized controlled trials are used increasingly to evaluate the quality, effectiveness, and cost of health care services.[13,14] The same arguments that are used to justify randomized controlled trials of clinical interventions (e.g., hydrocolloid dressings for pressure sores) apply to evaluations of organizational interventions (e.g., strategies to encourage implementation of a new clinical practice guideline for treatment of pressure sores).

In a randomized controlled trial, investigators randomly allocate study participants, practices, or service delivery organizations to receive or not receive the health services intervention and then follow participants forward in time to determine the effect of the intervention. The power of randomization is that intervention and control groups are likely to be balanced with respect to both known and unknown determinants of outcome. The limitations of randomized controlled trials in health services research relate to feasibility, external validity (generalizability), and their limited capacity to address the interaction of context, implementation, and impact of interventions. For a detailed description of randomized controlled trials, see Chapter 2, Finding the Evidence, and Chapter 4, Health Care Interventions.

The QI study[2,3] described earlier is an example of the use of a randomized controlled trial design to evaluate a health services intervention. Primary care clinics were randomly assigned to one of two QI programs or to usual care (mailing of practice guidelines) to determine if QI improved quality of care, mental health outcomes, and employment. Other examples include randomization of older postsurgical cancer patients to specialized home care or standard care to determine if the home care program improved survival;[15] randomization of high-risk older adults to an outpatient geriatric evaluation and management program or usual care to determine if the outpatient program prevented functional decline;[16] randomization of acute stroke patients to stroke unit care with early supported discharge or conventional stroke unit service to determine if stroke unit care with supported discharge increased independence;[17] and randomization of primary care patients to nurse practitioners or physicians to determine if patient satisfaction, health status, and service utilization differed between types of practitioners.[18]

In some circumstances, it is not advisable to randomize individual patients or clinicians to an intervention. For example, in a study of a new sex education intervention, if students within the same school are randomized to the new sex education program or to the conventional program, it is likely that students in the intervention group will discuss what they learn with students in the control group. As a result, an effective intervention could appear less effective or even ineffective because both groups have been exposed to the intervention. To avoid this problem, investigators use *cluster randomization* in which they randomize clusters such as primary care practices, schools, or communities, rather than individual patients or clinicians, to intervention and control groups. In the sex education example, schools rather than individual students could be randomized to receive or not receive the intervention.

The QI study[2,3] is an example of such a trial in which investigators randomized primary care clinics rather than individual patients or clinicians. If they had randomized individual patients, clinicians may have treated both intervention and control group patients and might apply their QI program learning to both groups rather than to the intervention group only. If they had randomized individual clinicians, those in the intervention group might have shared their learning with control group colleagues working closely with them in the same practice.

Observational Designs

Although randomized designs are sometimes used to evaluate health services interventions, observational study designs still predominate in the health services research literature. Many interventions that involve changes in policy, organizational structures, modes of practice, and health care personnel are not readily amenable to randomization and blinding.[13] Instead, the effects of such changes are evaluated using controlled before-and-after comparisons, interrupted time-series studies, cohort studies, and case-control studies. The strength of these observational designs lies in their potential to accommodate and assess the effects of contextual variation on processes and outcomes in a "natural" environment, thereby enhancing external validity. Their Achilles' heel is their vulnerability to threats to internal validity.

Controlled Before-and-After Studies

Before-and-after studies measure outcomes before and after the introduction of an intervention. Observed differences in outcomes, not otherwise explained, are assumed to be caused by the intervention. These studies are methodologically weak because secular trends (e.g., trends toward longer life expectancies) or other concurrent changes (e.g., hospital restructuring) make it difficult to attribute observed changes to the intervention being studied. In general, studies with before-and-after measures but no control group should not be used to evaluate the effects of health services, and the results of studies using such designs should be interpreted with great caution.[19,20] This design is commonly used to evaluate the impact of the implementation of new clinical practice guidelines. In implementing a new guideline for preventing pressure sores, investigators may record the number of pressure sores that occur over a specified time frame before and after guideline implementation. A reduction in the number of pressure sores may be incorrectly attributed to guideline implementation if, during the same time period, hospital restructuring resulted in lower patient-to-nurse ratios, decreased patient acuity, or shorter lengths of stay.

A modification is to introduce a comparison group or setting to act as a control. In *controlled before-and-after studies*, the investigator identifies a control group or setting that has similar characteristics to the intervention group but is not exposed to the intervention, and collects data from both groups before and after the intervention.[19] In the pressure sore guideline example, the investigator would identify two similar settings, collect baseline data from each about the incidence of pressure sores, implement the guideline in one setting, and then compare the incidence of pressure sores in the two settings after guideline implementation. If there were no secular trends or concurrent events or interventions affecting the occurrence of pressure sores, one would expect the number of pressure sores in the control setting to stay the same; if this was the case, any reductions in the number of pressure sores observed in the setting in which the guideline was implemented could more confidently be attributed to the guideline.

The systematic review of educational and organizational interventions to improve management of depression in primary care[1] included five controlled before-and-after studies. In one of these studies, investigators collected data about depression severity and satisfaction with care from depressed patients attending nine primary care clinics, three of which later implemented a continuous quality improvement (CQI) intervention. The remaining six clinics served as controls because they had similar on-site mental health resources, similar numbers of primary care clinicians, and similar geriatric populations. The CQI process consisted of a graded set of five care management options, ranging from watchful waiting to specialist care. Both patient groups completed follow-up surveys 3 months later, after the three clinics had implemented the CQI process. After 3 months, neither group (intervention nor control) experienced a significant change in depression symptoms or satisfaction with care from the preintervention levels.[21]

Although controlled before-and-after studies should protect against secular trends and concurrent interventions, it is often difficult to identify a comparable control group. Even in apparently well-matched intervention and control groups, preintervention measures of outcome may differ. For example, in a study of computerized reminders to clinicians to offer influenza vaccine, preintervention rates of vaccination differed in two practice settings, one of which received the intervention.[22] Such baseline imbalance may mean that the control group is not truly comparable and may not experience the same secular trends or concurrent interventions as the intervention group. Under these circumstances, differences between groups in changes from preintervention to postintervention should be interpreted with caution.[19]

Interrupted Time-Series Studies

Interrupted time-series studies attempt to detect whether an intervention has had an effect that is significantly greater than the underlying secular trend.[19,20] They are useful for evaluating the effects of interventions when it is difficult to randomize, such as the dissemination of national guidelines or mass media campaigns. Data are collected at several times both before and after the intervention; data collected before the intervention allow the underlying trend and cyclical (seasonal) effects to be estimated. Data collected after the intervention allow the intervention effect to be estimated, while accounting for underlying secular trends.[19,20]

An *interrupted time-series design* was used to evaluate the effectiveness of guidelines for cesarean section in Ontario, Canada.[23] Monthly data from hospitals from April 1982 to March 1986 provided preintervention information about antenatal practice. The guidelines were disseminated to all obstetricians in March 1986 to June 1986, and the effect was assessed by analyzing monthly data from April 1986 to March 1988. After release of the guidelines, there was no clear, dramatic decrease in cesarean section rates. However, statistical analysis revealed that during the 72 months before the guidelines, the average monthly increase in the underlying trend for the overall rate of cesarean section was 0.029%, whereas during the following 24 months, there was an average monthly decrease of 0.04%, a potential effect from the guidelines of 0.13 fewer cesarean sections per 100 deliveries each year [(0.04% − 0.029%) = 0.011% × 12 months = 0.13%].[23]

The greatest threat to the validity of a time-series design is the occurrence of another event at the same time as the intervention, both of which may be associated with the outcome.[24] To address this threat, investigators can incorporate a comparison group or setting; this is referred to as a *controlled interrupted time-series study*. In this design, multiple measures are taken in two groups, only one of which is exposed to the intervention. For example, the impact of a regional mass media campaign on smoking behavior in one region can be compared with another region in which no mass media campaign was carried out.[19]

Cohort Studies

In a *cohort study* (also known as a nonequivalent control group design[20]), the investigator identifies groups of patients, each a cohort, who are exposed and not exposed to the health services intervention and follows them forward in time to monitor the target outcome.[19] In the absence of randomization, it is possible that any observed differences in outcome might have nothing to do with the intervention being studied but may arise because of baseline differences between groups (confounding factors). Therefore, investigators must document the baseline characteristics of exposed and nonexposed participants and either demonstrate their comparability or use statistical techniques to adjust for differences.

However, even if investigators document the comparability of potentially confounding variables in exposed and nonexposed cohorts and even if they use statistical techniques to adjust for differences, important determinants of outcome that are unknown or unmeasured may be unbalanced between the groups and responsible for differences in outcome. Thus, the strength of inference from a cohort study will always be less than that of a rigorously conducted randomized trial, a controlled before-and-after study, or a controlled interrupted time-series study.[19] A systematic review of the effectiveness of interventions to prevent adolescent pregnancy provides an illustration of how less rigorous studies tend to overestimate the effectiveness of therapeutic and preventive interventions.[25] When estimates of the effect of the interventions on initiation of intercourse, use of birth control, and pregnancy were computed separately for 13 randomized trials and 17 cohort studies, the observational studies showed a significant intervention benefit, whereas the randomized trials found no benefit for any outcomes in either males or females. A possible explanation for this finding is that in cohort studies, schools that had lower baseline adolescent pregnancy rates might have been more likely to volunteer to participate in the intervention group (e.g., a new sex education program), whereas in randomized trials, these schools would have had an equal chance of being randomized to the intervention or control group. For a detailed description of cohort studies, see Chapter 2, Finding the Evidence, and Chapter 5, Harm.

A cohort study was used to assess the effect of helicopter ambulance services on patient outcomes in the United Kingdom. Two cohorts were recruited: patients attended by the helicopter emergency service during a 2-year period and those cared for by existing land ambulance paramedics over the same time period. All survivors were followed up for 2 and 6 months after their injury by means of mailed questionnaires. Comparison of outcomes was adjusted for possible confounding factors including age, sex, injury severity score, Glasgow Coma Score, Revised Trauma Score, Abbreviated Injury Scale, body region score, and type of incident. There was no evidence of reduced disability or better functional status in those attended by the helicopter service, despite the extra cost incurred.[26]

Historical cohort studies compare the outcomes of individuals or organizations exposed and not exposed to an intervention in the past. The practical advantage of a historical cohort study (also known as a *nonrandomized historical control study*) is that information on the long-term effects of the intervention (e.g., 10 or 20 years) can be assessed without having to wait the full time for the outcome to manifest itself. The disadvantages are that detailed information about the intervention received and potential confounding factors may be lacking (unless there are good historical records), and the investigator has no control over what information was collected in the past or how it was collected. Dependence on patients' or clinicians' recollection to fill information gaps may introduce serious biases.[19]

Case-Control Studies

In a *case-control study*, the starting point is the outcome of interest, such as an adverse event resulting from use or nonuse of a health services intervention. Those who experience the event are designated *cases*, and those who do not experience the event are designated *controls*. Investigators design case-control studies to ensure that controls are reasonably similar to cases with respect to important determinants of outcome such as age and sex, but who have not experienced the target outcome.[19] Using this case-control design, investigators then assess the relative frequency of exposure to the intervention in the cases and controls, adjusting for differences in known and measured determinants of outcome. For example, nursing home managers may want to compare elderly patients who have fall-related injuries (cases) to elderly patients matched for age and sex without fall-related injuries (controls) to compare exposure to a falls-prevention intervention.

As with cohort studies, case-control studies are susceptible to unmeasured confounding variables, particularly when exposure varies over time. Decision makers can draw inferences of only limited strength from the results of case-control studies because they only reveal whether an association exists and cannot determine whether such an association is causal.[19] For a detailed description of case-control studies, see Chapter 2, Finding the Evidence, and Chapter 5, Harm.

A case-control design was used to assess the effectiveness of a syringe exchange program in reducing the incidence of blood-borne viruses in injection drug users. The program had been implemented in the community 3 years before the evaluation. Within a study population of intravenous drug users, prior use of the exchange was compared in cases with confirmed hepatitis B or C and in appropriately matched controls without infection. The researchers demonstrated that use of the exchange was associated with a six-fold reduced risk of hepatitis B and a seven-fold reduced risk of hepatitis C, after adjustment for potential confounding factors.[27]

Mixed Methods

Mixed-methods studies combine data collection approaches, sometimes both qualitative and quantitative, into the study methodology[28] and are commonly used in the study of service delivery and organization. Some mixed-methods studies combine study designs (e.g., investigators may embed qualitative or quantitative process evaluations alongside quantitative evaluative designs to increase understanding of causal mechanisms, modifying factors, and findings). Some mixed-methods studies include a single overarching research design but use mixed methods for data collection (e.g., surveys, interviews, observation, and analysis of documentary material).

Bradley and colleagues[29] embedded a qualitative process evaluation into a pilot study of a secondary prevention program led by specialist nurses for patients with myocardial infarction or angina. The quantitative component revealed no important difference between the intervention and control groups in cardiovascular risk. The qualitative component, consisting of in-depth interviews of patients and practitioners, provided information to guide changes to the intervention, identify the tasks and processes needed to successfully operationalize the intervention, and confirm or question the evidence and theory on which the intervention was based.

Systematic Reviews

Systematic reviews of existing research can help to inform the decisions of policy makers, managers, clinicians, and health services users. They can be useful in choosing among competing policy alternatives (e.g., different models of community-based rehabilitation services or different ways of providing support to informal caregivers).[30]

In systematic reviews, investigators explicitly state inclusion and exclusion criteria for evidence, conduct a comprehensive search for the evidence, and summarize the results according to explicit rules that include examining how effects may vary in different subgroups. When a systematic review pools data from primary studies to provide a quantitative estimate of overall effect, we call it a *meta-analysis*. Systematic reviews provide strong evidence when the quality of primary study designs is high and sample sizes are large; they provide weaker evidence when study designs are poor and sample sizes are small. Because judgment is involved in many steps in a systematic review (including specifying inclusion and exclusion criteria, applying these criteria to potentially eligible studies, evaluating the methodological quality of the primary studies, and selecting an approach to data analysis), systematic reviews are not immune to bias. Nevertheless, in their rigorous approach to identifying and summarizing data, systematic reviews reduce the likelihood of bias in estimating causal links between health services intervention options and outcomes. For a detailed description of systematic reviews, see Chapter 9, Summarizing the Evidence Through Systematic Reviews.

Examples of systematic reviews of health services interventions include a meta-analysis that suggests that private for-profit ownership of hospitals results in a higher risk of death for patients compared with private not-for-profit ownership;[31] a meta-analysis that provides evidence that discharge planning may reduce length of hospital stay and readmissions and increase patient satisfaction;[32] and a meta-analysis that shows that nurse practitioners, when compared with physicians in primary care settings, had higher levels of patient satisfaction and quality of care, with no differences in patient health status.[6]

Our standard approach to using an article from the health care literature can be adapted for application to studies evaluating a health services intervention (Table 17-1). We ask (1) Are the results of this study valid? (2) What are the results? and (3) How do the results apply to health services decision making? This chapter builds on previously published Users' Guides that focused on reviewing articles reporting variations in outcomes of health services and clinical utilization reviews.[33,34]

ARE THE RESULTS VALID?

The extent to which a study will provide valid results depends on whether it was designed and conducted in a way that justifies claims about the benefits or risks of the health services intervention being evaluated. Table 17-2 outlines the validity criteria that apply to the main study designs that can be used to evaluate the effectiveness of health services interventions. In the next section, we describe each of these criteria. As when answering a clinical question, we should first attempt to identify a systematic review that can provide an objective summary of all available evidence (see Chapter 9, Summarizing the Evidence Through Systematic Reviews). However, interpreting systematic reviews requires an understanding of the rules of evidence for the studies that are included in the review.

Were Study Participants Randomized? If Yes, Was Randomization Concealed, and Were Study Participants Analyzed in the Groups to Which They Were Randomized?

The most objective way to evaluate an intervention is through random allocation of study participants to intervention and control groups. In health services research, study participants can be individuals, patients, practitioners, or organizations. Random allocation reduces the bias that can occur when investigators allocate study participants to comparison groups and increases the likelihood that intervention and control groups are balanced with respect to both known and unknown determinants of outcome.

The success of randomization depends on two interrelated processes.[35,36] The first entails generating an unpredictable sequence by which participants are allocated to intervention and control groups through the use of a random process (e.g., computer-generated numbers, random number tables, or coin flipping). The second process, *allocation concealment*, shields individuals recruiting study participants from knowing upcoming assignments in advance.[37,38] Without this protection, these individuals have been known to manipulate who gets the next assignment, compromising the balance

Table 17-1   Users' Guides for an Article Evaluating a Health Services Intervention

Are the Results Valid?

- Were study participants randomized? If yes, was randomization concealed, and were study participants analyzed in the groups to which they were randomized?
- Were groups shown to be similar in all known determinants of outcome, or were analyses adjusted for differences?
- Were valid determinant, process, and outcome measures used?
- Was assessment of exposure/outcome uniform and unbiased?
- Was ascertainment of exposure/outcome sufficiently complete?
- Were analyses adjusted for unit of assignment, if cluster assignment was used?
- Were rival plausible explanations considered for results of nonrandomized studies?

What Are the Results?

- How large was the intervention effect?
- How precise was the estimate of the intervention effect?

How Can I Apply the Results to Health Services Decision Making?

- Were the study setting and context similar to mine?
- Were all important processes and outcomes considered?

---

between treatment and control groups.[39] Careful investigators will ensure that randomization is concealed through, for example, remote randomization, in which the individual recruiting participants calls a central coordinating office to discover the group to which the participant is allocated, or ensuring that the envelope containing the code is opaque, sealed, and sequentially numbered. In cluster randomization, allocation concealment is not as critical because investigators commonly recruit all clusters before randomization and assign them to groups at the same time.

Investigators can also corrupt randomization by systematically omitting from the results study participants who do not receive their assigned intervention. Researchers need to include outcome data for all participants in the analysis—including those in the experimental group who do not adhere to the intervention—in order to arrive at an unbiased estimate of the intervention effect. For example, in a randomized controlled trial evaluating an education program for primary care physicians and nurses to improve their recognition and treatment of patients with depression, all 62 nurses attended the 4 hours of seminars, but 12 of 62 physicians in the intervention group did not attend all 4 hours of seminars; 9 attended at least 1 hour, and 3 attended none.[40] If the nonattending physicians were destined to do better than the other members of their group and were excluded from the analysis, this would result in a misleading underestimate of the true intervention effect. If, as is more often the case, the nonattending physicians were less likely to recognize depressive symptoms, omitting this group from the analysis would result in a misleading overestimate of the benefit of the intervention.

Table **17-2**   Assessing Validity of Research Designs to Evaluate Health Services Interventions

Criteria	Randomized Controlled Trial	Controlled Before-and-After Study, Controlled Interrupted Time-Series Study, Cohort Study	Interrupted Time-Series Study	Case-Control Study
Randomization of study participants	√			
Concealment of allocation	√			
Intention-to-treat analysis	√			
Similarity in all known determinants of outcome or adjustment for differences	√	√		√
Validity of determinant, process, and outcome measures	√	√	√	√
Uniform and unbiased assessment of exposure/outcome in comparison groups	√	√		√
Blinding of study participants and clinicians	Usually not possible	Not applicable	Not applicable	Not applicable
Completeness of ascertainment of exposure/outcome	√	√	√	√
Adjustment for cluster effect*	√	√		
Consideration of rival plausible explanations		√	√	√

*Only applicable to studies in which participants are grouped (clusters).

The principle that dictates counting all events in all randomized study participants, regardless of whether they received the intended intervention, is the *intention-to-treat principle*. When reviewing reports of randomized trials, look for evidence that the investigators analyzed all study participants in the groups to which they were assigned (see Chapter 15, The Principle of Intention to Treat). In the study described previously, Thompson conducted an intention-to-treat analysis retaining all practices in the study despite individual physician nonattendance at all seminars.[40] For a detailed description of randomization, allocation concealment, and the intention-to-treat principle, see Chapter 4, Health Care Interventions.

Were Groups Shown to Be Similar in All Known Determinants of Outcome, or Were Analyses Adjusted for Differences?

As mentioned before, the best way to ensure similar groups is through random allocation of participants to comparison groups. However, trials with small sample sizes will probably still have imbalances in baseline determinants of outcome. A determinant of outcome is a characteristic of participants that confers increased or decreased likelihood of experiencing the outcome. Demographic variables, such as age and sex, are examples of determinants. Studies that assign clusters, such as primary care practices, to receive or not receive a health services intervention tend to have relatively small sample sizes. For this reason, such studies are at higher risk of imbalances in baseline characteristics of the comparison groups. Therefore, it is important to compare baseline data and, if necessary, to adjust for baseline differences in the analysis.

Observational studies will also yield biased results if comparison groups differ in determinants of outcome. Although investigators can adjust for known differences, they will not necessarily know all of the determinants that interact with the intervention to influence outcomes. This is frequently more problematic in health services evaluations where our understanding of causal mechanisms and potential confounders may be poorer than in evaluations of clinical interventions.

How then, can you be assured that investigators have made the fairest possible outcome comparison? We summarize the steps in Table 17-3. First, did the investigators convince you, through their review of the literature and on the basis of what you know about the determinants of outcome, that they measured all of the important determinants? Second, because these measurements are only as good as the data that go into them, were the determinants measured in a reliable and valid manner?

Third, did they show the extent to which the groups being compared differed on the determinants they measured? Readers should look for a display of baseline characteristics of the intervention and control groups. Although we will never know whether similarity exists for unknown determinants, we are reassured when known determinants are well balanced between groups. The issue is not whether there are statistically significant differences in known determinants between groups but, rather, the size of these differences. If the differences are large, the validity of the study may be compromised. The stronger the relationship between the determinants and outcome, and the greater the differences in distribution of determinants between groups, the more the differences

Table **17-3**   Determining Whether Differences in Determinants of Outcome, Rather Than Differences in the Intervention, Explain Differences in Outcomes

- Were all important determinants measured?
- Were measures of determinants of outcome reliable and valid?
- To what extent were study participants similar with respect to these determinants?
- Was multivariate analysis used to adjust for imbalances in determinants?

will weaken the strength of any inference about the effect of the intervention (i.e., you will have less confidence in the study results). For example, in the QI study, relative to usual care patients, QI-Therapy patients were slightly older and more likely to be women; fewer QI-Meds patients were Hispanic; and more QI-Therapy and QI-Meds patients had some college education. More usual care patients had subthreshold depression rather than depressive disorder relative to intervention patients.[41]

Fourth, if substantial differences exist in baseline characteristics, did the researchers use *multivariate analyses* to adjust the results for these differences? Multivariate analyses are statistical procedures for analyzing the relationships among three or more variables simultaneously.[42] Examples of multivariate analyses include logistic regression, multiple regression, and multivariate analysis of covariance (see Chapter 31, Regression and Correlation). In the QI study, the investigators conducted multivariate analyses to adjust for differences between comparison groups in baseline determinants of outcome.[3]

Were Valid Determinant, Process, and Outcome Measures Used?

Evaluations of health services interventions can include three types of measures. *Determinants* are baseline characteristics of study participants or settings that confer an increased or decreased likelihood of a positive or adverse outcome. Ideally, these determinants are equally distributed among comparison groups. In the QI study, baseline characteristics of study sites that were compared included the number of provider groups, number of health maintenance organization (HMO) contracts, percentage of capitated patients, and percentage of uninsured patients. Baseline characteristics of patients included age, sex, marital status, education, ethnicity, and number of chronic conditions.[2]

Because it is not easy to determine whether an outcome is caused by some aspect of the care provided or attributable to a setting's unique characteristics or a patient's underlying health state, it is often more straightforward and valid in health services research to assess *processes of care*. For example, even exemplary care may be associated with bad outcomes if a patient's prognosis is inherently poor. Process-of-care criteria provide standards for assessing whether clinicians have made the right decisions. In some cases, studies are not large enough or of sufficient duration to detect differences in patient outcomes (e.g., mortality) and instead, investigators examine process measures, such as quality of care. In these instances, it is important that the process measure be directly linked through high-quality evidence to the outcome of interest. Process measures can also help to explain study results (e.g., possible reasons why no differences were found in outcome between comparison groups). In the QI study, the investigators measured several process-of-care variables, including antidepressant medication use, mental health specialty counseling visits, medical visits for mental health problems, and medical visits for any problem.[2]

Outcome measures are the study end points. These are the measures that the intervention is designed to improve. In the QI study, the outcomes included probable depression, health-related quality of life, and employment.[2]

The onus is on investigators to demonstrate that determinant, process, and outcome measures are *reliable* and *valid*. Three common sources of determinant, process, and outcome data in health services evaluations are administrative databases, clinical records, and participant self-report. These data sources can be combined (e.g., existing databases can be used as an important value-added feature of primary data collection efforts).[43] In the next section, we outline criteria for readers to keep in mind when reviewing studies that use administrative databases, clinical records (also referred to as chart audits), or self-reported data.

Administrative Databases

Evaluations of some health services interventions require large-scale assessments of practice patterns that would be prohibitively costly for investigators to collect.[43] In addition, to identify outcomes of interest that are rare, sample sizes need to be very large. As a result, many health services researchers rely on secondary analysis of existing databases. Databases may be organized by facility, health care provider, disease or organ, or sector. The types of data they contain include financial, utilization, demographic, and clinical data. Investigators can obtain data from the public or private sector or their own health care settings.[44] Use of these databases presents definite cost advantages, being less time-consuming, labor-intensive, and limiting in the number of cases and the number of organizations that can feasibly be examined.[43]

Huston and Naylor published a comprehensive summary of the potential limitations of studies using secondary data sources and proposed a checklist for studies using such data.[45] One of the most obvious disadvantages of using health administrative databases is that these systems were not created for research purposes and, consequently, often lack relevant detail.[43] Inaccuracy or incompleteness of routinely collected administrative data can be a problem.[44] Basic information on patient characteristics, diagnoses, and procedures, particularly subsidiary diagnoses and secondary procedures, may be miscoded. Data are generally available only for those who used the services or accessed the health care system during the period of interest. Patients could be miscounted if they had multiple sites of residence or underwent procedures out of province, state, or country.[45] Information about patients, clinicians, and interventions may be incomplete, with key clinical data on processes and outcomes missing, inconsistently recorded, miscoded, or coded according to broad definitions that are not clinically precise.[45]

When reading a report about the evaluation of a health services intervention based on secondary data sources, readers should ask the following questions about the appropriateness, accuracy, and precision of measures derived from these data (Table 17-4).

Did Investigators Provide a Detailed Description of the Secondary Data Source(s) and the Specific Information Obtained From Them? For example, in Canada (and many other jurisdictions), every hospital admission is recorded in computerized discharge abstracts that include codes for specific procedures, diagnoses, and complications. If a study uses hospital discharge abstracts, the report should describe the diagnosis or procedure codes that defined the study sample. The appropriateness of the data source should be substantiated by showing that it truly captures the process-of-care indicator or outcomes of interest.[45]

Did Investigators Report the Reliability and Validity of Secondary Data Sources? Researchers may cite relevant published work describing the reliability and validity of the data source, or they may incorporate validation of the secondary data source in their own study design. Methods for validating the quality of data sources vary.[46] Clinical experts may review original records to determine whether the information agrees with what is entered into the secondary data source or compare the consistency of two or more secondary data sources that address similar issues.[45]

Aiken and colleagues[47] linked data from surveys of 10,184 staff nurses, hospital discharge abstracts of 232,342 surgery patients, and administrative data from 168 non-federal adult general hospitals in Pennsylvania to determine whether risk-adjusted rates of surgical mortality and failure-to-rescue (deaths in surgical patients who develop serious complications) were lower in hospitals where nurses had smaller patient loads. Focusing on the administrative data, the investigators derived information about the characteristics of all 210 adult general hospitals in Pennsylvania using the 1999 American Hospital Association (AHA) Annual Survey and the 1999 Pennsylvania Department of Health Hospital Survey.[48,49] Because their study involved linking these administrative data with staff nurse surveys and hospital discharge abstracts, they ultimately included 168 of the 210 hospitals that had AHA data, discharge data for surgical patients in the targeted Diagnosis Related Groups (DRGs) during the study period, and survey data from 10 or more staff nurses.

Table 17-4 Criteria for Appraising the Use of Administrative Databases

- Did investigators provide a detailed description of the secondary data source(s) and the specific information obtained from them?
  - If they used hospital discharge abstracts, did they describe the diagnosis or procedure codes that defined the study sample?
  - Did they substantiate the appropriateness of the data source by showing that it captured the process-of-care indicator or outcomes of interest?
- Did investigators report the reliability and validity of secondary data sources?
  - Did they cite relevant published work describing the reliability and validity of the data source or incorporate validation of the secondary data source into their own study design?

They provided a fairly detailed description of data sources and references for additional information; however, they did not comment specifically on the reliability and validity of these data sources. With respect to hospital discharge abstracts, the investigators specified the diagnosis codes for the surgical patients included in the analyses. After adjusting for patient and hospital characteristics (i.e., size, teaching status, and technology), each additional patient per nurse was associated with a 7% increase in the likelihood of dying within 30 days of admission (odds ratio [OR], 1.07; 95% confidence interval [CI], 1.03 to 1.12) and a 7% increase in the odds of failure-to-rescue (OR, 1.07; 95% CI, 1.02 to 1.11). An OR of 1.07 indicates that the odds of patient mortality increased by 7% for every additional patient in the average nurse's workload and that the difference from four to six and from four to eight patients per nurse would be accompanied by 14% and 31% increased odds of dying, respectively. Using standardization techniques to predict excess deaths in all patients that would be expected if the staffing ratio in all hospitals was six patients rather than four patients per nurse, there would be 2.3 (95% CI, 1.1 to 3.5) additional deaths per 1000 patients.[47]

Clinical Records

Quality and patient safety concerns, together with the omnipresent focus on cost containment, have led a growing number of researchers, insurers, administrators, and policy makers to examine what clinicians do. In assessing clinical processes, researchers and managers seek to determine whether the right service is provided to the right type of patient for the right reasons at the right time and place. In evaluations of health services interventions, investigators often review clinical records to assess quality of care. This section will help readers to evaluate such research studies to determine if valid criteria were used to assess the clinical records (Table 17-5). Although this section pertains to clinical records, it is also applicable to administrative datasets if they are being used as a source of quality-of-care data.

Was There a Systematic Review and Summary of Evidence Linking Processes to Outcomes? The review of clinical records to assess quality of care must be done using explicit criteria based on the best evidence of optimal practice. Readers should look for a description

Table 17-5   Criteria for Appraising the Results of a Clinical Record Review

- Was there a systematic review and summary of evidence linking processes to outcomes?
- If necessary, was an explicit, systematic, and reliable process used to elicit expert opinion?
- Was there an explicit, appropriate specification of values or preferences associated with outcomes?
- Was the process of applying the criteria reliable, unbiased, and likely to yield robust conclusions?

of how review criteria were developed and whether they were based on current, high-quality systematic reviews. Any decision about whether a clinician has delivered quality care is only as strong as the evidentiary basis of the criteria, which may vary from blinded randomized trials with complete follow-up to weaker observational studies. Are the criteria based on trial evidence, observational evidence, inference, or expert opinion? The need to rely on weaker evidence reduces the validity of process-of-care criteria and confidence that adherence to the criteria will have a favorable impact on the outcome of interest.

If Necessary, Was an Explicit, Systematic, and Reliable Process Used to Elicit Expert Opinion? Commonly, criteria for reviewing clinical records are developed by researchers using unsystematic methods. However, the criteria are more likely to be valid if developed by a panel of clinical experts who use an explicit, sensible, systematic method for collating their judgments. The process should be informed by a comprehensive literature review and analysis of risks and benefits of the health care practice in various patient subgroups. When such evidence does not exist, the process for eliciting expert opinion from within and outside of the panel should be explicit and systematic. Readers should look for a clear description of how the panel was assembled, along with the members' specialties and any organizations they are representing, to ensure that personal interests do not jeopardize the objectivity of the process.

Was There an Explicit, Appropriate Specification of Values or Preferences Associated With Outcomes? Most treatment decisions involve trade-offs (e.g., one intervention may be associated with slightly lower early mortality, lower initial costs, and more rapid recovery, whereas another may be associated with better symptom relief, decreased use of medication, and fewer subsequent procedures). Although panelist ratings should reflect these types of trade-offs, we cannot be sure that patients would make the same choices. This issue is especially important when patients' preferences must be given special weight (e.g., types of chemotherapy where patients must trade off increased length of life against decreased quality of life). Unfortunately, reviews of clinical records using explicit criteria do not usually lend themselves to capturing patients' preferences and values.

Was the Process of Applying the Criteria Reliable, Unbiased, and Likely to Yield Robust Conclusions? Application of explicit process-of-care criteria often rests on data derived from retrospective review of clinical records by research staff (sometimes called chart abstractors). Evidence of the reliability of these ratings (e.g., if two or more research staff generate the same data from the same patients' records) and their validity (e.g., if the findings agree with those of a clinical expert) should increase confidence in their findings (see Chapter 30, Measuring Agreement Beyond Chance). Reliable and valid criteria require explicit definitions of the clinical variables to be incorporated into the criteria.

Ideally, chart abstractors should be blinded to institutional or clinician identity and to patient outcomes because they are more likely to rate care processes as inappropriate when severe adverse outcomes occur.[50] Reviews of clinical records are subject to errors resulting from poor legibility or incomplete documentation by clinicians.

In a trial of neonatal nurse practitioners, Mitchell-DiCenso and colleagues used indicator conditions to evaluate quality of care.[51] An *indicator condition* is a clinical situation (e.g., disease, symptom, injury, or health state) that occurs reasonably frequently and for which there is sound evidence that high-quality care is beneficial.[52] To identify and develop the indicator conditions, they reviewed the charts of all infants admitted to the neonatal intensive care unit (NICU) during a 6-month period, rank-ordered clinical problems by prevalence, and distributed the list to 14 neonatologists, who rated the problems with respect to their importance, evidence that good medical decisions regarding intervention made a difference in outcome, expected comprehensiveness of documentation in a tertiary NICU setting, and ease of extraction from patient charts.[51]

For the 14 highest-scoring indicator conditions, two neonatologists developed a list of investigations and interventions that would reflect good quality of care, and these were independently reviewed by a panel of neonatologists. A trained research nurse audited all charts and scored the indicator conditions when they arose. To evaluate the research nurse's accuracy in reviewing the charts, her scores were compared with those of a neonatologist who independently reviewed some of the same charts. To evaluate her reliability, she scored some of the same charts twice, separated by a 2-week period.[51]

Self-Reported Data

The validity of self-reports as measures of quality of care may be compromised by response biases. For example, when asked how they manage a certain condition, clinicians may provide a response that reflects ideal management rather than their actual performance in a busy clinical setting seeing patients with multiple problems. Adams and colleagues analyzed studies of clinician adherence to practice guidelines or other evidence-based recommendations and compared self-reported and objective adherence rates.[53] Of the 10 studies that used both self-reported and objective measures, eight supported the existence of response bias in all self-reported measures. In 87% of 37 comparisons, self-reported adherence rates exceeded the objective rates, resulting in a median overestimation of adherence of 27%.[53]

This overestimation may be explained by social desirability and interviewer bias. *Social desirability bias* occurs when an individual does not adhere to a social norm but reports the socially desirable behavior when questioned.[54,55] The process of guideline dissemination may produce social pressures that promote socially desirable responses that do not reflect actual practice. *Interviewer bias* occurs when respondents provide responses that they believe the interviewer wants to hear.[55] On the basis of their findings, Adams and colleagues recommended that self-report no longer be used as the sole measure of quality of care.[53]

Was Assessment of Exposure/Outcome Uniform and Unbiased?

Were the Same Measures Used to Collect Data from Comparison Groups?

Readers should ensure that the same measures and sources of exposure/outcome data are used for all comparison groups. Investigators have been known to collect data directly from study participants in the intervention group via interviews or surveys but to use administrative data or chart abstraction to gather the data for the comparison group.

Were Exposure/Outcome Assessors Blinded to Group Allocation?

It is often difficult, if not impossible, to blind participants to group allocation in studies that evaluate health services interventions. Usually, investigators compare a new health service intervention to usual care or compare alternative forms of a health service intervention. In these situations, patients know, for example, whether they are being seen by a nurse practitioner or a physician, whether they receive a nurse telehealth intervention in addition to usual care, or whether they receive supported early hospital discharge. It is not usually possible to duplicate the intervention in an inert form (i.e., placebo) as in a drug trial. However, some investigators may create an *attention placebo* for the control group; for example, for an intervention such as a social support group, those in the control group may be assigned to a social group that meets but does not receive the "active ingredient" of professional-mediated social support. It is also difficult, if not impossible, to blind those delivering the intervention in studies of health services.

Given the difficulty of blinding study participants and those delivering the intervention, it is important that those assessing exposures and/or outcomes (referred to as outcome assessors or data collectors) are unaware of which study participants are in which group. Study personnel assessing exposure and outcome can almost always be kept blind to group allocation, even if study participants cannot.

In case-control studies, ascertainment of exposure is a key issue. Cases may be more likely to recall exposure to a possible causal agent than would control group members because of greater probing by an interviewer (interviewer bias). Readers should note whether investigators used bias-minimizing strategies, such as blinding interviewers to which study participants were cases and which were controls.

Similarly, in randomized controlled trials and cohort studies, ascertainment of outcome is a key issue. If outcome assessors believe that certain individuals are at risk for developing an outcome, they may search more diligently for the outcome in those individuals. This could result in the exposed cohort having an apparent, but spurious, increase in risk—a situation we refer to as *surveillance bias*.

Investigators can take additional precautions by constructing a blinded adjudication committee to review health services data and decide on exposure and outcome-related issues. For example, the committee can evaluate study data to determine the reason for a hospital readmission and cause of a hospital death. The more that judgment is involved in determining whether a patient has been exposed or experienced a target outcome, the more important *blinding* becomes. Blinding is less crucial in studies with objective outcomes, such as all-cause mortality.

Was Ascertainment of Exposure/Outcome Sufficiently Complete?

The greater the number of study participants for whom outcome data are missing, the more a study's validity is potentially compromised. Data may be missing because participants are lost to follow-up or refuse to answer questions. Study participants who withdraw or disappear often have different prognoses than those who are retained; for example, patients may withdraw or disappear because they experience adverse outcomes (even death) or because they are doing well (and so do not return to be assessed).

The situation is completely analogous to the rationale for an intention-to-treat analysis: Participants who withdraw from an intervention may be less or more likely to experience the outcome of interest.

In cluster studies, data may be missing at the cluster level if an entire cluster withdraws. Administrative databases generally include data only for those who use the service; key clinical data on processes and outcomes may be missing, services or procedures may be miscoded, and outcomes of interest may not be captured.

One way to determine the seriousness of missing outcome data is to consider a worst-case scenario in which those in the intervention group who are lost to follow-up experience the target outcome (e.g., hospital readmission), whereas those lost to follow-up in the control group do not. For more details about this strategy, see Chapter 4, Health Care Interventions. When a worst-case scenario, if it were true, substantially alters the results, you must consider the plausibility of a markedly different outcome in intervention and control group participants who withdraw or disappear. The extent to which researchers can show that intervention and control participants who are lost to follow-up are similar with respect to important determinants of outcome reduces—but does not eliminate—the possibility of different rates of outcome in those who remain in the study and those who do not. An analogous worst-case scenario for case-control studies would involve assuming that all cases who are lost were not exposed to the exposure of interest, whereas those lost in the control group were exposed.

In conclusion, study participant withdrawal or failure to provide data and missing data in administrative datasets and clinical records potentially threaten a study's validity. If assuming a worst-case scenario does not change the inferences arising from study results, then this loss of data is not a problem. If such an assumption would significantly alter the results, validity is compromised.

Were Analyses Adjusted for Unit of Assignment, if Cluster Assignment Was Used?

Whereas in most clinical studies, the patient is the unit of assignment and analysis, in health services research, the unit of assignment and analysis may be the region, the hospital, a set of hospitals, the practice setting, the clinician, or the individual patient.[45] Although it is possible to conduct studies of organizational interventions in which individual participants are allocated to intervention and control groups, there is a danger that control group participants could unintentionally receive the experimental intervention because they share the same clinical or organizational environment with intervention group participants. This is known as *contamination*. Contamination occurs when the control group receives the intervention intended for the experimental group or vice versa. If contamination is likely, investigators will often randomize organizations, or groups of health care professionals or patients, rather than individuals. Similarly, organizations, geographically defined populations, or practices are often the unit of assignment in observational studies of health services interventions. In such circumstances, data are still often collected about the processes and outcomes of care at the individual level. Studies that assign participants to the intervention in groups, but collect data at the individual level, are said to employ *cluster assignment.*[56,57] Cluster assignment has important implications for the design, power, and analysis of studies.[19]

A fundamental assumption of standard statistics used to analyze studies of individuals is that the outcome for an individual is completely unrelated to that for any other individual; the outcomes are said to be *independent.* This assumption is violated, however, when cluster assignment is adopted because two individuals in any one cluster are more likely to respond in a similar manner than are two individuals in different clusters. For example, management of patients in a single hospital is more likely to be similar than management of patients in different hospitals.

In a cluster design, analyses at the individual level must incorporate an adjustment that accounts for the unit of assignment (the cluster) and the fact that individuals within a cluster will be more similar to each other than individuals in different clusters.[19] In a cluster randomized trial, Thompson and colleagues evaluated an educational program for primary care physicians and nurses to improve the recognition and treatment of patients with depression.[40] They randomized 29 primary care practices to the intervention group and 30 practices to the control group. Educators offered practice teams in the intervention group a 4-hour seminar supplemented by videotapes to demonstrate interview and counseling skills, small-group discussion of cases, and role-playing, and were available for the next 9 months to provide additional help as needed. The primary outcomes were recognition of depression and clinical improvement. Because data were also collected at the patient level, randomizing practices rather than individual physicians and nurses avoided the risk of contamination, which could have occurred in two ways: (1) if physicians and nurses randomized to the educational program shared their learning with physicians and nurses in their practice setting who were randomized to the control group; and (2) if physicians and nurses randomized to the intervention group provided care to patients who were usually cared for by their colleagues in the control group.[40] Because they used cluster assignment, the investigators adjusted for clustering in their analysis.

Another example of a cluster assignment is a study evaluating the effects of systematic implementation of an advance directive program in nursing homes on patient and family satisfaction and health care costs.[58] Investigators randomized three nursing homes to an advance directive program and three nursing homes to continue with usual advance directives policies. Although analysis was at the level of the nursing home resident, an adjustment was made in the analysis for the cluster effect, recognizing that residents in the same nursing home were likely to be more similar to one another than residents in different nursing homes.

Were Rival Plausible Explanations Considered for Results of Nonrandomized Studies?

The main limitation of nonrandomized designs is that the lack of randomized controls threatens *internal validity* and increases the likelihood of plausible rival hypotheses.[19] Cook and Campbell[20] identified eight possible threats to the internal validity of nonrandomized designs: (1) history (during the study period, an event occurs in addition to the intervention); (2) maturation (observed effect caused by changes in the passage of time rather than the intervention, e.g., growing older or more experienced); (3) testing (on repeat testing preintervention and postintervention, improvements may be a result of test familiarity rather than the intervention); (4) instrumentation (changes in the calibration of a measuring instrument or changes in exposure/outcome assessors may produce changes in obtained measurements); (5) statistical regression (when participants are selected on the basis of extreme results on preintervention measures); (6) selection bias (differential selection of participants for comparison groups resulting in unequal probabilities of experiencing the outcome of interest); (7) experimental mortality (differential loss of participants from comparison groups); and (8) interactions with selection, such as selection-maturation, selection-history, and selection-instrumentation (might be mistaken for the effect of the intervention).

According to Campbell and Stanley,[59] the controlled before-and-after design addresses all of these threats. In the absence of a concurrent control group, the interrupted time-series design may fail to control for history in that a concurrent event rather than the intervention may have produced the change, and it may fail to control for instrumentation if the measurement process changes over time. The cohort study design may fail to control for selection and regression.

Readers must systematically think through how each threat to internal validity may influence the study results. When all plausible threats can be reasonably discounted, readers can make confident conclusions about the relationship between the health services intervention and the outcome.[20]

USING THE GUIDE

How well did the QI study[2,3,41] meet the criteria for validity? The study is a randomized controlled trial in which investigators randomized primary care clinics (clusters) to intervention or control groups. Within each managed care organization, the investigators grouped primary care clinic clusters into matched blocks of three, based on patient demographics, clinician specialty, and distance to mental health providers. A clinic could be a single clinic, a cluster of small clinics, or a clinical care team within a large clinic. Within matched sets, they used a random number table to assign clinic clusters to the QI-Meds program, in which nurses provided medication follow-up (424 patients); the QI-Therapy program, in which trained psychotherapists provided individual or group cognitive behavioral therapy (489 patients); or usual care (443 patients). The investigators did not mention allocation concealment; however, randomizing all clusters at one time ensures concealment. They conducted an intention-to-treat analysis.

The investigators documented baseline characteristics in the three groups, including sex, mean age, marital status, education, ethnicity, depressive disorder status, mental health and physical health composite scores, number of chronic conditions, presence of an anxiety disorder, current alcohol abuse, and whether the patient had received treatment for depression in the preceding 6 months. Patients in the QI-Therapy group were older than control group patients (mean age 44.9 vs. 42.2 years) and were more likely to be women than control or QI-Meds patients (75.8% vs. 69.1% in the control group and 66.7% in the QI-Meds group). A lower percentage of QI-Meds patients were Hispanic (25.7% vs. 30.8% in the control group and 32% in the

Continued

QI-Therapy group), and a higher percentage of QI-Therapy and QI-Meds patients had some college education (21.6% in the QI-Therapy group and 22.9% in the QI-Meds group vs. 15% in the control group). A higher percentage of usual care patients had subthreshold depression rather than depressive disorder compared with intervention patients (48% vs. 36% in the QI-Meds group and 36% in the QI-Therapy group).[3,41] The investigators adjusted for these baseline differences in the analyses.

The primary outcomes included processes of care (use of antidepressant medication, mental health specialty counseling visits, medical visits for mental health problems, any medical visits), health outcomes (probable depression and health-related quality of life), and employment. Patients completed an interview including the affective disorders section of the Composite International Diagnostic Interview (CIDI) and the Center for Epidemiologic Studies Depression Scale (CES-D); a telephone interview on anxiety disorder, income, wealth, and employment; and a mail survey. Although some measures are well-established valid instruments, the investigators did not describe or test the validity of the mail survey or less-established data collection tools. Outcome assessment was uniform across the three groups. There was a potential for bias in that outcome assessors were not blinded.

At 24 months, 85% of patients completed the CIDI and the mailed surveys. The investigators did not provide attrition data by comparison group, and thus, it is difficult to determine if drop-out rates differed among groups. The investigators adjusted for the cluster effect.

The final assessment of validity is never a "yes" or "no" decision. Rather, think of validity as a continuum ranging from strong studies that are very likely to yield an accurate estimate of the intervention effect to weak studies that are very likely to yield a biased estimate of effect. Inevitably, judgment about where a study lies in this continuum involves some subjectivity. In this case, strengths of the study include cluster randomization to comparison groups; intention-to-treat analysis; adjustment for baseline differences; use of established, valid outcome measures; low overall lost-to-follow-up rate; and adjustment for cluster effect in the analysis. Limitations are three-fold: failure to demonstrate validity of process measures, lack of blinding of outcome assessors, and failure to provide attrition rates by comparison group. Our judgment is that although some of these limitations could bias the results, the validity is sufficiently high to warrant continued consideration.

WHAT ARE THE RESULTS?

How Large Was the Intervention Effect?

We have described the alternatives for expressing the strength of the association between an exposure and dichotomous or continuous outcomes in other chapters (see Chapter 4, Health Care Interventions, and Chapter 27, Measures of Association). The same measures that are used for reporting effect sizes in studies of clinical interventions are also used in studies evaluating health services interventions (e.g., means, medians, odds ratios, relative risks, absolute risk differences).

In interrupted time-series studies, the purpose of the analysis is to assess the magnitude and statistical significance of any shifts in the series after the interruption created by the introduction of the intervention.[20] Statistical methods to analyze interrupted time-series designs include *time-series regression techniques*[60] and *autoregressive integrated moving average (ARIMA) models.*[61] Factors that influence the analysis include the number of data points available and whether autocorrelation is present.[20] *Autocorrelation* refers to the situation whereby data points collected close in time are likely to be more similar to each other than to data points collected far apart. For example, for any given month, the waiting times in hospitals are likely to be more similar to waiting times in adjacent months than to waiting times in the previous 12 months.[19]

Analysis of cluster randomized trials involves three approaches: (1) analysis at the cluster level, (2) adjustment of standard tests for the clustering effect, and (3) advanced statistical techniques using data recorded at both individual and cluster levels.[57,62–64]

How Precise Was the Estimate of the Intervention Effect?

Clinicians can evaluate the precision of the estimate of effect by examining the confidence interval around the estimate (see Chapter 4, Health Care Interventions, and Chapter 29, Confidence Intervals). The larger the sample size and the number of outcome events, the narrower the confidence interval. The boundaries of the confidence interval can help us interpret study results. In a *positive study*—a study in which the authors conclude that an intervention is effective—one can look at the lower boundary of the confidence interval. If this intervention effect (the lowest effect that is consistent with the study results) is still important (i.e., large enough for you to recommend the intervention), then the investigators have enrolled sufficient study participants. If, on the other hand, you do not consider this intervention effect to be clinically important, then the study cannot be considered definitive, even if its results are statistically significant (i.e., they exclude a risk reduction of 0).

The confidence interval also helps us interpret *negative studies* in which the authors have concluded that the experimental intervention is no better than the control intervention. All we need to do is look at the upper boundary of the confidence interval. If the estimate of effect at this upper boundary would, if it was true, be important, the study has failed to exclude an important intervention effect. For information on determining whether a study was large enough, see Chapter 29, Confidence Intervals.

In the case of cluster studies, if the analysis does not adjust for clustering, it is likely to overestimate the statistical significance of the comparison, resulting in overly narrow confidence intervals or artificially low *P* values.[63]

USING THE GUIDE

At 24 months, control group patients had similar levels of current depressive disorder (34%) as QI-Meds patients (39%) and QI-Therapy patients (31%); the QI-Meds patients had a higher rate of disorder (39%) than did QI-Therapy patients (31%) ($P = .04$). Patients in the QI-Therapy group had better emotional well-being ($P = .04$) than did patients in the control group.

Continued

The investigators calculated a measure of overall poor outcome that classified patients as depressed if they scored in the depressed range on all three outcome measures (i.e., probable depression, Center for Epidemiologic Studies Depression Scale, and the mental health composite scale). At 24 months, QI-Therapy patients had reduced overall poor outcomes of 8% relative to control group patients, with borderline significance of $P = .06$. This translates into a relative reduction in overall poor outcome of 20%. QI-Therapy patients had reduced overall poor outcomes of 10% relative to QI-Meds patients ($P = .02$). This translates into a relative reduction in overall poor outcome of 27%.[3] Unfortunately, the investigators did not report confidence intervals around the differences between groups, limiting our interpretation of the precision of the estimate of intervention effects.

HOW CAN I APPLY THE RESULTS TO HEALTH SERVICES DECISION MAKING?

In health services research, determining the applicability of study findings to other settings can be challenging because health care settings differ in ways that may influence effective implementation of the intervention. Characteristics that may influence transferability of study findings include geographic location of the health care agency (e.g., rural versus urban), size of the agency, organizational culture, and method of funding.

For example, the first randomized controlled trial of primary care nurse practitioners was conducted more than 30 years ago and continues to be cited as a high-quality trial.[65] The investigators randomized more than 1000 families to the care of one of two family physicians or one of two nurse practitioners working collaboratively with the same family physicians. Critics of the study have correctly pointed out that the sample size of the study was not 1598 families but rather two nurse practitioners and two physicians in one primary care practice.[65] This raises questions about the similarity of these nurse practitioners and physicians to their professional colleagues, the similarity of this primary care practice to other practices, and ultimately, the generalizability of the study findings to nurse practitioners and family physicians in other primary care practices. Studies conducted in a single site or setting may not generalize to other sites or settings, particularly if components of the study intervention are highly idiosyncratic and depend on a clinical culture that is not readily transferable.[66]

Evaluations of health services interventions often use cluster assignment, in which a relatively small number of clusters are allocated to intervention or control groups. Although cluster allocation may strengthen the study design by reducing potential bias from contamination, the small number of clusters (and similarity within clusters) may limit the generalizability of study findings.

Were the Study Setting and Context Similar to Mine?

Health services interventions have effects within, and are influenced by, contexts and the local and regional health care system within which they operate.[67] Seemingly similar programs can have different effects depending on the local clinical culture and factors such as management structures and level and quality of staff.[30] These differences can limit the extent to which study findings can be generalized.

Generalizability of findings will also depend on the relevance of the comparison groups. In their systematic review of alternatives to conventional emergency department care, Roberts and Mays[68] found evidence suggesting that broadening access to primary care and employing primary care professionals in hospital emergency departments were effective strategies for reducing demand for expensive secondary care. However, they noted that the evidence was drawn from international research studies done in very different health settings and that transferring interventions that succeed in one setting (without understanding the process of change) would not necessarily have the same results in another setting. For example, they noted that in some U.S.-based studies, the deprived population in the control group had such low levels of access to primary care physicians that intervention effects (e.g., quality and timeliness of care, hospital admissions averted) were substantial. Applying the same intervention in the United Kingdom, they predicted, would have more modest effects because the deprived populations in the United Kingdom have higher levels of access to primary care services.[68]

The range of health services options perceived as feasible at any one time is conditioned by deep-rooted political and cultural assumptions and constrained by the institutional history of the jurisdiction in question.[30] Thus, the comparisons available in the empirical literature may not be politically practicable in the jurisdiction that wishes to use the research findings.[30] In a review of the impact of managed care on the cost and quality of health care, Robinson and Steiner[69] found that most research on managed care was from the United States and compared capitated managed care organizations of different types with fee-for-service medical practice under traditional third-party payer indemnity insurance. Although the use of capitation as one element in managed care was highly relevant to policy makers in publicly financed health systems such as in the United Kingdom and New Zealand, they concluded that the comparison with fee-for-service under traditional private medical insurance was not relevant.[69]

The timing of the research may also affect its relevance. For example, findings from a study evaluating the effect of a hospital-at-home scheme in reducing hospital length of stay is likely to be of far greater relevance to policy makers in a political era when shortening time spent in hospital is a priority.[30]

Readers should look for descriptions of the study setting and participants and consider the extent of similarity to their own setting. In studies of health systems, judging the extent to which to generalize study findings to other health systems will require examining similarities in features such as scope of practice, financial incentives for practice, governance models for health care, and health insurance.

Were All Important Processes and Outcomes Considered?

Even when investigators report favorable effects of a health services intervention on one or more important outcomes, readers should consider whether negative effects on other outcomes may not have been measured or reported. For example, a health services intervention may reduce length of hospital stay, but it may decrease quality of life or increase readmissions or out-of-hospital adverse events. An outcome that is often neglected is the resource implications of alternative health services interventions. The increasing resource constraints facing health care systems mandate careful attention to economic evaluation, particularly of resource-intense interventions (see Chapter 18, Economic Evaluation).

CLINICAL RESOLUTION

The six managed care organizations in the QI study were selected based on diversity of geography and organization. They included staff and network model multispecialty group practices and rural managed public health clinics. Patients had prepaid or managed fee-for-service (including Medicare and Medicaid) coverage. Managed fee-for-service is a type of health plan that has some restrictions, such as having to choose physicians from a specified list or requiring a referral before seeing a specialist. Of 48 primary care clinics with at least two clinicians, 46 participated. Patients were eligible for the study if they were depressed and intended to use the clinic as a source of care for the next 12 months. Patients were ineligible if they were younger than 18 years of age, had an acute medical emergency, did not speak English or Spanish, or did not have insurance or a public-pay arrangement that covered care delivered by the mental health specialists providing the interventions.[2]

As the administrative director of a primary care clinic in a managed care organization, you are intrigued by the results. There are numerous similarities between your setting and the primary care clinics in the study. Although many of the benefits were not sustained for 24 months, mental health–related quality-of-life effects persisted among patients in the QI-Therapy approach, and these patients had a lower rate of depressive disorder and reduced overall poor outcomes.

You return to the systematic review and note that the authors summarized a cost-effectiveness analysis of the QI program.[1] Relative to usual care, average health care costs increased US$485 per patient (13%) in QI-Therapy throughout 2 years ($P = 0.28$). Estimated costs per quality-adjusted life-year gained were between US$9478 and US$21,478 for the QI-Therapy group. Compared with patients in the usual care group, patients in the QI-Therapy group had 47 ($P = 0.01$) fewer days with depression burden (extrapolated number of days they experienced all three of probable major depressive disorder, significant depressive symptoms, and poor mental health–related quality of life) and were employed 20.9 ($P = 0.03$) more days during the study period.[70] You decide to hold a meeting with the clinicians in your clinic to share these findings and discuss the appropriateness of implementing the QI-Therapy program in the clinic.

REFERENCES

1. Gilbody S, Whitty P, Grimshaw J, Thomas R. Educational and organizational interventions to improve the management of depression in primary care: a systematic review. *JAMA*. 2003;289:3145-3151.
2. Wells KB, Sherbourne C, Schoenbaum M, et al. Impact of disseminating quality improvement programs for depression in managed primary care: a randomized controlled trial. *JAMA*. 2000;283:212-220.
3. Sherbourne CD, Wells KB, Duan N, et al. Long-term effectiveness of disseminating quality improvement for depression in primary care. *Arch Gen Psychiatry*. 2001;58:696-703.

4. Tyrer P, Coid J, Simmonds S, Joseph P, Marriott S. Community mental health teams (CMHTs) for people with severe mental illnesses and disordered personality. *Cochrane Database Syst Rev.* 2000;(2):CD000270.

5. Shepperd S, Iliffe S. Hospital at home versus in-patient hospital care. *Cochrane Database Syst Rev.* 2001;(3):CD000356.

6. Horrocks S, Anderson E, Salisbury C. Systematic review of whether nurse practitioners working in primary care can provide equivalent care to doctors. *BMJ.* 2002;324:819-823.

7. Szilagyi P, Vann J, Bordley C, et al. Interventions aimed at improving immunization rates. *Cochrane Database Syst Rev.* 2002;(4):CD003941.

8. Ploeg J, Biehler L, Willison K, Hutchison B, Blythe J. Perceived support needs of family caregivers and implications for a telephone support service. *Can J Nurs Res.* 2001;33:43-61.

9. Lohr KN, Steinwachs DM. Health services research: an evolving definition of the field. *Health Serv Res.* 2002;36:7-9.

10. American Association of Colleges of Nursing. A vision of baccalaureate and graduate nursing education: the next decade. Available at *http://www.aacn.nche.edu/Publications/positions/vision.htm.* Accessed January 9, 2004.

11. Black N. Health services research: saviour or chimera? *Lancet.* 1997;349:1834-1836.

12. Fulop N, Allen P, Clarke A, Black N. Issues in studying the organization and delivery of health services. In: Fulop N, Allen P, Clarke A, Black N, eds. *Studying the Organization and Delivery of Health Services: Research Methods.* New York: Routledge; 2001:1-23.

13. Balas EA, Austin SM, Ewigman BG, Brown GD, Mitchell JA. Methods of randomized controlled clinical trials in health services research. *Med Care.* 1995;33:687-699.

14. Weinberger M, Oddone EZ, Henderson WG, Smith DM, Huey J, Giobbie-Hurder A, Feussner JR. Multisite randomized controlled trials in health services research: scientific challenges and operational issues. *Med Care.* 2001;39:627-634.

15. McCorkle R, Strumpf NE, Nuamah IF, et al. A specialized home care intervention improves survival among older post-surgical cancer patients. *J Am Geriatr Soc.* 2000;48:1707-1713.

16. Boult C, Boult LB, Morishita L, et al. A randomized clinical trial of outpatient geriatric evaluation and management. *J Am Geriatr Soc.* 2001;49:351-359.

17. Fjaertoft H, Indredavik B, Lydersen S. Stroke unit care combined with early supported discharge: long-term follow-up of a randomized controlled trial. *Stroke.* 2003;34:2687-2691.

18. Mundinger MO, Kane RL, Lenz ER, et al. Primary care outcomes in patients treated by nurse practitioners or physicians: a randomized trial. *JAMA.* 2000;283:59-68.

19. Grimshaw J, Wilson B, Campbell M, Eccles M, Ramsay C. Epidemiological methods. In: Fulop N, Allen P, Clarke A, Black N, eds. *Studying the Organization and Delivery of Health Services: Research Methods.* New York: Routledge; 2001:56-72.

20. Cook TD, Campbell DT. *Quasi-experimentation: Design and Analysis Issues for Field Settings.* Chicago: Rand McNally; 1979.

21. Solberg LI, Fischer LR, Wei F, et al. A CQI intervention to change the care of depression: a controlled study. *Eff Clin Pract.* 2001;4:239-249.

22. Hutchison B. Effect of computer-generated nurse/physician reminders on influenza immunization among seniors. *Fam Med.* 1989;21:433-437.

23. Lomas J, Anderson GM, Dominick-Pierre K, Vayda E, Enkin MW, Hannah WJ. Do practice guidelines guide practice? The effect of a consensus statement on the practice of physicians. *N Engl J Med.* 1989;321:1306-1311.

24. Ramsay CR, Matowe L, Grilli R, Grimshaw JM, Thomas RE. Interrupted time series designs in health technology assessment: lessons from two systematic reviews of behaviour change strategies. *Int J Tech Assess in Health Care.* 2003;19:613-623.

25. Guyatt GH, DiCenso A, Farewell V, Willan A, Griffith L. Randomized trials versus observational studies in adolescent pregnancy prevention. *J Clin Epidemiol.* 2000;53:167-174.

26. Brazier J, Nicholls J, Snooks H. The cost and effectiveness of the London helicopter emergency medical service. *J Health Serv Res Policy.* 1996;1:232-237.

27. Hagan H, Des Jarlais DC, Friedman SR, Purchase D, Alter MJ. Reduced risk of hepatitis B and hepatitis C among injection drug users in the Tacoma Syringe Exchange Program. *Am J Public Health.* 1995;85:1531-1537.

28. Tashakkori A, Teddlie C. *Mixed Methodology: Combining Qualitative and Quantitative Approaches.* Newbury Park, CA: Sage Publications; 1998.

29. Bradley F, Wiles R, Kinmonth A-L, Mant D, Gantley M, for the SHIP Collaborative Group. Development and evaluation of complex interventions in health services research: case study of the Southampton heart integrated care project (SHIP). *BMJ.* 1999:318:711-715.

30. Mays N, Roberts E, Popay J. Synthesising research evidence. In: Fulop N, Allen P, Clarke A, Black N, eds. *Studying the Organization and Delivery of Health Services: Research Methods.* New York: Routledge; 2001:188–220.

31. Devereaux PJ, Choi PT, Lacchetti C, et al. A systematic review and meta-analysis of studies comparing mortality rates of private for-profit and private not-for-profit hospitals. *CMAJ.* 2002;166:1399-1406.

32. Parkes J, Shepperd S. Discharge planning from hospital to home. *Cochrane Database Syst Rev.* 2000;(4):CD000313.

33. Naylor CD, Guyatt GH. Users' guides to the medical literature. X. How to use an article reporting variations in the outcomes of health services. *JAMA.* 1996;275:554-558.

34. Naylor CD, Guyatt GH. Users' guides to the medical literature. XI. How to use an article about a clinical utilization review. *JAMA.* 1996;275:1435-1439.

35. Schulz KF. Subverting randomization in controlled trials. *JAMA.* 1995;274:1456-1458.

36. Schulz KF. Randomised trials, human nature, and reporting guidelines. *Lancet.* 1996;348:596-598.

37. Schulz KF. Assessing allocation concealment and blinding in randomised controlled trials: why bother? *Evid Based Nurs.* 2001;4:4-6.

38. Schulz KF, Chalmers I, Grimes DA, et al. Assessing the quality of randomization from reports of controlled trials published in obstetrics and gynecology journals. *JAMA.* 1994;272:125-128.

39. Schulz KF, Chalmers I, Hayes RJ, Altman DG. Empirical evidence of bias, dimensions of methodological quality associated with estimates of treatment effects in controlled trials. *JAMA.* 1995;273:408-412.

40. Thompson C, Kinmonth AL, Stevens L, et al. Effects of a clinical-practice guideline and practice-based education on detection and outcome of depression in primary care: Hampshire Depression Project randomised controlled trial. *Lancet.* 2000;355:185-191.

41. Wells KB. The design of Partners in Care: evaluating the cost-effectiveness of improving care for depression in primary care. *Soc Psychiatry Psychiatr Epidemiol.* 1999;34:20-29.

42. Polit DF. *Data Analysis & Statistics for Nursing Research.* Stamford, CT: Appleton & Lange; 1996.

43. Cowper DC, Hynes DM, Kubal JD, Murphy PA. Using administrative databases for outcomes research: select examples from VA health services research and development. *J Med Sys.* 1999;23:249-259.

44. Else BA, Armstrong EP, Cox ER. Data sources for pharmacoeconomic and health services research. *Am J Health-Syst Pharm.* 1997;54:2601-2608.

45. Huston P, Naylor D. Health services research: reporting on studies using secondary data sources. *CMAJ.* 1996;155:1697-1702.

46. Williams JI, Young W. A summary of studies on the quality of health care administrative databases in Canada. In: Goel V, Williams JI, Anderson GM, Blackstien-Hirsch P, Fooks C, Naylor CD, eds. *Patterns of Health Care in Ontario: The ICES Practice Atlas,* 2nd ed. Ottawa, ON: Canadian Medical Association; 1996:339-345.

47. Aiken LH, Clarke SP, Sloane DM, Sochalski J, Silber JH. Hospital nurse staffing and patient mortality, nurse burnout, and job dissatisfaction. *JAMA.* 2002;288:1987-1993.

48. *AHA Annual Survey Database.* Chicago: American Hospital Association; 1999.

49. Commonwealth of Pennsylvania. *Hospital Questionnaire: Reporting Period July 1, 1998-June 30, 1999.* Harrisburg, PA: Department of Health, Division of Statistics.

50. Caplan RA, Posner KL, Cheney FW. Effect of outcome on physician judgments of appropriateness of care. *JAMA.* 1991;265:1957-1960.

51. Mitchell-DiCenso A, Guyatt G, Marrin M, et al. A controlled trial of nurse practitioners in neonatal intensive care. *Pediatrics.* 1996;98:1143-1148.

52. Chambers LW, Sibley JC, Spitzer WO, Tugwell P. Quality of care assessment: how to set up and use an indicator condition. *Clin Invest Med.* 1981;4:41-50.

53. Adams AS, Soumerai SB, Lomas J, Ross-Degnan D. Evidence of self-report bias in assessing adherence to guidelines. *Int J Qual Health Care.* 1999;11:187-192.

54. Plous S. Social Influences. In: *The Psychology of Judgement and Decision Making*. New York: McGraw Hill; 1993:191-204.

55. Warwick DP, Lininger CA. *The Sample Survey: Theory and Practice*. New York: McGraw-Hill; 1975:201-202.

56. Donner A, Klar N. *Design and Analysis of Cluster Randomisation Trials in Health Research*. London: Arnold; 2000.

57. Murray DM. *The Design and Analysis of Group Randomised Trials*. Oxford: Oxford University Press; 1998.

58. Molloy DW, Guyatt GH, Russo R, et al. Systematic implementation of an advance directive program in nursing homes: a randomized controlled trial. *JAMA*. 2000;283:1437-1444.

59. Campbell DT, Stanley JC. *Experimental and Quasi-experimental Designs for Research*. Dallas: Houghton Mifflin Company; 1963.

60. Draper NR, Smith HF. *Applied Regression Analysis*. New York: Wiley; 1981.

61. Box GE, Jenkins GM. *Time-Series Analysis: Forecasting and Control*. San Francisco: Holden-Day; 1976.

62. Donner A. Some aspects of the design and analysis of cluster randomisation trials. *Applied Statistics*. 1998;47:95-113.

63. Campbell MK, Mollison J, Steen N, Grimshaw JM, Eccles M. Analysis of cluster randomized trials in primary care: a practical approach. *Fam Pract*. 2000;17:192-196.

64. Mollison J, Simpson JA, Campbell MK, Grimshaw JM. Comparison of analytical methods for cluster randomised trials: an example from a primary care setting. *J Epidemiol Biostat*. 2000;5:339-346.

65. Spitzer WO, Sackett DL, Sibley JC, et al. The Burlington randomized trial of the nurse practitioner. *N Eng J Med*. 1974;290:251-256.

66. Scott I, Campbell D. Health services research: what is it and what does it offer? *Intern Med J*. 2002;32:91-99.

67. Sheldon T. It ain't what you do but the way that you do it. *J Health Serv Res Policy*. 2001;6:3-5.

68. Roberts E, Mays N. Can primary care and community-based models of emergency care substitute for the hospital accident and emergency (A & E) department? *Health Policy*. 1998;44:191-214.

69. Robinson R, Steiner A. *Managed Health Care: US Evidence and Lessons for the National Health Service*. Buckingham, England: Open University Press, 1998.

70. Schoenbaum M, Unutzer J, Sherbourne C, et al. Cost-effectiveness of practice-initiated quality improvement for depression: results of a randomized controlled trial. *JAMA*. 2001;286:1325-1330.

18

Economic Evaluation

Deborah Marshall, Catherine Demers, Bernie O'Brien,
and Gordon Guyatt

Patricia Stone also made substantive contributions to this chapter.

*We gratefully acknowledge the work of Michael Drummond, Scott Richardson,
Mitchell Levine, and Daren Heyland on the original chapter that appears in the
Users' Guides to the Medical Literature, edited by Guyatt and Rennie.*

In This Chapter

Cost: Just Another Outcome?
   Costs Are More Variable Than Other Outcomes
   The Role of Costs in Clinical Decision Making Remains Controversial
   Using Cost Information to Inform Decisions Poses Special Challenges

Are the Results Valid?
   Did Investigators Adopt a Sufficiently Broad Viewpoint?
   Were Results Reported Separately for Patients With Different Baseline Risks?
   Were Costs Measured Accurately?
   Did Investigators Consider the Timing of Costs and Consequences?

What Are the Results?
   What Were the Incremental Costs and Effects of Each Strategy?
   Did Incremental Costs and Effects Differ Between Subgroups?
   How Much Did Allowance for Uncertainty Change the Results?

How Can I Apply the Results to Patient Care?
   Are the Treatment Benefits Worth the Risks and Costs?
   Can I Expect Similar Costs in My Setting?

As new health care interventions continue to be developed and evaluated, the cost of implementing all effective health and clinical services exceeds available resources. Because of the scarcity of resources, decisions about the implementation of new services frequently need to be based on economic analyses.[1] Once we are convinced about the benefits of a health care intervention, we must seek assurance that the societal resources (usually valued in dollars or other currency) consumed by implementing the intervention will be in keeping with the incremental benefit associated with the intervention.

Unfortunately, not all economic evidence is of high quality. In this chapter, we focus on how to critique a study that includes an economic evaluation and how to decide whether the results of the study can be applied in our practice setting. We begin by outlining some of the challenges of economic analysis, and we then use our three-step approach to using an article from the health care literature to guide patient care: Are the results valid? What are the results? How can I apply results to patient care?

Clinicians searching for the best economic evidence on a topic should begin by looking at the highest-level resource available. In Chapter 2, Finding the Evidence, we outline a hierarchy that progresses from the most to the least evolved preprocessed evidence-based information sources. The hierarchy begins with *systems* as the highest-level resource, followed by *synopses of syntheses* (systematic reviews), *syntheses*, *synopses of single studies*, and finally *studies* (see Chapter 2, Finding the Evidence, for details about this hierarchy).

In addition to the preprocessed resources outlined in Chapter 2, there is a synopsis-level resource that specifically summarizes economic evaluations. The United Kingdom National Health Service Economic Evaluation Database is available at no cost on the Internet *(www.york.ac.uk/inst/crd/nhsdhp.htm)*, and it summarizes the key methodological details and results of reviews and studies that include an economic evaluation.

For the purposes of illustrating how to critique a single study that includes an economic evaluation, we have selected a randomized controlled trial (RCT) of a multidisciplinary intervention to prevent readmission of elderly patients with congestive heart failure (HF). Although a systematic review (synthesis) summarizing cost-related data from eight RCTs on this topic does exist,[2] (and we would usually examine such a review as a first step), we will focus on a single study from the review.[3] The study is an RCT of the effect of a nurse-directed, multidisciplinary intervention on readmission rates, quality of life, and costs of care for high-risk patients 70 years of age or older who were hospitalized with congestive HF. Toward the end of the chapter, we return to the systematic review to examine the consistency of findings between the single study and the review.

COST: JUST ANOTHER OUTCOME?

In the course of their work, clinicians make many decisions about the care of individual patients. They may also participate in decisions for large groups of patients and may set clinical policy for an institution (e.g., Should our medical center implement a disease management strategy for HF patients discharged from hospital?) or at a more macrocosmic level (e.g., What model of care should our national or local health authority support for the management of patients with HF?). When making decisions for such patient groups, clinicians need not only weigh the benefits and risks, but they must also consider whether these benefits will be worth the health care resources consumed. Resources available to provide health care are not limitless. Thus, increasingly, clinicians have to convince colleagues and health policy makers that the benefits of interventions justify the costs.

To inform these resource allocation decisions, clinicians can use economic evaluations of clinical practices. Economic analyses, widely applied in the health care field, inform decisions at different levels, including managing major institutions such as hospitals and determining regional or national policy.[4,5] *Economic evaluation* is a set of formal, quantitative methods used to compare two or more treatments, programs, or strategies with respect to their resource use and their expected outcomes.[6,7] A comparison of two or more strategies that addresses just costs informs only the resource-use half of the decision and is termed a *cost analysis*. A comparison that addresses just their consequences (e.g., patient-important outcomes) informs only the outcomes half of the decision. A full economic comparison requires that both the costs and consequences be analyzed for each of the strategies being compared.

In one sense, like physiologic function, quality of life, morbid events (e.g., stroke and myocardial infarction), and death, cost is simply another outcome for clinicians to consider when assessing the effects of health care interventions. There are two fundamental strategies for discovering the impact of alternative management strategies on resource consumption. One is to conduct a single high-quality study, ideally an RCT, comparing two or more interventions. Such an approach asks "What does happen?" (on average, and limited by the precision of the estimate) when clinicians choose management strategy A versus strategy B. An example of this is a study that compared a specialist nurse intervention with usual care by general practitioners for patients discharged from hospital with HF.[8] At 1 year, patients in the intervention group had fewer readmissions for any reason, fewer readmissions for HF, and spent fewer days in hospital for HF than patients in the usual care group.[8]

The second approach is to construct a *decision tree* based on events that flow from a clinical decision, by using all available evidence to estimate the probabilities of all possible outcomes, including the costs generated. This second approach asks "What might happen?" if clinicians choose management strategy A versus strategy B.[9,10] The modeling approach using *decision analysis* allows investigators to deal with other problems, such as inadequate length of follow-up, by using available data to estimate what will happen over the long term. Decision analysis can also examine various cost assumptions and ways of organizing care and can calculate the sensitivity of the results to alternative assumptions.

A decision analytic model of alternative approaches to HF management was published by Stewart and colleagues[11] to examine what could happen if a national service based on three different models of specialist nurse management was established in the United Kingdom. The three models of care were home-based, clinic-based, or a combination of home-based plus clinic-based follow-up after discharge. The models incorporated estimates of the overall number of patients fulfilling the criteria as potential recipients of postdischarge management of HF, various assumptions about hospital activity related to HF, health care use after discharge, and health care costs from previous analyses done on the economic burden of HF in the United Kingdom. It was estimated that the relative thresholds at which cost savings generated from implementing these programs would equal the cost of applying these programs would be a 38% to 40% reduction in recurrent bed use resulting from reduced readmissions. Although there are fundamental similarities between cost and other outcomes, there are also important differences, which we now describe.

Costs Are More Variable Than Other Outcomes

Whether clinicians administer drug A or drug B to a particular patient with myocardial infarction in Toronto, Chicago, or Bangkok, the relative impact on mortality is likely to be the same. Indeed, treatment effects on conventional outcomes of quality of life, morbidity, and mortality are often similar not only across geographic locations, but also across patient groups and ways of administering the intervention (see Chapter 16, When to Believe a Subgroup Analysis).

In contrast to clinical end points, costs vary widely across jurisdictions, not only in absolute terms but also in the relative costs of different components of care, including nurses and physicians, other health care workers, drugs, services, and technologic devices. This geographic variation in costs can even lead to differing conclusions about the cost-effectiveness of an intervention. For example, outpatient treatment of deep venous thrombosis with low-molecular-weight heparin (LMWH) compared with inpatient treatment with unfractionated heparin is more cost-effective in the United States than in Canada, even though LMWH is more than double the price in the United States. The reason is that the price of reduced hospital days relative to the price of LMWH is much greater in the United States than in Canada.[12]

Costs also depend on how care is organized, and organization of care varies widely across jurisdictions. The same service may be delivered by a nurse practitioner or a physician, in an outpatient setting or in hospital, and with or without administrative costs related to adjudication of patient eligibility to receive the service. If care is delivered by a physician, in hospital, with maximal administrative costs—as the example of inpatient treatment of deep venous thrombosis in the United States suggests—the expense will be greater than if the service is delivered by a nurse practitioner, on an outpatient basis, or in an institution with lower administrative costs. When the intervention is a way of organizing health services, such as a nursing intervention for patients with HF, the argument may apply on the effect side as well as the cost side. In other words, not only may the cost of the nursing versus control intervention differ across jurisdictions according to health care organization, but the effects of the intervention on hospital readmission may also differ.

The substantial dependence of resource consumption on local costs and local organization of health care delivery means that most cost data are specific to a particular jurisdiction and have limited transferability. An additional problem with RCTs is that their conduct may alter practice patterns in a way that further limits generalizability to other settings, or even to their own setting, outside of the RCT context. For example, in an *economic evaluation* of misoprostol, a drug for prophylaxis against gastric ulcer in patients receiving high doses of nonsteroidal antiinflammatory drugs over long periods, Hillman and Bloom[13] used clinical data from a trial by Graham and colleagues.[14] This blinded RCT of 3 months' duration compared misoprostol (400 and 800 mg daily) with placebo. An important issue for economic analysis was that prevention of ulcers by misoprostol could generate savings in health care expenditures that could balance the cost of adding the drug. However, in this study, endoscopy was performed monthly. In regular clinical practice, endoscopy would be done only in response to symptoms. An unadjusted economic analysis of the results of this trial would have told clinicians of the cost implications of misoprostol administration when patients undergo routine monthly endoscopy. Such information would be useless, given how much these circumstances differ from regular clinical practice.

The what-could-happen modeling approach of decision analysis allows investigators to deal with such problems. Hillman and Bloom,[13] for instance, adjusted observed ulcer rates to reflect the finding that 40% of endoscopically determined lesions did not produce any symptoms. Noting that compliance of patients in the trial was greater than one would expect in clinical practice, these investigators also adjusted for lower compliance by using ulcer rates from the evaluable cohort and by assuming that only 60% of this efficacy would be achieved in practice.

The modeling approaches of decision analysis allow investigators to deal with other problems, such as inadequate length of follow-up, by using available data to estimate what will happen over the long term. Decision analysts can also examine various cost assumptions and ways of organizing care, and they can calculate the sensitivity of their results to these alternate assumptions.

The key limitation of the decision analytic approach is that if its assumptions are flawed, it will not provide an accurate picture. For instance, Schulman and colleagues[15] concluded that early use of zidovudine in asymptomatic persons with human immunodeficiency virus infection was cost-effective, based on projections of disease progression from a clinical trial with 1-year follow-up. However, a subsequent study with 3-year follow-up showed that the advantages of therapy in the first year decreased in subsequent years.[16] The ideal, then, may be a combination of the two approaches, in which the analysis is based on data from RCTs, with adjunctive analytic decision-based modeling to adapt the results to the real-life situations in which they will be applied.[17] However, even a combination approach must use average patient values, and these averages may be very different from values or preferences of individual patients (see Chapter 34, Incorporating Patient Values). These different values may affect the optimal management strategy. The extent to which the authors make their assumptions transparent will add to the credibility of any economic analysis.

The Role of Costs in Clinical Decision Making Remains Controversial

Although few would deny the importance of cost considerations in setting health care policy, the relevance of costs in making decisions about individual patients remains controversial. Some would argue, by taking an extreme of what can be called a *deontologic* approach to distributive justice, that a clinician's only responsibility should be to best meet the needs of the individual in his or her care. An alternate philosophical view, *consequentialist or utilitarian,* would contend that even when making decisions about individuals, clinicians should take a broader social view, which considers the effect on others of allocating resources to a particular patient's care.

As health care technologies proliferate, their potential benefits and their costs increase, but their marginal benefits over less resource-intensive approaches are often small. In such cases, the arguments for bedside rationing become more compelling because neglect of resource issues in one patient may affect resource availability for other patients.[18] On this basis, some have criticized evidence-based practice for not considering resource use and efficiency.[19,20]

Using Cost Information to Inform Decisions Poses Special Challenges

Typically, effective treatments help patients feel better, or they reduce the risk of major morbid or mortal events in the future. Moving from evidence to action involves trading off these benefits against common immediate side effects, long-term toxicity, and the inconvenience of complying with a treatment regimen. Individual patient values, ideally, will inform this trade-off (see Chapter 34, Incorporating Patient Values).

In health care policy decisions, we use cost information to allocate scarce resources efficiently. Let us assume that two treatments both cost, in comparison with conventional treatment and after consideration of all their consequences, $1,000,000 for each 100 patients treated for 1 year. For treatment A, the benefit achieved by this expenditure is the prevention of an average of two severe migraine headaches per patient, or 200 migraine headaches. For treatment B, the benefit is avoiding a single myocardial infarction. If, in a resource-constrained environment, one had to choose between A and B, which would be the better choice?

Choosing between competing beneficial treatments presents daunting logistic, ethical, and political challenges. The example demonstrates how, in economic analysis, we must trade off costs against benefits and deal with very different outcomes in very different people (in this case, migraine headaches in one patient group and myocardial infarction in another) in deciding how to allocate resources.

Economic analysis addresses the relative value of different outcomes and the trade-off of dollar values against health. Typically, health economists turn to one of three strategies. One is to report patient-important outcomes in physical or natural units, such as "life-years gained" or "migraine headaches prevented" or "myocardial infarctions prevented" (*cost-effectiveness analysis*). In a second approach, different types of outcomes are weighted to produce a composite index of outcome, such as the quality-adjusted life-year (QALY), or healthy years equivalent[21] (*cost-utility analysis,* sometimes classified as a subcategory of cost-effectiveness analysis). Quality adjustment involves placing a lower value on time spent with impaired physical and emotional function than time spent in full health. On a scale where 0 represents death and 1.0 represents full health, the greater the impairment is, the lower the value of a particular health state will be (see Chapter 12, Quality of Life). Finally, investigators may put a dollar value on years of life gained, migraine headaches prevented, or myocardial infarctions prevented. In these *cost-benefit analyses*, health care consumers consider what they would be willing to pay for programs or products that achieve particular outcomes, such as prolonging life or preventing adverse events.

Rich and colleagues[3] evaluated a nurse-directed, multidisciplinary intervention consisting of comprehensive education of patients and families, a prescribed diet, social service consultation and early discharge planning, medication review, and intensive follow-up. The investigators compared 142 patients who received the intervention with 140 patients who received conventional care comprising all standard treatments and services ordered by their primary physicians. The investigators chose survival for 90 days without readmission as the primary outcome measure, so the economic analysis was a cost-effectiveness analysis as previously defined. A secondary analysis was restricted to survivors of initial hospitalization.

The results showed a trend (not statistically significant) toward longer survival without readmission as well as lower costs for care in the group receiving the multidisciplinary, nurse-directed intervention. A finding of cost savings is not common for health care interventions, in which the incremental benefits of a new intervention often are achieved at additional cost. The authors also examined quality of life at baseline and 3 months using the Chronic Heart Failure Questionnaire[22] for a subset of patients and found greater improvement in quality of life in the intervention group.

Having outlined some of the challenges of economic analysis, we offer our usual structure for guides to the health care literature: Are the results valid? What are the results? How can I apply the results to patient care? (Table 18-1).

ARE THE RESULTS VALID?

Did Investigators Adopt a Sufficiently Broad Viewpoint?

Investigators can evaluate costs and consequences from the viewpoint of the patient, the hospital, the third-party payer (or national or local government in some countries), or society at large. Each viewpoint may be relevant depending on the question being asked, but broader viewpoints are most relevant to those allocating health care resources. For example, an evaluation adopting the viewpoint of the hospital is useful in estimating

Table **18-1**   Users' Guides for an Article About Economic Evaluation

Are the Results Valid?
- Did investigators adopt a sufficiently broad viewpoint?
- Were results reported separately for patients with different baseline risks?
- Were costs measured accurately?
- Did investigators consider the timing of costs and consequences?

What Are the Results?
- What were the incremental costs and effects of each strategy?
- Did incremental costs and effects differ between subgroups?
- How much did allowance for uncertainty change the results?

How Can I Apply the Results to Patient Care?
- Are the treatment benefits worth the risks and costs?
- Can I expect similar costs in my setting?

the budgetary impact of alternative therapies for that institution. However, *economic evaluation* is usually directed at informing policy from a broader societal perspective.[23,24]

For example, in an evaluation of an early-discharge program, reporting only hospital costs is not sufficient because patients discharged early may consume substantial community resources. These costs may not be borne by the hospital, but they are likely to have an impact on the third-party payer or the patient in some way or another. This was a limitation of a study by Topol and colleagues,[25] which assessed the feasibility and cost savings of hospital discharge 3 days after acute myocardial infarction and considered only hospital and professional charges. We have no knowledge of other community services consumed and whether these differed between early-discharge and conventional-discharge patients.

One of the main reasons for considering narrower viewpoints in an economic analysis is to assess the impact of change on the main budget holders because budgets may need to be adjusted before a new intervention can be adopted. This is often referred to as the *silo effect*. Weisbrod and colleagues[26] pointed out that, although a community-oriented mental illness program was worthwhile from the perspective of society as a whole, it would be more costly to the organization responsible for providing the care. Even within the same institution, narrow budgetary viewpoints can prevail. For example, if we compared two pharmacologic interventions for pain reduction, it would be wrong to focus exclusively on the relative costs of the drugs, which fall on the pharmacy budget, if there were also effects on other hospital resource use. In the example of deep venous thrombosis we used earlier,[12] use of outpatient LMWH would decrease costs related to hospital stays, but would increase costs accrued to the drug budget.

The patient's perspective may also merit specific consideration if costs (e.g., travel-related expenses) reduce access to care. In addition, some patients may not be able to participate in community care programs if these impose major costs for informal nursing support in the home. However, in general, the analysis integrates the patient's perspective by measuring the consequences of treatment, such as impact on quality of life.

From a societal viewpoint, determination of costs should include the impact of the intervention on patients' ability to work and hence to contribute to the nation's productivity. The issue of inclusion or exclusion of productivity changes remains a frequent topic of debate. Productivity costs represent resource-use changes similar to those occurring in the health care system. Conversely, production may not actually be lost if a worker is absent for a short period. For longer periods of absence, employers may hire a previously unemployed worker. Furthermore, depending on how productivity is measured (e.g., expected wages), inclusion of productivity changes biases evaluations in favor of programs for persons who are in full-time employment. Therefore, clinicians should be skeptical of any report of an economic analysis that does not fully discuss the reasons for inclusion or exclusion of productivity costs.

Table 18-2 presents a summary of how the study by Rich and colleagues[3] deals with these and other key methodological issues. The first major point to note about this study is that all data for outcomes and costs come from a single clinical trial rather than from multiple sources to construct a decision model. One disadvantage of this approach is that the time horizon was limited to 90 days after discharge.

Table 18-2 Key Methodological Features of the Study by Rich and Colleagues

Overall study design	Randomized controlled trial
Viewpoint for analysis	Hospital and caregiver
Alternatives compared	Nurse-directed, multidisciplinary intervention consisting of comprehensive education of patients and families, a prescribed diet, social service consultation and early discharge planning, medication review, and intensive follow-up compared with conventional care consisting of all standard treatments and services ordered by primary physicians
Benefit measures	Survival for 90 days without readmission, number of readmissions, quality of life
Time horizon	90 days after discharge from hospital
Source of effectiveness data	Randomized controlled trial (n = 282 patients)
Source of quality-of-life data	Baseline and 3-month scores on the Chronic Heart Failure Questionnaire[22] on a subset of patients (n = 126)
Estimates of resource use	Detailed data on all patients followed up for 90 days after discharge including baseline and all pertinent information pertaining to the hospital course
Sources of cost data	Cost logs for all medical and caregiver costs for 57 patients during the final year of the study; standard diagnosis-related group reimbursement costs for hospital admissions
Discounting	Not applied
Sensitivity analysis	None

Data from Rich MW, Beckham V, Wittenberg C, Leven CL, Freedland KE, Carney RM. A multidisciplinary intervention to prevent the readmission of elderly patients with congestive heart failure. N Engl J Med. 1995;333:1190–1195.

Rich and colleagues[3] recognized the importance of identifying and quantifying costs beyond direct medical care costs and included the cost of time spent by unpaid caregivers (e.g., spouses, family, friends) in the analysis. In fact, the costs for caregivers (valued at an hourly rate of US$6) constituted 15% to 25% of the total costs of care in both the control and intervention groups. However, these investigators failed to consider productivity costs of lost time from work that patients would have incurred as a result of HF.

Were Results Reported Separately for Patients With Different Baseline Risks?

The costs and consequences of treatment are likely to be related to the baseline risk of the condition in the population. For example, the cost-effectiveness of drug therapy for elevated cholesterol levels, compared with no treatment, will depend on age, sex, pretreatment cholesterol level, and other risk factors; the greater the patient's risk is, the lower will be the cost per unit of benefit.[27] In general, strategies that target services at populations with a high prevalence of disease are more cost-effective than those applied universally.[28]

Division of patients into risk categories is common in clinical practice. In a study of the cost-effectiveness of beta-blockers after acute myocardial infarction, Goldman and colleagues[29] found that the cost per life-year gained was US$2400 for patients at high risk compared with US$13,000 for those at low risk. The differences in the cost-effectiveness ratios were driven primarily by the extent to which patients could benefit from treatment, rather than by treatment cost (i.e., patients who are likely to do well without treatment will have a limited capacity to benefit).

The patients in the study by Rich and colleagues[3] were included only if their risk for early hospital readmission was high; in fact, these high-risk patients represented only 21.6% of hospitalized patients with congestive HF. The control group had almost double the overall readmission rate of the treatment group (control group = 67% and treatment group = 37%). Although Rich and colleagues[3] could not report costs for other risk groups, it is likely that costs and cost-effectiveness estimates would differ for a low-risk group because these patients are less likely to benefit from the intervention.

Were Costs Measured Accurately?

Although the viewpoint determines the relevant range of costs and consequences to be included in an *economic evaluation*, many issues relate to their measurement and evaluation. First, clinicians should look for the physical quantities of resources consumed or released by interventions separately from their prices or unit costs. Not only does this allow clinicians to scrutinize the method of assigning monetary values to resources, it also helps to extrapolate the study results to different settings that will have variable prices.

Second, there are different approaches to valuing costs or cost savings. One approach is to use published charges. However, charges may differ from real costs, depending on the sophistication of accounting systems and the relative bargaining power of health care institutions and third-party payers.[30] Where there is a systematic deviation between costs and charges, analysts may adjust the latter by a *cost-to-charge ratio*. However, because the relationship between charges and costs can vary markedly by institution, simple adjustments may not suffice. From a third-party payer perspective, charges will bear some relation to the amounts actually paid, although in some settings, payments vary by payer. From a societal perspective, we would like to know the real costs because these reflect what society is forgoing in benefits elsewhere to provide a given treatment.

For example, Cohen and colleagues[31] compared costs and charges for conventional angioplasty, directional atherectomy, stenting, and bypass surgery. Previous studies had suggested that total hospital charges for directional coronary atherectomy or intracoronary stenting were significantly higher than those for conventional angioplasty. However, when examining costs by adjusting itemized patient accounts by department-specific cost-to-charge ratios, the investigators found that the in-hospital costs of angioplasty and directional coronary atherectomy were similar. In addition, although the cost of coronary stenting was approximately US$2500 higher than that of conventional angioplasty, the magnitude of this difference was smaller than the US$6300 increment previously suggested by the analysis of hospital charges. Thus, the apparent cost difference based on the charges provided for each procedure may have been an artifact of hospital accounting systems, rather than a reflection of the real value to society of the resources consumed by those procedures, as represented by the cost.

Rich and colleagues[3] prospectively collected detailed costs for a subset of 57 patients enrolled in the study using cost logs. Study personnel also maintained logs to determine the cost of the intervention. Although collection of costs for all patients in a study is preferred, an accurate estimate for a subset of patients is preferable to a poor estimate for all patients. In the RCT by Rich and colleagues,[3] study nurses checked cost logs regularly for accuracy. As is common, but not ideal, the investigators estimated costs for hospital admissions by Medicare diagnosis-related group reimbursement rates. Sometimes the protocol requirements for RCTs generate additional costs of care beyond what would be incurred in routine practice. Rich and colleagues[3] were careful to exclude costs for research and monitoring, such as screening, randomization, data collection, and follow-up. The investigators used standard hourly wage rates to calculate costs of professional and unpaid caregivers and adjusted all costs to 1994 dollars.

Did Investigators Consider the Timing of Costs and Consequences?

A final issue in the measurement and valuation of costs and consequences relates to adjustments for differences in their timing. Generally, people prefer to receive benefits sooner and to postpone costs because of uncertainty about the future and because resources, if invested, usually yield a positive return. The accepted way of allowing for this in economic evaluations is to discount both costs and consequences occurring in the future to present values by assigning a lower weight to future costs and benefits. Based on a seminal paper by Weinstein and Stason in 1977,[32] *cost-effectiveness analysis* has usually used a 5% per annum discount rate. More recently, the United States Panel on Cost-Effectiveness in Health and Medicine[23] proposed a 3% discount rate based on the inflation-adjusted rate of return on United States government bonds. There are debates about the appropriate discount rate to use and whether health outcomes should be discounted at the same rate as costs.[33–37]

Rich and colleagues[3] did not use discounting because the time horizon was only 90 days. Discounting is most critical for long-term health care programs, comparisons of health care interventions with differing time profiles, and when the main expenditures occur at a different time from the benefits. For example, in evaluating the prevention of hepatitis B through a universal vaccination program, Krahn and Detsky[38] applied discount rates ranging from 2% to 8%, and the associated cost-effectiveness ratios ranged from cost saving to more than CDN$150,000 per life-year saved.

WHAT ARE THE RESULTS?

What Were the Incremental Costs and Effects of Each Strategy?

Let us start with the incremental costs. Look in the text and tables of the study report for listings of all the costs considered for each treatment option, and remember that costs are the product of the quantity of a resource used and its unit price. These should include the costs incurred to produce the treatment, such as physician's time, nurse's time, materials, and so forth, which we will refer to as *up-front costs,* as well as the *downstream costs* incurred by resources that will be consumed in the future in relation to clinical events attributable to the intervention.

For instance, in the article by Rich and colleagues,[3] the methods section includes information about the costs used in the cost analysis, and Table 5 provides a summary of the costs of care per patient broken down by component of care. Quantifying the resource use considered and providing a separate table on the unit price for specific resources would have improved their presentation. In Table 18-3, we see that the average cost of the study intervention was US$216 per patient. As anticipated, caregivers spent 33 more minutes per patient per day attending to patients in the intervention group than to those in the control group, for an estimated incremental cost of US$336 per patient. The main cost difference between the two groups at 90 days was the cost of readmissions (US$2178 for the intervention group and US$3236 for the control group; $P = 0.03$). Total costs per patient were US$4815 in the intervention group and US$5275 in the control group. The overall cost of care was higher in the control group by US$460 per patient over 90 days, an average of US$153 per patient per month.

The primary measure of effectiveness in the study by Rich and colleagues[3] was survival for 90 days without readmission. Survival for 90 days without readmission did not differ for the intervention and control groups (64.1% vs. 53.6%; absolute difference, 10.5%; 95% confidence interval, −0.9% to +21.9%; $P = 0.09$). When the analysis was

Table **18-3**   Costs, Effects, and Cost-Effectiveness Summary for Nurse-Directed Multidisciplinary Intervention Versus Conventional Care at 90 days

	Intervention Group	Control Group	Difference
Costs (US$ per patient)			
Intervention	$216	Not applicable	+$216
Caregivers	$1164	$828	+$336
Other medical care	$1257	$1211	+$46
Readmission	$2178	$3236	−$1058
Total costs	$4815	$5275	−$460
Survival without readmission	64.1%	53.6%	+19.6%*
Incremental cost-effectiveness of intervention	—	—	Cost saving

*Percent difference calculated by dividing the absolute percent difference between groups by the control group percentage.
Data from Rich MW, Beckham V, Wittenberg C, Leven CL, Freedland KE, Carney RM. A multidisciplinary intervention to prevent the readmission of elderly patients with congestive heart failure. N Engl J Med. 1995;333:1190–1195.

restricted to survivors of the initial hospitalization, survival for 90 days without readmission was significantly higher in the intervention group than in the control group (66.9% vs. 54.3%; absolute difference, 12.6%; 95% confidence interval, 1.1% to 24.1%; $P = 0.04$).

In an economic analysis, measuring effectiveness as a gain in life expectancy is optimal to allow comparison across different types of health care interventions and programs. If investigators measure outcomes in terms of years of life and collect data on preferences for survivors, they can combine these measures into a single metric.[39] One of the most popular approaches is the construction of QALYs, but health economists also use the healthy-years equivalents method.[40] Another measure, disability-adjusted life-years (DALYs), was used by the World Bank to compare outcomes of different interventions in the Global Burden of Disease Study and is particularly relevant to low-income countries.[41]

To derive QALYs, investigators assign utility weights (from death = 0 to healthy = 1) to patients who survive hospitalization with HF but sustain morbid events over time. These utility weights may be taken from the literature or collected in the trial directly by using specially designed methods such as the standard gamble[24] or indirectly by using surveys such as the Health Utilities Index[42] (see Chapter 12, Quality of Life). The study by Rich and colleagues[3] did not translate survival estimates into life expectancy gains or quality-adjusted life expectancy gains.

In summary, as shown in Table 18-3, Rich and colleagues[3] calculated both the incremental gain in survival without readmission for the intervention group (absolute difference, 10.5%; percentage difference, 19.6%) and the incremental cost per patient (absolute difference, −$460) over the 90-day time horizon of the study. In this instance, additional benefit was gained with the lower cost nursing intervention compared with conventional care, a situation referred to as cost saving. More typically, new interventions increase benefits at a higher cost compared with existing treatments, which generates an *incremental cost-effectiveness ratio* that can be interpreted as the price at which additional units of benefit can be obtained.

Did Incremental Costs and Effects Differ Between Subgroups?

The cost-effectiveness of the nurse-directed multidisciplinary intervention examined by Rich and colleagues[3] may depend on the patient group to whom it is applied. Some patients (e.g., those with prior history of HF) have a greater risk of mortality and hospital readmission, and thus the intervention will likely yield higher absolute risk reductions in these outcomes. Rich and colleagues[3] specifically included only patients with at least one risk factor for early readmission (e.g., prior history of HF, four or more hospitalizations for any reason in the preceding 5 years, or HF precipitated by either an acute myocardial infarction or uncontrolled hypertension).

How Much Did Allowance for Uncertainty Change the Results?

Uncertainty in *economic evaluation* can arise from lack of precision in estimation or from methodological controversy. The conventional way of allowing for uncertainty in economic analyses is to conduct a *sensitivity analysis*, in which the estimates for key variables are altered to assess their effect on the results.

Conducting economic evaluations concurrently with clinical trials provides an opportunity to apply conventional tests of statistical significance to resource quantities or costs.[43] When measurements from a clinical trial inform us of the distribution of cost variables, it is possible to set the range of estimates for sensitivity analysis based on the statistical properties of the distribution (e.g., two standard deviations from the mean). This raises certain important issues, such as the size of the economically important difference when comparing the cost or cost-effectiveness of two alternative interventions and the appropriateness of and methods for statistical tests applied to cost-effectiveness ratios.

Because economic evaluation methods are in their infancy compared with those for RCTs, investigators still debate many issues.[44] These include the appropriateness of alternative methods for valuing outcomes, the appropriateness of considering some types of consequences (e.g., the costs of lost production if persons are away from work because of illness), and the choice of discount rate.

A useful starting point for a sensitivity analysis is to examine the impact of variation in the effectiveness measure on the estimated cost-effectiveness. Investigators may assume the smallest plausible estimate of a treatment effect using, for instance, the lower boundary of a confidence interval generated in a meta-analysis of available RCTs (see Chapter 29, Confidence Intervals). They would then examine the impact of assuming this appreciably and plausibly smaller treatment effect on cost-effectiveness.

This analytical approach, however, only partially captures the uncertainty in the cost-effectiveness ratio because it assumes that the numerator (e.g., the cost) does not vary. Investigators are currently developing more formal procedures for estimating confidence intervals for cost-effectiveness ratios that permit both the numerator and the denominator to vary.[45,46]

The study by Rich and colleagues[3] did not include a sensitivity analysis. A sensitivity analysis would have demonstrated the degree of uncertainty around the point estimates for both costs and benefits. For example, although the point estimate of the absolute difference in the effect of the intervention was a 10.5% reduction in survival without hospital readmission, the 95% confidence interval ranged from −0.9% to +21.9%. If the intervention actually increased readmissions (as it would if the value of −0.9% represented the truth), the intervention would be harmful instead of beneficial and would increase costs appreciably.

HOW CAN I APPLY THE RESULTS TO PATIENT CARE?

Having established the results of the economic study, we now turn to two important issues of interpretation. The first is how to interpret incremental cost-effectiveness ratios to help in decision making; the second is the extent to which the data about costs and/or effects from the study can be applied to your practice setting.

Are the Treatment Benefits Worth the Risks and Costs?

In Figure 18-1, we present a framework for categorizing the results of economic studies. This 3 × 3 matrix categorizes studies into nine cells according to whether the new treatment is more costly than, less costly than, or of equivalent cost to the control and whether it is more effective, less effective, or equally effective.

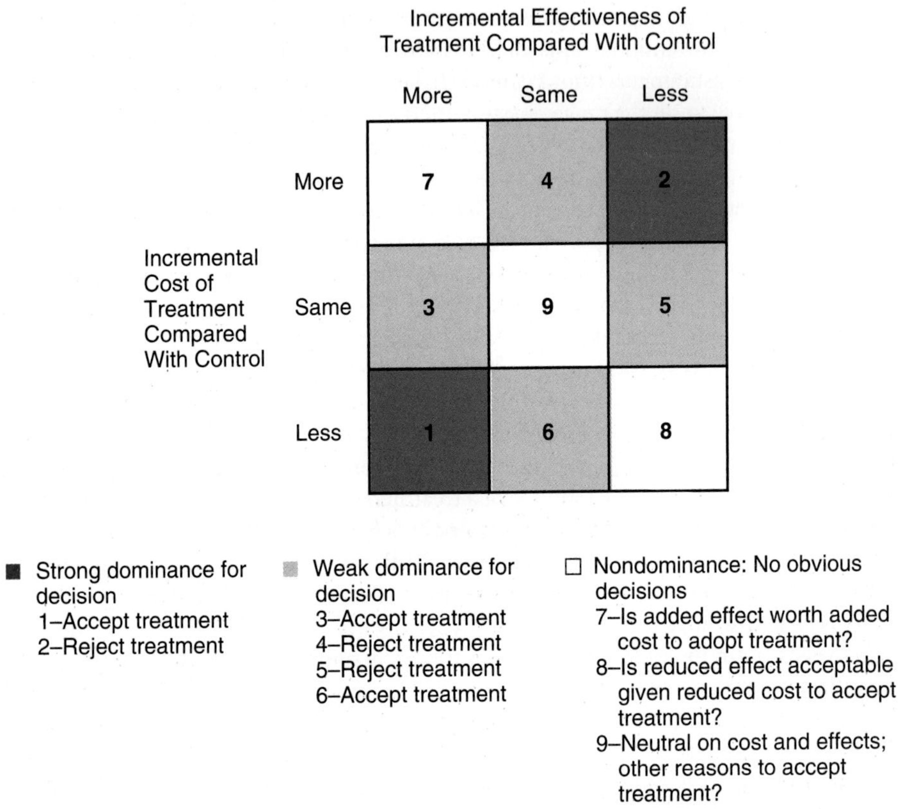

Incremental Effectiveness of
Treatment Compared With Control

		More	Same	Less
Incremental Cost of Treatment Compared With Control	More	7	4	2
	Same	3	9	5
	Less	1	6	8

■ Strong dominance for decision
1–Accept treatment
2–Reject treatment

▨ Weak dominance for decision
3–Accept treatment
4–Reject treatment
5–Reject treatment
6–Accept treatment

□ Nondominance: No obvious decisions
7–Is added effect worth added cost to adopt treatment?
8–Is reduced effect acceptable given reduced cost to accept treatment?
9–Neutral on cost and effects; other reasons to accept treatment?

Figure 18-1. Categorizing economic study results: Nine possible outcomes arising in the comparison of treatment and control groups in terms of incremental cost and incremental effectiveness.

In category 1, the new treatment is both less costly and more effective than the control, and so the new treatment is said to be strongly dominant. The study by Rich and colleagues[3] falls into this category because the nurse-directed multidisciplinary intervention was less costly and resulted in fewer deaths and hospital readmissions over a 90-day period. Category 2 represents strong dominance to reject a new treatment that has higher costs and lower effectiveness than the control. Four cases of so-called weak dominance follow, in which the two treatments have either equivalent cost or equivalent effectiveness: category 3 indicates weak dominance to accept the treatment (equivalent cost but better effectiveness); category 4 indicates weak dominance to reject the treatment (greater cost with equivalent effectiveness); and categories 5 and 6 indicate weak dominance to reject and accept, respectively.

All shaded cells in Figure 18-1 indicate comparative cost and effectiveness combinations that provide evidence of strong or weak dominance. No further analysis, such as calculation of cost-effectiveness ratios, is required for these shaded cells to inform decision making. However, further analysis is needed if results fall into the nondominance, unshaded cells of 7, 8, or 9. First, it may be that the treatment is associated with no statistically significant or clinically important difference in either effectiveness or cost, although the process of implementation and change of programs will generate costs not captured in the analysis.

The most common nondominance circumstance is category 7 (or its mirror image in category 8), in which the new intervention offers additional effectiveness but at increased cost. This situation describes the results of a study of beta-blocker therapy for HF in Canada,[47] which requires calculation of the incremental cost-effectiveness ratio of the new treatment. The study estimated the incremental cost-effectiveness ratio of carvedilol relative to metoprolol as CDN$8394 per life-year gained.

Having estimated the incremental cost-effectiveness of carvedilol relative to metoprolol, and assuming for the moment that these data apply to your practice setting, how do you decide whether approximately CDN$8000 is an acceptable price to pay for saving 1 additional year of life? The first important point is that this question involves a value judgment and cannot be resolved using only the study data. The study data can inform the decision, but do not indicate a clear choice. Some external criteria must be used to ascertain whether a jurisdiction or society is willing to pay this price for this improvement in outcome.

Numerous approaches can be used to interpret incremental cost-effectiveness ratios. In an ideal world of complete information, we would have data on the health (or other) outcomes we would be forgoing from other interventions and programs (within and outside of health care) that are not funded as a consequence of using carvedilol (the *opportunity cost* of carvedilol administration). Because data to accomplish this task are very limited, investigators have promulgated a variety of second-best interpretive strategies. One approach assumes that previous decisions to adopt new health care interventions of known cost-effectiveness reveal an underlying set of values with which to judge the acceptability of a new treatment.

A commonly cited acceptable cost-effectiveness threshold is $50,000 per life-year or QALY gained, but investigators have debated the validity of such interpretive strategies for incremental cost-effectiveness ratios at both theoretical[48,49] and practical[50] levels. For example, although Johannesson and Weinstein[48] maintained that prioritizing resource allocations based on rank orderings of interventions by incremental cost-effectiveness leads to an efficient allocation of resources, not all health economists agree. Most would agree that there are practical problems of comparisons among cost-effectiveness studies that may have used different methods, data, and assumptions.[43]

In summary, we should exercise caution when drawing conclusions from incremental cost-effectiveness ratios. The ultimate criterion is one of local opportunity cost: If the money for a new program will result in decreased ability to deliver other health care interventions, what are the health benefits you will no longer realize if the new health program is made available for all? The practical difficulty in applying this criterion is that many existing programs or services may not have been evaluated. Therefore, the opportunity cost of reducing or removing them is unknown or speculative.

Can I Expect Similar Costs in My Setting?

If costs or consequences differ in your setting, the cost-effectiveness, utility, and benefit ratios from a study will not apply. We deal with issues of whether you can anticipate the same consequences of treatment in your own setting in Chapter 33, Applying Results to Individual Patients, and focus here on costs. We note that in the trial by Rich and colleagues,[3] the economic data were collected for a subset of patients who had been discharged from one hospital medical center in St. Louis, Missouri, and inclusion criteria restricted study participation to patients at high risk for early readmission. The investigators excluded patients if they lived outside the hospital home care catchment area, planned discharge to a long-term care facility, had severe dementia or other serious psychiatric illness, or were anticipated to survive less than 3 months. Given the single hospital setting, the small sample on which economic data were collected, and the narrow inclusion and exclusion criteria, the study results are likely applicable only to a subset of patients hospitalized with HF.

In considering the transferability of cost estimates among jurisdictions (e.g., countries, states, regions, or even cities or institutions), remember that the cost of an intervention is the summation of the product of physical resources consumed (e.g., drugs and tests) and their unit prices. We noted earlier that cost data may not transfer well among jurisdictions because of differences in local prices and the organization of practice. A good *economic evaluation* should report prices and resource use separately so that readers can ascertain whether prices and practice patterns apply to their own jurisdictions.

The economic analysis by Rich and colleagues[3] provided the total number of hospital days for the treatment and control groups (556 vs. 865, respectively), and the total costs of hospital readmissions (US$2178 vs. US$3236 per patient over 3 months, respectively), although the per diem cost of hospital readmissions was not explicitly stated. A study conducted in Australia by Stewart and colleagues[51] reported total hospital-based costs of A$900 (US$583) per patient per month for the intervention and A$2200 (US$1424) for conventional care. Although both studies concluded that hospitalizations were reduced with the intervention, the additional cost of hospital care associated with conventional care was about US$350 per month in the study by Rich and colleagues[3] and US$840 per month in the study by Stewart and colleagues.[51] These results are clearly dependent on the relative per diem prices of hospitalization and the length of hospital stay.

Finally, countries (or social, cultural, or political groups within countries) may differ with respect to the value they place on health benefits versus other commodities. There is no reason why $50,000 per life-year, an acceptable cost-effectiveness threshold in the United States, should be applicable to, say, a less-industrialized country, where the *opportunity cost* of such resources will be much higher. The governments of various countries vary in their willingness to pay for health and health care.

In this chapter, we focused on a single RCT to illustrate the important concepts of economic evaluation. The results of the study by Rich and colleagues[3] are supported by other RCTs. In their systematic review of RCTs of multidisciplinary disease management programs in HF, McAlister and colleagues[2] searched multiple electronic databases, hand searched bibliographies of identified studies, and contacted content experts to identify additional studies. An independent review of the studies and independent data extraction by two of the investigators yielded a total of 11 RCTs eligible for inclusion. The authors examined mortality and hospitalization rates as the end points of interest. None of the six trials that assessed mortality found a significant difference between the intervention and control groups within the prespecified study period (risk ratio, 0.94; 95% confidence interval, 0.75 to 1.19). However, in the 11 trials that reported hospitalization rates, hospitalizations were reduced by the interventions (risk ratio, 0.87; 95% confidence interval, 0.79 to 0.96). Although the summary risk ratio for hospitalization suggests a beneficial effect of the disease management programs, there was significant heterogeneity in the results, mostly attributable to one study. Subgroup analysis found that the mechanism of follow-up with the patient was an important factor in the outcome. The two studies that used telephone contact and enhanced communication with primary care providers, rather than the multidisciplinary team visit, did not find any reduction in hospitalization (risk ratio, 1.15; 95% confidence interval, 0.96 to 1.37). The disease management programs for HF were shown to be cost saving in seven of the eight trials that reported cost data. Based on these findings, the results of the systematic review were consistent with those of the single study by Rich and colleagues.[3] However, the heterogeneity in findings among the studies in the systematic review emphasizes the importance of searching for the highest-quality, synthesized evidence before using a single study as an evidence base.

REFERENCES

1. Stone PW, Bakken S, Curran CR, Walker PH. Evaluation of studies of health economics. *Evid Based Nurs.* 2002;5:100-104.
2. McAlister FA, Lawson FME, Teo KK, Armstrong PW. A systematic review of randomized trials of disease management programs in heart failure. *Am J Med.* 2001;110:378-384.
3. Rich MW, Beckham V, Wittenberg C, Leven CL, Freedland KE, Carney RM. A multidisciplinary intervention to prevent the readmission of elderly patients with congestive heart failure. *N Engl J Med.* 1995;333:1190-1195.
4. Elixhauser A, Luce BR, Taylor WR, Reblando J. Health care CBA/CEA: an update on the growth and composition of the literature. *Med Care.* 1993;31:JS1-JS11, JS18-JS149.
5. Backhouse ME, Backhouse RJ, Edey SA. Economic evaluation bibliography. *Health Econ.* 1992;1:1-236.
6. Eisenberg JM. Clinical economics: a guide to the economic analysis of clinical practices. *JAMA.* 1989;262:2879-2886.
7. Detsky AS, Naglie IG. A clinician's guide to cost-effectiveness analysis. *Ann Intern Med.* 1990;113:147-154.
8. Blue L, Lang E, McMurray JJV, et al. Randomised controlled trial of specialist nurse intervention in heart failure. *BMJ.* 2001;323:715-718.
9. Weinstein MC, O'Brien B, Hornberger J, et al. Principles of good practice for decision analytic modeling in health-care evaluation: report of the ISPOR Task Force on Good Research Practices–Modeling Studies. *Value Health.* 2003;6:9-17.
10. Buxton MJ, Drummond MF, van Hout BA, et al. Modelling in economic evaluation: an unavoidable fact of life. *Health Econ.* 1997;6:217-227.
11. Stewart S, Blue L, Walker A, Morrison C, McMurray JJ. An economic analysis of specialist heart failure nurse management in the UK: can we afford not to implement it? *Eur Heart J.* 2002;23:1369-1378.
12. O'Brien B, Levine M, Willan A, et al. Economic evaluation of outpatient treatment with low-molecular-weight heparin for proximal vein thrombosis. *Arch Intern Med.* 1999;159:2298-2304.
13. Hillman AL, Bloom BS. Economic effects of prophylactic use of misoprostol to prevent gastric ulcer in patients taking nonsteroidal anti-inflammatory drugs. *Arch Intern Med.* 1989;149:2061-2065.
14. Graham DY, Agrawal NM, Roth SH. Prevention of NSAID-induced gastric ulcer with misoprostol: multicentre, double-blind, placebo-controlled trial. *Lancet.* 1988;2:1277-1280.

15. Schulman KA, Lynn LA, Glick HA, Eisenberg JM. Cost effectiveness of low-dose zidovudine therapy for asymptomatic patients with human immunodeficiency virus (HIV) infection. *Ann Intern Med.* 1991;114:798-802.

16. Concorde Coordinating Committee. Concorde: MRC/ANRS randomised double-blind controlled trial of immediate and deferred zidovudine in symptom-free HIV infection. *Lancet.* 1994;343:871-881.

17. O'Brien B. Economic evaluation of pharmaceuticals: Frankenstein's monster or vampire of trials? *Med Care.* 1996;34:DS99-DS108.

18. Ubel PA. The unbearable rightness of bedside rationing. In: *Pricing Life: Why It's Time for Health Care Rationing.* Cambridge, MA: MIT Press; 2000:137-151.

19. Williams A. Cochrane Lecture: all cost effective treatments should be free . . . or, how Archie Cochrane changed my life! *J Epidemiol Commun Health.* 1997;51:116-120.

20. Maynard A. Evidence-based medicine: cost effectiveness and equity are ignored. *BMJ.* 1996;313:170.

21. Mehrez A, Gafni A. Quality-adjusted life years, utility theory, and healthy-years equivalents. *Med Decis Making.* 1989;9:142-149.

22. Guyatt GH, Nogradi S, Halcrow S, Singer J, Sullivan MJ, Fallen EL. Development and testing of a new measure of health status for clinical trials in heart failure. *J Gen Intern Med.* 1989;4:101-107.

23. Gold MR, Siegel JE, Russell LB, Weinstein MC (eds). *Cost-Effectiveness in Health and Medicine.* Oxford: Oxford University Press; 1996.

24. Drummond MF, O'Brien BJ, Stoddart GL, Torrance GW. *Methods of the Economic Evaluation of Health Care Programmes.* Oxford, UK: Oxford University Press; 1997.

25. Topol EJ, Burek K, O'Neill WW, et al. A randomized controlled trial of hospital discharge three days after myocardial infarction in the era of reperfusion. *N Engl J Med.* 1988;318:1083-1088.

26. Weisbrod BA, Test MA, Stein LI. Alternative to mental hospital treatment. II. Economic benefit-cost analysis. *Arch Gen Psychiatry.* 1980;37:400-405.

27. Oster G, Epstein AM. Cost-effectiveness of antihyperlipemic therapy in the prevention of coronary heart disease: the case of cholestyramine. *JAMA.* 1987;258:2381-2387.

28. Stone PW, Teutsch S, Chapman RH, Bell C, Goldie SJ, Neumann PJ. Cost-utility analyses of clinical preventive services: published ratios, 1976-1997. *Am J Prev Med.* 2000;19:15-23.

29. Goldman L, Sia ST, Cook EF, Rutherford JD, Weinstein MC. Costs and effectiveness of routine therapy with long-term beta-adrenergic antagonists after acute myocardial infarction. *N Engl J Med.* 1988;319:152-157.

30. Finkler SA. The distinction between cost and charges. *Ann Intern Med.* 1982;96:102-109.

31. Cohen DJ, Breall JA, Ho KK, et al. Economics of elective coronary revascularization: comparison of costs and charges for conventional angioplasty, directional atherectomy, stenting and bypass surgery. *J Am Coll Cardiol.* 1993;22:1052-1059.

32. Weinstein MC, Stason WB. Foundations of cost-effectiveness analysis for health and medical practices. *N Engl J Med.* 1977;296:716-721.

33. Parsonage M, Neuburger H. Discounting and health benefits. *Health Econ.* 1992;1:71-76.

34. Cairns J. Discounting and health benefits: another perspective. *Health Econ.* 1992;1:76-79.

35. Krahn M, Gafni A. Discounting in the economic evaluation of health care interventions. *Med Care.* 1993;31:403-418.

36. van Hout BA. Discounting costs and effects: a reconsideration. *Health Econ.* 1998;7:581-594.

37. Smith DH, Gravelle H. The practice of discounting in economic evaluations of healthcare interventions. *Int J Technol Assess Health Care.* 2001;17:236-243.

38. Krahn M, Detsky AS. Should Canada and the United States universally vaccinate infants against hepatitis B? A cost-effectiveness analysis. *Med Decis Making.* 1993;13:4-20.

39. Torrance GW, Feeny D. Utilities and quality-adjusted life years. *Int J Technol Assess Health Care.* 1989;5:559-575.

40. Mehrez A, Gafni A. The healthy-years equivalents: how to measure them using the standard gamble approach. *Med Decis Making.* 1991;11:140-146.

41. World Bank World Development Report 1993: *Investing in Health.* Oxford: Oxford University Press; 1993.

42. Torrance GW, Furlong WJ, Feeney DH, Boyle M. Multi-attribute preference functions: Health Utilities Index. *Pharmacoeconomics*. 1995;7:503-520.

43. O'Brien BJ, Drummond MF, Labelle RJ, Willan A. In search of power and significance: issues in the design and analysis of stochastic cost-effectiveness studies in health care. *Med Care*. 1994;32:150-163.

44. Udvarhelyi IS, Colditz GA, Rai A, Epstein AM. Cost-effectiveness and cost-benefit analyses in the medical literature: are the methods being used correctly? *Ann Intern Med*. 1992;116:238-244.

45. Briggs AH, O'Brien BJ, Blackhouse G. Thinking outside the box: recent advances in the analysis and presentation of uncertainty in cost-effectiveness studies. *Annu Rev Public Health*. 2002;23:377-401.

46. Briggs AH, Goeree R, Blackhouse G, O'Brien BJ. Probabilistic analysis of cost-effectiveness models: choosing between treatment strategies for gastroesophageal reflux disease. *Med Decis Making*. 2002;22:290-308.

47. Levy AR, Briggs AH, Demers C, O'Brien BJ. Cost-effectiveness of beta-blocker therapy with metoprolol or with carvedilol for treatment of heart failure in Canada. *Am Heart J*. 2001;142:537-543.

48. Johannesson M, Weinstein MC. On the decision rules of cost-effectiveness analysis. *J Health Econ*. 1993;12:459-467.

49. Birch S, Gafni A. Changing the problem to fit the solution: Johannesson and Weinstein's (mis)application of economics to real world problems. *J Health Econ*. 1993;12:469-476.

50. Drummond M, Torrance G, Mason J. Cost-effectiveness league tables: more harm than good? *Soc Sci Med*. 1993;37:33-40.

51. Stewart S, Marley JE, Horowitz JD. Effects of a multidisciplinary, home-based intervention on unplanned readmissions and survival among patients with chronic congestive heart failure: a randomised controlled study. *Lancet*. 1999;354:1077-1083.

19

Computer Decision Support Systems

Carl Thompson, Dawn Dowding, and Gordon Guyatt

The following Editorial Board members also made substantive contributions to this chapter: Marie Driever and Annette Flanagin.

We gratefully acknowledge the work of Adrienne Randolph, Brian Haynes, Jeremy Wyatt, and Deborah Cook on the original chapter that appears in the Users' Guides to the Medical Literature, *edited by Guyatt and Rennie.*

In This Chapter

Finding the Evidence

Are the Results Valid?
Were Study Participants Randomized? If Not, Were Groups Shown to Be Similar in All Known Determinants of Outcome, or Were Analyses Adjusted for Differences?
Was the Control Group Uninfluenced by the Computer Decision Support System?
Were Interventions That Affect Outcome Similar in the Two Groups?
Was Outcome Assessed Uniformly in the Intervention and Control Groups?

What Are the Results?
How Large and Precise Was the Effect of the Computer Decision Support System?

How Can I Apply the Results to Patient Care?
What Elements of the Computer Decision Support System Are Required?
Is the Computer Decision Support System Exportable to a New Site?
Is the Computer Decision Support System Likely to Be Accepted by Clinicians in My Setting?
Do the Benefits of the Computer Decision Support System Justify the Risks and Costs?

Can a Computer Decision Support System Help Nurses Monitor Oral Anticoagulation in a Primary Care Setting?

As the nurse administrator of a large primary care organization, part of your role is to review the results of annual clinical audits submitted by your colleagues. In the past year, the nursing staff expended substantial effort on adherence to guidelines, particularly guidelines concerned with the monitoring and management of warfarin therapy in patients living in the community. You note significant variability in the results and, relative to other services, low satisfaction scores from patients. You think that part of the problem lies with the need for patients to visit hospital-based clinics. Patients have told staff members that they do not like attending both community-based and hospital-based clinics for the same problem and for what, to them, appears to be identical care. Moreover, you know that although a doctor ostensibly leads the hospital clinics, nurses usually deliver the care. Nursing colleagues also express concerns about their ability to make sense of international normalized ratios (INRs) in management decisions that occur within tight time constraints. Having spoken to medical colleagues in the primary care organization and local hospitals, you wonder whether a primary care–based approach to the management of anticoagulation regimens, coupled with a computer decision support system, could lead to greater concordance with guidelines. Your medical colleagues are broadly supportive of the idea as long as you can show that oral anticoagulation care provided by nurse-led primary care clinics will be at least as good as that provided in hospital clinics.

FINDING THE EVIDENCE

You decide to use the Internet to search for information on computer-assisted decision support for anticoagulation clinics run by nurses and go to PubMed at *www.pubmed.gov*. Because you do not know the exact search terms to use, you decide to have a look at the MeSH (Medical Subject Headings) database, located through a link on the left-hand side of the main PubMed screen. After you enter the term "decision" into the MeSH database search box and click on "go", you are presented with a list of MeSH terms and definitions. You peruse the list and check off "decision support techniques," "decision making, computer assisted," and "decision support systems, clinical," combining the terms with the "OR" command by choosing "Search Box with OR" from the "Send To" drop-down menu, and then clicking on the "Send To" feature. You can now see a box that has all the appropriate MeSH terms combined with OR, and you click the button underneath this box, "Search PubMed." Next, you clear the main search box, type in "nurses," and hit "go." Then, you clear the box again and type in "anticoagulation." To ensure that your results represent higher-quality research, you apply a limit to your final search by clicking on the "limits" tab and choosing "randomized controlled trial" from the "Publication Type" drop-down menu and again hit "go." Finally, you click on the "history" tab and have a look at the assigned numbers of the searches you have just performed. You combine the three major concepts, using their corresponding numbers and the "AND" command, by typing in a command such as #2 AND #3 AND #4.

The result of this search is a selection of three articles. On examination of the abstracts, two of the articles appear to be about the same study. You decide to retrieve the full text of the one entitled "Oral Anticoagulation Management in Primary Care With the Use of Computerized Decision Support and Near-Patient Testing: A Randomized, Controlled Trial."[1] Before logging off PubMed, you decide to try another search strategy to determine if there might have been an easier way to identify this paper. You return to the PubMed main page and simply type in the following terms: anticoagulation, nurses, computer decision support. This search results in the identification of the same three articles.

The study you have retrieved[1] was conducted in primary care practices in Birmingham, England, where patients requiring anticoagulant therapy were usually monitored at a local hospital. At the beginning of the study, the investigators randomly selected 12 practices, stratified by practice size, and randomized nine practices to the intervention group and three to the control group. Among practices in the intervention group, patients who were currently taking anticoagulation therapy were identified from practice lists and individually randomized to follow-up and monitoring from a nurse-led clinic that used on-site blood testing and a decision support system or to continue current hospital-based follow-up arrangements. All patients in practices randomized to the control group continued with current hospital-based follow-up arrangements. The clinical decision support system provided dosing recommendations based on each patient's current INR level in relation to therapeutic range. These recommendations were based on British Society of Haematology guidelines.[2] All of the recommendations made by the clinical decision support system could be overridden, and nurses were advised to check with medical staff if a change of dose was recommended.

Clinicians depend on computers. Laboratory data management software, pharmacy information management systems, applications for tracking patient location through admission and discharge, mechanical ventilators, and oxygen saturation measurement devices are among the many types of computerized devices and systems that have become an integral part of the health care system. These devices and systems capture, transform, display, or analyze data for use in clinical decision making. Of the available computer aids, we restrict the term *computer decision support system* (CDSS) to software designed to aid directly in clinical decision making about individual patients.

In CDSSs, detailed individual patient data are entered into a computer program and are matched to programs or algorithms in a computerized database, resulting in the generation of patient-specific assessments or recommendations for clinicians.[3] CDSSs must meet three key challenges if they are to be useful: (1) they must be based on the correct type of knowledge for the decision; (2) they must take into account natural variations in patients and thus work with individual patient profiles and data; and (3) they must offer tailored advice that informs decision making. Table 19-1 summarizes the functions of CDSSs developed for clinical purposes: alerting, reminding, critiquing, interpreting, predicting, diagnosing, assisting, suggesting, and facilitating.[4]

Many alerting, reminding, and critiquing systems are based on simple if/then rules, or *conditional probabilities* that tell the computer what to do when a certain event occurs. *Alerting systems* monitor a continuous signal or stream of data and generate a message (an alert) in response to items or patterns that may require action by a clinician.[5] Alerts

Table **19-1** Functions of Computer Decision Support Systems

Function	Example
Alerting	Highlighting out-of-range (either too high or too low) laboratory values
Reminding	Reminding the clinician to schedule a cervical smear
Critiquing	Rejecting an inappropriate order for a new drug
Interpreting	Analyzing an electrocardiogram
Predicting	Calculating the risk of mortality from a severity of illness score
Diagnosing	Listing a differential diagnosis for a patient with chest pain
Assisting	Tailoring the antibiotic choices for patients with sexually transmitted diseases
Suggesting	Generating suggestions for adjusting a mechanical ventilator in a critical care unit
Facilitating	Providing a forum for interaction, model building, and joint negotiation of treatment

can be found on computerized laboratory printouts and display screens that alert clinicians to values that are out of range with, for example, stars (*) or the letters H or L (denoting values that are either too high or too low). Alerting systems draw attention to events as they occur.

Reminder systems notify clinicians of important tasks that need to be done before an event occurs. An outpatient clinic reminder system may generate a list of immunizations required by each patient on the daily schedule. Although the rules behind alerts and reminders are often simple, alerting the correct person in a timely fashion is quite complex. For instance, clinicians may not notice or attend to reminders.

When a computer program evaluates a clinician's decision and generates an appropriateness rating or an alternative suggestion, the decision support approach is called *critiquing.* The distinction between assisting– and critiquing–decision support programs is that assisting programs help to formulate clinical decisions, whereas critiquing programs have no part in decision making, but evaluate an entered plan against an algorithm in the computer.[4] Critiquing systems are commonly applied to clinician order entry. For example, a clinician entering an order for a blood transfusion may receive a message stating that the patient's serum hemoglobin level is above the transfusion threshold, and the clinician must justify the order by stating an indication such as active bleeding.[6] Getting the attention of the person who can take action is one of the most difficult aspects of making alerting, reminding, and critiquing systems effective.

The automated interpretations of electrocardiogram readings[7] and the outcome predictions generated by severity of illness scoring systems[8] are examples of CDSSs used for interpreting and predicting, respectively. These systems filter and abstract detailed clinical data and generate a report characterizing the meaning of the data, such as "anterior myocardial infarction."[7]

Computer-aided diagnostic systems also can assist clinicians with the process of differential diagnosis.[9] When an electrocardiogram is not definitive, computer systems that try to distinguish between myocardial infarction and other sources of chest pain can sometimes outperform clinicians.[10] These types of systems require pertinent patient information, such as signs, symptoms, past medical history, laboratory values, and demographic characteristics. The program offers hypotheses, often prompts the user for more information, and ultimately provides a diagnosis or list of possible diagnoses ranked by probability.

Computerized patient management systems are complex programs that make suggestions about the optimal decision based on information currently known by the system. These types of systems are often integrated into the clinician ordering process. After collecting information on specific patient variables, the patient management program can tailor orders for interventions such as drug type and dosage or care protocols. For example, the Antibiotic Assistant[11] is a CDSS that implements guidelines to assist clinicians in ordering antibiotic agents. This system recommends the most cost-effective antibiotic regimen while taking into account the patient's renal function and drug allergies, site of infection, epidemiology of organisms in patients with this infection at the particular hospital, efficacy of the chosen antibiotic regimen, and cost of treatment. A system that instructs clinicians on how to manage the ventilation of patients with adult respiratory distress syndrome[12] is another example of a patient management program. Some of the more common CDSSs specific to nursing include Computer Aided Nursing Diagnosis and Intervention (CANDI) to help nurses form nursing diagnoses;[13] Urological Nursing Information Systems (UNIS) to assist nurses caring for elderly, incontinent patients living in nursing homes;[14] CAREPLAN for postpartum nursing care;[15] FLORENCE to advise on the identification of nursing diagnoses in new clients;[16] and Creighton Online Multiple Modular Expert System (COMMES) to provide computerized decision support.[17]

The primary reason to invest in computer support is to improve quality of care. If a computer system purports to aid in clinical decision making, enhance patient care, and improve outcomes, then it should be subject to the same rules of testing as any other health care intervention with similar claims. In this chapter, we describe how to use articles that evaluate the clinical impact of a CDSS. Many iterative steps are involved in developing, evaluating, and improving a CDSS before it is good enough to move beyond the laboratory environment and pilot-testing phase to broader clinical use. These steps involve the application of social science methods for evaluating human behavior and computer science methods for evaluating technologic safety and the ability of the system to deal with different situations. We limit our discussion to mature systems that have surpassed initial evaluation and are being implemented to change clinician behavior and patient outcomes.

ARE THE RESULTS VALID?

In keeping with the approach used in earlier chapters of this book, we consider three primary questions related to the validity of results, nature of results, and clinical application of results (Table 19-2). In so doing, we continue to refer back to the study by Fitzmaurice

Table 19-2   Users' Guides for an Article Evaluating a Computer Decision Support System

Are the Results Valid?

Did intervention and control groups begin the study with similar prognosis?

- Were study participants randomized? If not, were groups shown to be similar in all known determinants of outcome, or were analyses adjusted for differences?
- Was the control group uninfluenced by the CDSS?

Did intervention and control groups retain a similar prognosis after the study started?

- Were interventions that affect outcome similar in the two groups?
- Was outcome assessed uniformly in the intervention and control groups?

What Are the Results?

- How large and precise was the effect of the CDSS?

How Can I Apply the Results to Patient Care?

- What elements of the CDSS are required?
- Is the CDSS exportable to a new site?
- Is the CDSS likely to be accepted by clinicians in my setting?
- Do the benefits of the CDSS justify the risks and costs?

CDSS, *Computer decision support system.*

and colleagues,[1] which evaluated whether oral anticoagulation care provided in a nurse-led, primary care clinic involving on-site blood testing and a CDSS was at least as good as that provided by a hospital-based clinic.

When clinicians examine the effect of a CDSS on patient management or outcome, they should use the same criteria that are appropriate for any other intervention, whether it is a coping skills program, a home visiting program, or an approach to screening (see Chapter 4, Health Care Interventions). Thus, Table 19-2, which summarizes our approach to evaluating an article that examines the impact of a CDSS, includes the same validity criteria as our guides for evaluating studies of health care interventions. Table 19-2 also includes criteria from our guides for evaluating articles about harm (see Chapter 5, Harm). This is because randomization—and other strategies used to reduce bias in randomized trials—may not always be feasible in a CDSS evaluation.

Were Study Participants Randomized? If Not, Were Groups Shown to Be Similar in All Known Determinants of Outcome, or Were Analyses Adjusted for Differences?

The validity of the observational study designs often used to evaluate CDSSs is limited (see Chapter 3, Health Care Interventions and Harm: An Introduction; see also

Chapter 26, Bias and Random Error). The most common observational design, the *before-and-after design,* compares outcomes before a technology is implemented (by means of a historical control group) with those after the system is implemented. The validity of this approach is threatened by the risk that changes over time (*secular trends*) in patient mix or aspects of health care delivery may be responsible for changes in behavior or outcome that appear to be attributable to the CDSS.

Consider a CDSS assisting clinicians with the ordering of antibiotic drugs[11] that was implemented in the late 1980s and was associated with improvements in the cost-effectiveness of antibiotic ordering. This before-and-after study compared processes and outcomes for patients admitted to the unit before and after the CDSS was introduced. Changes in the health care system, including the advent of managed care, occurred simultaneously during that period. To control for secular trends, the investigators compared antibiotic prescribing practices with those of other acute-care hospitals in the United States for the duration of the study. Of course, these other hospitals differed in many ways aside from the CDSS, thereby limiting the validity of the comparison.

Investigators may strengthen the before-and-after design by turning the intervention on and off multiple times, a type of *time-series* design (see Chapter 17, Health Services Interventions). Although this makes it less likely that investigators will attribute changes independent of the intervention to the CDSS, random allocation of patients to a concurrent control group remains the strongest study design for evaluating therapeutic or preventive interventions (see Chapter 4, Health Care Interventions; see also Chapter 14, Surprising Results of Randomized Controlled Trials). Investigators have conducted successful randomized controlled trials of more than 70 CDSSs.[18-20]

A special issue for CDSS evaluation is the *unit of allocation.* Usually, investigators in clinical trials randomize patients. When evaluating the effect of a CDSS on patient care, the intervention is usually aimed at having an impact on the decisions made by clinicians. Hence investigators may randomize clinician clusters, such as health care teams, hospital wards, or outpatient practices.[21] A common mistake made by investigators is to analyze their data as if they had randomized individuals rather than clusters such as practices.[22] Chapter 17, Health Services Interventions includes a detailed discussion about cluster assignment and analysis.

To highlight the problem, we use an extreme example. Consider a study in which a researcher randomizes one team of nurses to use a CDSS and another team to standard practice. Over the course of the study, each team cares for 10,000 patients. If the investigator analyzes the data as though patients were individually randomized, the sample size will appear huge. However, it is plausible, perhaps even likely, that the two teams of nurses differed in their performance from the start (e.g., in educational background or years of nursing experience), and that this difference continued throughout the study, independent of the CDSS. Because the sample size in this study is really only two (teams), the likelihood of imbalance despite randomization is large.

Obtaining a sample of sufficient size can be difficult when randomizing health care teams. If only a few health care teams are available, investigators can pair them according to their similarities on several factors and randomly allocate each team in a matched pair to the intervention or control group.[23] In addition, investigators can use statistical methods developed specifically for analyzing studies using *cluster randomization,* which allow investigators to take full advantage of the available data.[24]

One other issue regarding randomization should be considered. If some patients assigned to the CDSS fail to receive the intervention, should these patients be included in the analysis? The answer, counterintuitive to some, is yes. Randomization can accomplish the goal of balancing groups with respect to both known and unknown determinants of outcome only if patients (or clinicians) are analyzed in the groups to which they are randomized. Dropping patients (or clinicians) who fail to receive the intervention or re-assigning them to the control group after randomization, compromises or destroys the balance that randomization is designed to achieve. *Intention to treat* is the technical term for an analysis in which patients (or clinicians) are included in the groups to which they were randomized, regardless of whether they received the intervention (see Chapter 15, The Principle of Intention to Treat).

Was the Control Group Uninfluenced by the Computer Decision Support System?

The possibility that patients in the control group could receive all or part of the therapeutic intervention (in this case, anticoagulation management in nurse-led primary care clinics) threatens the integrity of randomized trials. Studies to evaluate CDSSs are particularly vulnerable to this problem of *contamination.* For example, Strickland and Hasson[25] randomly allocated patients with complex medical problems on mechanical ventilation to automatic, computer-directed weaning or physician-controlled weaning. Because the same physicians and respiratory therapists using the computer protocol also managed the care of patients not assigned to the protocol, it is possible that clinicians could remember and apply protocol algorithms to control patients. When the control group is influenced by the intervention, the effect of a CDSS may be diluted. Contamination may spuriously decrease, or even eliminate, a true intervention effect.

One method of preventing exposure of the control group to the CDSS is to assign individual clinicians to use or not use the CDSS. This is often problematic because when covering for one another, clinicians in the intervention group could be responsible for patients of clinicians in the control group. Comparisons of the performance of wards or hospitals that do and do not use the CDSS is another possibility. Unfortunately, it is usually not feasible to enroll a sufficient number of hospitals and when sample size is small, randomization may fail to ensure prognostically similar groups.

Were Interventions That Affect Outcome Similar in the Two Groups?

The results of studies evaluating interventions aimed at treatment or prevention are more believable if patients, their clinicians, and the study personnel are blinded to the treatment (see Chapter 4, Health Care Interventions). *Blinding* also diminishes the *placebo effect,* which, in the case of CDSSs, may be the tendency of patients to ascribe positive outcomes to use of a computer decision system. Although blinding clinicians, patients, and study personnel to the presence of a CDSS may prevent this type of bias, blinding is sometimes not possible.

Lack of blinding can result in bias if interventions other than the treatment are differentially applied to treatment and control groups, particularly if the use of effective nonstudy treatments is permitted at the discretion of clinicians. Concerns about lack of blinding are ameliorated if investigators describe permissible cointerventions and their differential use or standardize cointerventions,[26] or both, to ensure that their application is similar in both treatment and control groups.

Was Outcome Assessed Uniformly in the Intervention and Control Groups?

Unblinded study personnel who measure outcomes may provide different interpretations of marginal findings or differential encouragement during performance tests.[27] In some studies, the computer system may be used as a data collection tool to evaluate outcomes in the CDSS group. Using the information system to log episodes in the treatment group and using a manual system in the non-CDSS group can create a *data completeness bias.*[5] If the computer logs more episodes than the manual system, it may appear that the CDSS had more events, and this could bias the outcome in favor of or against the CDSS group. To prevent such bias, investigators should log outcomes similarly in both groups.

Using the Guide

How well did the study by Fitzmaurice and colleagues[1] meet the criteria for validity? The study is a randomized controlled trial in which investigators randomized nine practices to the intervention group (Anticoagulation Management CDSS) and three to control services (hospital-based clinics). Because practices varied from small to large, randomization was stratified by practice size. The investigators used two control populations: patients individually randomly allocated as controls in the intervention practices and all patients in the control practices. This allowed investigators to determine whether clinicians in the intervention practices influenced the care received by patients randomized to the control group; that is, it is plausible that clinicians, aware of which patients were in the control group and concerned that these patients were not receiving the new intervention, provided more vigilant care than usual to this group. In the intervention practices, individual patients taking warfarin were randomized, using computer-generated random codes, to be monitored within the practice by nurses using on-site blood testing and the CDSS or to continue existing follow-up arrangements (hospital management).

To determine which control group to use in the analysis, the investigators tested whether outcomes differed between the two control populations (i.e., those allocated as controls within intervention practices and all patients in the control practices). This analysis would have had to be based on the unit of allocation (practices), with a sample size of only three in the control group. If the investigators found differences, there could have been two possible explanations: the control and intervention practices differed from the start or the study influenced practice. Differences between the two control populations would support comparing patients receiving the intervention with patients in the control practices rather than with control patients in the intervention practices. If this were the case, the unit of randomization, and thus the unit of analysis, would be by practice, and the control sample size would be three. Alternatively, if the investigators found that success of monitoring was similar in the two control groups, they could discard the control data from the three control practices and compare intervention and control group patients within practices. In this case, the unit of randomization, and thus the unit of analysis, would be patients.

Over the year, 122 patients in intervention practices were randomized to on-site blood testing and CDSS, and 102 patients were randomized to usual hospital-based care. Another 143 patients were followed-up from control practices. Because the investigators stated that practices were stratified by size before randomization, it seems odd that the three control practices had more than half as many patients as the nine intervention practices (one would have expected about a third). The authors provided no explanation for this apparent discrepancy.

Because outcomes in the two control groups were similar (e.g., 53% of control patients in the intervention practices were in the target INR range, as were 62% of patients in the control practices), the investigators discarded the data from the three control practices and analyzed by patient (because the patient was the unit of randomization within intervention practices). Furthermore, 11 patients randomized to CDSS-driven care actually returned to hospital care. However, the data from these patients were appropriately analyzed within the CDSS group, that is, on an intention-to-treat basis, thus reducing the risk of bias.

The risk of contamination would have been high if all patients had been attending primary care clinics for oral anticoagulation monitoring by nurses and if these nurses had been instructed to use the CDSS with patients allocated to the intervention group and a different intervention, say a paper-based guideline, with patients allocated to the control group. If this had been the case, the performance of nurses with control patients could have been improved as a result of exposure to the CDSS. Instead, the control group received oral anticoagulation monitoring in the hospital setting rather than the clinic setting. The disadvantage of this arrangement is that the investigators are comparing more than the CDSS. To the extent that outcomes in the two settings differ, we are uncertain about how much of this difference is attributable to the CDSS and how much to differences in the clinicians and practice setting. If the outcomes are the same, we are uncertain whether the similarity would be maintained if the nurse-led clinic care did not include use of the CDSS.

With respect to cointervention, nurses could override the dosing recommendations provided by the CDSS and were advised to check with medical staff if a change of medication dose was recommended. This meant that patients in the intervention group could have received treatment that was not recommended by the CDSS. The authors did not provide data on the number of times CDSS advice was overridden in the intervention group, and thus it is not possible to assess the role of clinical judgment independent of the CDSS on care in the intervention group. Moreover, during the study, one of the hospital sites attended by patients in the control group began to use a CDSS with patients seen by a technician at this site.

The primary outcome was INR control. Blood samples of patients in the intervention group were tested on site by practice staff using Thrombotrak (INR blood testing

Continued

device), whereas blood samples of patients in the control group were tested at one of three local hospital laboratories. Although it is unlikely that hospital laboratory staff would be aware of which patients were participating in the study, practice staff in the clinic had to be aware of INRs to use the CDSS to make dosing recommendations. Thrombotrak proved difficult to use because of the need for pipetting skills to reconstitute reagents. Despite this problem, the authors noted that practice staff overcame these difficulties and performed within the external quality assurance scheme. Such assurances are unconvincing. To the extent that nurses in the intervention group were invested in the success of their approach, they may have been inclined to report better INR control. Furthermore, the number of INR results available may have influenced the outcome of proportion of time in range. The authors of the study did not report the distribution of frequency of INR measurements in the intervention and control groups.

In summary, the validity of the results of the study by Fitzmaurice and colleagues[1] was demonstrated by randomization of patients, inclusion of two control populations to demonstrate that intervention effects in the control group were unlikely, and analysis of all patients in the groups to which they were randomized even if they did not receive the intervention. Different ways of measuring the outcome in the intervention and control groups compromise the validity of the study.

WHAT ARE THE RESULTS?

How Large and Precise Was the Effect of the Computer Decision Support System?

We have described the alternatives for summarizing intervention effects such as relative risks, relative risk reductions, risk differences, and absolute risk reductions in other chapters (see Chapter 4, Health Care Interventions, and Chapter 27, Measures of Association). Clinicians can evaluate the precision of the estimate of effect by examining the confidence interval around the estimate (see Chapter 4, Health Care Interventions, and Chapter 29, Confidence Intervals). The larger the sample size and the number of outcome events, the narrower the confidence interval. The boundaries of the confidence interval can help us interpret study results. In a *positive study* in which the authors conclude that an intervention is effective, one can look at the lower boundary of the confidence interval. If this intervention effect (the lowest effect that is consistent with the study results) is still important (i.e., large enough for you to recommend the intervention), then the investigators have enrolled a sufficient number of study participants. In a *negative study* in which the authors conclude that the experimental intervention is no better than the control intervention, one can look at the upper boundary of the confidence interval. If the estimate of effect at this upper boundary would, if it was true, be important, the study has failed to exclude an important intervention effect. For information on determining whether a study was large enough, see Chapter 29, Confidence Intervals.

In the case of cluster studies, if the analysis does not adjust for clustering, it is likely to overestimate the statistical significance of the comparison, resulting in overly narrow confidence intervals or artificially low *P* values (see Chapter 17, Health Services Interventions).

Using the Guide

In the study by Fitzmaurice and colleagues,[1] the intervention and control groups did not differ in the proportion of patients who achieved appropriate INR control. Patients in the nurse-led group spent a higher percentage of time in the therapeutic INR range than did patients in the hospital group (69% vs. 57%; *P* < 0.001). The authors did not provide confidence intervals around this difference of 12%, but the low *P* value suggests that the lower boundary of the confidence interval is not close to zero (no difference). There were also no significant differences between the groups in overall death rates or serious adverse events.

The intervention cost, on average, was approximately $160 (in equivalent United States dollars) per patient per year more than for controls, primarily because of the capital costs of setting up the practice-based clinics and the increased frequency of testing within the practices. The practice-based costs averaged $270 per patient per year, whereas the mean hospital costs were $110 per patient per year.

HOW CAN I APPLY THE RESULTS TO PATIENT CARE?

Many of the issues specific to a CDSS arise in its application. Implementing a CDSS within your own environment can be challenging.

What Elements of the Computer Decision Support System Are Required?

It is important to understand which aspects of a particular CDSS were evaluated. Investigators can evaluate, separately, two of the major elements comprising a CDSS: the logic that has been incorporated and the computer interface used to present the logic. However, sometimes it is not possible to separate these two elements and achieve the same impact. For example, a randomized controlled trial of patients with adult respiratory distress syndrome found that patients managed with a computerized protocol did as well as those managed with standard clinical care with extracorporeal carbon dioxide removal used as a rescue therapy.[12] Was this result caused by the logic in the protocol, the use of the computer, or an interaction of these two components? To test whether a computer is a necessary component of the intervention, investigators could have one group apply the protocol logic as written on paper and the other group apply the same logic using a computer. Sometimes, however, the logic is so complex that use of a computer is required for implementation.

The CDSS may have a positive impact for unintended reasons. The effects of structured data collection forms and *performance* evaluations (called the *checklist effect* and the *feedback effect*,[5] respectively) on decision making can equal that of computer-generated advice.[28] The CDSS intervention itself may be administered by research personnel or paid clinical staff (despite scant mention in the published study report), without whom the impact of the system would be seriously undermined.

The CDSS used in the study by Fitzmaurice and colleagues[1] had three components: (1) a knowledge base consisting of British Society of Haematology guidelines[2] as a basis for anticoagulant dosage recommendations; (2) a database that stored INR results and dosing decisions; and (3) an inference engine that compared the database with the knowledge base and sent a dosing recommendation to the computer terminal for display.

Is the Computer Decision Support System Exportable to a New Site?

For a CDSS to be exported to a new site, it must have the ability to be integrated with existing software. In addition, users at the new site must be able to maintain the system, and they must accept the system. *Double charting* occurs when systems require staff to enter the data once into the computer and once again on a flow sheet. Systems that require double charting increase staff time for documentation, frustrate users, and divert time that could be spent on patient care. In general, experience suggests that systems that require double entry of data fail in clinical use and are ultimately abandoned.

Therefore, it is important to assess how the information necessary to run the decision support system is entered. In general, successful systems are ones with automatic electronic interfaces to existing data producing systems. Unfortunately, building interfaces to diverse computer systems is often extremely challenging and sometimes impossible.

The CDSS in the study by Fitzmaurice and colleagues[1] was the Anticoagulation Management Support System developed by Softop Information Systems in Warwick, England and validated in primary[29] and secondary[30] care settings. Although this CDSS stores all dosing decisions within the practice-based clinic, it is independent of the existing clinical data systems in the primary care practices. This means that data cannot be imported or exported from existing systems into the CDSS, thus resulting in duplication of data entry and the extra time this entails. The dosing recommendations made by the CDSS were based on individual therapeutic ranges from the British Society of Haematology guidelines.[2] Depending on whether these guidelines are internationally accepted, it may be possible to take the knowledge built into the system and use it in another health care environment. If, after critically appraising a study describing the impact of a CDSS, you are convinced that the CDSS would be useful, you will need to have sufficient resources to rebuild the system at your own site.

Is the Computer Decision Support System Likely to Be Accepted by Clinicians in My Setting?

Clinicians who differ in important ways from those in the study may not accept the CDSS. The choice of evaluative group may limit the generalizability of a study's conclusions if recruitment is based on enthusiasm, demographics, or a zest for new technology. Managers promoting use of a CDSS in a new setting may be surprised when their colleagues do not use the CDSS with the same enthusiasm as the original participants.

The user interface is an important component of the effectiveness of a CDSS. The CDSS interface should be developed on the basis of potential users' capabilities and limitations, the users' tasks, and the environment in which those tasks are performed.[28] One of the main difficulties with alerting systems is sending information about a potential problem (e.g., an abnormal laboratory value) as quickly as possible to the person with decision-making capability. A group of investigators tried numerous different alerting methods, from a highlighted icon on the computer screen to a flashing yellow light placed on the top of the computer.[31] These investigators later used pagers to alert nurses about abnormal laboratory values.[32] The nurses could then decide how to act on the information and when to alert the physician.

To ensure user acceptance, users must believe that they can count on the system to be available whenever they need it. The amount of down time needed for data backup, troubleshooting, and upgrading should be minimal. The response time must be fast, data integrity must be maintained, and data redundancy must be minimized. If systems have been functioning at other sites for a period of time, major problems may have been eradicated, thus decreasing down time and improving acceptance. It is also important to assess the amount of training required for users to feel comfortable with the system. If users become frustrated with the system, system performance will be suboptimal.

Many computer programs may function well at the site where the program was developed. Unfortunately, the staff at your own institution may disagree with the approaches taken elsewhere. For example, an expert system for managing patients who have adult respiratory distress syndrome and are receiving mechanical ventilation may use trials of continuous positive airway pressure to wean patients from the ventilator, whereas clinicians at your institution may prefer pressure-support weaning. Syntax, laboratory coding, and phrasing of diagnoses and therapeutic interventions can vary markedly across institutions. Customizing the application to the environment may not be feasible, and additional expense may be invoked when mapping vocabulary to synonyms unless a mechanism to do so has already been incorporated into the programming. To ensure user acceptance, the needs and concerns of users should be considered, and users should be included in decision making and implementation stages.

The Anticoagulation Management Support System[1] uses the British Society of Haematology guidelines[2] for anticoagulation. This use of established guidelines could enhance clinician acceptance by convincing them that the recommendations will positively influence patient outcomes. However, such practices do not ensure acceptance, and you will likely need a method for gaining consensus in your local clinical area. Furthermore, clinicians will need time to become familiar with any new system.

When the study by Fitzmaurice and colleagues[1] began, none of the practice nurses had used the CDSS system before, and they required training to use it. The system was designed for large hospital clinics and did not link with existing data management systems. It was therefore not adapted to the needs of the nurses in the primary care practices. The authors did not report on the nurses' satisfaction with the system. This information would have been helpful in determining how easily this system would be accepted in other primary care settings.

Do the Benefits of the Computer Decision Support System Justify the Risks and Costs?

The real cost of a CDSS is usually much higher than the initial hardware, software, interface, training, maintenance fees, and upgrade costs (which may not be included in the study report). Often, a CDSS is designed and maintained by staff whose actions are critical to the success of the intervention. Your institution may not want to pay for the time of such people in addition to the cost of the computer software and hardware. Indeed, it can be very difficult to estimate the costs of purchasing or building and implementing an integrated CDSS.

Are CDSSs beneficial? Human performance may improve when people are aware that their behavior is being observed *(the Hawthorne effect)*[33] or evaluated *(the sentinel effect)*. The same behavior may not be exhibited when monitoring of outcomes has stopped. Taking into account the influence of a study environment, a published systematic review of studies assessing CDSSs used in inpatient and outpatient clinical settings by clinicians,[3] that was subsequently updated,[20] showed that most CDSSs studied were beneficial. The outcomes assessed were patient-related outcomes (e.g., mortality, length of hospital stay, and decrease in infections) or health care process measures (e.g., compliance with reminders or with evidence-based processes of care). A total of 68 prospective trials that included concurrent control groups reported the effects of using CDSSs related to drug dosing, diagnosis, preventive care, and active medical care. Sixty-six percent of studies (43/65) showed that CDSSs improved physician performance. These included nine of 15 studies on drug dosing systems, one of five studies on diagnostic aids, 14 of 19 studies on preventive care systems, and 19 of 26 studies evaluating CDSSs for active medical care. Forty-three percent of studies (6/14) showed that CDSSs improved patient outcomes, three studies showed no benefit, and the remaining studies lacked sufficient power to detect a clinically important effect. Of the three studies that examined CDSSs involving nurses,[14,34,35] one showed an improvement in patient outcomes (decreased urinary incontinence in elderly patients living in a nursing home).[14]

Investigators evaluate health care processes more often than patient health outcomes because process events occur more frequently than do major health outcomes. For example, a trial designed to show a 25% improvement (from 50% to 62.5%) in the proportion of patients who are compliant with a certain medication (a process measure) would need to enroll 246 patients per group. A trial designed to show that the same medication reduces mortality (an outcome measure) by 25% (from 5% to 3.75%) would need to enroll 4177 patients per group. Furthermore, long follow-up periods are required to show that preventive interventions improve patient outcomes.

Fortunately, evaluation of health care processes will be adequate to infer benefit if the care processes are already known to improve outcomes. For example, randomized controlled trials have shown that tighter control of blood pressure reduces cardiovascular event rates. Unfortunately, however, the link between processes and outcomes is often unknown or weak.

A computer-based CDSS evaluation involves the interplay of three complex elements:

1. One or more human intermediaries
2. An integrated computerized system and its interface
3. Knowledge of the decision support

This interplay makes evaluation of a computer-based CDSS a complex undertaking. Systematic reviews of the effects of CDSSs on clinician behavior and patient outcomes have shown evidence of benefit.[3,18-20] It is difficult to compare the results of these reviews because the evaluation process used in the reviews was not standard.

In this chapter, we describe a process of evaluating studies that measure the impact of a CDSS on clinician decisions or patient outcomes. Despite the complexity of evaluation, clinicians can use basic principles of evidence-based care to evaluate a CDSS. A study evaluating a CDSS is more believable if there is a concurrent control group with random allocation of participants. Randomization by clusters avoids contamination, a bias that occurs when the control group receives the intervention intended for the experimental group. Contamination can mask the effect of a CDSS because both groups have been exposed to the intervention. When randomizing clusters (e.g., practices or hospitals and their respective patients), it is important to consider the practice or hospital, rather than the patients, as the unit of analysis. Because most studies evaluating a CDSS are not blinded, controlling for cointerventions that could bias the outcome is particularly important.

Even if a study is valid and a positive effect is shown, CDSSs have special applicability issues that clinicians and managers must consider. Is the computer essential to deployment of the knowledge in the CDSS? Can the CDSS be exported to a new site? Will clinicians at your site accept the CDSS? Finally, is it possible to evaluate the cost of the CDSS accurately when assessing risks and benefits?

The development of CDSSs could be something of a turning point in health care delivery. However, the effects are uncertain, and the design of evaluations is challenging. The demystifying effect of a structured appraisal approach can help clinicians seeking to establish the risks and benefits on a case-by-case basis.

CLINICAL RESOLUTION

The study by Fitzmaurice and colleagues[1] suggested that nurse-led primary care clinics with on-site blood testing and a CDSS may be at least as effective as usual, hospital-based follow-up for patients requiring anticoagulation therapy. However, differences in the way outcomes were monitored in intervention and control groups limit the strength of any inferences. Those interested in the specific impact of the CDSS will be troubled by uncertainty about how many times the CDSS recommendations were overridden and how well the nurses would have done in monitoring INR in the absence of the CDSS.

Furthermore, installing the system would require special training, and the dual entry of data may limit its acceptance by nurses working in other clinical areas. The authors of the study suggested that the cost of setting up and using the system varied by practice size, from $128 to $560 (in equivalent United States dollars) per patient per year (mean, $270), compared with a mean hospital cost of $110 per patient per year. Therefore, because patient-important outcomes were similar in the two groups, it seems unlikely that the benefits are worth the cost of purchasing, installing, training for, and maintaining the CDSS, particularly when the contribution of the CDSS to the nurses' apparent success remains uncertain. Ultimately, decisions about adopting a CDSS will depend on local values and politics.

REFERENCES

1. Fitzmaurice DA, Hobbs FDR, Murray ET, Holder RL, Allan TF, Rose PE. Oral anticoagulation management in primary care with the use of computerized decision support and near-patient testing: a randomized controlled trial. *Arch Intern Med.* 2000;160:2343-2348.

2. British Society of Haematology, British Committee for Standards in Haematology Haemostasis and Thrombosis Task Force. Audit of oral anticoagulant treatment. *J Clin Pathol.* 1993;46:1069-1070.

3. Johnston M, Langton K, Haynes R, Mathieu A. Effects of computer-based clinical decision support systems on clinician performance and patient outcome: a critical appraisal of research. *Ann Intern Med.* 1994;120:135-142.

4. Pryor TA. Development of decision support systems. *Int J Clin Monit Comput.* 1990;7:137-146.

5. Friedman CP, Wyatt JC. *Evaluation Methods in Medical Informatics.* New York: Springer-Verlag; 1997.

6. Lepage E, Gardner R, Laub R, Golubjatnikov O. Improving blood transfusion practice: role of a computerized hospital information system. *Transfusion.* 1992;32:253-259.

7. Weinfurt PT. Electrocardiographic monitoring: an overview. *J Clin Monit.* 1990;6:132-138.

8. Knaus WA, Wagner DP, Draper EA, et al. The APACHE III prognostic system: risk prediction of hospital mortality for critically ill hospitalized adults. *Chest.* 1991;100:1619-1636.

9. Berner E, Webster G, Shugerman A, et al. Performance of four computer-based diagnostic systems. *N Engl J Med.* 1994;330:1792-1796.

10. Kennedy R, Harrison R, Burton A, et al. An artificial neural network system for diagnosis of acute myocardial infarction (AMI) in the accident and emergency department: evaluation and comparison with serum myoglobin measurements. *Comput Methods Programs Biomed.* 1997;52:93-103.

11. Evans RS, Pestotnik SL, Classen DC, et al. A computer-assisted management program for antibiotics and other antiinfective agents. *N Engl J Med.* 1998;38:232-238.

12. Morris AH, Wallace CJ, Menlove RL, et al. Randomized clinical trial of pressure-controlled inverse ratio ventilation and extracorporeal CO_2 removal for adult respiratory distress syndrome. *Am J Respir Crit Care Med.* 1994;149:295-305.

13. Roth K, DiStefano JJ, Chang BL. CANDI. Development of the automated nursing assessment tool. *Comput Nurs.* 1989;7:222-227.

14. Petrucci K, Petrucci P, Canfield K, McCormick KA, Kjerulff K, Parks P. Evaluation of UNIS: urological nursing information systems. *Proc Annu Symp Comput Appl Med Care.* 1991:43-47.

15. Probst CL, Rush J. The CAREPLAN knowledge base: a prototype expert system for postpartum nursing care. *Comput Nurs.* 1990;8:206-213.

16. Bradburn C, Zeleznikow J, Adams A. FLORENCE: synthesis of case-based and model-based reasoning in a nursing care planning system. *Comput Nurs.* 1993;11:20-24.

17. Lappe JM, Dixon B, Lazure L, Nilsson P, Thielen J, Norris J. Nursing education application of a computerized nursing expert system. *J Nurs Educ.* 1990;29:244-248.

18. Shea S, DuMouchel W, Bahamonde L. A meta-analysis of 16 randomized controlled trials to evaluate computer-based clinical reminder systems for preventive care in the ambulatory setting. *J Am Med Inform Assoc.* 1996;3:399-409.

19. Balas E, Austin S, Mitchell J, Ewigman B, Bopp K, Brown G. The clinical value of computerized information services: a review of 98 randomized clinical trials. *Arch Fam Med.* 1996;5:271-278.

20. Hunt D, Haynes R, Hanna S. Effects of computer-based clinical decision support systems on physician performance and patient outcomes: a systematic review. *JAMA.* 1998;280:1339-1346.

21. Cornfield J. Randomization by group: a formal analysis. *Am J Epidemiol.* 1978:108;100-102.

22. Whiting-O'Keefe Q, Henke C, Simborg D. Choosing the correct unit of analysis in medical care experiments. *Med Care.* 1984;22:1101-1114.

23. Klar N, Donner A. The merits of matching in community intervention trials: a cautionary tale. *Stat Med.* 1997;16:1753-1764.

24. Thompson SG, Pyke SD, Hardy RJ. The design and analysis of paired cluster randomized trials: an application of meta-analysis techniques. *Stat Med.* 1997;16:2063-2079.

25. Strickland JH, Hasson JH. A computer-controlled ventilator weaning system: a clinical trial. *Chest.* 1993;103:1220-1226.

26. Morris AH, East TD, Wallace CJ, et al. Standardization of clinical decision making for the conduct of credible clinical research in complicated medical environments. *Proc AMIA Annu Fall Symp.* 1996:418-422.
27. Guyatt GH, Pugsley SO, Sullivan MJ, et al. Effect of encouragement on walking test performance. *Thorax.* 1984;39:818-822.
28. Adams ID, Chan M, Clifford PC, et al. Computer aided diagnosis of acute abdominal pain: a multicentre study. *BMJ.* 1986;293:800-804.
29. Fitzmaurice DA, Hobbs FDR, Murray ET, Bradley CP, Holder R. Evaluation of computerised decision support for oral anticoagulation management in primary care. *Br J Gen Pract.* 1996;46:533-535.
30. Ryan P, Gilbert M, Rose PE. Computer control of anticoagulant dose for therapeutic management. *BMJ.* 1989;299:1207-1209.
31. Bradshaw K, Gardner R, Pryor T. Development of a computerized laboratory alerting system. *Comput Biomed Res.* 1989;22:575-587.
32. Tate K, Gardner R, Scherting K. Nurses, pagers, and patient-specific criteria: three keys to improved critical value reporting. *Proc Annu Symp Comput Appl Med Care.* 1995:164-168.
33. Roethligsburger FJ, Dickson WJ. *Management and the Worker.* Cambridge, MA: Harvard University Press; 1939.
34. Keller LS, McDermott S, Alt-White A. Effects of computerized nurse careplanning on selected health care effectiveness measures. *Proc Annu Symp Comput Appl Med Care.* 1991;38-42.
35. Vadher BD, Patterson DLH, Leaning M. Comparison of oral anticoagulant control by a nurse practitioner using a computer decision-support system with that by clinicians. *Clin Lab Haematol.* 1997;19:203-207.

Diagnosis

Chapter 20   Clinical Manifestations
of Disease

Chapter 21   Differential Diagnosis

Chapter 22   Clinical Prediction Rules

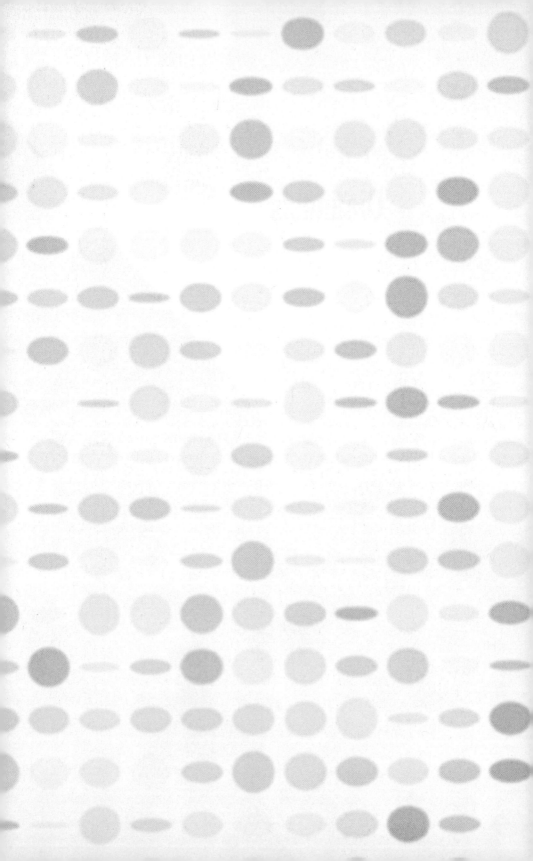

20

Clinical Manifestations of Disease

Andrew Jull, Alba DiCenso, and Gordon Guyatt

The following Editorial Board members also made substantive contributions to this chapter: Rien de Vos, Teresa Icart Isern, and Mary van Soeren.

We gratefully acknowledge the work of Scott Richardson, Mark Wilson, John Williams, Virginia Moyer, and David Naylor on the original chapter that appears in the Users' Guides to the Medical Literature, *edited by Guyatt and Rennie.*

In This Chapter

Are the Results Valid?
    Were the Right Patients Enrolled? Was the Patient Sample Representative of Those With the Disorder?
    Was the Definitive Diagnostic Standard Appropriate? Was the Diagnosis Verified Using Credible Criteria That Were Independent of the Clinical Manifestations Under Study?
    Were Clinical Manifestations Sought Thoroughly, Carefully, and Consistently?
    Were Clinical Manifestations Classified by When and How They Occurred?

What Are the Results?
    How Frequently Did the Clinical Manifestations of Disease Occur?
    How Precise Were These Estimates of Frequency?
    When and How Did These Clinical Manifestations Occur in the Course of Disease?

How Can I Apply the Results to Patient Care?
    Are the Study Patients Similar to Those in My Clinical Setting?
    Is It Unlikely That the Disease Manifestations Have Changed Since This Evidence Was Gathered?
    How Can I Use the Results in Generating a Differential Diagnosis?

CLINICAL SCENARIO

Do Equal Bilateral Pulses Rule Out Aortic Dissection in a Man With Chest Pain?

After several years' absence, you have returned to nursing, are working in the emergency department at a community hospital, and are orientating with the triage nurse. A 58-year-old man arrives by car with chest pain that started about an hour ago. The patient describes the sudden onset of severe pain in the center of his chest that radiates to his neck and midback, and he is anxious. The patient is triaged as category 2 (imminently life-threatening and requiring medical attention within 10 minutes), and the on-call physician is paged. Thinking that myocardial infarction may be the cause of these symptoms, you follow the patient to the examination room and begin a nursing assessment while awaiting the physician. You learn that he has essential hypertension, for which he takes a diuretic.

When she arrives, the physician focuses on the patient's thorax and cardiovascular system. She finds clear lungs; present and bilaterally equal carotid, radial, and femoral pulses; a diastolic murmur of aortic regurgitation; and diastolic hypotension, with blood pressure of 162/56 mm Hg. The electrocardiogram shows left ventricular hypertrophy, but no signs of ischemia or infarction. The initial set of cardiac enzymes is normal. An arterial blood gas study shows mild respiratory alkalosis and normal oxygenation. The physician explains to the patient and family that she suspects acute aortic dissection and wants to arrange definitive testing and a consultation with the surgical team. The surgeons advise giving the patient esmolol and a very low dose of sodium nitroprusside until they can review the patient's case.

While the patient is off having further tests, you ask the physician whether the absence of pulse deficit (asymmetry) would rule out the possibility of aortic dissection in this patient. The physician tells you that she has an interesting article on the clinical features and differential diagnosis of aortic dissection in her office and offers to share it with you. The article, by Spittell and colleagues[1] describes the clinical presentation in 235 patients who were ultimately diagnosed as having aortic dissection. It is the end of your shift, and you go home to read the article.

Two types of systematic investigations can inform the process of generating a differential diagnosis. One type of study addresses the presenting manifestations of a disease or condition. The second, and more important, type of study directly addresses the underlying causes of a presenting symptom, sign, or constellation of symptoms and signs. This chapter focuses on how to critique studies that address the former. Chapter 21 focuses on how to critique studies that address the latter. Table 20-1 summarizes the criteria for interpreting an article about the clinical manifestations of disease.

ARE THE RESULTS VALID?

Were the Right Patients Enrolled? Was the Patient Sample Representative of Those With the Disorder?

Ideally, a study sample will mirror the population of patients with the target condition so that the frequency of clinical manifestations in the sample approximates that in the

Table 20-1   Users' Guides for an Article About the Clinical
Manifestations of Disease

Are the Results Valid?

- Were the right patients enrolled? Was the patient sample representative of those with the disorder?
- Was the definitive diagnostic standard appropriate? Was the diagnosis verified using credible criteria that were independent of the clinical manifestations under study?
- Were clinical manifestations sought thoroughly, carefully, and consistently?
- Were clinical manifestations classified by when and how they occurred?

What Are the Results?

- How frequently did the clinical manifestations of disease occur?
- How precise were these estimates of frequency?
- When and how did these clinical manifestations occur in the course of disease?

How Can I Apply the Results to Patient Care?

- Are the study patients similar to those in my clinical setting?
- Is it unlikely that the disease manifestations have changed since this evidence was gathered?
- How can I use the results in generating a differential diagnosis?

underlying population. Such a patient sample is termed *representative.* The more representative a sample is, the more accurate the resulting frequencies of clinical findings will be.[2]

To judge the representativeness of a study sample, we suggest three tactics. First, examine the study setting. Patients seen in referral care settings may have higher proportions of unusual findings or illnesses that are harder to diagnose and thus will have different frequencies of clinical manifestations than patients diagnosed in community practice.[3] Second, examine the methods used to identify and include study patients and to exclude others. Ask yourself if they included all important demographic groups (e.g., those characterized by age, sex, and race) or excluded important subgroups. Third, examine the description of study patients' illnesses. Are patients with mild, moderate, and severe symptoms included? If different clinical patterns of disease are known, does the sample include patients with each pattern?

Combining these three considerations, you can judge whether the spectrum of included patients is broad enough for the study to yield valid results about the clinical manifestations of the disease. For instance, a study of the clinical findings in patients with thyrotoxic periodic paralysis included 19 patients who were hospitalized during an episode of paralysis and excluded 11 patients who were diagnosed during the study period but were not admitted.[4] To the extent that clinical manifestations differed in hospitalized and nonhospitalized patients, such a restriction could introduce bias into the study.

Investigators may deliberately choose to describe the manifestations of a disease in a purposefully narrow target population defined by demographics (e.g., a study of the findings of myocardial infarction in elderly patients[5]), prognosis (e.g., a study of the clinical findings before death in patients with fatal pulmonary embolism[6]), or site of care (e.g., a study of the findings in patients with ruptured abdominal aortic aneurysm who present to internists in their offices, rather than to emergency departments[7]). In such situations, you can assess whether the study sample is representative of the limited target population.

Was the Definitive Diagnostic Standard Appropriate? Was the Diagnosis Verified Using Credible Criteria That Were Independent of the Clinical Manifestations Under Study?

These questions address two closely linked issues. First, how sure are the investigators that patients in the study really did have this particular disease, rather than another disease? Clinicians often encounter patients with tentative diagnoses. However, in studies of disease manifestations, such diagnostic uncertainty could introduce bias because the sample could include patients with other diseases. To minimize this threat, investigators can use a set of explicit diagnostic criteria and include only patients who meet these criteria. Ideally, for every disease, there would be a set of published, widely accepted, diagnostic criteria, including one or more well-established *reference, gold,* or *criterion standard* tests that could be applied in a reproducible way. Reference standards can be anatomic, physiologic, radiographic, or genetic, to name a few. To judge how the presence of disease was verified, identify the standards that were used for disease verification, how they were used, and whether the standards were clinically credible.

When no reference standards exist, the degree of diagnostic certainty is much lower. In such situations, known sometimes as *syndrome diagnosis,*[8] diagnostic criteria usually rely on a list of clinical features required for diagnosis. For example, the definition of chronic fatigue syndrome uses an explicit set of clinical features as diagnostic criteria.[9] Such explicit criteria represent an advance over an implicit, haphazard approach.

However, problems arise when investigators use these clinical manifestations to make the syndrome diagnosis, select the patient sample, and then examine the frequency of these same clinical findings in the study patients. This situation creates a form of circular reasoning that can bias upward the frequencies of these findings in the study sample. For example, a study of the clinical features of 36 patients with relapsing polychondritis had this *incorporation bias,* because the investigators used diagnostic criteria that were based primarily on characteristic clinical findings.[10] Although this may be the best available method for clinical diagnosis, incorporation bias limits the inferences we can draw about the frequency of clinical manifestations. To judge the independence of verifying criteria, compare the list of these criteria with the list of clinical manifestations studied.

Were Clinical Manifestations Sought Thoroughly, Carefully, and Consistently?

This criterion addresses three closely related issues. First, were study patients evaluated thoroughly enough to detect clinical findings if they were present? Within reason, the more comprehensive the workup is, the lower the chance of missing findings and drawing invalid conclusions about their frequency. Second, how did the investigators ensure that the information they collected was correct and free of distortion? Were patients asked about symptoms in neutral, nonjudgmental ways, or were leading questions asked that could have suggested symptoms? Were patients examined by skilled examiners? The more carefully data are gathered, the more credible the resulting frequencies will be. Third, how consistently was the evaluation performed? Variable assessments could yield erroneous frequencies of disease manifestations.

You may find it relatively easy to judge the thoroughness, care, and consistency of the search for manifestations if clinicians evaluated patients prospectively using a standardized diagnostic approach. It becomes harder to judge when investigators use information previously collected by unstandardized methods. For example, a retrospective analysis of disease manifestations in 68 patients with lumbar spinal stenosis did not include a description of the search for clinical findings in sufficient detail to judge how well the investigators protected against biased ascertainment.[11] Ordinarily, a prospective study of clinical manifestations of disease provides more credible results than a retrospective study.

Were Clinical Manifestations Classified by When and How They Occurred?

Clinical manifestations of disease can range from permanent to fleeting. They can occur early, late, or throughout the course of disease. Investigators would obtain the most complete information about the timing of disease manifestations if they could begin collecting data the instant the disease begins and continue to the end of the illness. Because knowing this "zero time" with certainty is impossible for most diseases, investigators can use the next strongest approach of targeting all findings that occur from the onset of first symptoms of an illness episode. Studies that do not start collecting information at the beginning of the episode or do not report the timing of evaluation relative to symptom onset may miss transient findings, and our confidence in their validity decreases. For instance, in a study of the clinical manifestations before death in 92 patients with fatal pulmonary embolism, investigators recorded findings for only the final 24 hours before death and thus may have missed transient but important diagnostic clues that occurred before that time.[6]

Sometimes, studies describe qualitative findings that may be useful in clinical diagnosis, particularly in triggering initial diagnostic hypotheses. For instance, patients often describe the pain of aortic dissection as a "tearing" or "ripping" sensation located in the center of the torso and reaching maximal intensity quite quickly.[12] Just as with the temporal aspects, these qualitative descriptions are more credible if practitioners gathered them deliberately and carefully.

Using the Guide

Spittell and colleagues[1] studied patients from the Mayo Clinic in Rochester, Minnesota, which provides both community hospital care and tertiary referral care. The sample included 158 patients (67%) with acute aortic dissection (duration less than 2 weeks) and 78 patients (33%) with chronic aortic dissection (duration at least 2 weeks). In 60 patients, the initial clinical impression was a diagnosis other

Continued

than aortic dissection. The sample included patients who had died suddenly, including 10 patients with out-of-hospital cardiac arrests and five deaths that occurred in hospital. It also included 11 patients without pain but with other symptoms and 33 patients without pain or other symptoms, who had abnormal chest radiographs. Thus, the sample displays a wide array of clinical presentations likely to be representative of the full spectrum of this disorder.

The investigators studied 235 patients who had 236 aortic dissections confirmed by surgical intervention (in 162), autopsy (in 27), or radiographic studies (in 47). They excluded patients with aortic dissection that occurred intraoperatively or during invasive catheterization procedures. Thus, the diagnoses of study patients appear to have been verified using clinically credible methods that were independent of the clinical manifestations.

Spittell and colleagues[1] retrospectively reviewed patient charts after clinical evaluations were completed. They did not explicitly describe the diagnostic evaluation. The tables of results include detailed information about the clinical examination, which suggests a careful approach. Uncertainty remains, however, about the extent of standardization during the workup.

The investigators described the clinical manifestations of aortic dissection at presentation for patients with acute (duration less than 2 weeks) and chronic (duration at least 2 weeks) illness from aortic dissection. They also described the location of pain in relation to the site of dissection and clustering of pain with other findings, along with unusual findings, such as hoarseness and dysphagia. Thus, despite the retrospective study design, the investigators classified the temporal and qualitative features sufficiently to provide valid results for patients with acute aortic dissection. We may be less confident of the results for chronic dissection because early transient findings may not have been detected.

WHAT ARE THE RESULTS?

How Frequently Did the Clinical Manifestations of Disease Occur?

Studies of clinical manifestations of disease often display the main results in a table listing the clinical findings and the number and percentages of patients with each of those manifestations. Because patients usually have more than one finding, these proportions are not mutually exclusive. Some studies also report the number of patients with any of the findings, either as a total or separately by particular group.

Textbook descriptions can emphasize the presence of particular classic findings that are proved uncommon by systematic study. If clinicians rely on such findings, they will miss many cases. For example, although experts previously considered hemoptysis to be a hallmark of acute pulmonary embolism, only 30% of 327 patients with angiographically proved pulmonary emboli had hemoptysis.[13] Thus, it would be unwise to use the absence of hemoptysis to exclude a diagnosis of pulmonary embolism.

Systematic studies of disease manifestations may also prove some findings to be more common than expected. For instance, murmur of aortic regurgitation was detected in

40 (32%) of 124 patients with confirmed aortic dissection, a finding suggesting that clinicians should purposefully seek this finding in suspected cases.[12]

How Precise Were These Estimates of Frequency?

Even when valid, frequencies of clinical manifestations are only estimates of the true frequencies. You can determine the precision of these estimates by examining their confidence intervals (CIs). If the authors do not provide CIs, you can calculate them using the following formula (for 95% CI):

$$95\% \ CI = P \pm 1.96 \times \sqrt{(P\{1 - P\}/n)}$$

where P is the proportion of patients with the finding of interest and n is the number of patients in the sample. This formula becomes inaccurate when the number of cases is five or fewer, so approximations have been developed for this situation.[14,15]

For example, consider the clinical finding of pulse deficit found in 14 (6%) of 217 patients in the study by Spittell and colleagues.[1] Using the formula, we would start with $P = 0.06$ (14/217), $(1 - P) = 0.94$, and n = 217. Working through the arithmetic, we find the CI to be 0.06 ± 0.03. Thus, although the most likely frequency of pulse deficit is 6%, it may range from 3% (i.e., 6% − 3%) to 9% (i.e., 6% + 3%).

Whether you consider the CI sufficiently precise depends on how you expect to use the information. For example, if a finding occurs in 50% of cases, you may plan to look for it on examination but not to use the presence or absence of this finding to exclude the diagnosis. If the CI for this estimate ranged from 30% to 70%, it would not change your expected use of the information, so the result may be precise enough. Conversely, if a finding occurs in 97% of patients, you may hope to use its absence to help you rule out the diagnosis. If the CI for this estimate ranged from 60% to 100% (the same 40-point range as before), using this finding to exclude the diagnosis could lead you to miss up to 40% of patients with the disorder. Such a result would be too imprecise to be used to rule out the disorder of interest.

When and How Did These Clinical Manifestations Occur in the Course of Disease?

Some studies report the temporal sequence of symptoms in sufficient detail to characterize symptoms as presenting (i.e., the symptoms prompted patients to seek care), concurring (i.e., the symptoms did not prompt patients to seek care but were present initially), or eventual (i.e., the symptoms were not present initially but were found subsequently). For example, in 100 patients with pancreatic cancer, investigators described weight loss and abdominal pain as presenting manifestations in 75 and 72 patients, respectively, whereas jaundice, commonly taught as a key presenting sign, was found in only 24 patients.[16] In addition to reporting the chronology of events, such studies can also describe the location, quality, intensity, situational context, aggravating and alleviating factors, and associated findings for important features of the disorder.

> ### USING THE GUIDE
>
> Spittell and colleagues[1] reported that 168 (74%) patients initially had acute onset of severe pain, 33 (15%) patients were asymptomatic but had abnormal chest radiographs, and 15 (6%) patients experienced cardiac arrest or sudden death. Of the 217 of 235 (92%) patients with a record of the cardiac examination, murmurs of aortic regurgitation were detected in 22 (10%). Pulse deficits were uncommon, occurring in 14 (6%) patients.
>
> The investigators did not provide the 95% CIs for the probabilities they found. However, as illustrated, if you are concerned about how close the probabilities are to your thresholds, you can calculate the 95% CIs.
>
> Spittell and colleagues[1] described in detail the symptoms at initial assessment, both as individual findings and in clusters. They also described the location of pain and its association with the site of aortic dissection. They did not describe delayed manifestations in as much detail.

HOW CAN I APPLY THE RESULTS TO PATIENT CARE?

Are the Study Patients Similar to Those in My Clinical Setting?

The closer the match is between patients in your clinical setting and those in the study, the more confident you can be in applying the results. We suggest that you ask yourself whether the setting or the patients are so different from yours that you cannot use the results.[17] You could consider whether patients in your clinical setting come from a geographic, demographic, cultural, socioeconomic, or clinical group that could be expected to differ substantively in the ways in which the disorder is expressed. For instance, the presenting symptoms of acute myocardial infarction were found to differ with advancing patient age. A study of 777 elderly hospitalized patients with myocardial infarction found that syncope, stroke, and acute confusion were common and sometimes the sole presenting symptoms.[5]

Is It Unlikely That the Disease Manifestations Have Changed Since This Evidence Was Gathered?

As time passes, evidence about the clinical manifestations of disease can become obsolete. New diseases can emerge, and old diseases can present in new ways. New disease taxonomies can be built, thus changing the distinctions between disease states. Such events can so alter the clinical manifestations of disease that previously valid studies may no longer be applicable to current practice. For example, the arrival of acquired immunodeficiency syndrome dramatically changed our concept of pneumonia caused by *Pneumocystis carinii*, a fungus that causes disease most commonly when cell-mediated immunity is depressed.[18,19]

Similar changes can occur as the result of progress in health science or medical practice. For instance, early descriptions of *Clostridium difficile* infection emphasized severe cases of life-threatening colitis. As diagnostic testing improved and awareness of the infection became widespread, milder cases were documented, and the presenting manifestations were recognized to vary widely.[20] Treatment advances can change the course of disease, so previously common eventual clinical manifestations may occur with less frequency. Moreover, new treatments bring the possibility of new iatrogenic disease, which may coexist and combine with underlying diseases in new ways.

How Can I Use the Results in Generating a Differential Diagnosis?

For studies that prove valid and applicable to your patients, knowing the clinical manifestations of possible conditions will help you to generate a differential diagnosis. A few findings may occur in almost all patients with the disease. As this proportion nears 100%, the absence of these findings allows you to omit the disease from your differential diagnosis. The presence of findings that occur in the range of 10% to 90% of patients with the disease suggests that the condition should remain among those you are considering as an explanation for your patient's presentation. Some manifestations occur seldom enough—in fewer than 10% of patients—that their presence would not prompt consideration of the illness in your differential diagnosis.

USING THE GUIDE

Spittell and colleagues[1] did not describe the referral filters through which their patients arrived. However, the Mayo Clinic provides community hospital care for 125,000 local residents along with referred care for many others. Of the 235 patients, 158 (67%) were men, and their mean age was close to that of the patient presenting in the emergency department. The authors did not describe patients' comorbid conditions, socioeconomic status, race, or cultural background. Thus, although some uncertainty remains, these patients are sufficiently similar to the patient presenting in the emergency department to allow application of the results.

The study was published in 1993 and reported on patients seen from 1980 to 1990. You know of no new diseases emerging since then that would change the clinical features of aortic dissection. Both diagnostic testing for suspected dissection and treatment of hypertension (a major risk factor for aortic dissection) have changed during this period, but you expect that they would not change the presenting clinical features of acute dissection.

CLINICAL RESOLUTION

Based on the evidence from Spittell and colleagues,[1] you realize that absence of pulse asymmetry does not rule out a diagnosis of aortic dissection. Given the presence of the aortic regurgitation murmur and diastolic hypotension, along with the patient's known risk and the absence of findings for myocardial infarction, you become more confident that the patient's diagnosis may be proximal aortic dissection. Indeed, when you return to work the next day, you learn that the patient's aortogram confirmed aortic dissection of the ascending aorta and arch, complicated by aortic regurgitation and that the patient was taken to the operating room for emergency surgery.

References

1. Spittell PC, Spittell JA Jr, Joyce JW, et al. Clinical features and differential diagnosis of aortic dissection: experience with 236 cases (1980 through 1990). *Mayo Clin Proc.* 1993;68:642-651.
2. Ransohoff DF, Feinstein AR. Problems of spectrum and bias in evaluating the efficacy of diagnostic tests. *N Engl J Med.* 1978;299:926-930.
3. Fletcher RH, Fletcher SW, Wagner EH. *Clinical Epidemiology: The Essentials.* 3rd ed. Baltimore: Williams & Wilkins; 1996.
4. Manoukian MA, Foote JA, Crapo LM. Clinical and metabolic features of thyrotoxic periodic paralysis in 24 episodes. *Arch Intern Med.* 1999;159:601-606.
5. Bayer AJ, Chadha JS, Farag RR, Pathy MS. Changing presentation of myocardial infarction with increasing old age. *J Am Geriatr Soc.* 1986;34:263-266.
6. Morgenthaler TI, Ryu JH. Clinical characteristics of fatal pulmonary embolism in a referral hospital. *Mayo Clin Proc.* 1995;70:417-424.
7. Lederle FA, Parenti CM, Chute EP. Ruptured abdominal aortic aneurysm: the internist as diagnostician. *Am J Med.* 1994;96:163-167.
8. Wulff HR. *Rational Diagnosis and Treatment: An Introduction to Clinical Decision-Making.* 2nd ed. Oxford: Blackwell Scientific Publications; 1981.
9. Fukuda K, Straus SE, Hickie I, et al. The chronic fatigue syndrome: a comprehensive approach to its definition and study. *Ann Intern Med.* 1994;121:953-959.
10. Trentham DE, Le CH. Relapsing polychondritis. *Ann Intern Med.* 1998;129:114-122.
11. Hall S, Bartleson JD, Onofrio BM, Baker HL Jr, Okazaki H, O'Duffy JD. Lumbar spinal stenosis: clinical features, diagnostic procedures, and results of surgical treatment in 68 patients. *Ann Intern Med.* 1985;103:271-275.
12. Slater EE, DeSanctis RW. The clinical recognition of dissecting aortic aneurysm. *Am J Med.* 1976;60:625-633.
13. Bell WR, Simon TL, DeMets DL. The clinical features of submassive and massive pulmonary emboli. *Am J Med.* 1977;62:355-360.
14. Hanley JA, Lippman-Hand A. If nothing goes wrong, is everything all right? Interpreting zero numerators. *JAMA.* 1983;249:1743-1745.
15. Newman TB. If almost nothing goes wrong, is almost everything all right? Interpreting small numerators. *JAMA.* 1995;274:1013.
16. Gudjonsson B, Livstone EM, Spiro HM. Cancer of the pancreas: diagnostic accuracy and survival statistics. *Cancer.* 1978;42:2494-2506.
17. Glasziou P, Guyatt GH, Dans LF, Straus SE, Sackett DL. Applying the results of trials and systematic reviews to patients (editorial). *ACP J Club.* 1998;129:A15-A16.
18. Walzer PD, Perl DP, Krogstad DJ, Rawson PG, Schultz MG. *Pneumocystis carinii* pneumonia in the United States: epidemiologic, diagnostic, and clinical features. *Ann Intern Med.* 1974;80:83-93.
19. Kovacs JA, Hiemenz JW, Macher AM, et al. *Pneumocystis carinii* pneumonia: a comparison between patients with the acquired immunodeficiency syndrome and patients with other immunodeficiencies. *Ann Intern Med.* 1984;100:663-671.
20. Caputo GM, Weitekamp MR, Bacon AE III, Whitener C. *Clostridium difficile* infection: a common clinical problem for the general internist. *J Gen Intern Med.* 1994;9:528-533.

Differential Diagnosis

21

Andrew Jull and Gordon Guyatt

The following Editorial Board members also made substantive contributions to this chapter: Rien de Vos, Sharon Lock, and Ania Willman.

We gratefully acknowledge the work of Scott Richardson, Mark Wilson, Jeroen Lijmer, and Deborah Cook on the original chapter that appears in the Users' Guides to the Medical Literature, *edited by Guyatt and Rennie.*

In This Chapter

Finding the Evidence

Are the Results Valid?
   Were the Right Patients Enrolled? Was the Patient Sample Representative of
      Those With the Clinical Problem?
   Was the Definitive Diagnostic Standard Appropriate? Was the Diagnostic
      Process Credible?
   For Initially Undiagnosed Patients, Was Follow-up Sufficiently Long and
      Complete?

What Are the Results?
   What Were the Diagnoses and Their Probabilities?
   How Precise Were the Estimates of Disease Probability?

How Can I Apply the Results to Patient Care?
   Are the Study Patients Similar to Those in My Clinical Setting?
   Is It Unlikely That the Disease Possibilities or Probabilities Have Changed
      Since This Evidence Was Gathered?

Clinical Scenario

A 33-Year-Old Man With Palpitations: What Is the Cause?

You are training as an emergency department nurse practitioner. Your instructor presents the following clinical scenario to you. A 33-year-old man arrives in the emergency department with heart palpitations. He describes the new onset as episodes of fast, regular chest pounding that come on gradually, last from 1 to 2 minutes, and occur several times per day. There is no relationship between symptoms and activity and no change in exercise tolerance. The patient works as a teacher and tends to have anxiety related to role demands. He has no other symptoms, no personal or family history of heart disease, and takes no medications. Physical examination reveals a regular heart rate of 90 beats per minute and normal eyes, thyroid gland, and lungs. His heart sounds also are normal, without click, murmur, or gallop, and his 12-lead electrocardiogram is normal, without arrhythmia or signs of pre-excitation. You are asked to list the likely causes of this man's palpitations.

You suspect that this patient's palpitations may be explained by anxiety, mediated by hyperventilation, and that they may be part of a panic attack. Cardiac arrhythmia and hyperthyroidism are also possibilities, although you wonder whether these disorders are common enough in this type of patient to warrant serious consideration. You reject pheochromocytoma (tumor of adrenal gland that causes excess production of adrenaline) as too unlikely to consider further. Thus, although you can identify several possible causes of palpitations, you want more information about the frequency of these causes as a basis for choosing a diagnostic workup. You ask the following question: In patients presenting with heart palpitations, what are the potential causes, and how do they guide the diagnostic workup?

FINDING THE EVIDENCE

Your computer networks with the health sciences library, where PubMed is online. In the left hand column, under "PubMed Services," you click onto "Clinical Queries," which has built-in research methodology filters. You then click on the category "diagnosis," with an emphasis on "sensitivity." In the "Enter Subject Search" field, you type in the following keywords: palpitations, causes, outcomes. On pressing "Go," you are presented with four citations, one of which explicitly addresses differential diagnosis in patients presenting with palpitations.[1] With a keystroke and a mouse click, you review the full text of the article by Weber and Kapoor.[1]

A *differential diagnosis* considers the active alternatives that can plausibly explain a patient's presentation. As clinicians learn and incorporate new information, they may modify the differential diagnosis. Two types of systematic investigations can inform the process of generating a differential diagnosis. One type of study addresses the presenting manifestations of a disease or condition (see Chapter 20, Clinical Manifestations of Disease). The second, and more important, type of study directly addresses the underlying causes of a presenting symptom, sign, or constellation of symptoms and signs. This chapter will focus on the second type of study. Table 21-1 summarizes the criteria for assessing a study about diagnostic possibilities.

Table **21-1**   Users' Guides for an Article About Differential Diagnosis

Are the Results Valid?

- Were the right patients enrolled? Was the patient sample representative of those with the clinical problem?
- Was the definitive diagnostic standard appropriate? Was the diagnostic process credible?
- For initially undiagnosed patients, was follow-up sufficiently long and complete?

What Are the Results?

- What were the diagnoses and their probabilities?
- How precise were the estimates of disease probability?

How Can I Apply the Results to Patient Care?

- Are the study patients similar to those in my clinical setting?
- Is it unlikely that the disease possibilities or probabilities have changed since this evidence was gathered?

ARE THE RESULTS VALID?

Were the Right Patients Enrolled? Was the Patient Sample Representative of Those With the Clinical Problem?

These questions address two related issues: defining the clinical problem and ensuring a representative population. First, how do the investigators define the clinical problem? The definition of the clinical problem determines the population from which the study patients should be drawn. Thus, investigators studying hematuria could include patients with microscopic and gross hematuria, with or without symptoms. Conversely, investigators studying asymptomatic, microscopic hematuria would exclude patients with symptoms or with gross hematuria. Differing definitions of a clinical problem will yield different frequencies of underlying diseases. Including patients with gross hematuria or urinary symptoms increases the frequency of acute infection as the underlying cause relative to patients without symptoms. Therefore, assessing the validity of a study about differential diagnosis begins with a search for a clear definition of the clinical problem.

Having identified the target population by first defining the clinical problem, investigators next assemble a patient sample. Ideally, the sample mirrors the target population in all important ways so the frequency of underlying diseases in the sample approximates that of the target population. A *representative* patient sample mirrors the underlying target population. The more representative a sample is, the more accurate the resulting disease probabilities will be.

Investigators seldom use the strongest method of ensuring representativeness, which is to obtain a random sample of the entire population of patients with the clinical problem. The next strongest methods are to include all patients with the clinical problem from a defined geographic area or to include a consecutive series of all patients with the clinical problem who receive care at the investigator's institution. Using a nonconsecutive case series opens the study to differential inclusion of patients with different underlying disorders or disease states and thus compromises the study's validity.

You can judge the representativeness of a sample by examining the setting from which patients are identified. Patients with ostensibly the same clinical problem can present to different clinical settings; as a result, different services see different types of patients. Typically, patients in secondary or tertiary care settings have higher proportions of more serious or uncommon diseases than do patients seen in primary care settings. For instance, in a study of patients presenting with chest pain, a higher proportion of patients from referral practices had coronary artery disease than did patients from primary care practices, even among those with similar clinical histories.[2]

To evaluate representativeness further, you can note how patients were identified, what measures were used to avoid missing patients, and which patients were included and excluded. The wider is the spectrum of patients in a sample, the more representative the sample should be of the whole population, and the more valid the results will be. For example, in a study of *Clostridium difficile* colitis in 609 patients with diarrhea, the sample comprised adult inpatients whose diarrheal stools were tested for cytotoxin, an approach that excluded patients whose clinicians chose not to perform this test.[3] Inclusion of only patients who had cytotoxin testing of stools is likely to increase the probability of *C. difficile* infection in relation to the entire population of patients with diarrhea.

Was the Definitive Diagnostic Standard Appropriate? Was the Diagnostic Process Credible?

An article about differential diagnosis will provide valid evidence only if the investigators arrive at a correct final diagnosis. To do so, they must develop and apply explicit criteria for assigning a final diagnosis to each patient. The criteria should include not only findings needed to confirm each diagnosis, but also findings useful for rejecting each diagnosis. For example, published diagnostic criteria for group A streptococcal pharyngitis include criteria for verifying the infection and criteria for rejecting it.[4,5] Investigators can then classify patients into diagnostic groups that are mutually exclusive, with the exception of patients whose symptoms stem from more than one etiologic factor. This approach allows clinicians to understand which diagnoses remain possible for any patients whose conditions are undiagnosed.

Diagnostic criteria should include a search that is sufficiently comprehensive to ensure detection of all important causes of the clinical problem. The more comprehensive the investigation is, the smaller the chance that investigators will reach invalid conclusions about disease frequency. For example, a retrospective study of stroke in 127 patients with mental status changes failed to include a comprehensive search for all causes of delirium, and 118 cases remained unexplained.[6] Because the investigators did not describe a complete and systematic search for causes of delirium, the disease probabilities appear less credible.

The goal of developing and applying explicit, credible criteria is to ensure a reproducible diagnosis, and the ultimate test of reproducibility is a formal evaluation of agreement.

Your confidence in a study's findings will increase if investigators formally demonstrate the extent to which they achieved agreement in diagnosis. In a study by Kroenke and colleagues,[7] all study patients underwent a comprehensive assessment of their dizziness, including a history, physical examination, neuro-ophthalmologist examination, health status measurement, psychiatric assessment, and laboratory tests. All data for each patient were abstracted onto a standard form, and these data abstract forms were independently reviewed by three investigators: a general internist, a neurologist, and a neuro-ophthalmologist. Each recorded their opinion about the primary cause of a patient's dizziness. Disagreements were discussed, and a final cause was determined by consensus. The overall kappa of 0.39 approached only moderate agreement. Agreement was best for vertigo (0.52), followed by agreement for psychiatric disorders (0.42), presyncope (0.41), disequilibrium (0.31), and unknown cause (-0.06) (see Chapter 30, Measuring Agreement Beyond Chance). Raters tended to have diagnostic preferences, with the neurologist diagnosing vertigo more often than the other two raters, the neuro-ophthalmologist diagnosing presyncope more often, and the general internist diagnosing psychiatric disorders more frequently. The investigators concluded that multiple raters and a consensus process should be used in studies of diagnostic possibilities to counterbalance diagnostic biases.

When reviewing diagnostic criteria, keep in mind that "lesion finding" is not necessarily the same as "illness explaining." In other words, by using explicit and credible criteria, investigators may find that patients have two or more disorders that could explain the clinical problem, and this can cause some doubt about which disorder is the culprit. Better studies of disease probability include some assurance that the disorders found actually did account for the patients' illnesses. For example, in a sequence of studies of syncope, investigators required that the symptoms occur simultaneously with an arrhythmia before that arrhythmia was judged to be the cause.[8] In a study of chronic cough, investigators gave cause-specific therapy and used positive responses to this therapy to strengthen the case that these disorders actually caused the chronic cough.[9]

Explicit diagnostic criteria are of little use unless they are applied consistently. This does not mean that every patient must undergo every test. Instead, for many clinical problems, a clinician can take a detailed, focused history and perform a problem-oriented physical examination of the involved organ systems, along with a few initial tests. Then, depending on the diagnostic clues from this information, further inquiry will proceed down one of several branching pathways. Ideally, investigators would evaluate all patients with the same initial workup and then follow the clues using prespecified testing sequences. Once a definitive test result confirms a final diagnosis, further confirmatory testing is unnecessary and costly. It is also unethical because it may delay treatment and cause unnecessary discomfort.

It may be easier to judge whether patients' illnesses have been well investigated when investigators prospectively evaluate patients using a predetermined diagnostic approach than when they use an unstandardized approach. For example, in a study of precipitating factors in 101 patients with symptomatic heart failure, although all patients had a history and physical examination, subsequent testing was not standardized, making it difficult to judge the accuracy of the disease probabilities.[10]

For Initially Undiagnosed Patients, Was Follow-up Sufficiently Long and Complete?

Even when investigators consistently apply explicit and comprehensive diagnostic criteria, some patients' clinical problems may remain unexplained. The higher the number of undiagnosed patients, the greater is the chance of error in the estimates of disease probability. For example, in a retrospective study of various causes of dizziness in 1194 patients in an otolaryngology clinic, about 27% were not assigned a diagnosis.[11] With more than one quarter of patients' illnesses unexplained, the disease probabilities for the overall sample could be inaccurate.

If the study evaluation leaves patients' conditions undiagnosed, investigators can follow up these patients and search for additional clues leading to eventual diagnoses and observe the prognosis. The longer and more complete this follow-up is, the greater will be our confidence in the benign nature of the condition in patients whose illnesses remain undiagnosed yet who are unharmed at the end of the study. How long is long enough? No single answer applies to all clinical problems, but we suggest 1 to 6 months for acute and self-limited symptoms and 1 to 5 years for chronically recurring or progressive symptoms. For example, in a study of nonacute abdominal complaints in family practice, 933 patients were followed-up for at least 1 year (mean, 18 months) before a final diagnosis was assigned.[12]

USING THE GUIDE

Weber and Kapoor[1] defined palpitations broadly as any one of several patient complaints (e.g., fast heartbeat, skipped heartbeats) and included patients with new and recurring palpitations. The investigators identified patients from three clinical settings (an emergency department, inpatient floors, and a medical clinic) in a university medical center in a mid-sized North American city. Of 229 adult patients presenting consecutively for care of palpitations, 39 refused participation; the investigators included the remaining 190 patients, including 62 from the emergency department. No important subgroups appear to have been excluded, so the sample likely represents the full spectrum of patients presenting with palpitations.

The investigators developed a priori, explicit, and credible criteria for confirming each possible disorder that caused palpitations and listed their criteria in an appendix, along with supporting citations. They evaluated patients prospectively and assigned final diagnoses based on structured interviews completed by one of the investigators and the combined diagnostic evaluation (i.e., history, examination, and testing) chosen by the individual physician who saw the patient at the index visit. In addition, all patients completed self-administered questionnaires designed to assist in detecting various psychiatric disorders. Electrocardiograms were obtained in most patients (166 of 190), and many patients had other testing for cardiac disease as well. When relevant, the investigators required that the palpitations occurred at the same time as the arrhythmias before they would attribute the symptoms to that arrhythmia. However, the investigators did not report on agreement for the ultimate decisions about the diagnoses attributed to each patient.

Thus, the diagnostic workup was reasonably comprehensive—although not exhaustive—for common disease categories. Because subsequent tests ordered by individual physicians were not fully standardized, some inconsistency may have been introduced, although it does not appear likely to have distorted the probabilities of common disease categories such as psychiatric or cardiac causes.

Weber and Kapoor[1] identified a diagnosable cause of palpitations in all but 31 (16.3%) of 190 patients. The investigators followed up 96% of patients for at least 1 year, during which time an additional diagnosis (symptomatic correlation with ventricular premature beats) was made in patients with initially undiagnosed conditions. None of the 31 patients with undiagnosed conditions had a stroke or died.

WHAT ARE THE RESULTS?

What Were the Diagnoses and Their Probabilities?

In many studies of disease probability, the authors display the main results in a table listing the diagnoses made and the numbers and percentages of patients with those diagnoses. For some symptoms, patients may have more than one underlying disease coexisting with and, presumably, contributing to the clinical problem. In these situations, authors often identify the major diagnosis for such patients and separately tabulate contributing causes. Alternatively, authors sometimes identify a separate, multiple-etiology group.

How Precise Were the Estimates of Disease Probability?

Even when valid, disease probabilities are only estimates of the true frequencies. You can examine the precision of these estimates using the confidence intervals (CIs) presented by the authors. If the authors do not report them, you can calculate them yourself by using the following formula:

$$95\% \text{ CI} = P \pm 1.96 \times \sqrt{(P\{1-P\}/n)}$$

where P is the proportion of patients with the cause of interest and n is the number of patients in the sample. This formula becomes inaccurate when the number of cases is five or fewer, and approximations are available for such situations.[13,14]

For instance, consider the study by Weber and Kapoor in which 58 patients (31%) were diagnosed with psychiatric causes of palpitations.[1] Using the formula, we would start with $P = 0.31$, $(1 - P) = 0.69$, and n = 190. Working through the arithmetic, we find the CI to be 0.31 ± 0.07. Thus, although the most likely true proportion is 31%, it may range from 24% (31% – 7%) to 38% (31% + 7%).

Whether you deem the CIs sufficiently precise depends on where the estimated proportion and CIs fall in relation to your test or treatment thresholds (see Chapter 6, Diagnosis). If both the estimated proportion and the entire 95% CI are on the same side of your threshold, the result will be precise enough to permit firm conclusions about disease probability for use in planning tests or treatments. Conversely, if the confidence interval around the estimate crosses your threshold, the result may not be precise enough for definitive conclusions about disease probability. You may still use a valid but imprecise probability result, but keep in mind the uncertainty and its implications for testing or treatment.

USING THE GUIDE

In the study by Weber and Kapoor,[1] 58 patients (31%) were diagnosed with psychiatric causes, 82 (43%) had cardiac disorders, five (2.6%) had thyrotoxicosis, and none had pheochromocytoma. This distribution differed across clinical settings. For instance, cardiac disorders were more than twice as likely to occur in patients presenting to the emergency department than in patients presenting to the outpatient clinic.

The investigators did not provide the 95% CIs for the probabilities they found. However, as illustrated, if you are concerned about how close the probabilities are to your thresholds, you can calculate the 95% CIs.

HOW CAN I APPLY THE RESULTS TO PATIENT CARE?

Are the Study Patients Similar to Those in My Clinical Setting?

As mentioned previously, we suggest that you ask yourself whether the setting and patients are so different from your own that you should disregard the results.[15] For instance, consider whether the patients in your clinical setting come from areas where one or more of the underlying disorders are endemic, a factor that could result in higher frequencies of disorders in your setting than were found in the study.

Is It Unlikely That the Disease Possibilities or Probabilities Have Changed Since This Evidence Was Gathered?

As time passes, evidence about disease frequencies can become obsolete. Old diseases can be controlled or even eradicated. New diseases and new epidemics of disease can arise. Such events can so alter the spectrum of possible diseases or their likelihood that previously valid and applicable studies may lose their relevance. For example, the emergence of human immunodeficiency virus dramatically transformed the list of diagnostic possibilities for such clinical problems as generalized lymphadenopathy, chronic diarrhea, and unexplained weight loss. More recently, severe acute respiratory syndrome has been added to the list of potential diagnoses for a traveler arriving with a fever of more than 38° C and a dry cough.

Similar changes can occur as the result of progress in medical science or public health. For instance, in studies of fever of unknown origin, newer diagnostic technologies have substantially altered the proportions of patients who are found to have malignancy or whose fevers remain unexplained.[16-18] Treatment advances that improve survival, such as chemotherapy for childhood leukemia, can bring about shifts in disease likelihood because the treatment may cause complications, such as secondary malignant disease, years after the initial disease is cured. Public health measures that control such diseases as cholera can alter the likelihood of the remaining causes of the clinical problems that the disease would have caused—in this example, acute diarrhea.

USING THE GUIDE

Weber and Kapoor[1] recruited 190 patients with palpitations from those presenting to outpatient clinics, inpatient medical and surgical services, and an emergency department (62 patients) in a university medical center in a mid-sized North American city. Thus, the study patients are likely to be similar to the patients seen in your hospital emergency department, and you can use the study results to help inform the pretest probabilities for the presenting patient.

Considering the results reported in the study, you know of no new developments likely to cause a change in the spectrum or probabilities of disease in patients with palpitations.

CLINICAL RESOLUTION

Considering the possible causes of the patient's palpitations, your leading hypothesis is that acute anxiety is the cause. However, you do not believe that the diagnosis of anxiety is so certain that you can rule out other disorders (i.e., the pretest probability is below your threshold for treatment without testing). See Chapter 6, Diagnosis, for a discussion of pretest probabilities. After reviewing the study on palpitations by Weber and Kapoor,[1] you decide to include in your list of active alternatives cardiac arrhythmias (common, serious, and treatable) and hyperthyroidism (less common but serious and treatable), and you suggest testing to exclude these disorders (i.e., these alternatives are above your threshold for treatment without testing). Finally, given that none of the 190 study patients had pheochromocytoma, and because the presenting patient has none of the other clinical features of this disorder, you place it into your "other hypotheses" category (i.e., below your test threshold), which would delay testing for this condition.

REFERENCES

1. Weber BE, Kapoor WN. Evaluation and outcomes of patients with palpitations. *Am J Med*. 1996;100:138-148.
2. Sox HC, Hickam DH, Marton KI, et al. Using the patient's history to estimate the probability of coronary artery disease: a comparison of primary care and referral practices. *Am J Med*. 1990;89:7-14.
3. Katz DA, Bates DW, Rittenberg E, et al. Predicting *Clostridium difficile* stool cytotoxin results in hospitalized patients with diarrhea. *J Gen Intern Med*. 1997;12:57-62.
4. McIsaac WJ, White D, Tannenbaum D, Low DE. A clinical score to reduce unnecessary antibiotic use in patients with sore throat. *CMAJ*. 1998;158:75-83.

5. McIsaac WJ, Goel V, To T, Low DE. The validity of a sore throat score in family practice. *CMAJ.* 2000;163:811-815.

6. Benbadis SR, Sila CA, Cristea RL. Mental status changes and stroke. *J Gen Intern Med.* 1994;9:485-487.

7. Kroenke K, Lucas CA, Rosenberg ML, et al. Causes of persistent dizziness: a prospective study of 100 patients in ambulatory care. *Ann Intern Med.* 1992;117:898-904.

8. Kapoor WN. Evaluation and outcome of patients with syncope. *Medicine (Baltimore).* 1990;69:160-175.

9. Pratter MR, Bartter T, Akers S, et al. An algorithmic approach to chronic cough. *Ann Intern Med.* 1993;119:977-983.

10. Ghali JK, Kadakia S, Cooper R, Ferlinz J. Precipitating factors leading to decompensation of heart failure: traits among urban blacks. *Arch Intern Med.* 1988;148:2013-2016.

11. Katsarkas A. Dizziness in aging: a retrospective study of 1194 cases. *Otolaryngol Head Neck Surg.* 1994;110:296-301.

12. Muris JW, Starmans R, Fijten GH, Crebolder HFJM, Schouten HJA, Knotterus JA. Non-acute abdominal complaints in general practice: diagnostic value of signs and symptoms. *Br J Gen Pract.* 1995;45:313-316.

13. Hanley JA, Lippman-Hand A. If nothing goes wrong, is everything all right? Interpreting zero numerators. *JAMA.* 1983;249:1743–1745.

14. Newman TB. If almost nothing goes wrong, is almost everything all right? Interpreting small numerators. *JAMA.* 1995;274:1013.

15. Glasziou P, Guyatt GH, Dans AL, Dans LF, Straus SE, Sackett DL. Applying the results of trials and systematic reviews to individual patients (editorial). *ACP J Club.* 1998;129:A15-A16.

16. Petersdorf RG, Beeson PB. Fever of unexplained origin: report on 100 cases. *Medicine (Baltimore).* 1961;40:1–30.

17. Larson EB, Featherstone HJ, Petersdorf RG. Fever of undetermined origin: diagnosis and follow up of 105 cases, 1970-1980. *Medicine (Baltimore).* 1982;61:269-292.

18. Knockaert DC, Vanneste LJ, Vanneste SB, Bobbaers HJ. Fever of unknown origin in the 1980s: an update of the diagnostic spectrum. *Arch Intern Med.* 1992;152:51-55.

Clinical Prediction Rules

22

Andrew Jull, Alba DiCenso, and Gordon Guyatt

The following Editorial Board members also made substantive contributions to this chapter: Rien de Vos and Mary van Soeren.

We gratefully acknowledge the work of Thomas McGinn, Peter Wyer, David Naylor, and Ian Stiell on the original chapter that appears in the Users' Guides to the Medical Literature, *edited by Guyatt and Rennie.*

In This Chapter

Clinical Prediction Rules

Developing a Clinical Prediction Rule

Validation

Interpreting the Results

Testing the Rule's Impact

CLINICAL SCENARIO

Can a Clinical Prediction Rule Reduce Unnecessary Ankle Radiographs?

You are a nurse educator responsible for the continuing nursing education program for nurse practitioners in outpost settings. You have been conducting a series on how to best use research evidence to guide practice. The nurse practitioners are interested in strategies that minimize the need to send patients out for consultations and diagnostic tests because of the associated inconvenience to patients and costs to the health care system. Some of the nurses are using clinical prediction guides to assist with this process, but they are not confident in their ability to identify high-quality clinical prediction guides. In planning your education session, you decide to identify a clinical prediction guide that is relevant to nurse practitioners and has been shown to be useful. From your own clinical practice, you are familiar with the Ottawa ankle rules (Figure 22-1), and you recently came across a systematic review on the accuracy of these rules in *BMJ*.[1] You have a careful look at the review and are confident that it is methodologically sound. The review concludes that this clinical prediction rule is accurate for excluding fractures of the ankle and midfoot. The clinical prediction rule has a sensitivity of almost 100% and modest specificity. The authors estimated that use of the Ottawa ankle rules would reduce the number of unnecessary radiographs by 30% to 40%. You decide to search for the original studies on the development and validation of the Ottawa ankle rules to help illustrate the criteria for evaluating clinical prediction rules. In the systematic review, you find references to the original articles that described the development of the Ottawa ankle rules in 1992[2] and their validation.[3]

This chapter outlines the criteria for deciding on the strength of inferences you can make about the accuracy and impact of clinical prediction rules. Examples of clinical prediction rules of interest to nurses include an antenatal index to predict postpartum depression,[4] a risk assessment tool (STRATIFY) to predict which elderly inpatients will fall,[5] a prediction rule to identify patients in whom venous leg ulcers will heal with limb compression bandages,[6] and a risk index to predict, at the point of initial triage, mortality at 30 days in patients with ST-elevation myocardial infarction.[7]

CLINICAL PREDICTION RULES

Establishing a patient's diagnosis and determining the prognosis are closely linked activities. Diagnoses and assessments of patients' prognoses often determine the recommendations we make to patients. Clinical experience provides us with an intuitive sense of which findings on history, physical examination, and laboratory or radiologic investigation are critical in making an accurate diagnosis or assessment of a patient's prognosis. Although intuition can often be extraordinarily accurate, it can also be misleading. Clinical prediction rules attempt to test, simplify, and increase the accuracy of clinicians' diagnostic and prognostic assessments.

A *clinical prediction rule* can be defined as a clinical tool that quantifies the individual contributions of various components of the history, physical examination, and basic laboratory results toward the diagnosis, prognosis, or likely response to treatment of

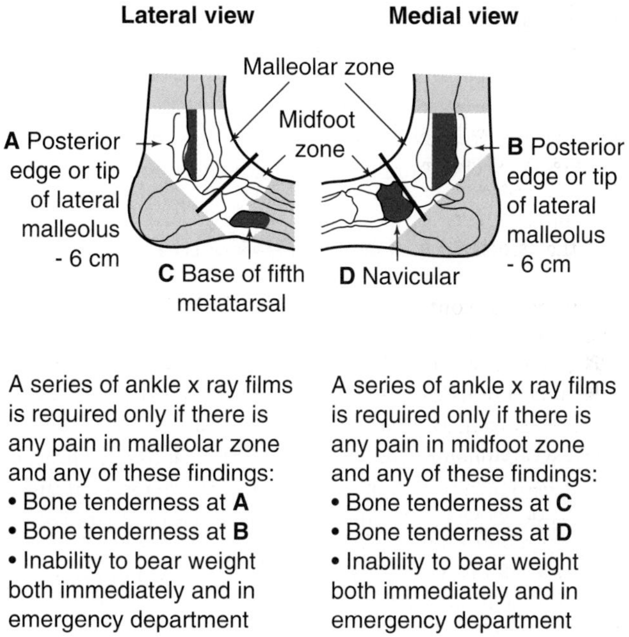

Lateral view   **Medial view**

A Posterior edge or tip of lateral malleolus - 6 cm

B Posterior edge or tip of lateral malleolus - 6 cm

C Base of fifth metatarsal

D Navicular

Malleolar zone

Midfoot zone

A series of ankle x ray films is required only if there is any pain in malleolar zone and any of these findings:
• Bone tenderness at **A**
• Bone tenderness at **B**
• Inability to bear weight both immediately and in emergency department

A series of ankle x ray films is required only if there is any pain in midfoot zone and any of these findings:
• Bone tenderness at **C**
• Bone tenderness at **D**
• Inability to bear weight both immediately and in emergency department

Figure 22-1. Ottawa ankle rules. *(Modified and reproduced with permission of the BMJ Publishing Group from Bachmann LM, Kolb E, Koller MT, Steurer J, ter Riet G. Accuracy of Ottawa ankle rules to exclude fractures of the ankle and mid-foot: systematic review.* BMJ. *2003;326:417.)*

individual patients.[8] This definition also applies to what have been called clinical prediction guides and clinical decision rules.

Prediction implies helping clinicians to determine a future clinical event more accurately. *Decision* implies directing clinicians to a specific course of action. As you will see, application of clinical prediction rules sometimes results in a decision and other times in a prediction. It can also result in a probability or likelihood ratio (LR) that a clinician can apply to a current diagnostic problem. In this last application, the term *clinical diagnosis rule* or *clinical diagnosis guide* may be more accurate. We use the term *clinical prediction rule* regardless of whether the output of the rule is a suggested clinical course of action, the probability of a future event, or an increase or decrease in the likelihood of a particular diagnosis.

Whatever the clinical prediction rule generates—a decision, a prediction, or a change in diagnostic probability—it is most likely to be useful when decision making is complex, the clinical stakes are high, or opportunities exist to achieve cost savings without compromising patient care.

Developing and testing a clinical prediction rule involves three steps: (1) creation or derivation of the rule, (2) testing or validation of the rule, and (3) assessment of the impact of the rule on clinical behavior—the *impact analysis.* The validation process may require several studies to test the accuracy of the rule fully at different clinical sites

(Figure 22-2). Each step in the development of a clinical prediction rule may be published separately by different authors, or all three steps may be included in one article. Table 22-1 presents a hierarchy of evidence that can guide clinicians in assessing the full range of evidence supporting the use of a clinical prediction rule in their practice. We now review the steps in the development and testing of a clinical prediction rule and relate each stage of the process to the hierarchy of evidence presented in Table 22-1.

DEVELOPING A CLINICAL PREDICTION RULE

The development of the Ottawa ankle rules was described in an article by Stiell and colleagues that was published in 1992.[2] Developers of clinical prediction rules begin by constructing a list of potential predictors of the outcome of interest—in this case, ankle fractures demonstrated on ankle radiograph. The list typically includes items from the history, physical examination, and basic laboratory tests. The investigators then examine a group of patients and determine (1) whether the candidate clinical predictors are present and (2) each patient's status on the outcome of interest—in this case, the result of the ankle radiograph. Statistical analysis reveals which predictors are most powerful and which predictors can be omitted from the rule without loss of predictive power. Typically, the statistical techniques used in this process are based on *logistic regression* (see Chapter 31, Regression and Correlation). Other techniques include *discriminant analysis*, which produces equations similar to regression analysis[9]; *recursive partitioning analysis*, which divides the patient population into smaller and smaller groups based on discriminating risk factors[10]; and *artificial neural networks*, which apply non-linear statistics to pattern recognition problems.[11]

Clinical prediction rules that have been derived but not validated should not be considered ready for clinical application (see Table 22-1). Although these rules have predicted the outcome in one sample, it does not necessarily mean that they will predict the outcome in another sample or in the same sample when applied by clinicians in

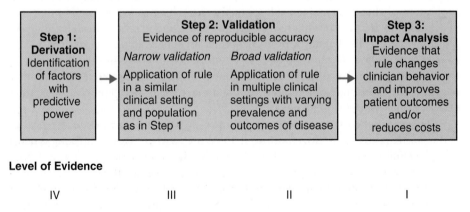

Level of Evidence

IV	III	II	I

Figure 22-2. Development and testing of a clinical prediction rule.

Table **22-1**   Hierarchy of Evidence for Clinical Prediction Rules

Level IV: **Rules that need further evaluation before they can be applied clinically**

These rules have been derived but not validated or have been validated only in split samples, large retrospective databases, or by means of statistical techniques.

Level III: **Rules that clinicians may consider using with caution and only if patients in the study are similar to those in their clinical setting**

These rules have been validated in only one narrow prospective sample.

Level II: **Rules that can be used in various settings with confidence in their accuracy**

At this level, rules must have demonstrated accuracy either by one large prospective study including a broad spectrum of patients and clinicians or by validation in several smaller settings that differ from one another.

Level I: **Rules that can be used in a wide variety of settings with confidence that they can change clinician behavior and improve patient outcomes**

At this level, rules must have at least one prospective validation in a different population plus one impact analysis, along with a demonstration of change in clinician behavior with beneficial consequences.

practice. However, investigators interested in validating a clinical prediction rule first need to determine whether the derivation process has been well done and whether the rule meets certain criteria. Table 22-2 summarizes criteria for determining whether the derivation process was well done. Interested readers can find a complete discussion of the derivation process and criteria for assessing the process in an article by Laupacis and colleagues.[8]

VALIDATION

There are three reasons that even rigorously derived clinical prediction rules are not ready for application in clinical practice without further validation. First, prediction rules derived from one set of patients may reflect associations between given predictors and outcomes that occur primarily because of the play of chance. If that is so, a different set of predictors will emerge in a different group of patients, even if these patients come from the same setting. Second, predictors may be idiosyncratic to the population, the clinicians using the rule, or other aspects of study design. If that is so, the rule may fail in different settings. Finally, because of problems with the feasibility of rule application in clinical settings, clinicians may fail to implement a rule comprehensively or accurately. The result would be that a rule succeeds in theory but fails in practice.

Table **22-2** Methodological Standards for Derivation of a Clinical
Prediction Rule

- Were all important predictors included in the derivation process?
- Were all important predictors present in a significant proportion of the study
  population?
- Were the outcome event and predictors clearly defined?
- Were those assessing the outcome event blinded to the presence of the
  predictors, and were those assessing the presence of predictors blinded to the
  outcome event?
- Was the sample size adequate (including an adequate number of outcome
  events)?
- Does the rule make clinical sense?

Statistical methods can deal with the first of these problems. For instance, investigators can split a population into two groups and use one to develop the rule and the other to test it. Alternatively, investigators can use more sophisticated statistical methods built on the same logic. Conceptually, these approaches involve removing one patient from the sample, generating the rule using the remainder of patients, and testing the rule on the patient who was removed from the sample. One repeats this procedure, sometimes referred to as a *bootstrap technique*, in sequence for every patient under study.

Although statistical validations within the same setting or group of patients reduce the likelihood that the rule reflects the play of chance rather than true associations, they fail to address the other two threats to validity. The success of a clinical prediction rule may be peculiar to the particular populations of patients and clinicians involved in the derivation study. Even if this is not so, clinicians may have difficulties using the rule in practice, compromising its predictive power. Thus, to ascend from level IV in our hierarchy of evidence, studies must test the use of the rule by clinicians in clinical practice.

A clinical prediction rule developed to predict serious outcomes (e.g., heart failure or ventricular arrhythmia) in patients with syncope highlights the importance of validation.[12] Investigators derived the rule using data from 252 patients who presented to an emergency department; subsequently, the investigators attempted to validate it prospectively in a sample of 374 patients. The prediction rule assigned patients a score from 0 to 4, depending on the number of clinical predictors present. The probability of poor outcomes corresponding to almost every score in the derivation set was approximately twice that of the validation set. For example, in the derivation set, the risk of a poor outcome in a patient with a score of 3 was estimated to be 52%. By contrast, a patient with the same score in the validation set had a probability of a poor outcome of only 27%. This variation in results may have been caused by differences in the severity of syncope cases in the two studies or differences in criteria for generating a score of 3. Because there is a risk that a clinical prediction rule will provide misleading information when applied in real-world clinical settings, rules that have been developed but not validated are designated as level IV in our hierarchy (see Table 22-1).

Despite this major limitation, clinicians can still extract clinically relevant messages from an article describing the development of a clinical prediction rule. Clinicians can identify the most important predictors and consider them more carefully in their own practice. They can also consider giving less importance to variables that failed to show predictive power. For instance, in developing a clinical prediction rule to predict mortality from pneumonia, investigators found that the white blood cell count had no bearing on subsequent mortality.[13] Hence, clinicians could put less weight on the white blood cell count when they make decisions about admitting patients with pneumonia to hospital.

To move up the hierarchy, clinical prediction rules must provide additional evidence of validity. After developing the Ottawa ankle rules, Stiell and colleagues refined and prospectively validated them.[3] Validation of a clinical prediction rule involves demonstrating that its repeated application as part of the process of clinical care leads to the same results. Ideally, validation entails application of the rule prospectively in a new population with a prevalence and spectrum of disease that differ from those of patients in the derivation set. It is important to be sure that a clinical prediction rule performs similarly in different populations and with different clinicians who work in numerous institutions. It is also important to be sure that it works well when clinicians consciously apply it as a rule, rather than as a statistical derivation from a large number of potential predictors.

If the setting in which a prediction rule was originally developed was limited and its validation was confined to this setting, application by clinicians in other settings will be less secure. Validation in a similar setting can take several forms. Most simply, after developing the prediction rule, the investigators return to their population, identify a new sample of patients, and test the rule's performance. Thus, we classify rules that have been validated in the same— or very similar—limited or narrow population as was used in the development phase as level III on our hierarchy, and we recommend that clinicians use the result cautiously (see Table 22-1). If patients in the derivation set are from a sufficiently heterogeneous population across various institutions, testing the rule in the same population provides strong validation. Validation in a new population provides clinicians with strong inferences about the usefulness of the rule, corresponding to level II in our hierarchy (see Table 22-1). The more numerous and diverse the settings in which the rule is tested and found to be accurate, the more likely it is that it will generalize to untested settings.[14]

The Ottawa ankle rules were derived in two large, university-based emergency departments in Ottawa, Canada[2] and then prospectively validated in a large sample of patients from the same emergency departments.[3] At this stage, the rules would be classified as level II in our hierarchy because of the large number and diversity of patients and physicians involved in the study. Since that initial validation, the rules have been validated in many different clinical settings, with relatively consistent results.[1] This evidence further strengthens our inference about its predictive power.

Many clinical prediction rules are derived and then validated in a small, narrowly selected group of patients (level III). One such rule was derived to predict preserved left ventricular function after myocardial infarction.[15] The initial derivation and validation were performed on 314 patients who had been admitted to a tertiary care center. The prediction rule was derived using 162 patients and then validated using 152 patients in the same setting. When the rule predicted that left ventricular function had been preserved, this was, in fact, true in 99% of patients. At this stage in the rule development, the rule would be considered to be level III, to be used only in settings similar to those of the validation study (i.e., in similar cardiac care units). The rule was further validated in two larger trials, one involving 213 patients[16] from one site and a larger trial involving 1891 patients from several different institutions.[17] In both settings, of patients predicted to have preserved left ventricular function, 11% actually had abnormal left ventricular function. This drop in accuracy changes the potential use and implications of the rule in clinical practice. At this point in development, the rule would be designated as level II, meaning that the rule could be used in clinical settings with a high degree of confidence, but with adjusted results. This example highlights the importance of validating a clinical prediction rule on a diverse patient population before applying it broadly.

Regardless of whether investigators validated a rule in a similar, narrow (level III) population or a broad, heterogeneous, or different (level II) population, the results allow stronger inferences if the investigators adhered to certain methodological standards (Table 22-3). Interested readers can find a complete discussion of the validation process and criteria for assessing this process in an article by Laupacis and colleagues.[8]

If investigators evaluating predictor status of study patients are aware of the outcome, or if those assessing the outcome are aware of patients' status with respect to predictors, the assessments may be biased. For instance, in a clinical prediction rule developed to predict the presence of pneumonia in patients presenting with cough,[18] the authors did not mention blinding during either the derivation process or the validation process. Knowledge of history or physical examination findings could have influenced the judgments of the unblinded radiologists.

The investigators testing the Ottawa ankle rules enrolled consecutive patients, obtained radiographs for all of them, and ensured that clinicians assessing the clinical predictors were unaware of the radiologic results and that radiologists assessing ankle fractures had no knowledge of the clinical data.

INTERPRETING THE RESULTS

Regardless of the level of evidence associated with a clinical prediction rule, its usefulness depends on its predictive power. Investigators may report their results in various ways. First, the results may dictate a specific course of action. The ankle component of the

Table **22-3**   Methodological Standards for Validation of a Clinical
Prediction Rule

- Were the patients chosen in an unbiased fashion, and do they represent a wide spectrum of severity of disease?
- Was there a blinded assessment of the criterion standard for all patients?
- Was there an explicit and accurate interpretation of the predictor variables and the actual rule without knowledge of the outcome?
- Was there 100% follow-up of those enrolled?

Ottawa ankle rules states that an ankle series of radiographs is indicated only for patients with pain near the malleoli plus either localized bone tenderness at the posterior edge or tip of either malleolus or inability to bear weight (see Figure 22-1). Underlying this decision are the sensitivity and specificity of the rule as a diagnostic test (see Chapter 6, Diagnosis). In the development process, all patients with fractures had a positive result (sensitivity of 100%), but only 40% of those without fractures had a negative result (specificity of 40%).[2] These results suggest that if clinicians order radiographs only for patients with a positive result, they will not miss any fractures and will avoid the test in 40% of patients without a fracture.

The validation study confirmed these results;[3] in particular, the test maintained a sensitivity of 100%. This is particularly reassuring because the sample size was sufficiently large to result in a narrow confidence interval (CI) around the estimate of sensitivity (95% CI, 93% to 100%). Thus, clinicians adopting the rule would miss very few, if any, fractures.

Another way of reporting clinical prediction rule results is in terms of probability of the target condition being present given a particular result. For example, a prediction rule for pulmonary embolus derived and validated by Wells and colleagues[19] accurately placed patients into low (3.4%; 95% CI, 2.2% to 5%), intermediate (28%; 95% CI, 23.4% to 32.2%), or high (78%; 95% CI, 69.2% to 89.6%) probability categories. When investigators report prediction rule results in this fashion, they are implicitly incorporating all clinical information. In doing so, they remove the need for clinicians to consider independent information when deciding about the likelihood of a diagnosis or about a patient's prognosis.

Finally, prediction rules may report their results as likelihood ratios (LRs) or as absolute or relative risks. For example, the CAGE (Cut down, Annoyed, Guilty, Eye-opener), a prediction rule for detecting alcoholism, has been reported as likelihood ratios (e.g., for a CAGE score of 0/4, LR = 0.14; for a score of 1/4, LR = 1.5; for a score of 2/4, LR = 4.5; for a score of 3/4, LR = 13; and for a score of 4/4, LR = 100). To interpret these data, remember that likelihood ratios greater than 1.0 increase the probability that the target condition (i.e., alcoholism) is present, and the greater is the likelihood ratio, the greater is the increase in probability. Likelihood ratios less than 1.0 decrease the probability that the target condition is present, and the smaller is the likelihood ratio, the greater is the decrease in probability. In this example, the probability of alcoholism depends on a combination of the prevalence of alcoholism in the community and score on the CAGE prediction rule.[20] When investigators report their results as likelihood ratios, they are implicitly suggesting that clinicians should use other, independent information to generate a pretest (or prerule) probability. Clinicians can then use the likelihood ratios generated by the rule to establish a posttest probability. (For approaches to using likelihood ratios, see Chapter 6, Diagnosis.)

TESTING THE RULE'S IMPACT

Given that the Ottawa ankle rules were developed in 1992, numerous studies have been conducted to examine their impact. The systematic review identified at the beginning of this chapter[1] included 32 studies that investigated the accuracy of the Ottawa ankle rules. Meta-analysis included 27 studies (reporting on 15,581 patients) that had prospective data collection and blinded assessment of radiographs. The clinical prediction rules had a sensitivity of almost 100%, a modest specificity (median of 31.5%), and a pooled LR for a negative result of the ankle rule of 0.08 (95% CI, 0.03 to 0.18).

This review tells us about the accuracy of the rule. However, demonstration of accuracy is insufficient to warrant a confident recommendation for use of the rule in clinical practice. Use of clinical prediction rules involves remembering predictor variables and often entails making calculations to determine a patient's probability of having the target outcome. Pocket cards and computer algorithms can facilitate the task of using complex clinical prediction rules. Nonetheless, they demand time and energy, and their use is warranted only if they change clinicians' behavior and only if that behavior change results in improved patient outcomes or reduced costs while maintaining quality. If these conditions are not met, attempts to use a clinical prediction rule systematically will be a waste of time, regardless of its accuracy.

An accurate prediction rule may not change behavior or improve outcomes for several reasons. First, clinicians' intuitive estimation of probabilities may be as good as, if not better than, the rule. If this is so, use of a clinical prediction rule will not improve their practice. Second, clinicians may not use the rule because the calculations involved are cumbersome. Even worse, they could make errors in the calculations. Third, practical barriers could impede acting on the results of the clinical prediction rule. For instance, in the case of the Ottawa ankle rules, clinicians may be sufficiently concerned about protecting themselves against litigation that they may order radiographs despite a prediction rule result suggesting a negligible probability of fracture. These considerations lead us to classify a clinical prediction rule with evidence of accuracy in diverse populations as level II and to insist on a positive result from a study of impact before the rule ascends to level I.

Ideally, an impact study would randomize patients or larger administrative units to apply or not apply the clinical prediction rule and would follow up patients for all relevant outcomes (including quality of life, morbidity, and resource utilization). Randomization of individual patients is unlikely to be appropriate because one would expect participating clinicians to incorporate the rule into the care of all patients. A suitable alternative is to randomize institutions or practice settings and conduct analyses appropriate to these larger units of randomization. Another potential design is to assess the outcomes of a single group before and after clinicians begin to use the clinical prediction rule, but the choice of a before/after study substantially reduces the strength of inference.

With respect to the Ottawa ankle rules, investigators conducted a randomized trial to examine outcomes associated with application of the decision rules. Six emergency departments were randomized to use or not use the decision rules.[21] One center dropped out before the study began, leaving a total of five emergency departments: two in the intervention group and three in the usual-care group. The intervention consisted of the following: (1) introducing the prediction rules at a general meeting, (2) distributing pocket cards summarizing the rules, (3) posting the rules throughout the emergency department, and (4) applying preprinted data collection forms to each patient chart. In the control group, the only intervention was the introduction of preprinted data collection forms without the Ottawa rules attached to each chart. The investigators entered a total of 1911 eligible patients into the study, 1005 in the control group and 906 in the intervention group. There were 691 radiographs requested for intervention group patients and 996 requested for control group patients. In an analysis focused on the ordering physician, the investigators found that the mean proportion of patients referred for radiography was 78.9% in the intervention group and 99.6% in the control group ($P = 0.03$). The investigators noted three missed fractures in the intervention group, none of which led to adverse outcomes. Thus, the investigators demonstrated a positive resource utilization impact of the Ottawa ankle rules (decreased test ordering) without an increase in adverse outcomes, thus moving the clinical prediction rule to level I in the hierarchy (see Table 22-1).

CLINICAL RESOLUTION

You conduct the continuing nurse education program for outpost nurse practitioners, and they are enthusiastic about using the Ottawa ankle rules at their sites with the objective of sending fewer patients for unnecessary radiographs. In addition, the nurses note in their evaluations that the session has armed them with the knowledge they need to critique studies that describe other clinical prediction rules that may be applicable to their practice.

The next day, as you reflect on the session, you wonder whether the nurse practitioners will indeed use the Ottawa ankle rules. In preparing for the session, you came across a study by Cameron and Naylor that reported an initiative in which clinicians who were expert in the use of the Ottawa ankle rules trained 16 other workers to teach the use of the rules.[22] These persons used slides, overhead projections, and a 13-minute instructional video to train their colleagues locally and regionally in the use of the rules. Surprisingly, this program led to no change in the use of ankle radiography. You are also aware that little research has been done on evaluating practice change in nursing. You decide to work more closely with this group of nurse practitioners to identify and implement strategies to reinforce their learning and evaluate changes in their clinical practice.

Clinical prediction rules inform our clinical judgment and have the potential to change clinical behavior and reduce unnecessary costs while maintaining quality of care and patient satisfaction. The challenge for clinicians is to evaluate the strength of a rule and its likely impact, as well as to find ways of incorporating level I rules efficiently into their daily practice. Clinicians can access a summary of clinical prediction rules and associated levels of evidence on the Internet (*http://www.mssm.edu/medicine/general-medicine/ebm*).

REFERENCES

1. Bachmann LM, Kolb E, Koller MT, Steurer J, ter Riet G. Accuracy of Ottawa ankle rules to exclude fractures of the ankle and mid-foot: systematic review. *BMJ*. 2003;326:417.
2. Stiell IG, Greenberg GH, McKnight RD, Nair RC, McDowell I, Worthington JR. A study to develop clinical decision rules for the use of radiography in acute ankle injuries. *Ann Emerg Med*. 1992;21:384-390.
3. Stiell IG, Greenberg GH, McKnight RD, et al. Decision rules for the use of radiography in acute ankle injuries: refinement and prospective validation. *JAMA*. 1993;269:1127-1132.

4. Nielsen Forman D, Videbech P, Hedegaard M, et al. Postpartum depression: identification of women at risk. *Br J Obstet Gynaecol.* 2000;107:1210-1217.

5. Oliver D, Britton M, Seed P, et al. Development and evaluation of evidence based risk assessment tool (STRATIFY) to predict which elderly inpatients will fall: case-control and cohort studies. *BMJ.* 1997;315:1049-1053.

6. Margolis DJ, Berlin JA, Strom BL. Which venous leg ulcers will heal with limb compression bandages? *Am J Med.* 2000;109:15-19.

7. Morrow DA, Antman EM, Giugliano RP, et al. A simple risk index for rapid initial triage of patients with ST-elevation myocardial infarction: an InTIME II substudy. *Lancet.* 2001;358:1571-1575.

8. Laupacis A, Sekar N, Stiell IG. Clinical prediction rules: a review and suggested modifications of methodological standards. *JAMA.* 1997;277:488-494.

9. Rudy TE, Kubinski JA, Boston JR. Multivariate analysis and repeated measurements: a primer. *J Crit Care.* 1992;7:30-41.

10. Cook EF, Goldman L. Empiric comparison of multivariate analytic techniques: advantages and disadvantages of recursive partitioning analysis. *J Chronic Dis.* 1984;37:721-731.

11. Baxt WG. Application of artificial neural networks to clinical medicine. *Lancet.* 1995;346:1135-1138.

12. Martin TP, Hanusa BH, Kapoor WN. Risk stratification of patients with syncope. *Ann Emerg Med.* 1997;29:459-466.

13. Fine MJ, Auble TE, Yealy DM, et al. A prediction rule to identify low-risk patients with community-acquired pneumonia. *N Engl J Med.* 1997;336:243-250.

14. Justice AC, Covinsky KE, Berlin JA. Assessing the generalizability of prognostic information. *Ann Intern Med.* 1999;130:515-524.

15. Silver MT, Rose GA, Paul SD, O'Donnell CJ, O'Gara PT, Eagle KA. A clinical rule to predict preserved left ventricular ejection fraction in patients after myocardial infarction. *Ann Intern Med.* 1994;121:750-756.

16. Tobin K, Stomel R, Harber D, Karavite D, Sievers J, Eagle K. Validation in a community hospital setting of a clinical rule to predict preserved left ventricular ejection fraction in patients after myocardial infarction. *Arch Intern Med.* 1999;159:353-357.

17. Krumholz HM, Howes CJ, Murillo JE, Vaccarino LV, Radford MJ, Ellerbeck EF. Validation of a clinical prediction rule for left ventricular ejection fraction after myocardial infarction in patients > or = 65 years old. *Am J Cardiol.* 1997;80:11-15.

18. Heckerling PS, Tape TG, Wigton RS, et al. Clinical prediction rule for pulmonary infiltrates. *Ann Intern Med.* 1990;113:664-670.

19. Wells PS, Ginsberg JS, Anderson DR, et al. Use of a clinical model for safe management of patients with suspected pulmonary embolism. *Ann Intern Med.* 1998;129:997-1005.

20. Buchsbaum DG, Buchanan RG, Centor RM, Schnoll SH, Lawton MJ. Screening for alcohol abuse using CAGE scores and likelihood ratios. *Ann Intern Med.* 1991;115:774-777.

21. Auleley GR, Ravaud P, Giraudeau B, et al. Implementation of the Ottawa ankle rules in France: a multicenter randomized controlled trial. *JAMA.* 1997;277:1935-1939.

22. Cameron C, Naylor CD. No impact from active dissemination of the Ottawa Ankle Rules: further evidence of the need for local implementation of practice guidelines. *CMAJ.* 1999;160:1165-1168.

Summarizing the Evidence Through Systematic Reviews

Chapter **23** Publication Bias

Chapter **24** Evaluating Differences in Study Results

Chapter **25** Fixed-Effects and Random-Effects Models

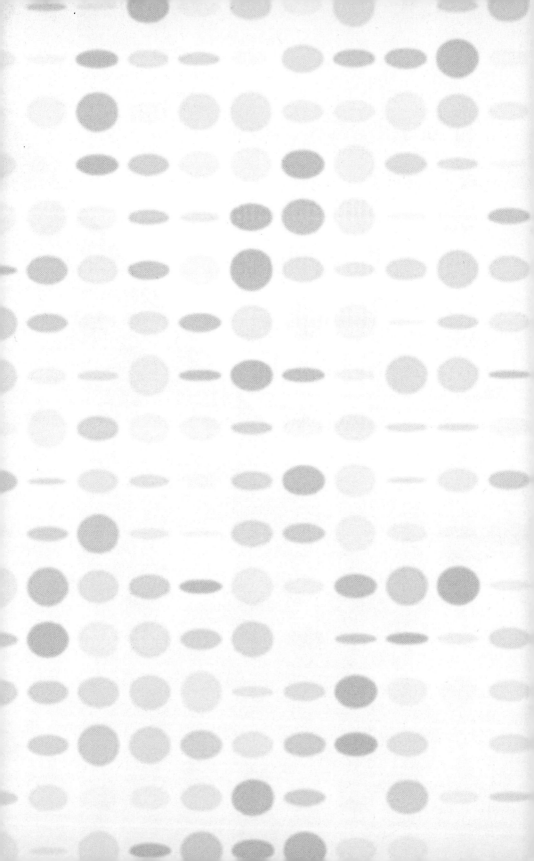

23

Publication Bias

Donna Ciliska and Gordon Guyatt

We gratefully acknowledge the work of Victor Montori on the original chapter that appears in the Users' Guides to the Medical Literature, *edited by Guyatt and Rennie.*

In This Chapter

Bias in Systematic Reviews

Sources of Publication Bias

Publication Bias and Size of Trials

How Researchers Contribute to Publication Bias

Strategies to Identify Likely Publication Bias

A Strategy to Reduce Publication Bias

BIAS IN SYSTEMATIC REVIEWS

In designing a systematic review, researchers specify the research question, criteria for inclusion and exclusion of primary studies, a search strategy, the data extraction process, quality assessment procedures, and data analysis plans (see Chapter 9, Summarizing the Evidence Through Systematic Reviews). Systematic error leading to bias can be introduced at any of these steps. Perhaps the most difficult type of bias for those conducting reviews to overcome is *publication bias,* the selective publication of manuscripts based on the magnitude, direction, or statistical significance of the study results.

SOURCES OF PUBLICATION BIAS

Excluding unpublished studies from a systematic review will not bias the results of a review if the unpublished studies show, on average, the same magnitude of effect as the published reports. Unfortunately, studies that fail to reject the *null hypothesis* (those without statistically significant results, also called *negative studies*) are less likely to be published than studies that show apparent differences between experimental and control interventions, or *positive studies.* The magnitude and direction of a study's results may be more important determinants of publication than study design, relevance, or quality.[1,2] Positive studies may be up to three times more likely to be published than negative studies.[3] Journal editors' naive belief that the peer review process guarantees the validity, quality, or representativeness of the published literature may lead them to reject systematic reviews that include unpublished data.[4] Even when negative studies are ultimately accepted for publication, their publication is often delayed.[2,5] Indeed, publication bias can affect virtually all stages of planning, implementing, and disseminating research (Table 23-1).

PUBLICATION BIAS AND SIZE OF TRIALS

When those conducting the review fail to identify and include unpublished studies in a systematic review, they risk presenting an overly optimistic estimate of a health care intervention's effectiveness (Figure 23-1). The risk is higher for reviews that include small studies than for those that do not include such studies.[6] Studies with large sample sizes are less likely to remain unpublished or ignored and tend to provide more precise estimates of treatment effects, whether positive or negative. Egger and colleagues offered examples of meta-analyses of small trials that showed larger treatment effects than subsequent large trials.[7] Discrepancies between results of a meta-analysis and subsequent large trials may occur as often as 20% of the time,[8] and publication bias may be a major contributor to the discrepancies. Sutton and colleagues estimated that publication bias affected 23 of 48 meta-analyses examined and may have changed the conclusions of four meta-analyses.[9]

HOW RESEARCHERS CONTRIBUTE TO PUBLICATION BIAS

Publication bias usually occurs because investigators do not submit their studies for publication rather than because journals reject the submissions, although journal publishing policies may also play a role.[10] Researchers may fail to submit negative studies because of lack of time or because they believe that their results are uninteresting.[11]

Table 23-1 Sources of Publication Bias

Phases of Research Publication	Actions Contributing to or Resulting in Publication Bias
Preliminary and pilot studies	Small studies, which are more likely to be negative (e.g., those with discarded failed hypotheses) are unpublished; some are classified as proprietary information.
Trial design, organization, and funding	Proposal selectively cites positive studies.
Institutional/ethics review board approval	No registries are kept of approved trials.
Study completion	Interim analysis shows that a study is likely to be negative, and the project is dropped.
Report completion	Authors decide that reporting a negative study is worthless and uninteresting, and no time or effort is assigned.
Report submission	Authors decide to forgo submission of the negative study.
Journal selection	Authors decide to submit the report of the negative study to a nonindexed, non-English, limited-circulation journal.
Editorial consideration	The editor decides that the negative study is not worth the peer review process and rejects the manuscript; if the editor decides it is worth reviewing, the manuscript goes to a lower-priority list.
Peer review	Peer reviewers conclude that the negative study does not contribute to the field and recommend rejecting the manuscript.
Author revision and resubmission	The author of a rejected manuscript decides to forgo the revision of the negative study or submit it to another journal (see Journal selection above).
Report publication	The journal delays publication of the negative study.
Lay press report	The negative study is not considered newsworthy.
Electronic database indexing	MEDLINE and EMBASE do not scan or index articles in the journal or language of publication of the negative study.
Decision-maker retrieval	Health managers and policymakers do not retrieve the negative study to dictate policy.
Further trial evidence	New trial reports discuss their findings but do not cite the findings of the negative study.
Narrative review	Experts draft a review, but the negative study is never cited.

Continued

Table 23-1   Sources of Publication Bias—cont'd

Phases of Research Publication	Actions Contributing to or Resulting in Publication Bias
Systematic review	Reviewers go to extremes to identify negative reports, but miss the negative study; industry-associated reviewers use arbitrarily selected unpublished data"on file"; this further discredits incorporation of unpublished reports in systematic reviews.
Systematic review submission	Journal editors reject the systematic review because it included unpublished reports not exposed to the rigor of peer review; review then follows the same path described here for the negative study.
Practice guidelines	Evidence-based guidelines are produced based on a systematic review that missed the negative study.
Funding opportunities	Further funding opportunities are identified without consideration of the negative study.

Funding sources also influence investigators' decisions regarding submission. Negative studies funded by pharmaceutical companies are less likely to be published than negative studies funded by nonprofit organizations or government agencies.[1,12,13] Cultural or political factors may also influence publication decisions; one report suggests that investigators from certain countries never publish negative studies.[14]

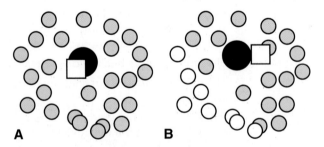

Figure 23-1. Intervention effectiveness and publication bias. **A,** The black circle represents the underlying truth. The white square represents the pooled estimate from a systematic review of all the evidence. The small shaded circles represent the results of individual studies. **B,** The white circles represent the results of the studies that were not included because they were not published. Note the error in the pooled estimate represented by the gap between the pooled estimate (white square) and the underlying truth (black circle).

Electronic databases, including MEDLINE, limit the type and number of journals indexed. For example, 20% to 70% of randomized trials may not be identified using MEDLINE.[15] Researchers' decisions about where to submit their work are based on journal prestige and readership, as well as the perceived likelihood of manuscript acceptance. Accordingly, they may send positive studies to more visible journals and negative studies to less readily available journals.[16] Non-English-language authors may publish positive studies in English-language journals and negative studies (of equivalent methodological quality)[17] in local non-English-language journals that are less likely to be indexed in MEDLINE.[18] Thus, reviews that do not seek studies from more obscure journals may produce the same exaggerated estimates of intervention effect as reviews that are subject to publication bias, a phenomenon known as *postpublication bias*.

Systematic reviews are less likely to be affected by postpublication bias if those conducting the review search several different databases, include studies published in all languages, hand search pertinent journals, and review the reference lists of all relevant articles. Clinicians considering use of the results of a systematic review to guide practice can be concerned less about publication bias if those conducting the review contacted experts (in one study, 24% of references would have been missed without expert input[19]), reviewed conference proceedings,[20] and searched databases of dissertations and registries that collect studies at their inception. The Cochrane Collaboration has encouraged a rigorous search for unpublished data. In general, Cochrane reviews are more likely to include a comprehensive search than are reviews found elsewhere.

STRATEGIES TO IDENTIFY LIKELY PUBLICATION BIAS

Because even comprehensive efforts may fail to identify all unpublished studies, those conducting reviews can use procedures to determine the likelihood that publication bias is influencing their results. In a figure that relates the precision (as measured by sample size and the inverse of the standard error) of studies included in a meta-analysis to the magnitude of treatment effect (as measured by the effect size, relative risk reduction, and odds ratio), the resulting display should resemble an inverted funnel. Such *funnel plots* should be symmetric around the point estimate (dominated by the largest trials) or the results of the largest trials themselves (Figure 23-2A). *Asymmetry,* judged by inspection, may indicate publication bias (Figure 23-2B). Statistical testing[6] also may reveal publication bias, although some investigators have questioned the proposed statistical methods.[21-23] It is important to keep in mind, however, that funnel plots and statistical tests have low power for detecting publication bias in systematic reviews with a small number of trials. Reasons for asymmetry may include publication bias, post-publication bias (including English-language bias), inclusion of multiple publications of the same study, poor design of small studies, fraud, and true larger effects in small studies (e.g., if compliance is higher or the intervention is more consistently delivered[7]).

Those conducting reviews may attempt to estimate the true treatment effect in the presence of what they believe is publication bias. They begin by removing, or trimming, small positive studies that do not have a negative study counterpart and then calculate a supposed true effect from the resulting symmetric funnel plot. They then replace the positive studies they have removed and add hypothetical studies that mirror these

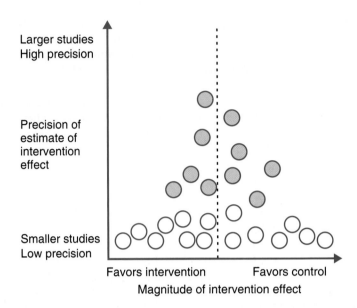

Figure 23-2A. Funnel plot. The circles represent the point estimates of the trials. The pattern of distribution resembles an inverted funnel. Larger studies (shaded circles) tend to be closer to the pooled estimate (the dashed line). In this case, the effect sizes of the larger (shaded circles) and the smaller studies (white circles) are more or less symmetrically distributed around the pooled estimate.

positive studies to create a symmetric funnel plot that retains the new pooled effect estimate. This *trim-and-fill method* allows the calculation of an adjusted confidence interval and an estimate of the number of missing trials.[9]

Another method is to calculate a *fail-safe N*, which represents the number of undetected negative studies that would be needed to change the conclusions of a meta-analysis.[24] A small fail-safe N suggests that the conclusion of the meta-analysis may be susceptible to publication bias. If those conducting a systematic review have obtained the results of some unpublished studies and if published and unpublished data show different results, they have definitively established publication bias.[25,26] Perhaps the most powerful test of publication bias comes from a comparison of prospectively registered trials with published study results.[27] Because registration of trials is completed before the results are available, the results do not influence study inclusion. Indeed, prospective registration of all trials represents the ultimate solution to the problem of publication bias. Alternative suggestions include amnesty for unpublished trials (invitation to researchers to register unreported trial data) and electronic publishing of all studies[28] regardless of prior or future journal publication. These suggestions face apathy on the part of authors,[29] resistance from journal editors,[30] and the possibility of misleading presentation of data from methodologically flawed studies.[31]

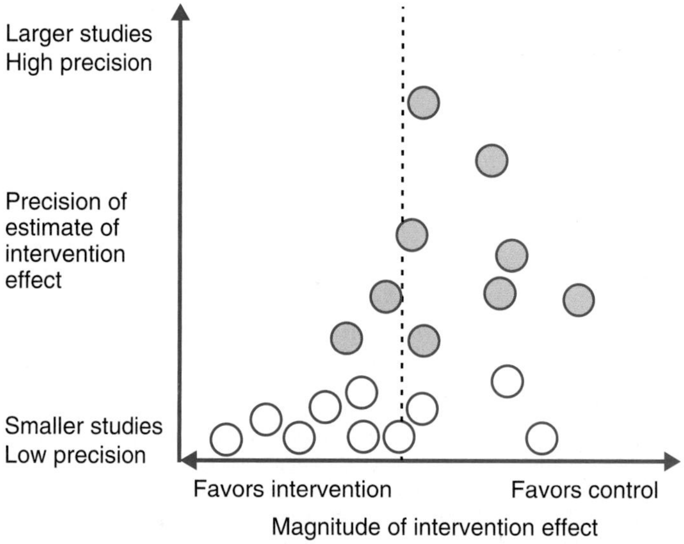

Figure 23-2B. Publication bias. This funnel plot shows that the smaller studies (white circles) are not symmetrically distributed around either the pooled estimate (dominated by the larger trials) or the results of the larger trials (shaded circles) themselves. The trials expected in the bottom right quadrant are missing. This suggests publication bias—and an overestimation of the intervention effect relative to the underlying truth.

A STRATEGY TO REDUCE PUBLICATION BIAS

Prospective study registration with accessible results is likely to represent the best solution to publication bias. Proposals exist to link prospective trial registration to the work of institutional or ethics review boards,[32] or to the editorial process of health care journals and publishing societies.[33] Some pharmaceutical companies have made their research information available online.[34] Some journals, such as *The Lancet*, have established Web sites for posting study protocols and reports of completed studies undergoing peer review.[35] Until prospective registration and complete reporting become a reality, clinicians using systematic reviews to guide their practice must remain aware of the dangers of publication bias.

REFERENCES

1. Easterbrook PJ, Berlin JA, Gopalan R, Matthews DR. Publication bias in clinical research. *Lancet*. 1991;337:867-872.
2. Misakian AL, Bero LA. Publication bias and research on passive smoking: comparison of published and unpublished studies. *JAMA*. 1998;280:250-253.
3. Egger M, Smith GD. Bias in location and selection of studies. *BMJ*. 1998;316:61-66.
4. Cook DJ, Guyatt GH, Ryan G, et al. Should unpublished data be included in meta-analyses? Current convictions and controversies. *JAMA*. 1993;269:2749-2753.
5. Stern JM, Simes RJ. Publication bias: evidence of delayed publication in a cohort study of clinical research projects. *BMJ*. 1997;315:640-645.

6. Begg C, Berlin J. Publication bias: a problem in interpreting medical data. *J R Stat Soc A*. 1988;151:419-463.

7. Egger M, Davey Smith G, Schneider M, Minder C. Bias in meta-analysis detected by a simple, graphical test. *BMJ*. 1997;315:629-634.

8. Cappelleri JC, Ioannidis JP, Schmid CH, et al. Large trials vs meta-analysis of smaller trials: how do their results compare? *JAMA*. 1996;276:1332-1338.

9. Sutton AJ, Duval SJ, Tweedie RL, Abrams KR, Jones DR. Empirical assessment of effect of publication bias on meta-analyses. *BMJ*. 2000;320:1574-1577.

10. Callaham ML, Wears RL, Weber EJ, Barton C, Young G. Positive-outcome bias and other limitations in the outcome of research abstracts submitted to a scientific meeting. *JAMA*. 1998;280:254-257.

11. Dickersin K, Min YI. NIH clinical trials and publication bias. *Online J Curr Clin Trials*. 1993;Document 50.

12. Dickersin K, Min YI, Meinert CL. Factors influencing publication of research results: follow-up of applications submitted to two institutional review boards. *JAMA*. 1992;267:374-378.

13. Friedberg M, Saffran B, Stinson TJ, Nelson W, Bennett CL. Evaluation of conflict of interest in economic analyses of new drugs used in oncology. *JAMA*. 1999;282:1453-1457.

14. Vickers A, Goyal N, Harland R, Rees R. Do certain countries produce only positive results? A systematic review of controlled trials. *Control Clin Trials*. 1998;19:159-166.

15. Alderson P, Green S, Higgins JPT, eds. *Cochrane Reviewers' Handbook, 4.2.2* [updated December 2003]. In: The Cochrane Library, Issue 1, 2004. Chichester, UK: John Wiley & Sons Ltd.

16. Frank E. Authors' criteria for selecting journals. *JAMA*. 1994;272:163-164.

17. Moher D, Fortin P, Jadad AR, et al. Completeness of reporting of trials published in languages other than English: implications for conduct and reporting of systematic reviews. *Lancet*. 1996;347:363-366.

18. Gregoire G, Derderian F, Le Lorier J. Selecting the language of the publications included in a meta-analysis: is there a Tower of Babel bias? *J Clin Epidemiol*. 1995;48:159-163.

19. McManus RJ, Wilson S, Delaney BC, et al. Review of the usefulness of contacting other experts when conducting a literature search for systematic reviews. *BMJ*. 1998;317:1562-1563.

20. Scherer RW, Dickersin K, Langenberg P. Full publication of results initially presented in abstracts: a meta-analysis. *JAMA*. 1994;272:158-162.

21. Irwig L, Macaskill P, Berry G, Glasziou P. Bias in meta-analysis detected by a simple, graphical test: graphical test is itself biased. *BMJ*. 1998;316:470; discussion, 470-471.

22. Stuck AE, Rubenstein LZ, Wieland D. Bias in meta-analysis detected by a simple, graphical test: asymmetry detected in funnel plot was probably due to true heterogeneity. *BMJ*. 1998;316:469; discussion, 470-471.

23. Seagroatt V, Stratton I. Bias in meta-analysis detected by a simple, graphical test: test had 10% false positive rate. *BMJ*. 1998;316:470; discussion 470-471.

24. Gleser LJ, Olkin I. Models for estimating the number of unpublished studies. *Stat Med*. 1996;15:2493-2507.

25. Man-Son-Hing M, Wells G, Lau A. Quinine for nocturnal leg cramps: a meta-analysis including unpublished data. *J Gen Intern Med*. 1998;13:600-606.

26. Simes RJ. Confronting publication bias: a cohort design for meta-analysis. *Stat Med*. 1987;6:11-29.

27. Langhorne P. Bias in meta-analysis detected by a simple, graphical test: prospectively identified trials could be used for comparison with meta-analyses. *BMJ*. 1998;316:471.

28. Varmus H. E-Biomed: a proposal for electronic publications in the biomedical sciences (PubMed Central Web site). 1999. Available at: *www.nih.gov/welcome/director/ebiomed/ebi.htm*. Accessed February 1, 2001.

29. Roberts I. An amnesty for unpublished trials: one year on, many trials are unregistered and the amnesty remains open. *BMJ*. 1998;317:763-764.

30. Relman AS. The NIH "E-biomed" proposal: a potential threat to the evaluation and orderly dissemination of new clinical studies. *N Engl J Med*. 1999;340:1828-1829.

31. Taubes G. A plan to register unpublished studies. *Science*. 1997;277:1754.

32. Boissel JP, Haugh MC. Clinical trial registries and ethics review boards: the results of a survey by the FICHTRE project. *Fundam Clin Pharmacol*. 1997;11:281-284.

33. Horton R, Smith R. Time to register randomised trials: the case is now unanswerable. *BMJ*. 1999;319:865-866.

34. Levy MD. A new register for clinical trial information. *Can Med Assoc J*. 2000;162:970-971.

35. McConnell J, Horton R. Lancet electronic research archive in international health and eprint server. *Lancet*. 1999;354:2-3.

24

Evaluating Differences
in Study Results

Donna Ciliska and Gordon Guyatt

We gratefully acknowledge the work of Victor Montori and Rose Hatala on the original chapter that appears in the Users' Guides to the Medical Literature, *edited by Guyatt and Rennie.*

In This Chapter

Arriving at a Single Estimate of Treatment Effect

The Problem of Variability in Study Results: To Pool or Not to Pool?

The Formal Statistical Test of Heterogeneity

What to Do When Pooling May Not Be Appropriate

ARRIVING AT A SINGLE ESTIMATE OF TREATMENT EFFECT

The goal of a *systematic review* is to provide, when possible, a single best estimate of a treatment effect (or the harmful effect of an exposure, the power of a diagnostic test, or a patient's prognosis) to guide clinical practice. The starting assumption of a systematic review of a focused clinical question is that the effect of the intervention is more or less the same across the range of patients, interventions, and outcomes in the studies included in the review (see Chapter 9, Summarizing the Evidence Through Systematic Reviews). This chapter focuses on systematic reviews in which the goal of those conducting the review is to produce a quantitative summary by statistically pooling results across studies included in the review (a *meta-analysis*). The decision about whether the results of individual studies should be combined statistically rests on the degree of similarity of the results of the individual studies.

In Chapter 9, Summarizing the Evidence Through Systematic Reviews, we framed the dilemma faced by those conducting reviews and by clinicians evaluating reviews. On the one hand, framing the question to include a broad range of patients, interventions, and ways of measuring outcome has advantages. This strategy of formulating broad eligibility criteria helps to avoid the bias that may occur when one focuses on a subgroup of patients (perhaps chosen because their results differ from those of other subgroups) (see Chapter 16, When to Believe a Subgroup Analysis). In addition, pooling the results of multiple studies reduces random error and increases applicability across a broad range of patients. At the same time, however, pooling the results of multiple studies risks violating the starting assumption of the analysis—that the magnitude of effect is more or less the same across patients, interventions, outcomes, and methodology. The solution to this dilemma is to evaluate the extent to which the results of individual studies differ from one another. We refer to this difference in magnitude of effect as *heterogeneity* of study results. This chapter expands on the brief discussion of how readers should critically appraise the assessment of study-to-study variability presented in Chapter 9, Summarizing the Evidence Through Systematic Reviews.

THE PROBLEM OF VARIABILITY IN STUDY RESULTS: TO POOL OR NOT TO POOL?

Two studies seldom yield point estimates (e.g., odds ratios, relative risks) that are extremely close to one another, and they virtually never yield identical point estimates. Thus, in any meta-analysis that pools multiple studies, there will inevitably be some heterogeneity of results. The question is whether the heterogeneity is sufficiently large to make us uncomfortable with the systematic reviewer's decision to pool the results of the individual studies.

The graphical display of results from individual studies allows a visual examination of the degree of heterogeneity between studies.[1] The more results differ from study to study, the more the reader should question the decision to combine the results of studies. Consider the results of two meta-analyses shown in Figure 24-1 and Figure 24-2. Reviewing the results of these studies, are we comfortable with pooling the results?

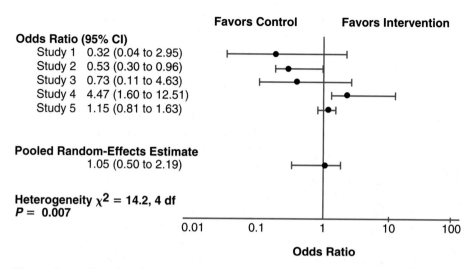

Figure 24-1. Results of meta-analysis A.

Most readers would be uncomfortable with the decision to pool the results in Figure 24-1 but would be comfortable with the decision to pool the results in Figure 24-2.

When reviewing graphical displays such as Figures 24-1 and 24-2, readers should make two observations: are the point estimates of individual studies on the same side of the line of no effect, and more importantly, do confidence intervals around the point

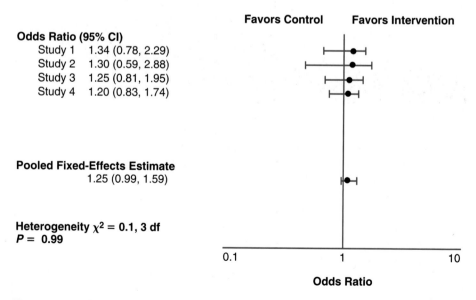

Figure 24-2. Results of meta-analysis B.

estimates of individual studies overlap? Figure 24-1 presents the results of five studies, the first three of which suggest harm (odds ratios favor the control group) and the last two of which suggest benefit (odds ratios favor the intervention group). Figure 24-2 presents the results of four studies, all of which suggest benefit (odds ratios favor the intervention group).

While comfort with pooling may increase when the point estimates of all studies are on the same side of the line of no effect (that is, all studies suggest benefit, or all studies suggest harm), Figure 24-3 gives us reason to question this rule. This meta-analysis also shows point estimates on both sides of the line of no effect (odds ratio = 1.0), but in this case, because the between-study differences are small and because confidence intervals around point estimates of individual studies overlap, most readers would be comfortable with pooling the results. This leads us to reject a rule that focuses exclusively on study results suggesting benefit or harm. Rather, readers should consider the magnitude of the differences in the point estimates of the studies. The large between-study differences in point estimates make readers uncomfortable with pooling in Figure 24-1 (e.g., difference between point estimates of study 1 (odds ratio, 0.32; 95% CI, 0.04 to 2.95) and study 4 (odds ratio, 4.47; 95% CI, 1.60 to 12.51)); the similarity of point estimates leads to comfort with pooling in Figure 24-2.

Readers should also apply a second criterion when judging whether pooling is appropriate. If confidence intervals around the point estimates of individual studies overlap with one another (as in Figure 24-2), chance remains a plausible explanation of the differences in the point estimates. If the confidence intervals around the point estimates of individual studies do not overlap with one another (as in studies 2 and 4 in Figure 24-1), then chance becomes an unlikely explanation for differences in apparent treatment

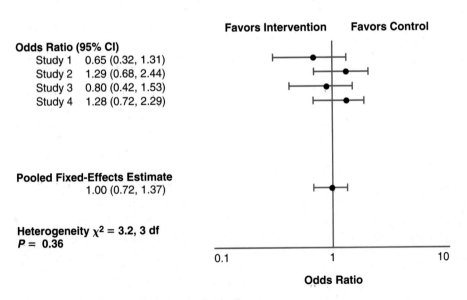

Figure 24-3. Results of meta-analysis C.

effect across studies. The greater is the overlap in confidence intervals, the more comfortable one can be with combining results. Widely separated confidence intervals flag the presence of important variability that requires explanation.

THE FORMAL STATISTICAL TEST OF HETEROGENEITY

Clinicians can also consider the results of formal statistical tests to help evaluate the validity of pooling studies in a meta-analysis. The null hypothesis of a test of heterogeneity is that the underlying effect is the same in each study (e.g., the odds ratio in study 1 is the same as the odds ratios in studies 2, 3, and 4) (see Chapter 28, Hypothesis Testing), and the observed effects differ because of sampling variation only. A test of heterogeneity is performed to determine whether the effect sizes of the individual studies included in the systematic review differ significantly from one another. The test (often a chi-square test) provides a P value that represents how often one would obtain differences in study results as large or larger than those observed if the null hypothesis were true, and we repeated the studies over and over.[1] A low P value in the test for heterogeneity (e.g., $P < 0.05$) means that chance is an unlikely explanation of the differences in results from study to study and would raise doubts about the wisdom of pooling results across studies.

We generally use the traditional cut point for statistical significance, which is that significant heterogeneity exists if the P value is less than 0.05, although investigators sometimes choose 0.1 as the threshold value.[2] In Figure 24-1, the P value is very small ($P = 0.007$) because it would be very unlikely to see results this disparate if all studies had the same underlying effect. In other words, chance is an unlikely explanation of the differences in results from study to study. The P value in Figure 24-2 is large ($P = 0.99$) because, if the null hypothesis were true, we would observe differences in study results as large as in these studies on most repetitions of the experiment. In other words, chance, rather than true differences, is a likely explanation of the differences in results from study to study.

The test of heterogeneity is limited in that a nonsignificant result does not rule out important underlying heterogeneity of treatment effect. This test is underpowered when the meta-analysis includes relatively few studies, all with small sample sizes. Under these circumstances, we may be unable to exclude chance as an explanation of differences, but we would remain suspicious that other factors (e.g., differences in populations, interventions, or measurement of outcomes) are responsible for differences in study results (see Chapter 16, When to Believe a Subgroup Analysis). This situation emphasizes the need for visual inspection of, first, differences in point estimates and, second, the extent to which confidence intervals overlap. Large differences in point estimates dictate caution in interpreting the overall findings, even in the presence of a nonsignificant test of heterogeneity.

The test of heterogeneity may also provide potentially misleading results when it has very high power. This will occur when a meta-analysis includes many studies with very large sample sizes. Under these circumstances, one may see small and unimportant differences in point estimates, but because of narrow confidence intervals, the statistical test of heterogeneity will be positive (i.e., $P < 0.05$).

WHAT TO DO WHEN POOLING MAY NOT BE APPROPRIATE

What should clinicians expect of systematic reviewers when study-to-study differences in results suggest that pooling may not be appropriate? When chance becomes an unlikely explanation for differences in the magnitude of effect between studies, those conducting the review must examine other possible explanations. In particular, differences in study participants, interventions, outcomes, and study methodology (ideally specified before the data analysis began) may explain variations in treatment effect. For example, in a systematic review of the effectiveness of interventions to reduce unintended pregnancies among adolescents, DiCenso and colleagues tested 10 a priori hypotheses that might explain heterogeneity of study results: publication type (published and unpublished), control group intervention (alternate intervention or none), year of publication (before 1995 and 1995 or later), randomization (appropriate and inappropriate), data collection (biased and unbiased), loss to follow-up ($\geq 80\%$ and $< 80\%$), difference in loss to follow-up between groups ($\leq 2\%$ and $> 2\%$), follow-up period (≥ 12 months and < 12 months), baseline differences (none, favoring control, and favoring intervention), and type of intervention (school-based sex education, multifaceted program, family planning clinic, and abstinence program).[3] For an explanation of the principles for exploring sources of heterogeneity, see Chapter 16, When to Believe a Subgroup Analysis.

The optimal statistical approach to arriving at a best estimate of treatment effect and a corresponding confidence interval in a systematic review is controversial. Some argue that the presence of heterogeneity influences which of two common statistical approaches, fixed-effects or random-effects models, is best used to combine study results.[4] Some investigators use *fixed-effects models* when no significant heterogeneity exists among studies. The goal of this model is to provide the best estimate of the treatment effect in the studies that are part of the analysis.[5] The error term for a fixed-effects model comes only from within-study variation (study variance), and the model ignores between-study variation or heterogeneity. The goal of the *random-effects model* is to provide the best estimate of treatment effect in a hypothetical set of all possible studies of the relevant question and assumes the available studies are a random sample of those studies. The calculation of the summary statistic (e.g., relative risk or odds ratio) in the random-effects model incorporates both within-study and between-study variation (heterogeneity)[6] (see Chapter 25, Fixed-Effects and Random-Effects Models). Some argue that the random-effects model is, except under unusual circumstances, the optimal statistical approach to pooling.

When there is heterogeneity among studies, the between-study variation is large, and differences between fixed-effects and random-effects models can be substantial. While both random-effects and fixed-effects models give greater weight to large studies than to smaller studies, the fixed-effects model uses a larger gradient in weight between large and small studies than does the random-effects model. When there is not much heterogeneity, the fixed-effects and the random-effects models will yield essentially identical results.[7]

What if, in the end, we are left with a large degree of unexplained between-study heterogeneity that is not adequately explained by chance? Presumably, some underlying differences in patients, interventions, outcome measurement, or methodology are responsible for these differences. Some argue that investigators should refrain from pooling when unexplained heterogeneity exists. Investigators who subscribe to this approach can systematically summarize (but not meta-analyze) the study findings.[1] Others believe that pending further studies that explain differences between study results, the pooled result remains the best available estimate of the treatment effect. Clinicians must nevertheless be cautious in recommending interventions on the basis of pooled estimates associated with unexplained heterogeneity.

REFERENCES

1. Egger M, Davey Smith G, Phillips AN. Meta-analysis: principles and procedures. *BMJ.*1997;315:1533-1537.
2. Bailey KR. Inter-study differences: how should they influence the interpretation and analysis of results? *Stat Med* 1987;6:351-360.
3. DiCenso A, Guyatt G, Willan A, Griffith L. Interventions to reduce unintended pregnancies among adolescents: systematic review of randomised controlled trials. *BMJ.* 2002;324:1426.
4. Fleiss JL. The statistical basis of meta-analysis. *Stat Methods Med Res.* 1993;2:121-145.
5. Lau J, Ioannidis JP, Schmid CH. Summing up evidence: one answer is not always enough. *Lancet.* 1998;351:123-127.
6. DerSimonian R, Laird N. Meta-analysis in clinical trials. *Control Clin Trials.* 1986;7:177-188.
7. Petitti DB. *Meta-analysis, decision analysis, and cost-effectiveness analysis.* New York: Oxford University Press, 1994.

25

Fixed-Effects and Random-Effects Models

Donna Ciliska and Gordon Guyatt

We gratefully acknowledge the work of Victor Montori, Andrew Oxman, and Deborah Cook on the original chapter that appears in the Users' Guides to the Medical Literature, *edited by Guyatt and Rennie.*

In This Chapter

Models for Pooling Data for Meta-Analysis

Differences in Results From Fixed-Effects and Random-Effects Models

Examples of Differences in Summary Point Estimates and Confidence Intervals From Fixed-Effects and Random-Effects Models

MODELS FOR POOLING DATA FOR META-ANALYSIS

In a meta-analysis, results from two or more primary studies are combined statistically. Methods for pooling primary study results include fixed-effects and random-effects models.[1]

The *fixed-effects model* restricts inferences to the set of studies included in the meta-analysis,[2] and it assumes that a single true value underlies all of the primary study results. In other words, the assumption is that if all studies were infinitely large, they would yield identical estimates of effect. Thus, observed estimates of effect differ from each other only because of random error.[3] The error term for a fixed-effects model comes only from within-study variation (study variance); the model ignores between-study variation, or heterogeneity (see Chapter 24, Evaluating Differences in Study Results).

By contrast, the *random-effects model* assumes that the studies included are a random sample of a population of studies addressing the question posed in the meta-analysis.[4] Each study estimates a different underlying true effect, and the distribution of these effects is assumed to be normal around a mean value.[3] The random-effects model takes into account both within-study variation and between-study variation (heterogeneity) (see Chapter 24, Evaluating Differences in Study Results).

When there is not much heterogeneity, fixed-effects and random-effects models will both weight studies according to sample size, and they will yield essentially identical results. If studies are markedly heterogeneous, fixed-effects and random-effects models are likely to yield results that differ considerably.

DIFFERENCES IN RESULTS FROM FIXED-EFFECTS AND RANDOM-EFFECTS MODELS

The fixed-effects model is usually used when no significant heterogeneity exists among studies. When there is heterogeneity among studies, the between-study variation is large, and this variation dominates the weights assigned to the studies in the random-effects model. Compared with the fixed-effects model, the random-effects model gives smaller studies proportionally greater weight in the pooled estimate. Consequently, the direction and magnitude of the pooled estimate are influenced more by smaller studies.

For the random-effects pooled estimate to be closer to the *null result* (i.e., no treatment effect) than the fixed-effects pooled estimate, two conditions are required. First, the results of smaller studies must be closer to the null result than those of larger studies; second, the variability in study results must be greater than that explained by within-study variability. If the smaller studies are farther from the null result, the random-effects model will tend to produce larger estimates of beneficial or harmful effects than the fixed-effects model. A pooled estimate derived from the random-effects model is more susceptible to publication bias, a phenomenon that primarily affects smaller studies (see Chapter 23, Publication Bias).[5]

Between-study variability beyond that explained by within-study variability can inflate a random-effects estimate of random error. An important effect of this larger error term in the analysis is that the random-effects model generally produces wider confidence intervals around pooled estimates than does the fixed-effects model. In this sense, the random-effects model generally produces a more conservative assessment of the precision of the pooled estimate than does the fixed-effects model.

EXAMPLES OF DIFFERENCES IN SUMMARY POINT ESTIMATES AND CONFIDENCE INTERVALS FROM FIXED-EFFECTS AND RANDOM-EFFECTS MODELS

Which model is preferred? Consider Figure 25-1, which shows eight randomized controlled trials of interventions designed to improve birth control use by adolescent girls.[6] We see that four studies have point estimates to the right of the vertical line of no effect (i.e., odds ratios greater than 1), favoring the intervention group and suggesting that the interventions are beneficial in increasing the odds of birth control use.[7–10]

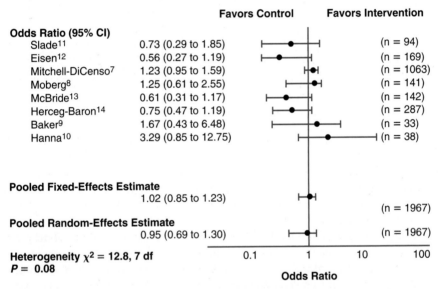

Figure 25-1. Impact of the meta-analysis model on the pooled estimate of efficacy: effect of pregnancy prevention interventions on birth control use by adolescent girls. This meta-analysis includes seven small studies (n <300) and one larger study, with point estimates on both sides of the vertical line of no effect (odds ratio = 1) and some confidence intervals with little overlap (i.e., confidence intervals around estimates in different studies have few shared values). Using the fixed-effects model, the confidence interval is very narrow, underestimating the uncertainty about the magnitude of the effect. The random-effects model provides a more conservative estimate of the level of uncertainty about the intervention effect.

Four studies have point estimates to the left of the vertical line of no effect (i.e., odds ratios less than 1.0), favoring the control group and suggesting that the interventions had the opposite to their intended effect and actually reduced the odds of birth control use.[11-14] There are large differences between the point estimates, and the confidence intervals for the studies by Eisen and colleagues[12] and Mitchell-DiCenso and colleagues[7] do not overlap much. Despite these appreciable differences in study results, the formal test of heterogeneity did not reach the conventional, relatively strict, 0.05 criterion for statistical significance ($P = .08$) (see Chapter 24, Evaluating Differences in Study Results). Consider the pooled estimate derived using the fixed-effects model (OR = 1.02; 95% CI, 0.85 to 1.23). This pooled estimate reflects the results of the larger studies, and it slightly favors the intervention group. Because the smaller studies have a greater impact on the random-effects model results, the pooled estimate slightly favors the control group (OR = 0.95; 95% CI, 0.69 to 1.30). However, neither result is statistically significant (given that the confidence intervals around both pooled estimates include an odds ratio of 1.0 representing no effect).

Which confidence interval around these pooled estimates better reflects the level of uncertainty we have about the true effect of the intervention? We suggest that the narrower confidence interval provided by the fixed-effects model overestimates the strength of inference that we can make about the true effect of the intervention, whereas the confidence interval provided by the random-effects model provides a more realistic estimate of the range of plausible true values (see Chapter 29, Confidence Intervals).

Figure 25-2 presents the results of a meta-analysis of two randomized controlled trials of raloxifene for secondary prevention of osteoporotic vertebral fractures. The two studies had very different sample sizes: the trial by Ettinger and colleagues[15] included 7705 participants, whereas the trial by Lufkin and colleagues[16] included 143 participants. The contradictory results of these two studies are reflected in the large difference between the point estimates and the nonoverlapping confidence intervals. In this instance, one would intuitively rely on the much larger of the two studies to suggest the magnitude and precision of the estimates of the underlying effect. We find that the extent to which the random-effects model moves the point estimate toward the smaller study and inflates the confidence interval is counterintuitive.

How should readers judge whether the appropriate model was used in a given meta-analysis? There is always some heterogeneity of results of studies included in a meta-analysis (see Chapter 24, Evaluating Differences in Study Results), and it is unlikely that true effects are identical in varying populations of patients. Furthermore, we are always interested in extrapolating results beyond a study sample to patients in our clinical settings. These considerations draw us toward the random-effects model. As well, the wisdom of a conservative estimate of confidence intervals is supported by instances in which subsequent large studies have contradicted the results of meta-analyses of small studies.

Conversely, the increased susceptibility of the random-effects model to publication bias as a result of increased weighting of small trials is a disadvantage. It is difficult to defend the use of the random-effects model in the rare instances (see Figure 25-2) in which it generates counterintuitive results. Fortunately, these are likely to be restricted to situations in which there are only a few studies in the review, one study is much larger than the others, and the point estimates differ greatly.

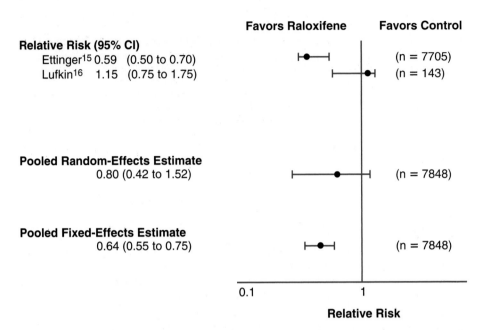

Figure 25-2. Impact of the meta-analysis model on the pooled estimate of efficacy: effect of raloxifene on vertebral fractures. This meta-analysis pools results from one large study and one small study. In this case, the fixed-effects model seems to provide a sensible estimate of the uncertainty about the magnitude of the effect, whereas the random-effects model over-estimates this uncertainty.

We do not think it appropriate to be dogmatic about the choice of an analytic model. Understanding the implications associated with the choice of model allows clinicians to identify instances in which uncertainty exists about the appropriateness of the selected model. In such instances of uncertainty, readers should consider the results of both analytic approaches.

REFERENCES

1. Fleiss JL. The statistical basis of meta-analysis. *Stat Methods Med Res.* 1993;2:121-145.
2. Anello C, Fleiss JL. Exploratory or analytic meta-analysis: should we distinguish between them? *J Clin Epidemiol.* 1995;48:109-116.
3. Lau J, Ioannidis JP, Schmid CH. Summing up evidence: one answer is not always enough. *Lancet.* 1998;351:123-127.
4. DerSimonian R, Laird N. Meta-analysis in clinical trials. *Control Clin Trials.* 1986;7:177-188.
5. Poole C, Greenland S. Random-effects meta-analyses are not always conservative. *Am J Epidemiol.* 1999;150:469-475.
6. DiCenso A, Guyatt G, Willan A, Griffith L. Interventions to reduce unintended pregnancies among adolescents: systematic review of randomised controlled trials. *BMJ.* 2002;324:1426.

7. Mitchell-DiCenso A, Thomas BH, Devlin MC, et al. Evaluation of an educational program to prevent adolescent pregnancy. *Health Educ Behav.* 1997;24:300-312.

8. Moberg DP, Piper DL. The Healthy for Life project: sexual risk behavior outcomes. *AIDS Educ Prev.* 1998;10:128-148.

9. Baker C. Self-efficacy training: its impact upon contraception and depression among a sample of urban adolescent females [doctoral dissertation]. South Orange, NJ: Seton Hall University; 1990.

10. Hanna KM. Effect of nurse-client transaction on female adolescents' contraceptive perceptions and adherence [doctoral dissertation]. Pittsburgh: University of Pittsburgh; 1990.

11. Slade LN. Life-outcome perceptions and adolescent contraceptive use [doctoral dissertation]. Atlanta: Emory University; 1989.

12. Eisen M, Zellman GL, McAlister AL. Evaluating the impact of a theory-based sexuality and contraceptive education program. *Fam Plann Perspect.* 1990;22:261-271.

13. McBride D, Gienapp A. Using randomized designs to evaluate client-centered programs to prevent adolescent pregnancy. *Fam Plann Perspect.* 2000;32:227-235.

14. Herceg-Baron R, Furstenberg FF Jr, Shea J, Harris KM. Supporting teenagers' use of contraceptives: a comparison of clinic services. *Fam Plann Perspect.* 1986;18:61-66.

15. Ettinger B, Black DM, Mitlak BH, et al. Reduction of vertebral fracture risk in postmenopausal women with osteoporosis treated with raloxifene: results from a 3-year randomized clinical trial. Multiple Outcomes of Raloxifene Evaluation (MORE) Investigators (published erratum appears in *JAMA* 1999;282:2124). *JAMA.* 1999;282:637-645.

16. Lufkin EG, Whitaker MD, Nickelsen T, et al. Treatment of established postmenopausal osteoporosis with raloxifene: a randomized trial. *J Bone Miner Res.* 1998;13:1747-1754.

UNIT V

Understanding
the Results

Chapter 26   Bias and Random Error

Chapter 27   Measures of Association

Chapter 28   Hypothesis Testing

Chapter 29   Confidence Intervals

Chapter 30   Measuring Agreement Beyond
              Chance

Chapter 31   Regression and Correlation

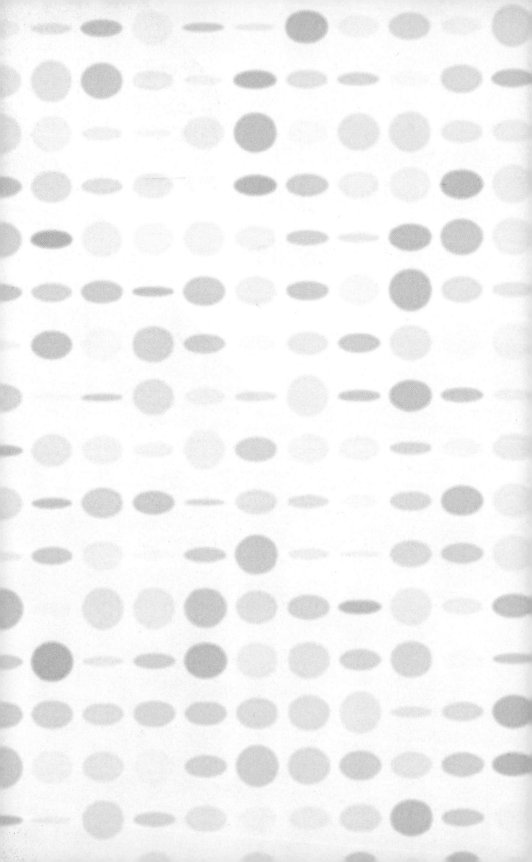

26

Bias and Random Error

Alba DiCenso and Gordon Guyatt

The following Editorial Board members also made substantive contributions to this chapter: Heather Arthur and Annette Flanagin.

In This Chapter

Random Error
　　Application to Health Research

Bias
　　Prognostic Differences Between Intervention and Control Patients
　　Placebo Effect
　　Differential Administration of Interventions
　　Differential Measurement of the Target Outcome
　　Loss to Follow-up

Differentiating Degrees of Bias and Random Error

Strategies for Reducing Bias in Studies of Health Care Interventions and Harm

RANDOM ERROR

Our clinical questions have correct answers that correspond to an underlying reality or truth. For instance, there is a true underlying magnitude of the effect of hip protectors on hip fractures after falls in elderly people living in institutions, of the effect of active or passive mobilization on deep venous thrombosis in hospitalized patients, and of the effect of warming patients before surgical procedures on the incidence of postoperative wound infections. Unfortunately, however, we will never know what that true effect really is. Why is this so?

Consider a perfectly balanced, or true, coin. Every time we flip the coin, the probability that it will land with heads up or tails up is equal—50%. Assume that we, as investigators, do not know that the coin is perfectly balanced. In fact, we have no idea how well balanced it is, and we would like to find the answer. We can state our question formally: What is the true underlying probability of a resulting head or tail on any given coin flip? Our first experiment addressing this question is a series of 10 coin flips. The result: eight heads and two tails. What are we to conclude? Taking our result at face value, we infer that the coin is very unbalanced (i.e., biased in such a way that it yields heads more often than tails) and that the probability of heads on any given flip is 80%.

Few would be happy with this conclusion. The reason for our discomfort is that we know that the world is not constructed so that a perfectly balanced, or true, coin will always yield five heads and five tails in any given set of 10 coin flips. Rather, the result is subject to the play of chance, otherwise known as *random error*. Some of the time, 10 flips of a perfectly balanced coin will yield eight heads. On occasion, nine of 10 flips will turn up heads. On rare occasions, we will find heads on all 10 flips.

What if the 10 coin flips yield five heads and five tails? Our awareness of the play of chance makes us hesitant to conclude that the coin is truly balanced. We know that not only may we get eight heads and two tails when the real probability of a head is 0.5, but also that a series of 10 coin flips with a very biased coin (a true probability of heads of 0.8, for instance) could yield five heads and five tails.

Let us say that a funding agency, intrigued by the results of our first small experiment, provides us with resources to conduct a larger study. This time, we increase the sample size of our experiment markedly and conduct a series of 1000 coin flips. When we end up with 500 heads and 500 tails, are we ready to conclude that we are dealing with a perfectly balanced coin? Not quite. We know that if the true underlying probability of heads were 51%, we would sometimes see 1000 coin flips yield the very same result we have just observed.

Application to Health Research

We can apply the foregoing logic to the results of experiments addressing health care issues in human beings. A randomized controlled trial (RCT) shows that five of 100 adolescents allocated to receive sex education become pregnant within 1 year and that 10 of 100 adolescents in the control group who do not receive sex education become pregnant within 1 year. Does sex education really reduce the adolescent pregnancy rate by 50%? Maybe, but awareness of chance will leave us with considerable uncertainty about the magnitude of the intervention effect and perhaps about whether the intervention helps at all. To use a real-world example, 26 (32%) of 81 patients with heart failure allocated to usual care were readmitted to hospital for heart failure within 1 year, as were 12 (14%) of 84 patients allocated to a specialist nurse intervention of planned home visits and telephone contact.[1] Although the true underlying reduction in the relative risk of readmission for heart failure is likely to be about 56% (i.e., $1 - [0.14/0.32] = 0.56 \times 100 = 56\%$), we must acknowledge that considerable uncertainty remains about the true magnitude of the effect. Let us remember the question with which we started: Why is it that, no matter how powerful and well designed our experiment, we will never be sure of the true intervention effect? The answer is chance.

BIAS

What do we mean when we say that a study is valid, believable, or credible? *Validity* is the degree to which a study accurately answers the question being asked or accurately measures what it intends to measure. In this book, we use validity as a technical term that relates to the magnitude of *bias*. In contrast to random error, in which the direction of deviation from the truth is unpredictable (i.e., it can result in either over-estimation or under-estimation), bias leads to systematic deviation from the underlying truth (i.e., the error is not random but has direction). In studies of interventions or harm, bias leads to either an underestimate or an overestimate of the underlying beneficial or harmful effect.

Bias may intrude as a result of differences between patients in intervention and control groups at the beginning of the study (also called baseline differences). Alternatively, it may reflect differences that develop after the study begins.

Prognostic Differences Between Intervention and Control Patients

At the start of a study, each patient, if left untreated, is destined to do well or poorly. To do poorly means to have an adverse event—say, a stroke—during the course of the study. We often refer to the adverse event that is the focus of a study as the *target outcome* or event. Many factors are associated with or causally related to the likelihood that a patient will experience the target outcome. Consider a trial of patients at risk for a cerebrovascular event. Patients who are male, elderly, have severe underlying disease (atherosclerosis), or high blood pressure are more likely than other patients to have a stroke.[2] We call each of these patient characteristics *prognostic factors* or *determinants of outcome*. These prognostic factors determine patients' destiny with respect to whether they will experience the target adverse event.

We can contrast these patient characteristics with other characteristics, such as eye color or shoe size. Eye color and shoe size differ from the first set of characteristics in that they are seldom, if ever, related to the likelihood of having a stroke. Patients with blue eyes are no more or less likely to have a stroke than those with brown eyes. Those with size 12 shoes are at no greater or lesser risk than those with size 8 shoes.

Bias will intrude if patients in the intervention and control groups differ in substantive outcome-associated ways at the start of the study. Differences in eye color or shoe size will not create bias because they are not associated with the target outcome, but differences in important prognostic factors will lead to bias. For example, if treated patients have more severe atherosclerosis or are older than control patients, their destiny will be to experience a greater proportion of adverse events than those in the control group, and the results of the study will be biased against the intervention group. In other words, the study will yield a systematically lower estimate of the intervention effect than if the study groups were prognostically alike. Thus, the study results will not reflect the underlying truth.

What if the control group has a higher mean blood pressure or a greater proportion of men than the intervention group? In these cases, the bias will be in the opposite direction (i.e., it will be against the control group). If control patients begin the study with a greater stroke risk, the results will be biased in favor of the intervention group, and the intervention will appear to benefit patients more than it really does. Thus, one source of bias is prognostic differences between treated and control patients at the start of a study.

Placebo Effect

Even if treated and control patients initially have the same expected outcome, the study may still produce a biased estimate of the intervention effect. One reason for this is the placebo effect. The *placebo effect* is an improvement in outcome that occurs when patients believe in the intervention they are receiving and therefore anticipate a positive outcome. Such anticipation may have a profound effect on how patients actually feel and, furthermore, on how they function. Placebo effect may bias the results toward suggesting a greater effect of treatment than is really the case because two components contribute to the intervention effect: the true effect of the intervention and the effect of the patient's belief that the intervention is effective.

To isolate the true effect of an intervention, investigators need to control for the placebo effect, that is, determine the true effect of the intervention over and above the placebo effect. The ideal strategies for controlling for the placebo effect involve administering a placebo to patients in the control group and keeping the intervention and control group unaware of whether they are receiving the active intervention or placebo. Any intervention effect in the control group can be totally attributed to placebo effect, and any treatment effect in the intervention group will be that over and above the placebo effect experienced by the control group.

Differential Administration of Interventions

Another potential source of bias is differential administration of interventions (other than that under study) to patients in the intervention and control groups. For example, in a study of a new intervention for stroke in which more patients in the intervention group receive aspirin than those in the control group, the results will overestimate the treatment effect. This will not be true if more patients in the intervention group receive saline eye drops or antacid medications. The reason is that saline eye drops and antacids have no effect on the frequency of stroke, whereas aspirin reduces stroke incidence.[3] *Cointervention* is a technical term used to describe a situation in which interventions that affect the incidence of the target outcome (over and above the one being studied) are differentially administered to intervention and control groups.

Note some parallels: we are not concerned about imbalances of eye color or shoe size when patients start the study (we often call these *baseline characteristics*), nor are we concerned about imbalances of saline eye drops or antacid administration after the study starts. We are concerned about the imbalance in disease severity in intervention and control patients and about differential administration of aspirin to the two groups because these factors may affect the likelihood of stroke. Study results will be biased if factors that affect prognosis, either baseline characteristics or subsequent treatment, are unequal in the groups being compared. A *confounding variable* is any prognostic factor or effective intervention that is not equally distributed in the groups being compared. For a study to be unbiased, the groups must start the same (with respect to their likelihood of experiencing the target outcome) and stay the same.

Differential Measurement of the Target Outcome

Differential measurement of the target outcome can also introduce bias. For instance, whether a patient has had a transient ischemic attack or a small stroke may be a matter of judgment. If all such events are identified and recorded as strokes in the control group but as transient ischemic attacks in the intervention group, the study will overestimate the effect of the intervention on stroke reduction.

Loss to Follow-up

Studies may introduce bias related to measurement of outcome when large numbers of patients are *lost to follow-up*. The reason is that patients who are lost to follow-up often have different prognoses from those who are retained; these patients may disappear because they experience adverse outcomes (even death) or because they are doing well (and so did not return to be assessed). Loss to follow-up is particularly problematic if intervention patients lost to follow-up did poorly, while control patients lost to follow-up did well. If rates of adverse outcomes differ in patients lost to follow-up, the necessity of relying on data from patients who were followed up will result in findings that differ from the underlying truth.

DIFFERENTIATING DEGREES OF BIAS AND RANDOM ERROR

When asked what makes a study valid, students often respond, "large sample size." Small sample size does not produce bias (and thus compromise validity), but it can increase the likelihood of a misleading result through *random error*. You may find the following exercise helpful in clarifying notions of bias and random error.

Consider a set of studies with identical designs and sample sizes that recruit from the same patient pool. Just as an experiment of 10 coin flips will not always yield five heads and five tails, the play of chance will ensure that despite their identical designs, each study will have different results.

Consider four sets of such studies. Within each set, the design and sample size of each individual trial are identical. Two of the four sets of studies have small sample sizes, and two have large sample sizes. Two sets include only RCTs in which patients, clinicians, and outcome assessors are all blinded. Two sets use only an observational design (e.g., patients are in intervention or control groups on the basis of their choice, their clinician's choice, or happenstance), a design that is far more vulnerable to bias. In this exercise, we are in the unique position of knowing the true intervention effect. In Figure 26-1, each of the bull's-eyes in the center of the four squares of the figure represents the truth. Each blue dot represents not a single patient, but the results of one repetition of the study. The farther a smaller dot lies from the central bull's-eye, the larger is the difference between the study result and the underlying true effect of the intervention.

Each set of studies represents the results of RCTs or observational studies and studies with large or small sample sizes. Before reading further, examine Figure 26-1 and draw your own conclusions about the study designs and number of patients in each of the four components (*A* through *D*).

Figure 26-1*A* represents the results of a series of RCTs with large sample sizes. The results are valid because of the strong study design and thus are distributed around the true effect, represented by the central bull's-eye. The results do not fall exactly on target because of chance, or random error. However, the large sample size, which minimizes random error, ensures that the result of any individual study is relatively close to the truth. Contrast this set of results with those depicted in Figure 26-1*B*. Again, because of the strong study design, individual study results are distributed around the truth. However, because the sample sizes are small and random error is large, the results of individual studies may be far from the truth.

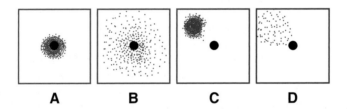

A   **B**   **C**   **D**

Figure 26-1. Representation of four sets of identically conducted studies demonstrating varying degrees of bias and random error. Black dots represent true effect; each blue dot represents the results of a single study.
A, A series of randomized controlled trials with large sample sizes. Strong study design results in distribution around true effect (validity). Large sample sizes → small random error → similar results of individual studies.
B, A series of randomized controlled trials with small sample sizes. Strong study design results in distribution around true effect (validity). Small sample sizes → large random error → dissimilar results of individual studies.
C, A series of observational studies with large sample sizes. Weaker study design results in systematic deviation from the truth (bias). Large sample sizes → small random error → similar results of individual studies. **D,** A series of observational studies with small sample sizes. Weaker study design results in systematic deviation from the truth (bias). Small sample sizes → large random error → dissimilar results of individual studies.

If we think back to our coin flip experiments, this clarifies the difference between the studies in Figure 26-1*A* and *B*. In a series of experiments in which each study involves 10 flips of a perfectly balanced coin, individual results may fall far from the truth, and findings of 70%, or even 80%, heads (or tails) will not be unusual. This situation is analogous to Figure 26-1*B*. If our experiments each involve 1000 coin flips, analogous to Figure 26-1*A*, we will seldom see distributions more extreme than, say, 540, or a 54% probability of heads or tails. With smaller sample sizes, individual results are far from the truth; with larger sample sizes, they are all close to the truth.

Figure 26-1 illustrates the rationale for pooling results of different studies, a process called *meta-analysis*. Assume that the available evidence about therapeutic effectiveness comes from a series of small RCTs. However, there is a problem. Chance will ensure that the study results vary widely, and we will not know which one to believe. Because of the strong study design (i.e., RCT), the distribution of the results is centered around the truth. As a result of this favorable situation, we can pool the results of the studies to decrease random error and increase the strength of our inferences from the uncertainty of Figure 26-1*B* to the confidence of Figure 26-1*A*.

In Figure 26-1*C*, the center of the set of dots is far from the truth. This is because studies with observational designs, even large ones, are vulnerable to bias. Because the studies share an identical design, each one will be subject to the same magnitude and direction of bias. The results are very precise, with minimal random error, but they are incorrect.

A real-world example of this phenomenon is the apparent benefit of vitamin E on reducing mortality from coronary artery disease suggested by the results of some large observational studies.[4] By contrast, a subsequent, very large, well-conducted RCT failed to demonstrate any impact of vitamin E on coronary deaths.[5]

A second example comes from the many large observational studies suggesting a 35% relative risk reduction for coronary death in women taking postmenopausal hormone replacement therapy.[6] Notably, the first RCT comparing hormone replacement therapy to placebo in women at high risk for coronary events showed no benefit.[7] In both of these situations, the likely explanation is that people with a lower underlying risk of coronary artery disease are the ones who tend to take vitamin E and hormone replacement therapy. Their lower initial risk resulted in a consistently biased estimate of effectiveness when compared with people who chose not to take these drugs.

The situation depicted in Figure 26-1*C* is particularly dangerous because the large size of the studies instills confidence in clinicians that the results are accurate. For example, many clinicians, aware of the consistent results of large observational studies, still believe the prevailing dogma of the beneficial effect of hormone replacement therapy on coronary artery disease mortality.

Like Figure 26-1*C*, Figure 26-1*D* depicts a series of observational studies leading to biased results that are far from the truth. However, because the sample sizes are all small, the results vary widely from study to study. One could be tempted to conduct a meta-analysis of these data. This would be dangerous because we risk converting imprecise estimates with large random error to precise estimates with small random error; both, however, are biased.

STRATEGIES FOR REDUCING BIAS IN STUDIES OF HEALTH CARE INTERVENTIONS AND HARM

We have noted that bias arises from differences in prognostic factors in intervention and control groups at the start of a study or from differences in prognosis that arise as a study proceeds. What can investigators do to reduce these biases? Table 26-1 summarizes the available strategies.

When studying new health care interventions, investigators often have a great deal of control. They can reduce the likelihood of differences in the distribution of prognostic features in treated and untreated patients at baseline by randomly allocating patients to the two groups. They can markedly reduce placebo effects by administering placebos to patients in the control group and by blinding patients to whether they have been assigned to the active treatment or the placebo. Blinding clinicians to whether patients are receiving active or placebo treatment can eliminate the risk of important cointervention, and blinding outcome assessors minimizes bias in the assessment of event rates.

In medication trials, investigators achieve blinding by giving control group patients pills that are biologically inert but otherwise identical to the active medication that treated patients receive. For instance, in a recent RCT that suggested that combined

Table **26-1**   Strategies to Reduce Bias in Studies of Health Care Interventions and Harm

Source of Bias	Health Care Interventions: Strategies for Reducing Bias	Harm: Strategies for Reducing Bias
Differences Noted at the Start of the Study		
Treatment and control patients differ in prognosis	Randomization	Statistical adjustment for prognostic differences in the analysis of data
Differences that Arise as the Study Proceeds		
Placebo effects	Administration of placebo to control group Blinding of patients	Choice of outcomes that are less subject to placebo effects (e.g., mortality)
Cointervention	Blinding of clinicians	Documentation of treatment differences and statistical adjustment
Bias in assessment of outcome	Blinding of outcome assessors	Choice of outcomes that are less subject to observer bias (e.g., mortality)
Loss to follow-up	Ensuring complete follow-up	Ensuring complete follow-up

estrogen and progestin may increase coronary heart disease events and breast cancer, women were allocated to the active drug or placebo.[8] However, because some women experienced persistent vaginal bleeding, the investigators had to break the code for 3444 (40%) of the women in the estrogen plus progestin group and 548 (7%) of the women in the placebo group, thus unblinding these patients and their clinicians. As a result, in this study, placebo effects were only minimized rather than eliminated.

The use of placebos is not limited to drug trials. For example, in a trial of respiratory muscle training using a hand-held plastic resistance device, control patients were trained on an identical device that provided minimal resistance.[9] Investigators will sometimes create attention placebos in which patients in the control group are given a similar amount of attention as the intervention group but do not receive the "active" part of the intervention. For example, in a study evaluating the efficacy of two Internet interventions for community-dwelling individuals with symptoms of depression, Christensen and colleagues[10] randomized one group of participants to weekly contact with an interviewer who directed their use of a Web site offering evidence-based information on depression and its treatment, one group of participants to weekly contact with an interviewer who directed their use of a Web site offering cognitive behavior therapy for the prevention of depression, and one group to an attention placebo, which provided weekly contact with a lay interviewer to discuss lifestyle factors such as exercise, education, and health habits. The use of the attention placebo allowed the investigators to determine the true effect of the Web sites over and above the attention effect of weekly contact with the lay interviewer.

For certain interventions, including surgical and most nursing interventions, it is challenging, if not impossible, to create appropriate placebo interventions. How, for instance, would you create placebos for hand washing, shaving patients before surgical procedures, or a nurse-led asthma education program? In most evaluations of nursing interventions, therefore, the control group receives usual care. For example, in the RCT evaluating a specialist nurse intervention for patients with chronic heart failure, patients in the intervention group received home visits and telephone contacts, whereas those in the control group received usual care, consisting of follow-up by their general practitioner.[1] In a trial evaluating the effect of enteral nutrition on postoperative complications in patients with gastrointestinal cancer, patients in the control group received parenteral nutrition, the existing standard of care.[11] In a trial assessing the effect of a preoperative smoking cessation intervention on postoperative complications in patients having elective knee or hip replacement, patients in the intervention group received a smoking cessation program delivered by a nurse, whereas patients in the control group received little or no information or counseling on smoking cessation.[12]

Given that the control groups in most studies of nursing interventions do not receive placebos, patients and clinicians are seldom blinded to which patients are receiving active treatment. As a result, there is a risk of cointervention, especially by clinicians who may feel compelled to act in some way to reduce target events in control group patients. Blinding the monitoring and recording of target outcomes, if possible, and blinding the adjudication of those outcomes (which is virtually always possible) are particularly important in such studies.

In general, investigators studying the effects of potentially harmful exposures have far less control than those investigating the effects of potentially beneficial treatments. They must be content to compare patients whose exposures are determined by their choice or by circumstance, and they can address potential differences in patients' fate only by statistical adjustment for known prognostic factors. Blinding is impossible, so their best defense against placebo effects and bias in outcome assessment is to choose end points that are less subject to these biases (e.g., death). Investigators addressing both sets of questions can reduce bias by minimizing loss to follow-up (see Table 26-1).

These general rules do not always apply. Sometimes, investigators find it difficult or impossible to randomize patients to intervention and control groups. Under such circumstances, they choose observational study designs, and clinicians must apply the validity criteria developed for questions of harm to such studies (see Chapter 5, Harm). Similarly, if the potentially harmful exposure is a drug with beneficial effects, investigators may be able to randomize patients to intervention and control groups. In this case, clinicians can apply the validity criteria designed for health care intervention questions (see Chapter 4, Health Care Interventions). Whether for issues of intervention or harm, the strength of inference from RCTs will almost invariably be far greater than the strength of inference from observational studies.

REFERENCES

1. Blue L, Lang E, McMurray JJ, et al. Randomised controlled trial of specialist nurse intervention in heart failure. *BMJ*. 2001;323:715-718.
2. Goldstein LB, Adams R, Becker K, et al. Primary prevention of ischemic stroke: a statement for healthcare professionals from the Stroke Council of the American Heart Association. *Stroke*. 2001;32:280-299.
3. Sandercock P, Gubitz G, Foley P, Counsell C. Antiplatelet therapy for acute ischaemic stroke. *Cochrane Database Syst Rev*. 2003;(2):CD000029.
4. Knekt P, Reunanen A, Jarvinen R, Seppanen R, Heliovaara M, Aromaa A. Antioxidant vitamin intake and coronary mortality in a longitudinal population study. *Am J Epidemiol*. 1994;139:1180-1189.
5. Yusuf S, Dagenais G, Pogue J, Bosch J, Sleight P. Vitamin E supplementation and cardiovascular events in high-risk patients: the Heart Outcomes Prevention Evaluation study investigators. *N Engl J Med*. 2000;342:154-160.
6. Stampfer MJ, Colditz GA. Estrogen replacement therapy and coronary heart disease: a quantitative assessment of the epidemiologic evidence. *Prev Med*. 1991;20:47-63.
7. Hulley S, Grady D, Bush T, et al. Randomized trial of estrogen plus progestin for secondary prevention of coronary heart disease in postmenopausal women: Heart and Estrogen/progestin Replacement Study (HERS) research group. *JAMA*. 1998;280:605-613.
8. Rossouw JE, Anderson GL, Prentice RL, et al. Risks and benefits of estrogen plus progestin in healthy postmenopausal women: principal results from the Women's Health Initiative randomized controlled trial. *JAMA*. 2002;288:321-333.
9. Guyatt GH, Keller J, Singer J, Halcrow S, Newhouse M. Controlled trial of respiratory muscle training in chronic airflow limitation. *Thorax*. 1992;47:598-602.
10. Christensen H, Griffiths KM, Jorm AF. Delivering interventions for depression by using the internet: randomised controlled trial. *BMJ*. 2004;328:265.
11. Bozzetti F, Braga M, Gianotti L, et al. Postoperative enteral versus parenteral nutrition in malnourished patients with gastrointestinal cancer: a randomised multicentre trial. *Lancet*. 2001;358:1487-1492.
12. Moller AM, Villebro N, Pedersen T, et al. Effect of preoperative smoking intervention on postoperative complications: a randomised clinical trial. *Lancet*. 2002;359:114-117.

Measures of Association

27

Alba DiCenso and Gordon Guyatt

The following Editorial Board members also made substantive contributions to this chapter: Sharon Lock and Susan Marks.

We gratefully acknowledge the work of Roman Jaeschke, Alexandra Barratt, Stephen Walter, Deborah Cook, Finlay McAlister, and John Attia on the original chapter that appears in the Users' Guides to the Medical Literature, *edited by Guyatt and Rennie.*

In This Chapter

Dichotomous and Continuous Outcomes

The 2 × 2 Table

Absolute Risk

Absolute Risk Reduction

Relative Risk

Relative Risk Reduction

Odds Ratio

Relative Risk and Odds Ratio Versus Absolute Risk Reduction: Why the Fuss?

Number Needed to Treat

Number Needed to Harm

Back to the 2 × 2 Table

Confidence Intervals

Continued

Survival Data

Case-Control Studies

Which Measure of Association Is Best?

When clinicians consider the results of studies designed to evaluate health care interventions, they are interested in the association between the intervention and the target outcome. The study under consideration may or may not demonstrate an association between the intervention and the outcome.

The focus of this chapter is on yes/no or dichotomous outcomes, such as wound infection, functional disability, depression, readmission to hospital, or death. In presenting the results of studies assessing the effects of an intervention on dichotomous outcomes, authors generally include the proportion of patients in each group who experienced the target outcome. As depicted in Figure 27-1, consider three different interventions that were administered to three different populations and reduced readmission to hospital. The first intervention was administered to a population with a 30% risk of readmission and reduced the risk to 20%. The second intervention was administered to a population with a 10% risk of readmission and reduced the risk to 6.7%. The third intervention reduced the risk of readmission from 1% to 0.67%.

Although all three interventions reduced the risk of readmission by a third, this piece of information does not fully capture the impact of the intervention. Expressing the strength of an association as a *relative risk* (RR), a *relative risk reduction* (RRR),

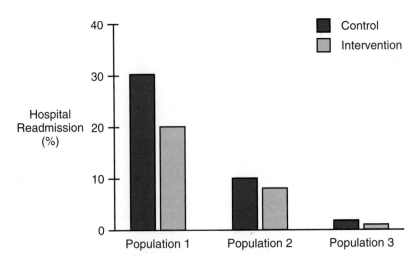

Figure 27-1. Constant relative risk with varying risk differences.

an *absolute risk reduction* (ARR) or *risk difference* (RD), an *odds ratio* (OR), a *number needed to treat* (NNT), or a *number needed to harm* (NNH) conveys different information.

DICHOTOMOUS AND CONTINUOUS OUTCOMES

A study's primary analysis often is concerned with the proportion of patients who experience a particular target outcome, end point, or event in the intervention and control groups. This is true whenever the outcome captures the presence or absence of negative events, such as depression, infection, readmission to hospital, functional disability, or death. It is also true for positive events, such as ulcer healing or resolution of symptoms. Even if an outcome is not a dichotomous variable, investigators sometimes elect to present the results as if this were the case. For example, investigators may present end points such as change in quality of life, number of episodes of hyperglycemia per month, change in pulmonary function, or number of visits to the emergency department as the mean values for intervention and control groups. Alternatively, they may transform these variables into dichotomous data by specifying a threshold or degree of change that constitutes an important improvement or deterioration and then examine the proportion of patients above and below this threshold. For example, a study of the efficacy of oral corticosteroids in patients with chronic stable airflow limitation assessed forced expiratory volume in 1 second (FEV_1), a continuous outcome. The investigators, however, defined an event as an improvement in baseline FEV_1 of more than 20%, a dichotomous outcome.[1] In another study of patients with chronic lung disease, investigators examined the difference in the proportion of patients who achieved an important improvement in health-related quality of life.[2] The investigators' choice of the magnitude of change required to designate an improvement as "important" can affect the apparent effectiveness of an intervention (although less so for odds ratios than for other measures of association, as discussed later in this chapter).

THE 2 × 2 TABLE

Table 27-1 depicts a 2 × 2 table that captures the information for a dichotomous outcome. For instance, in a randomized controlled trial, investigators compared hospital readmission rates in patients with chronic heart failure who received a specialist nurse intervention consisting of home visits and telephone contact with similar patients who received usual care by their general practitioner.[3] After follow-up of 1 year, 12 of 84 patients assigned to the specialist nurse intervention were readmitted with heart failure, as were 26 of 81 patients assigned to usual care (Table 27-2).

ABSOLUTE RISK

The simplest measure of association to understand is the *absolute risk* which is the proportion of patients who experience the outcome in each group. The absolute risk of readmission in the specialist nurse group is 14.3% [(12/84), or a/(a+b)], and the absolute risk of readmission in the usual care group is 32.1% [(26/81), or c/(c+d)].

Table **27-1** The 2 × 2 Table

		Outcome Yes	No	Total
Exposure to Intervention	**Yes**	a	b	a+b
	No	c	d	c+d
	Total	a+c	b+d	

Absolute Risk Reduction (ARR)	=	$\dfrac{c}{c+d} - \dfrac{a}{a+b}$
Relative Risk (RR)	=	$\dfrac{a/(a+b)}{c/(c+d)}$
Relative Risk Reduction (RRR)	=	$\dfrac{c/(c+d) - a/(a+b)}{c/(c+d)}$
Odds Ratio (OR)	=	$\dfrac{a/b}{c/d} = \dfrac{ad}{bc}$
Number Needed to Treat (NNT)	=	$\dfrac{1}{ARR}$

We often refer to the risk of the adverse outcome in the control group as the *baseline risk* or *control event rate*.

ABSOLUTE RISK REDUCTION

One can relate these two absolute risks by calculating the difference between them. We refer to this difference as the *absolute risk reduction* (ARR) or the *risk difference* (RD). Algebraically, the formula for calculating the ARR or RD is [c/(c+d)] − [a/(a+b)] (see Table 27-1). This measure of effect tells us what percent of patients will be spared the adverse outcome if they receive the experimental intervention, rather than the control intervention. In our example, the ARR is 32.1% − 14.3% = 17.8% (or stated as a proportion, ARR = 0.178).

RELATIVE RISK

Another way to relate the absolute risks in the two groups is to take the ratio of the two; this is called the *relative risk* also known as the *risk ratio* (RR). The relative risk tells us the proportion of the original risk (in this case, the risk of hospital readmission with usual care) that is still present when patients receive the experimental intervention (in this case, the specialist nurse intervention). Looking at our 2 × 2 tables, the formula for this calculation is [a/(a+b)]/[c/(c+d)] (see Table 27-1 and the Appendix). In our example, the relative risk of readmission after receiving the specialist nurse intervention versus usual care is 12/84 or 14.3% (the risk in the specialist nurse group) divided by 26/81 or

Table **27-2**   Results From a Randomized Controlled Trial of a
Specialist Nurse Intervention Compared With Usual Care
for Patients With Chronic Heart Failure

		Outcome		
		Readmitted to Hospital With Chronic Heart Failure	Not Readmitted to Hospital With Chronic Heart Failure	Total
Exposure	Specialist Nurse	12	72	84
	Usual Care	26	55	81

Absolute risk reduction	$=$	$(26/81 - 12/84)$	$= 0.178$
Relative risk	$=$	$(12/84 \div 26/81)$	$= 0.45$
Relative risk reduction	$=$	$(26/81 - 12/84) \div 26/81$	$= 0.55$
Odds ratio	$=$	$(12 \times 55)/(72 \times 26)$	$= 0.35$
Number needed to treat	$=$	$(1/0.178)$	$= 6$

*Data from Blue L, Lang E, McMurray JJ, et al. Randomised controlled trial of specialist nurse interven-
tion in heart failure. BMJ. 2001;323:715-718.*

32.1% (the risk in the usual care group), which equals 0.45 or 45%. In other words, we
would say that the risk of hospital readmission with a specialist nurse intervention is a
little less than half of that with usual care.

RELATIVE RISK REDUCTION

Another measure used when assessing effectiveness of an intervention is the *relative risk
reduction* (RRR), which is an estimate of the proportion of baseline risk that is reduced
by the intervention. The relative risk reduction is calculated by dividing the absolute risk
reduction by the absolute risk in the control group (see Table 27-1 and the Appendix).
In our example of patients with chronic heart failure, the calculation for RRR is 17.8%
(the ARR) divided by 32.1% (the risk in the usual care group), or 55% (also expressed
as 0.55). One may also derive the RRR as $(1.0 - \text{RR})$. In the example, we have RRR = 1.0
$- 0.45 = 0.55$, or 55%. Using nontechnical language, we would say that the specialist
nurse intervention decreased the relative risk of hospital readmission by 55% compared
with usual care.

ODDS RATIO

Instead of looking at the risk of an event, we could estimate the odds of having an event
versus not having an event. You may be most familiar with odds in the context of sporting
events, when bookies or newspaper commentators quote the chances for and against a
horse's, boxer's, or tennis player's winning a particular event. In terms of health care, the
odds ratio (OR) represents the proportion of patients with the target event divided by
the proportion without the target event. In most clinical investigations, odds and risks

are approximately equal, and many authors calculate relative odds and then report the results as if they had calculated relative risks. The following discussion will help clinicians to understand what an odds ratio is and to identify those circumstances in which treating an odds ratio as a relative risk will be misleading.

The following is a numerical example: if one of five patients in a study develops a wound infection, the odds of having a wound infection are (1/5)/(4/5) or 0.20/0.80, or 0.25. It is easy to see that because the denominator is the same in both the top and bottom expressions, it is canceled out, leaving the number of patients with the event (1) divided by the number of patients without the event (4). To convert from odds to risk, divide the odds by 1 plus the odds. For instance, if the odds of a wound infection is 0.25, the risk is 0.25/(1 + 0.25), or 0.20. Table 27-3 presents the relationship between risk and odds. The greater the magnitude of the risk is, the greater is the divergence between the risk and odds.

In our example, the odds of hospital readmission in the nurse specialist group are 12 (readmitted) versus 72 (not readmitted), or 12 to 72 or 12/72 (a/b), and the odds of hospital readmission in the usual care group are 26/55 (c/d). The formula for the ratio of these odds is (a/b)/(c/d) (see Table 27-1); in our example, this yields (12/72)/(26/55), or 0.35. If one were formulating a terminology parallel to risk (in which we call a ratio of risks a relative risk), one would call the ratio of odds a *relative odds*. Epidemiologists, who have been averse to simplifying parallel terminology, have chosen relative risk as the preferred term for a ratio of risks and odds ratio for a ratio of odds.

Clinicians have a good intuitive understanding of risk and even of a ratio of risks. Gamblers have a good intuitive understanding of odds. No one (with the possible exception of certain statisticians) intuitively understands a ratio of odds.[4,5] Nevertheless, until recently, the odds ratio has been the predominant measure of association.[6] The reason is that the odds ratio has a statistical advantage in that it is essentially independent of the arbitrary choice between a comparison of the risks of an event (e.g., death) and a comparison of the corresponding nonevent (e.g., survival), a situation that is not true of the relative risk.[7]

As clinicians, we would like to be able to substitute the relative risk, which we intuitively understand, for the odds ratio, which we do not understand. Looking back at our 2 × 2 table (see Table 27-1), we see that the validity of this substitution requires that

Table **27-3** Risks and Odds*

Risk (%)	Odds
80	4
60	1.5
50	1
40	0.67
33	0.50
25	0.33
20	0.25
10	0.11
5	0.053

*Risk is equal to odds/(1 + odds); odds are equal to risk/(1 − risk).

[a/(a+b)]/[c/(c+d)]—the RR—be more or less equal to (a/b)/(c/d)—the OR. For this to be the case, a must be much less than b, and c much less than d; in other words, the outcome must occur infrequently in both the intervention and the control groups. As we have noted, Table 27-3 demonstrates that as the risk decreases, the odds and risk become more similar. If event rates are low, as is common in most randomized trials, the odds ratio and relative risk are very close. The relative risk and odds ratio are also closer together when the magnitude of the intervention effect is small (i.e., OR and RR are close to 1.0) than when the intervention effect is large.

When event rates are high and effect sizes are large, there are ways of converting odds ratios to relative risks.[8,9] Fortunately, clinicians rarely need to consult such conversion tables. Consider a randomized controlled trial of enteral nutrition versus parenteral nutrition for postoperative complications in malnourished patients having surgical procedures for gastrointestinal cancer.[10] This trial found an overall postoperative complication rate of 49% with parenteral nutrition—as high an event rate as one is likely to find in most trials. The OR associated with enteral nutrition was 0.54, a large effect. Despite the high event rate and large effect, the RR of 0.69 is not very different from the OR. The two are close enough—and this is the crucial point—that choosing one measure or the other is unlikely to have an important influence on intervention decisions.

RELATIVE RISK AND ODDS RATIO VERSUS ABSOLUTE RISK REDUCTION: WHY THE FUSS?

Having decided that distinguishing between odds ratios and relative risks seldom has major importance, we can introduce hypothetical changes to the 2 × 2 table (see Table 27-2) to understand why it is important to distinguish between odds ratios or relative risks and absolute risk reductions. Let us assume that the number of patients readmitted to hospital with heart failure decreased by approximately 50% in both groups. We now have six readmissions among 84 patients in the specialist nurse group and 13 readmissions among 81 patients in the usual care group. The risk of readmission decreases from 14.3% (12/84) to 7.15% (6/84) in the nurse specialist group and from 32.1% (26/81) to 16% (13/81) in the usual care group. The RR becomes 6/84 (the risk in the specialist nurse group) divided by 13/81 (the risk in the usual care group), or 45%, the same as before. The OR becomes (6/78)/(13/68) or 0.40, moderately different from 0.35 in our original example and closer to the RR. The absolute risk reduction decreases quite dramatically from 17.8% to 8.9%. Thus, the decrease in the proportion of those readmitted in both groups by a factor of 2 leaves the RR unchanged, results in a moderate increase in the OR, and reduces the absolute risk reduction by a factor of 2. This example (see Figure 27-1) shows how the same relative risk can be associated with quite different absolute risk reduction and that although the relative risk does not reflect changes in the baseline risk in the control group, the absolute risk reduction can change markedly with changes in this baseline risk.

Thus, an RR of 0.67, for example, may represent a situation in which treatment reduces the risk of readmission from 1% to 0.67% or from 30% to 20% (see Figure 27-1). Assume that the frequency of severe side effects associated with such an intervention was 10%—we may encounter this situation in offering chemotherapy to patients with cancer, for instance. Under these circumstances, we would probably not recommend the treatment to most patients if it reduced the probability of dying by 0.33% (from 1% to 0.67%), but we might be willing to recommend this treatment if the probability of an adverse outcome dropped from 30% to 20%. In the latter situation, 10 patients per 100 would benefit, whereas one would experience adverse effects, a trade-off that most patients would consider worthwhile.

The relative risk reduction behaves in the same way as the relative risk and does not reflect the change in the underlying risk in the control population. In our example, the RRR will be of the same magnitude if the frequency of events decreases by approximately half in both groups: $[(6/84) - (13/81)] / (13/81)$, or 55%.

NUMBER NEEDED TO TREAT

One can also express the impact of an intervention by the number of patients one would need to treat to prevent one adverse event, the *number needed to treat* (NNT).[11,12] Table 27-2 shows that the risk of readmission was 14.3% in the specialist nurse group, and 32.1% in the usual care group. Using these estimates, we can calculate the ARR (control event rate minus intervention event rate or 32.1% − 14.3%), which would show that if 100 patients received the specialist nurse intervention rather than usual care, 18 patients would avoid readmission. If we need to treat 100 patients to avoid 18 readmissions, how many patients would we need to treat to avoid one readmission? The answer, 100 divided by 18, or approximately 6 (i.e., 100 divided by the risk difference, 18, expressed as a percentage), is the number needed to treat. One can also calculate the NNT by taking the reciprocal of the absolute risk reduction expressed as a proportion (i.e., 1/ARR or 1/0.18; see Table 27-1). You will note that both the number needed to treat and the absolute risk reduction change with the difference in the underlying risk. This is not surprising because the number needed to treat is the reciprocal of the absolute risk reduction. Given knowledge of the baseline risk and relative risk reduction, a nomogram presents a third way of arriving at the number needed to treat (Figure 27-2).[13]

The number needed to treat is inversely related to the proportion of patients in the control group who have an adverse event. If the risk of an adverse event doubles, we need treat only half as many patients to prevent an adverse event. If the risk decreases by a factor of 4, we will need to treat four times as many patients. In our example, if the frequency of events (the baseline risk) decreases by a factor of 2 while the relative risk reduction remains constant, providing 100 patients with a specialist nurse intervention would result in nine patients avoiding readmission (ARR = 16% − 7.15% = 9%), and the NNT would approximately double, to 11 (100/9% or 1/0.09).

The number needed to treat is also inversely related to the relative risk reduction. A more effective treatment with twice the relative risk reduction will reduce the number needed to treat by half. If the relative risk reduction with a new treatment is only one fourth of that achieved by an alternative strategy, the number needed to treat will be four times greater. Table 27-4 presents hypothetical data that illustrate these relationships.

By using absolute risk reduction and its reciprocal, the number needed to treat, we incorporate the influence of the changing baseline risk. If we only know the absolute risk reduction or number needed to treat, however, we will not know the size

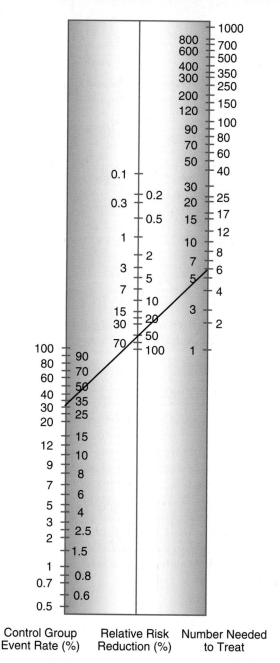

Control Group Event Rate (%)	Relative Risk Reduction (%)	Number Needed to Treat

Figure 27-2. Nomogram for calculating the number needed to treat. A straight line is drawn from the point corresponding to the control group event rate in the left hand column to the point corresponding to the relative risk reduction on the middle scale. The point of intercept of this line with the right hand scale gives the number needed to treat (NNT). Using estimates from Table 27-2 to illustrate, the control group event rate is 32.1% (26/81), the relative risk reduction is 55%, and the NNT is 6. *(Modified and reproduced with permission from the BMJ Publishing Group from Chatellier G, Zapletal E, Lemaitre D, Menard J, Degoulet P. The number needed to treat: a clinically useful nomogram in its proper context. BMJ. 1996;312:426-429.)*

Table **27-4** Relationship Between the Baseline Risk, the Relative Risk Reduction, and the Number Needed to Treat*

Control Event Rate	Intervention Event Rate	Relative Risk	Relative Risk Reduction	Risk Difference	Number Needed to Treat
0.02	0.01	50%	50%	0.01	100
0.4	0.2	50%	50%	0.2	5
0.04	0.02	50%	50%	0.02	50
0.04	0.03	75%	25%	0.01	100
0.4	0.3	75%	25%	0.1	10
0.01	0.005	50%	50%	0.005	200

*Relative risk = intervention event rate/control event rate; relative risk reduction = 1 – relative risk; risk difference = control event rate – intervention event rate; number needed to treat = 1/risk difference.

of the baseline risk. For example, an ARR of 5% (and a corresponding NNT of 20) may represent reduction of the risk of death from 10% to 5% (an RRR of 50%) or from 50% to 45% (an RRR of 10%).

NUMBER NEEDED TO HARM

Clinicians can calculate the *number needed to harm* (NNH) in exactly the same way. If one expects that five of 100 patients will develop groin pain when pressure bandages are applied immediately after coronary angiography to prevent bleeding, for every 20 patients with pressure bandages, one patient will develop groin pain (i.e., NNH = 20).

In this discussion we have not mentioned the problem that investigators may report odds ratios instead of relative risks. As we have mentioned, the best way of dealing with this situation when event rates are low is to assume the relative risk will be very close to the odds ratio. The higher the risk is, the less secure is the assumption. Tables 27-5 and 27-6 provide a guide for making an accurate estimate of the number needed to treat and number needed to harm when you know a patient's baseline risk and the investigator has provided only an odds ratio.

BACK TO THE 2 × 2 TABLE

Regardless of the way we choose to express the magnitude of an intervention effect, the 2 × 2 table reflects results at a given point in time. Therefore, our comments on relative risk, absolute risk reduction, relative risk reduction, odds ratio, and number needed to treat or number needed to harm must be qualified by imposing a time frame on them. For example, we have to say that providing a specialist nurse intervention rather than usual care resulted in an ARR of readmission of 18% and an NNT of six *over 1 year*. The results might have been different if the duration of observation had been very short (if there was no time to develop an event) or very long (after all, if the outcome is death, after 100 years of follow-up, everybody will die).

Table 27-5 Deriving the Number Needed to Treat From the Odds Ratio

Control Event Rate	Therapeutic Intervention (Odds Ratio)								
	0.5	0.55	0.6	0.65	0.7	0.75	0.8	0.85	0.9
0.05	41	46	52	59	69	83	104	139	209
0.1	21	24	27	31	36	43	54	73	110
0.2	11	13	14	17	20	24	30	40	61
0.3	8	9	10	12	14	18	22	30	46
0.4	7	8	9	10	12	15	19	26	40
0.5	6	7	8	9	11	14	18	25	38
0.7	6	7	9	10	13	16	20	28	44
0.9	12	15	18	22	27	34	46	64	101

Modified from Hux JE, Levinton CM, Naylor CD. Prescribing propensity: influence of life-expectancy gains and drug costs. J Gen Intern Med. 1994;9:195-201.
The formula for determining the NNT is:

$$NNT = \frac{1 - CER\,(1 - OR)}{CER\,(1 - CER)\,(1 - OR)}$$

CER, Control event rate; NNT, number needed to treat; OR, odds ratio.

Table 27-6 Deriving the Number Needed to Harm From the Odds Ratio

Control Event Rate	Therapeutic Intervention (Odds Ratio)								
	1.1	1.2	1.3	1.4	1.5	2	2.5	3	3.5
0.05	212	106	71	54	43	22	15	12	9
0.1	112	57	38	29	23	12	9	7	6
0.2	64	33	22	17	14	8	5	4	4
0.3	49	25	17	13	11	6	5	4	3
0.4	43	23	16	12	10	6	4	4	3
0.5	42	22	15	12	10	6	5	4	4
0.7	51	27	19	15	13	8	7	6	5
0.9	121	66	47	38	32	21	17	16	14

Modified from Hux JE, Levinton CM, Naylor CD. Prescribing propensity: influence of life-expectancy gains and drug costs. J Gen Intern Med. 1994;9:195-201.
The formula for determining the NNH is:

$$NNH = \frac{1 + CER(OR - 1)}{CER\,(1 - CER)\,(OR - 1)}$$

CER, Control event rate; NNH, number needed to harm; OR, odds ratio.

CONFIDENCE INTERVALS

We have presented all the measures of association for comparing a specialist nurse intervention with usual care as if they represented the true effect. The results of any study, however, represent only an estimate of the truth. The true effect of an intervention may actually be somewhat greater—or less—than what we observed. The *confidence interval* tells us, within the bounds of plausibility, how much greater or smaller the true effect is likely to be (see Chapter 29, Confidence Intervals). Statistical programs permit computation of confidence intervals for each of the measures of association we have discussed.

SURVIVAL DATA

As previously stated, the analysis of a 2×2 table implies an examination of data at a specific point in time. This analysis is satisfactory if we are looking for events that occur within relatively short time periods and if all patients have the same duration of follow-up. In longer-term studies, however, we are interested not only in the total number of events, but in their timing as well. For example, we may focus on whether group psychosocial support for patients with metastatic breast cancer delays death.[14]

When the timing of events is important, investigators can present the results in the form of several 2×2 tables constructed at different times during a study. For example, Table 27-2 represents the situation after 12 months of follow-up. Similar tables could be constructed describing the fate of all patients available for analysis after enrollment at 1 week, 1 month, 3 months, or whatever time frame we choose to examine. The analysis of accumulated data that takes into account the timing of events is called *survival analysis*. Do not infer from the name, however, that such an analysis is restricted to deaths; in fact, any dichotomous outcome will qualify.

A survival curve describes the status of a group of patients at different time points after a defined starting point.[15] Figure 27-3 shows the Kaplan-Meier survival curve for the specialist nurse trial, which graphs the time to first event, in this case either death from any cause or readmission to hospital with worsening heart failure.[3] This end point (readmission or death) is different from the end point we have discussed previously (readmission). The survival curve begins at time 0 with 100% of patients in both groups event free (81 in the usual care group and 84 in the intervention group). It then splits into two lines, one showing the percentage of patients in the specialist nurse intervention group *(dotted line)* who died or were admitted to hospital for heart failure over 12 months and one showing the same outcome in the usual care control group *(solid line)*. The number of patients at risk at each time point includes all those who have not yet experienced the outcome (death or readmission to hospital for heart failure) and who have been followed up for at least this duration of time. At some point, prediction becomes very imprecise because few patients are available to estimate the probability of survival. Confidence intervals around the survival curves (not shown in this example) capture the precision of the estimate.

Even if the true relative risk or relative risk reduction is the same for each duration of follow-up, the play of chance will ensure that the point estimates differ. Ideally then, we would estimate the overall relative risk reduction by applying an average, weighted for the

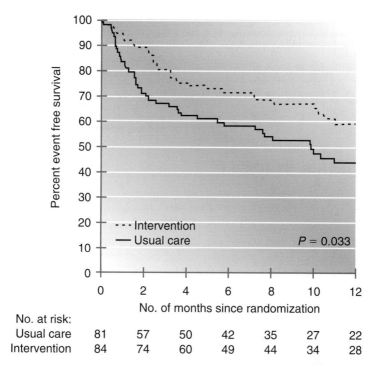

Figure 27-3. Survival curves for specialist nurse intervention and usual care. *(Modified and reproduced with permission of the BMJ Publishing Group from Blue L, Lang E, McMurray JJ, et al. Randomised controlled trial of specialist nurse intervention in heart failure. BMJ. 2001;323;715-718.)*

number of patients available, for the entire survival experience. Statistical methods allow just such an estimate. The weighted relative risk over the entire study is known as the *hazard ratio*. In the specialist nurse trial, fewer patients had events in the intervention group than in the usual care group (hazard ratio = 0.61; 95% confidence interval, 0.38 to 0.96).

Assuming the null hypothesis (i.e., that no difference exists between two survival curves), we can generate a *P* value that informs us about the likelihood that chance explains the differences in results. Statistical techniques (most commonly, the *Cox regression model*) allow the results to be adjusted or corrected for differences in the two groups at baseline (see Chapter 29, Confidence Intervals). If one group were older (and thus at higher risk) or had less severe disease (and thus at lower risk), the investigators could have conducted an analysis that took these differences into account. This, in effect, tells us what would have happened if the two groups had comparable risk factors for the adverse outcome at the start of the trial. In the nurse specialist trial, treatment was the sole covariate in the Cox proportional hazards model. However, in a trial evaluating the effect of group psychosocial support on survival of patients with metastatic breast cancer,[14] the Cox regression model included factors that differed between groups at baseline, such as age at diagnosis, nodal stage, presence or absence of estrogen and progesterone receptors, use or nonuse of adjuvant chemotherapy, and time from first metastasis to randomization.

Another way of reading survival curves is to plot the points at which a chosen percentage of patients in each group has reached an end point. The difference between these points is a reflection of the delay in outcomes in the intervention group. For example, although angiotensin-converting enzyme inhibitors may decrease the risk of mortality up to 25% in patients after myocardial infarction, this decrease translates into a few extra months of life, a result that may not seem as impressive.[16]

CASE-CONTROL STUDIES

Our previous examples have come from prospective randomized controlled trials. In these trials, we start with a group of patients who are exposed to an intervention and a group of patients who are not exposed to the intervention. The investigators follow the patients over time and record the frequency of events. The process is similar in observational studies called *prospective cohort studies*, although in this study design, the exposure or treatment is not controlled by the investigators. For randomized trials and prospective cohort studies we can calculate risks, absolute risk reductions, and relative risks.

In *case-control studies*, investigators choose or sample participants on the basis of whether they have experienced a target outcome rather than on whether they have been exposed to an intervention or risk factor. Participants start the study with or without the event, rather than with or without the exposure or intervention. Investigators compare patients with the adverse outcome—be it hyperactivity, depression, leukemia, asthma, or hip fracture—with control patients without the outcome. The usual question is whether any factors seem to be more commonly present in one group than the other.

In a case-control study, investigators examined whether sunbeds or sunlamps increased the risk of skin melanoma.[17] The investigators identified 583 patients with melanoma (cases) and 608 controls. The case and control patients had similar distributions of age, sex, and residence. Table 27-7 presents the findings for men who participated in this study.

If the information in Table 27-7 had come from a prospective cohort study or randomized controlled trial, we could begin by calculating the risk of an event in the exposed and control groups. This would not make sense in the case-control study because the number of patients who did not have melanoma was chosen by the investigators. We need to know the population at risk to calculate a relative risk, and a case-control study does not provide this information.

The odds ratio provides the only sensible measure of association in a case-control study. One can ask whether the odds of exposure to sunbeds or sunlamps among people with melanoma were the same as the odds of exposure among the control patients. In the study, the odds of exposure were 67/210 in patients with melanoma and 41/242 in control patients. The OR is therefore (67/210)/(41/242), or 1.88 (95% confidence interval, 1.20 to 2.98), suggesting an association between exposure to sunbeds or sunlamps and developing melanoma. Since the confidence interval does not overlap or include 1.0, it suggests that the association is unlikely to have resulted from chance.

Table 27-7   Results From a Case-Control Study Examining the Association of Cutaneous Melanoma and the Use of Sunbeds and Sunlamps

	Exposure	Cases	Controls
Sunbeds or sunlamps	Yes	67	41
	No	210	242

Data from Walter SD, Marrett LD, From L, Hertzman C, Shannon HS, Roy P. The association of cutaneous malignant melanoma with the use of sunbeds and sunlamps. Am J Epidemiol. 1990;131: 232-243.

Even if the association did not occur by chance, it does not necessarily mean that sunbeds or sunlamps caused melanoma. Potential explanations could include greater recollection of using these devices among people with melanoma *(recall bias)*, longer sun exposure among these people, and different skin color; the investigators addressed many of these explanations. Additional confirmatory studies would be required to be confident that exposure to sunbeds or sunlamps was the cause of melanoma.

WHICH MEASURE OF ASSOCIATION IS BEST?

As evidence-based practitioners, we must decide which measure of association deserves our focus. Does it matter? The answer is "yes." The same results, when presented in different ways, may lead to different intervention decisions.[18-22] For example, Forrow and colleagues[18] demonstrated that clinicians were less inclined to treat patients when they were shown the results of trials in terms of absolute changes in outcomes compared with relative changes in outcomes. In a similar study, Naylor and colleagues[19] found that clinicians rated the effectiveness of an intervention lower when events were presented in absolute terms rather than using relative risk reductions. Moreover, effectiveness was rated lower when results were expressed in terms of numbers needed to treat than when the same data were presented as relative risk reductions or absolute risk reductions.

Patients are as susceptible as clinicians to the mode in which results are communicated.[13,23-25] In one study, when researchers presented patients with a hypothetical life-threatening illness, patients were more likely to choose an intervention described in terms of relative risk reductions than in terms of equivalent absolute risk reductions.[13]

Aware that they will perceive results differently depending on how they are presented, what are clinicians to do? We believe that the best option is to consider all the data (either as a 2 × 2 table or as a survival analysis) and then consider both the relative and absolute figures. As you examine the results, you will find that if you can calculate the absolute risk reduction and its reciprocal, the number needed to treat, these will be most useful in deciding whether to offer an intervention to an individual patient (see Chapter 32, Number Needed to Treat). The conscientious evidence-based practitioner will use all available information to formulate the likely risks and benefits for an individual patient (see Chapter 33, Applying Results to Individual Patients).

REFERENCES

1. Callahan CM, Dittus RS, Katz BP. Oral corticosteroid therapy for patients with stable chronic obstructive pulmonary disease: a meta-analysis. *Ann Intern Med.* 1991;114:216-223.
2. Guyatt GH, Juniper EF, Walter SD, Griffith LE, Goldstein RS. Interpreting treatment effects in randomised trials. *BMJ.* 1998;316:690-693.
3. Blue L, Lang E, McMurray JJ, et al. Randomised controlled trial of specialist nurse intervention in heart failure. *BMJ.* 2001;323:715-718.
4. Sinclair JC, Bracken MB. Clinically useful measures of effect in binary analyses of randomized trials. *J Clin Epidemiol.* 1994;47:881-889.
5. Sackett DL. Down with odds ratios! *Evid Based Med.* 1996;1:164-166.
6. Laird NM, Mosteller F. Some statistical methods for combining experimental results. *Int J Technol Assess Health Care.* 1990;6:5-30
7. Walter SD. Choice of effect measure for epidemiological data. *J Clin Epidemiol.* 2000;53:931-939.
8. Davies HT, Crombie IK, Tavakoli M. When can odds ratios mislead? *BMJ.* 1998;316:989-991.
9. Zhang J, Yu KF. What's the relative risk? A method of correcting the odds ratio in cohort studies of common outcomes. *JAMA.* 1998;280:1690-1691.
10. Bozzetti F, Braga M, Gianotti L, et al. Postoperative enteral versus parenteral nutrition in malnourished patients with gastrointestinal cancer: a randomised multicentre trial. *Lancet.* 2001;358:1487-1492.
11. Laupacis A, Sackett DL, Roberts RS. An assessment of clinically useful measures of the consequences of treatment. *N Engl J Med.* 1988;318:1728-1733.
12. DiCenso A. Clinically useful measures of the effects of treatment. *Evid Based Nurs.* 2001;4:36-39.
13. Chatellier G, Zapletal E, Lemaitre D, Menard J, Degoulet P. The number needed to treat: a clinically useful nomogram in its proper context. *BMJ.* 1996;312:426-429.
14. Goodwin PJ, Leszcz M, Ennis M, et al. The effect of group psychosocial support on survival in metastatic breast cancer. *N Engl J Med.* 2001;345:1719-1726.
15. Coldman AJ, Elwood JM. Examining survival data. *Can Med Assoc J.* 1979;121:1065-1068, 1071.
16. Tan LB, Murphy R. Shifts in mortality curves: saving or extending lives? *Lancet.* 1999;354:1378-1381.
17. Walter SD, Marrett LD, From L, Hertzman C, Shannon HS, Roy P. The association of cutaneous malignant melanoma with the use of sunbeds and sunlamps. *Am J Epidemiol.* 1990;131:232-243.
18. Forrow L, Taylor WC, Arnold RM. Absolutely relative: how research results are summarized can affect treatment decisions. *Am J Med.* 1992;92:121-124.
19. Naylor CD, Chen E, Strauss B. Measured enthusiasm: does the method of reporting trial results alter perceptions of therapeutic effectiveness? *Ann Intern Med.* 1992;117:916-921.
20. Hux JE, Levinton CM, Naylor CD. Prescribing propensity: influence of life-expectancy gains and drug costs. *J Gen Intern Med.* 1994;9:195-201.
21. Redelmeier DA, Tversky A. Discrepancy between medical decisions for individual patients and for groups. *N Engl J Med.* 1990;322:1162-1164.
22. Bobbio M, Demichelis B, Giustetto G. Completeness of reporting trial results: effect on physicians' willingness to prescribe. *Lancet.* 1994;343:1209-1211.
23. Malenka DJ, Baron JA, Johansen S, Wahrenberger JW, Ross JM. The framing effect of relative and absolute risk. *J Gen Intern Med.* 1993;8:543-548.
24. McNeil BJ, Pauker SG, Sox HC Jr, Tversky A. On the elicitation of preferences for alternative therapies. *N Engl J Med.* 1982;306:1259-1262.
25. Hux JE, Naylor CD. Communicating the benefits of chronic preventive therapy: does the format of efficacy data determine patients' acceptance of treatment? *Med Decis Making.* 1995;15:152-157.

28

Hypothesis Testing

Cathy Kessenich, Alba DiCenso, and Gordon Guyatt

The following Editorial Board members also made substantive contributions to this chapter: Rien de Vos, Teresa Icart Isern, and Ann Mohide.

We gratefully acknowledge the work of Roman Jaeschke, Deborah Cook, and Stephen Walter on the original chapter that appears in the Users' Guides to the Medical Literature, *edited by Guyatt and Rennie.*

In This Chapter

The Role of Chance

The *P* Value

The Risk of a False-Negative Result

An Example Using a Continuous Measure of Outcome

Taking Account of Baseline Differences

Multiple Tests

Limitations of Hypothesis Testing

Individual studies can only estimate the true underlying relationship between an exposure and an outcome (see Chapter 26, Bias and Random Error). Exposure can be to an intervention, risk factor, diagnostic test, or prognostic factor, depending on the study question. For illustrative purposes, we will focus on exposures to nursing interventions.

Investigators use statistical methods to advance their understanding of the true effect between an exposure and an outcome. For some time, hypothesis testing has been the essential model for statistical inference in the health care literature. The investigator starts with a *null hypothesis* that the statistical test is designed to consider and possibly disprove. Typically, the null hypothesis is that there is no difference between the interventions being compared. In a randomized trial that compares an experimental nursing intervention with a placebo control, one can state the null hypothesis as follows: the true difference between the experimental and control group interventions in their effect on the outcome of interest is zero. For instance, in a study of 321 patients who had acute respiratory failure and required mechanical ventilation, investigators compared the mean duration of mechanical ventilation in those who received a nurse-directed sedation protocol with those who received traditional, nonprotocol, physician-directed sedation.[1] We start with the assumption that the interventions are equally effective, and we maintain this position unless the data make it untenable. In the sedation protocol trial, the null hypothesis could be stated as follows: the true difference in the mean duration of mechanical ventilation between patients who receive nurse-directed sedation and those who receive physician-directed sedation is zero.

In this hypothesis-testing framework, the statistical analysis addresses whether the observed data are consistent with the null hypothesis. The logic of the approach is as follows: even if the intervention truly has no positive or negative impact on the outcome (i.e., the effect size is zero), the results observed will seldom show exact equivalence; that is, absolutely no difference between the intervention and control groups. As the results diverge farther and farther from the finding of "no difference," the null hypothesis that there is no difference between intervention effects becomes less and less credible. If the difference between the results of the intervention and control groups becomes large enough, clinicians must abandon belief in the null hypothesis. We develop the underlying logic further by describing the role of chance in clinical research.

THE ROLE OF CHANCE

In Chapter 26, Bias and Random Error, we considered a balanced coin with which the true probability of obtaining either heads or tails in any individual coin toss was 0.5. We noted that if we tossed this coin 10 times, we would not be surprised if we did not see exactly five heads and five tails. Occasionally, the results would be quite divergent from the 5:5 split, such as 8:2 or even 9:1. Furthermore, very infrequently the 10 coin tosses would result in 10 consecutive heads or tails.

Chance is responsible for this variability in results, and certain recreational games illustrate how chance operates. On occasion, a roll of two unbiased dice (dice with an equal probability of rolling any number between one and six) will yield two ones or two sixes. On occasion (much to the delight of the recipient), the dealer at a poker game will dispense a hand consisting of five cards of a single suit. Even less frequently, the five cards will not only belong to a single suit, but will also have consecutive face value.

Chance is not restricted to the world of coin tosses, dice, and card games. If we take a sample of patients from a community, chance may result in unusual distributions of chronic disease. Chance also may be responsible for substantial imbalances in the event rates in two groups of patients who receive different interventions that are, in fact, equally effective. Much statistical inquiry focuses on determining the extent to which unbalanced distributions could be attributed to chance and the extent to which one should invoke other explanations (e.g., intervention effects). As we will show, the conclusions of statistical inquiry are determined to a large extent by the size of the study.

THE *P* VALUE

One way that an investigator can err is to conclude that there is a difference between an intervention group and a control group when, in fact, no such difference exists. In statistical terminology, making the mistake of erroneously concluding such a difference exists is called a *type I error,* and the probability of making such an error is referred to as the *alpha level.* Imagine a situation in which we are uncertain whether a coin is biased; that is, we suspect that a coin toss is more likely to result in either heads or tails. One could construct a null hypothesis that the true proportions of heads and tails are equal (i.e., the coin is unbiased). In this situation, the *probability* that any given toss will land heads is 50%, as is the probability that any given toss will land tails. We could test this hypothesis by an experiment that comprises a series of coin tosses. Statistical analysis of the results of the experiment would address whether the results observed were consistent with chance.

Let us conduct a hypothetical experiment in which the suspected coin is tossed 10 times, and the result is heads on all 10 occasions. How likely is this to have occurred if the coin was indeed unbiased? Most people would conclude that it is highly unlikely that chance could explain this extreme result. We would therefore be ready to reject the hypothesis that the coin is unbiased (the null hypothesis) and conclude that the coin is biased. Statistical methods allow us to be more precise by ascertaining just how unlikely the result is to have occurred as a result of chance if the null hypothesis is true. The law of multiplicative probabilities for independent events (in which one event in no way influences the other) tells us that the probability of 10 consecutive heads can be found by multiplying the probability of a single head (1/2) 10 times over; that is, $1/2 \times 1/2 \times 1/2$, and so on. The probability of getting 10 consecutive heads is then slightly less than 1 in 1000. In a research publication, one would likely see this probability expressed as a *P* value, such as $P < 0.001$. What is the precise meaning of this *P* value? If the coin were unbiased (i.e., if the null hypothesis were true) and one repeated the experiment of 10 coin tosses many times, 10 consecutive heads would be expected to occur by chance less than once in 1000 times.

In the hypothesis testing framework, the experiment would not be over because one has to make a decision. Are we willing to reject the null hypothesis and conclude that the coin is biased? This decision has to do with how much faith we have in concluding that the coin is biased when, in fact, it is not. In other words, what risk or chance of making a type I error are we willing to accept? The reasoning implies a threshold value that demarcates a boundary. On one side of this boundary we are unwilling to reject the null hypothesis; on the other side we are ready to conclude that chance is no longer a plausible explanation for the results. To return to the example of 10 consecutive heads, most people would be ready to reject the null hypothesis when the observed results would be expected to occur by chance alone less than once in 1000 times.

Let us repeat the coin toss experiment. This time we obtain nine tails and one head. Again, it is unlikely that the result is because of chance alone. This time the P value is 0.02. That is, if the coin were unbiased and the null hypothesis were true, results as extreme as those observed (i.e., nine heads and one tail, or nine tails and one head) would be expected to occur by chance alone two times per 100 repetitions of the experiment.

Given this result, are we willing to reject the null hypothesis? The decision is arbitrary and is a matter of judgment. Statistical tradition, however, suggests that the answer is "yes," because the conventional boundary or threshold that separates the plausible from the implausible is five times per 100, which is represented by a P value of 0.05. This boundary is dignified by long tradition, although other choices of boundary could be equally reasonable. We call results that fall beyond this boundary (i.e., P value < 0.05) *statistically significant.* The meaning of statistically significant, therefore, is as follows: sufficiently unlikely to result from chance alone that we are ready to reject the null hypothesis.

Let us repeat our experiment twice more, both times with a new coin. On the first repetition, we obtain eight heads and two tails. Calculation of the P value associated with an 8/2 split tells us that if the coin were unbiased, results as extreme as or more extreme than 8/2 (or 2/8) would occur solely as a result of chance 11 times per 100 tosses ($P = 0.11$). We have crossed to the other side of the conventional boundary between what is plausible and what is implausible. If we accept the convention, the results are not statistically significant, and we will not reject the null hypothesis.

On our final repetition of the experiment, we obtain seven tails and three heads. Experience tells us that such a result, although not the most common, would not be unusual even if the coin were unbiased. The P value confirms our intuition: results as extreme as or more extreme than this 7/3 split would occur under the null hypothesis 34 times per 100 ($P = 0.34$). Again, we will not reject the null hypothesis.

Although health care research is concerned with questions other than determining whether coins are unbiased, the reasoning is applicable to the P values reported in journal articles. When investigators compare two nursing interventions, they want to know the likelihood that the observed difference is the result of chance alone. If we accept the conventional boundary of $P < 0.05$, we will reject the null hypothesis and conclude that the nursing intervention has some effect when repetitions of the experiment would yield differences as extreme as or more extreme than those observed less than 5% of the time.

Let us return to the example of the randomized trial comparing nurse-directed with physician-directed sedation in patients with acute respiratory failure who were receiving mechanical ventilation. As well as examining the duration of mechanical ventilation, the investigators also compared mortality rates in the two groups. The mortality data illustrate hypothesis testing using a dichotomous (yes/no) outcome.[1] During the study, 49 of 162 patients (30%) assigned to nurse-directed sedation died, as did 57 of 159 (36%) of those assigned to physician-directed sedation. Application of a statistical test that compares proportions (the *chi-square test*) reveals that if there were actually no difference in mortality between the two groups, differences as large as or larger than those actually seen (6%) would be expected 34 times per 100 ($P = 0.34$). Using the hypothesis testing framework and the conventional threshold of $P < 0.05$, we would conclude that we cannot reject the null hypothesis and that the difference observed is compatible with chance.

THE RISK OF A FALSE-NEGATIVE RESULT

A clinician could comment on the results of the comparison of nurse-directed sedation with that of physician-directed sedation as follows: although I accept the 5% threshold and agree that we cannot reject the null hypothesis, I am still suspicious that nurse-directed sedation results in a lower mortality than does physician-directed sedation. The experiment still leaves me in a state of uncertainty. In making these statements, the clinician recognizes a second type of error that an investigator can make: falsely concluding that an effective intervention does not have an important clinical effect on a specified outcome. A *type II error* occurs when one erroneously concludes that an actual intervention or treatment effect does not exist.

In the comparison of nurse-directed and physician-directed sedation, the possibility exists of erroneously concluding that there is no difference in mortality between the two interventions. The investigators found that 6% fewer patients receiving nurse-directed sedation died than those receiving physician-directed sedation. If the true difference in mortality really were 6%, we would readily conclude that patients would receive an important benefit if we used nurse-directed sedation. Despite this, we were unable to reject the null hypothesis, which, in this case, states that the true difference in the proportion of deaths between patients receiving nurse-directed sedation and those receiving physician-directed sedation is zero.

Failure to reject the null hypothesis may have to do with the study sample size. Important differences between intervention and placebo groups are sometimes missed by a statistical test because investigators do not enroll enough patients to warrant confidence that the important difference observed is a real difference. The likelihood of missing an important difference (and therefore of making a type II error) decreases as the sample size increases. When a high risk of making a type II error exists, we say the study has inadequate *power*. The larger the sample size is, the greater the power and the lower the risk of type II error will be. Although the sedation trial included 321 patients, very large sample sizes are often required to detect small differences in dichotomous variables such as mortality. For example, researchers conducting the trials that established the optimal treatment of acute myocardial infarction with thrombolytic agents both anticipated and found absolute differences between treatment and control mortality of less than 5%. Because of this small absolute difference between treatment and control groups, these investigators recruited thousands of patients to ensure adequate power.

When a trial has failed to reject the null hypothesis (i.e., when $P > 0.05$), the investigators may have missed a true intervention effect, and you should consider whether the *power* of the trial was adequate. In these negative studies, the stronger the nonsignificant trend in favor of the experimental intervention, the more likely it is that the investigators missed a true intervention effect.[2] Chapter 29, Confidence Intervals, describes how to decide whether a study is sufficiently large.

Some studies are not designed to determine whether a new intervention is more effective than the current one, but focus on whether the new intervention is equally effective but less expensive, easier to administer, or less toxic. Such studies are often referred to as *equivalence studies.*[3] In equivalence studies, it is even more important to consider whether investigators recruited an adequate sample size to ensure that small but important intervention effects are not missed. If the sample size of an equivalence study is inadequate, investigators risk concluding that the interventions are equivalent when, in fact, patients given standard therapy derive important benefits compared with the easier, less expensive, or less toxic alternative.

AN EXAMPLE USING A CONTINUOUS MEASURE OF OUTCOME

To this point, our examples have used dichotomous outcomes such as yes or no, heads or tails, or dying or not dying, all of which can be expressed as proportions. Often, however, investigators compare the effects of two or more interventions using variables such as length of hospital stay, glycosylated hemoglobin concentrations, or scores on quality of life or patient satisfaction questionnaires. These *continuous variables* can take on a large range of values (e.g., scores of 1 to 50), with small differences between values.

The study of nurse-directed versus physician-directed sedation in patients with acute respiratory failure who required mechanical ventilation[1] provides an example of the use of a continuous variable as an outcome in a hypothesis test. The investigators compared the effect of the two approaches to sedation on mean duration of mechanical ventilation. Mean duration of mechanical ventilation was 89.1 hours for patients who received nurse-directed sedation and 124.0 hours for those who received physician-directed sedation. Using a test appropriate for continuous variables (the *t test*), the investigators compared the mean duration of mechanical ventilation between the two groups and found that the difference between the groups was unlikely to have occurred by chance ($P = 0.003$). Using the hypothesis testing framework, we can reject the null hypothesis and conclude that nurse-directed sedation reduced the duration of mechanical ventilation in patients with acute respiratory failure.

TAKING ACCOUNT OF BASELINE DIFFERENCES

Investigators conducting hypothesis tests must also account for baseline differences in groups, an *adjusted analysis. Randomization,* a process whereby chance alone dictates to which groups patients are allocated, generally produces comparable groups. Sometimes, however, prognostic factors that determine outcome may have substantially different distributions in the two groups. For example, in a trial in which it is known that older patients have a poorer outcome, a larger proportion of older patients may be randomly allocated to one of two interventions being compared. Because older patients are at greater risk of adverse events, an imbalance in age could threaten the validity of an analysis that did not take age into account. The adjusted test yields a P value corrected for differences in the age distribution of the two groups. In this instance, readers can consider that investigators are providing them with the probability that would have been generated had the age distribution in the two groups been the same. Investigators can make adjustments for several variables at once, and you can interpret the P value as previously described.

MULTIPLE TESTS

University students are popular subjects for all sorts of experiments. In keeping with this tradition, we chose nursing students as the subjects for our next hypothetical experiment. Picture a nursing school in which two instructors teach an introductory course on statistics. One instructor is more popular than the other instructor. The dean of the nursing school has a particular passion for fairness and decides that she will deal with the situation by assigning the 200 nursing students in the first-year class to one instructor or the other by a process of random allocation in which each student has an equal chance (50%) of being allocated to one of the two instructors.

The instructors decide to take advantage of this decision and illustrate some important principles of statistics. They therefore ask the following question: are there characteristics of the two groups of students that differ beyond a level that could be explained by the play of chance? The characteristics they choose include sex distribution, eye color, height, grade-point average in the last year of high school, socioeconomic status, and favorite type of music. The instructors formulate null hypotheses for each of their tests. For instance, the null hypothesis associated with sex distribution is as follows: the students are drawn from the same group of people, and therefore the true proportion of females in the two groups is identical. You note that, in fact, the students were drawn from the same underlying population and were assigned to the two groups by random allocation. The null hypothesis in each case is true; therefore, any time the hypothesis is rejected in this experiment will represent a false-positive result.

The instructors survey their students to determine their status on each of the six variables of interest. For five of these variables, they find similar distributions in the two groups, and all P values associated with formal tests of the differences between groups are > 0.10. The instructors find that for eye color, however, 25 of 100 students in one group have blue eyes, whereas 38 of 100 students in the other group have blue eyes. A formal statistical analysis reveals that if the null hypothesis were true (which it is), then differences in the proportion of students with blue eyes in the two groups as large as or larger than the difference observed would occur slightly less than five times per 100 repetitions of the experiment. Using the conventional boundary, the instructors would reject the null hypothesis.

How likely is it that in testing six independent hypotheses on the same two groups of students, the instructors would have found at least one result that crossed the threshold of 0.05 by chance alone? By *independent* we mean that the result of a test of a single hypothesis does not depend in any way on the results of tests of any other hypotheses. Because our likelihood of crossing the significance threshold for any one characteristic is 0.05, the likelihood of not crossing the threshold for that same characteristic is 1.0 minus 0.05 or 0.95. When two hypotheses are tested, the probability that neither crosses the threshold would be 0.95×0.95, or 0.95^2, or 90%; when six hypotheses are tested, the probability that not a single hypothesis would cross the 5% threshold is 0.95^6, or 74%. When six independent hypotheses are tested, the probability that at least one result is statistically significant is therefore 26% (100% minus 74%), or approximately 1 in 4, rather than 1 in 20. If we want to maintain our overall standard of 0.05, we would have to divide the threshold P value by six, so that each of the six tests would use a boundary value of 0.008.

The message here is twofold. First, rare findings do occasionally happen by chance. Even with a single test, a finding with a P value of 0.01 will happen 1% of the time. Second, one should beware of multiple hypothesis testing that may yield misleading results. Examples of this phenomenon abound in the clinical literature. For example, in a survey of 45 trials from three leading health care journals, Pocock and colleagues found that the median number of end points mentioned was six, and most were tested for statistical significance.[4]

We find a specific example of the dangers of use of multiple end points in a randomized trial of the effect of rehabilitation on quality of life after myocardial infarction. In this study, investigators randomized patients to standard care, an exercise program, or a counseling program. Outcomes included patient reports on work, leisure, sexual activity, satisfaction with outcome, compliance with advice, quality of leisure and work, psychiatric symptoms, cardiac symptoms, and general health.[5] The three groups did not differ for most variables. However, at 18 months of follow-up, patients were more satisfied with the exercise regimen than the other two regimens, families in the counseling group were less protective than in the other groups, and patients in the counseling group worked more hours and had sexual intercourse more frequently. Should the exercise and counseling programs be implemented on the basis of the small number of outcomes that changed in their favor, or should they be rejected because most of the outcomes did not differ from standard care? The authors concluded that their results did not support the effectiveness of rehabilitation for improving quality of life. However, a program's advocate could argue that if even some of the ratings favored treatment, the intervention would be worthwhile. The use of multiple instruments opens the door to such potential controversy.

Certain statistical strategies can deal with the issue of testing multiple hypotheses on the same data set. We illustrated one of these in a previous example: dividing the P value by the number of tests. One can also specify, before the study begins, a single primary outcome on which the major conclusions of the study will hinge. A third approach is to derive a single global test statistic (e.g., a pooled effect size) that effectively combines the multiple outcomes into a single measure. Full discussion of strategies for dealing with multiple outcomes is beyond the scope of this book, but interested readers can find a cogent discussion elsewhere.[4]

LIMITATIONS OF HYPOTHESIS TESTING

Some clinicians may have several questions about hypothesis testing that leave them uneasy. Why, for example, use a single cut point when the choice of a cut point is arbitrary? Why dichotomize the question of whether an intervention is effective into a yes/no issue, when it may be viewed more appropriately as a continuum (e.g., from very unlikely to be effective to almost certainly effective)?

We believe that clinicians asking these questions are on the right track. They can refer to Chapter 29, Confidence Intervals, for an explanation of why we consider an alternative to hypothesis testing a superior approach.

REFERENCES

1. Brook AD, Ahrens TS, Schaiff R, et al. Effect of a nursing-implemented sedation protocol on the duration of mechanical ventilation. *Crit Care Med.* 1999;27:2609-2615.
2. Detsky AS, Sackett DL. When was a "negative" trial big enough? How many patients you needed depends on what you found. *Arch Intern Med.* 1985;145:709-715.
3. Kirshner B. Methodological standards for assessing therapeutic equivalence. *J Clin Epidemiol.* 1991;44: 839-849.
4. Pocock SJ, Geller NL, Tsiatis AA. The analysis of multiple end points in clinical trials. *Biometrics.* 1987;43:487-498.
5. Mayou R, MacMahon D, Sleight P, Florencio MJ. Early rehabilitation after myocardial infarction. *Lancet.* 1981;2:1399-1401.

29

Confidence Intervals

Alba DiCenso and Gordon Guyatt

The following Editorial Board members also made substantive contributions to this chapter: Phyllis Brenner, Andrew Jull, and Cathy Kessenich.

We gratefully acknowledge the work of Stephen Walter, Deborah Cook, and Roman Jaeschke on the original chapter that appears in the Users' Guides to the Medical Literature, *edited by Guyatt and Rennie.*

In This Chapter

What Are Confidence Intervals?

Using Confidence Intervals to Interpret the Results of Clinical Trials

Interpreting Apparently "Negative" Trials

Interpreting Apparently "Positive" Trials

Was the Trial Large Enough?

Hypothesis testing involves estimating the probability that observed results would have occurred by chance if a *null hypothesis*, which most commonly states that there is no difference between an intervention condition and a control condition, were true (see Chapter 28, Hypothesis Testing). In nursing research, we are accustomed to the reporting of probability *(P)* values and recognize the conventional threshold of $P < 0.05$ as one that signals a "significant difference" between groups. In other words, we can reject the null hypothesis and conclude that the difference observed is not compatible with chance. When we see values such as $P < 0.01$ and $P < 0.001$, we feel even more confident in rejecting the null hypothesis and sometimes describe the differences as "highly significant."

However, use of the hypothesis testing framework and *P* values has limitations. First, when a trial fails to reject the null hypothesis (i.e., when $P > 0.05$), the investigators may have missed an important intervention effect if the study was not large enough; a *P* value does not provide us with the information we need to determine the likelihood that, despite the lack of a statistically significant difference, a patient-important differ-ence is still present. Second, use of a hypothesis testing framework produces a single value most likely to represent the true difference between the intervention and control groups. This value is only an estimate of the true difference, however, and the *P* value provides no information about the plausible range within which the true difference falls.

Consequently, an alternative approach, estimation through the use of *confidence intervals,* is becoming more popular. In this chapter, we define confidence intervals, illustrate how to interpret them, and outline the advantages of confidence intervals in determining whether the sample size of a study is large enough and in determining the importance of the results to patients. Numerous authors[1–5] have outlined the concepts that we introduce here, and you may find their discussions helpful in supplementing this chapter.

WHAT ARE CONFIDENCE INTERVALS?

The use of confidence intervals is an alternative approach that does not ask how compatible the results are with the null hypothesis. Rather, this approach poses the following question: Given the observed difference between the intervention and control groups, what is the plausible range of differences between the two groups within which the true difference may actually lie? We illustrate the use of confidence intervals with a coin-toss experiment.

Suppose we have a coin that may or may not be balanced. In other words, although the true probability of heads on any individual coin toss may be 0.5, the true probability may be as high as 1.0 in favor of heads (every toss will yield heads) or 1.0 in favor of tails (every toss will yield tails). We conduct an experiment to determine the true nature of the coin.

We begin by tossing the coin twice, observing one head and one tail. At this point, what is our best estimate of the probability of heads on any given coin toss? Our best estimate is the value we have obtained (otherwise known as the *point estimate*), which is 0.5. What is the plausible range within which the true probability of finding a head on

Desire a Narrow confidence interval

any individual coin toss may lie? This range is very wide, and most people would think that the probability may still be as high as or higher than 0.9 or as low as or lower than 0.1. In other words, if the true probability of heads on any given coin toss is 0.9, it would not be surprising if any sample of two coin tosses resulted in one head and one tail. Hence, after two coin tosses, we are not much further ahead in determining the true nature of the coin.

We proceed with eight additional coin tosses. After a total of 10 tosses, we have observed five heads and five tails. Our best estimate of the true probability of heads on any given coin toss remains 0.5, the point estimate. The range within which the true probability of heads may plausibly lie has narrowed, however. It is no longer plausible that the true probability of heads is as great as 0.9. In other words, if the true probability were 0.9, it would be very unlikely that a sample of 10 coin tosses would result in five tails. Although people's sense of the range of plausible probabilities may differ, most would agree that probabilities greater than 0.8 or less than 0.2 are very unlikely.

After 10 coin tosses, all values between 0.2 and 0.8 are not equally plausible. The most likely value for the probability is the point estimate, 0.5, but probabilities close to that point estimate (e.g., 0.4 or 0.6) are also quite likely. The further the probability is from the point estimate, the less likely it is that the value represents the truth.

Ten coin tosses have still left us with considerable uncertainty about our coin, so we conduct another 40 repetitions. After 50 coin tosses, we have observed 25 heads and 25 tails, and our point estimate remains 0.5. We are now beginning to believe that the coin is very unlikely to be extremely biased, and our estimate of the range of probabilities, which is still reasonably consistent with 25 heads in 50 coin tosses, may be 0.35 to 0.65. This range still is quite wide, and we may persist with another 50 repetitions. If after 100 tosses, we observed 50 heads, we may guess that the true probability is unlikely to be more extreme than 0.40 or 0.60. If we were willing to endure the tedium of 1000 coin tosses and if we observed 500 heads, we would be very confident (but still not certain) that our coin is minimally, if at all, biased.

What we have done through this experiment is to use common sense to generate confidence intervals around an observed proportion, 0.5. In each case, the confidence interval represents the range within which the truth plausibly lies. The smaller the sample size is, the wider the confidence interval will be. As the sample size becomes very large, the confidence interval narrows, and we become increasingly certain that the truth is not far from the point estimate we have calculated from our experiment.

Because people's common sense differs considerably, we can turn to statistical techniques for precise estimation of confidence intervals. To use these techniques, we must first be more specific about what we mean by "plausible". In our coin-toss example, we could ask the following question: What is the range of probabilities within which the truth would lie 95% of the time? Table 29-1[6] presents the actual 95% confidence intervals around the observed proportion of 0.5 for our experiment. If we need not be quite so certain, we could ask about the range within which the true value would lie 90% of the time. This 90% confidence interval, also presented in Table 29-1, is somewhat narrower.

The coin-toss example also illustrates how the confidence interval tells you whether the study is large enough to answer the research question. If you wanted to be reasonably

Table **29-1**   Confidence Intervals Around a Proportion of 0.5 in a
Coin-Toss Experiment

Number of Coin Tosses	Observed Result	95% Confidence Interval	90% Confidence Interval
2	1 head, 1 tail	0.01 to 0.99	0.03 to 0.98
10	5 heads, 5 tails	0.19 to 0.81	0.22 to 0.78
50	25 heads, 25 tails	0.36 to 0.65	0.38 to 0.62
100	50 heads, 50 tails	0.40 to 0.60	0.41 to 0.59
1000	500 heads, 500 tails	0.47 to 0.53	0.47 to 0.53

Modified and reproduced with permission of the Canadian Medical Association from Guyatt G, Jaeschke R, Heddle N, Cook D, Shannon H, Walter S. Basic statistics for clinicians. Interpreting study results: confidence intervals. Can Med Assoc J. 1995;152:169-173.

certain that the true value was no more than 10% greater or smaller than the point estimate (i.e., the ends of the confidence interval are within 10% of the point estimate), you would need approximately 100 coin tosses. If you needed greater precision—with 3% in either direction—1000 coin tosses would be required. All you have to do to obtain greater precision is to make more measurements. In clinical research, this involves enrolling more patients.

USING CONFIDENCE INTERVALS TO INTERPRET THE RESULTS OF CLINICAL TRIALS

How do confidence intervals help us to interpret the results of a trial? In a randomized controlled trial of 821 infants in a tertiary level neonatal intensive care unit, we compared care delivered by a team of clinical nurse specialists/neonatal practitioners (CNS/NPs) with that delivered by a team of pediatric residents.[7] During their stay in the neonatal unit, 19 of 414 infants (4.6%) assigned to the CNS/NP team died, as did 24 of 407 infants (5.9%) assigned to the pediatric resident team. The absolute difference of −1.3% is the *point estimate,* our best single estimate of the mortality benefit from using CNS/NPs. The 95% confidence interval around this difference is −4.4% to 1.7% (Table 29-2).

How can we interpret these results? The most likely value for the absolute mortality difference between the two teams is 1.3% in favor of the CNS/NP team, but the true difference may be as high as 1.7% in favor of the pediatric resident team (i.e., in 100 patients, 1.7 fewer deaths in the pediatric resident team) or as high as 4.4% in favor of the CNS/NP team (i.e., in 100 patients, 4.4 fewer deaths in the CNS/NP team). In other words, the 95% confidence interval is consistent with the CNS/NP team having a reduction in mortality as high as 4.4% or an increase in mortality as high as 1.7% when compared with the pediatric resident team. Values progressively farther from 1.3% will be less and less probable. We can conclude that although we have failed to show important differences between the two teams, important differences in mortality in favor of the

Table 29-2 Comparison of Outcomes in Clinical Nurse Specialist/Neonatal Practitioner and Pediatric Resident Trial

	CNS/NP Group n = 414	Pediatric Resident Group n = 407	Absolute Difference	95% CI Around Difference	Relative Risk	95% CI Around Relative Risk	Relative Risk Reduction	95% CI Around Relative Risk Reduction	P Value
Mortality	19 (4.6%)	24 (5.9%)	−1.3%	−4.4% to 1.7%	0.78	0.43 to 1.40	22.2%	−40.0% to 56.7%	0.40
Mean Length of Hospital Stay	12.5 days	11.7 days	0.8 days	−1.1 to 2.7					0.42

Data from Mitchell-DiCenso A, Guyatt G, Marrin M, et al. A controlled trial of nurse practitioners in neonatal intensive care. Pediatrics. 1996;98:1143-1148. CI, Confidence interval; CNS/NP, clinical nurse specialist/neonatal practitioner.

CNS/NP team and in favor of the resident team remain plausible. To that extent, the sample size of this trial was not adequate to answer definitively the question of the relative mortality of the two approaches to care.

This way of understanding the results avoids the yes/no dichotomy of hypothesis testing and obviates the need to argue whether a study should be considered positive or negative. One can conclude that, although it is most likely that the difference in mortality between the two approaches to care is small, an important difference in mortality remains plausible.

In the same trial, we also compared mean length of hospital stay in infants cared for by the CNS/NP team and those cared for by the pediatric resident team. The mean length of stay was 12.5 days in the CNS/NP group and 11.7 days in the pediatric resident group. The absolute difference of 0.8 days is our best single estimate of the benefit of being cared for by the pediatric resident team. The 95% confidence interval around this difference in means is −1.1 to 2.7 (see Table 29-2).

How do we interpret these study results? The most likely value for the mean difference in hospital stay between the two teams is 0.8 days favoring the pediatric resident team, but the true difference may be as high as 2.7 days longer with the CNS/NP team (i.e., favoring the pediatric resident team). Alternatively, it remains plausible that care from the CNS/NP team results in average hospital stays up to 1.1 days shorter than the pediatric resident team (i.e., favoring the CNS/NP team).

In interpreting the results, you must ask yourself the following: If the CNS/NP team really results in longer hospital stays by an average of 2.7 days, would that represent an important benefit of using pediatric residents? Most of us would think a mean difference of 2.7 days is quite important. As a result, one must conclude that although we have failed to show an important difference in length of stay favoring either approach, the study has not excluded an important difference in length of stay in favor of the pediatric resident team.

The 95% confidence interval of −1.1 to 2.7 also includes a difference in mean number of hospital days of zero, signifying that it remains plausible that no difference actually exists in length of hospital stay between the two groups, (i.e., there was no statistically significant difference in length of hospital stay between the two groups). Indeed, people typically believe that studies that fail to show statistically significant differences have demonstrated that the groups did not differ. If you have understood what we have said about confidence intervals, you can see how badly mistaken it is to assume that the truth is "no difference."

When we understand confidence intervals, we realize just how much uncertainty exists, even when we have the results of randomized trials to inform us of important issues in managing patients or the health care system. At the same time, we must make choices, even in the face of uncertainty. It may be reasonable, then, to acknowledge that there may still be important differences between infants cared for by a CNS/NP team and those cared for by a pediatric resident team, but the results have failed to show such differences. Knowing that we may be wrong, and pending further evidence, we may operate under the assumption that the two approaches do not differ and make our choices accordingly.

To summarize the study findings, our best estimate of the difference in mean length of stay indicates that infants cared for by the pediatric resident team were in hospital 0.8 days less than infants cared for by the CNS/NP team. The 95% confidence interval around this mean difference of −1.1 to 2.7 tells us that the true difference could be somewhere between a 2.7-day longer hospital stay with the CNS/NP team and a 1.1-day shorter hospital stay with the CNS/NP and could in fact be zero, reflecting no difference between groups. The width of this confidence interval is determined by the sample size of the study. Given that a difference in hospital stay as high as 2.7 days may be important, we conclude that the sample size of this trial was not adequate to answer definitively the question of the relative length of hospital stay in the two groups.

When examining confidence intervals around *absolute risk differences* in dichotomous variables (e.g., mortality) or continuous variables (e.g., length of hospital stay, quality of life scores, or patient satisfaction scores), a confidence interval around the difference that includes *zero* signifies that no difference between groups remains a plausible estimate of the true effect. In the CNS/NP trial, the confidence interval around the absolute risk difference for mortality of −1.3% (−4.4% to 1.7%) and the confidence interval around the mean difference in length of hospital stay of 0.8 days (−1.1 to 2.7) both include zero, indicating that no difference between groups is a plausible estimate of the true effects. Confidence intervals that include no difference between groups as a plausible estimate of the true effects are consistent with a value of $P > 0.05$, signifying no statistically significant difference between groups.

Conversely, when we use *odds ratios* or *relative risks* to determine differences between groups for dichotomous variables such as death, no difference between groups is a plausible estimate of the true effect if the confidence interval includes 1.0. For example, in the CNS/NP trial, the relative risk of mortality was 0.78 with a 95% confidence interval of 0.43 to 1.40 (see Table 29-2), indicating there may be no difference in mortality between groups.

INTERPRETING APPARENTLY "NEGATIVE" TRIALS

When you see an apparently negative trial (one that fails to exclude the null hypothesis in the hypothesis testing framework), the confidence interval around the difference between groups will help you to determine whether the trial was indeed large enough to exclude a patient-important benefit. The CNS/NP trial provided a good example. Although the trial failed to show differences between the two groups (thus, it was a negative trial), it also failed to exclude the possibility of important differences in mortality and length of hospital stay.

We will use another example to further illustrate this issue. Until 1999, only four randomized controlled trials had compared magnesium sulfate with placebo or no anticonvulsant for prevention of eclampsia in women with preeclampsia.[8-11] The four trials were small, including a total of 1112 women. Three (0.5%) of the 558 women allocated to magnesium sulfate had convulsions compared with 11 (2%) of the 554 women allocated to placebo or no anticonvulsant. The point estimate from these results is a 1.5% (2% minus 0.5%) absolute reduction in convulsions in the magnesium sulfate group. Meta-analysis of these four trials revealed a relative risk of 0.33 and a 95% confidence interval of 0.11 to 1.02.[12]

This meta-analysis may appear to exclude a possible benefit from magnesium sulfate because the confidence interval includes a relative risk of 1.0, which means that the underlying possible truth still includes no difference in convulsions between the two groups. However, the confidence interval is wide. By subtracting the lower and upper boundaries of the confidence interval from 1.0, we can calculate the relative risk reduction that accompanies each boundary. We find that the truth lies somewhere between an 89% (1.00 minus 0.11) risk reduction of convulsions favoring the magnesium sulfate group (using the lower boundary of the confidence interval, i.e., 0.11) and a 2% (1.00 minus 1.02) increase in the risk of convulsions with magnesium sulfate favoring the control group (using the upper boundary of the confidence interval, i.e., 1.02). Note that subtracting 1.02 from 1.00 results in a negative risk reduction which translates into a risk increase. With the truth lying somewhere between an 89% risk reduction and a 2% risk increase, we can conclude that the trials individually or combined did not exclude a patient-important benefit and, in that sense, were not large enough.

This example emphasizes that many patients must participate if trials are to generate precise estimates of intervention effects. In 2002, a very large randomized controlled trial was published in which investigators allocated 5071 women in 33 countries to magnesium sulfate and 5070 women to placebo.[13] Fewer eclamptic convulsions occurred among women allocated to magnesium sulfate than among those allocated to placebo (0.8% versus 1.9%), resulting in a relative risk of 0.42 and a 95% confidence interval of 0.29 to 0.60, clearly favoring the intervention. Not surprisingly, when this large trial was included in an update of the systematic review described earlier,[14] the 95% confidence interval around the relative risk (0.41) was much tighter (0.29 to 0.58 compared with 0.11 to 1.02) and now excluded the possibility of no difference between groups. The relative risk and the accompanying confidence interval clearly favored magnesium sulfate over placebo in the prevention of eclamptic convulsions.

A confidence interval around a difference in an apparently negative trial can help to determine whether the trial is definitely negative. If the boundary of the confidence interval most in favor of the intervention excludes any important benefit of the intervention, you can indeed conclude the trial is definitely negative. Conversely, if the confidence interval includes an important benefit (as did the original meta-analysis of the four trials described earlier,[12] with a 95% confidence interval of 0.11 to 1.02), the trial has not ruled out the possibility that the intervention may still be worthwhile.

This logic of the negative trial is crucial in the interpretation of studies designed to help determine whether we should substitute an intervention that is less expensive, easier to administer, or less toxic for an existing intervention. In an *equivalence study*, such as the CNS/NP trial described earlier,[7] we will be ready to make the substitution only if we are sure that the standard intervention does not have important additional benefits beyond the less expensive or more convenient substitute. We will be confident that we have excluded the possibility of important additional benefits of the standard intervention if the upper boundary of the confidence interval around the difference is below our threshold. As we have shown, if we consider a mortality increase of 1.7%

or an increase in length of stay of 2.7 days to be important, then the CNS/NP trial failed definitively to establish the CNS/NP team as an acceptable alternative to pediatric residents.

INTERPRETING APPARENTLY "POSITIVE" TRIALS

How can confidence intervals be informative in a positive trial (one that, in a hypothesis testing framework, makes chance an unlikely explanation for observed differences between interventions)? In a blinded (health care providers, data collectors, and data analysts) randomized controlled trial of mothers whose 6- to 12-month old infants had severe sleep problems, investigators compared a behavioral sleep intervention with a mailed fact sheet describing normal infant sleep patterns.[15] Twenty-three (30%) of 76 mothers in the behavioral sleep intervention group reported unresolved infant sleep problems at 2 months compared with 40 (53%) of 76 mothers in the mailed fact sheet (control) group. Expressing the results another way, the intervention reduced residual sleep problems from 53% to 30%. The relative risk of sleep problems is 30%/53% = 57%, and the 95% confidence interval around this relative risk is 38% to 86% (Table 29-3). In other words, the risk of residual sleep problems in the behavioral sleep intervention group is a little over half (57%) of that in the mailed fact sheet group. Although our point estimate is 57%, the 95% confidence interval indicates that the true relative risk could be as low as 38% or as high as 86%. The relative risk reduction is 43% (1.0 minus relative risk or 1.0 minus 0.57). Using nontechnical language, we would say that the behavioral sleep intervention decreases the relative risk of sleep problems by 43% compared with the mailed fact sheet (see Chapter 27, Measures of Association). The 95% confidence interval around the relative risk reduction of 43% is 14% to 62%, a finding indicating that although our point estimate is 43%, the true relative risk reduction could be as low as 14% or as high as 62% (see Table 29-3).

The point estimate of the absolute difference in infant sleep problem resolution is −23% (30% minus 53%), and the 95% confidence interval around this difference is −8% to −38% (see Appendix for calculation of a confidence interval around a difference between two proportions) (see Table 29-3). Thus, the smallest effect of the behavioral sleep intervention that is compatible with the data is an 8% reduction in the absolute number of infants with sleep problems. If, as a clinician in a maternal and child health center, you consider it worthwhile to provide the sleep intervention to 12 mothers to resolve a single infant's sleep problems (8% is equivalent to about 1 in 12), then this represents a definitive trial.

What could you tell a mother who is considering participating in the sleep intervention? It would be reasonable to focus first on the point estimate of the intervention effect. You could inform the mother that if she does not participate, her chances of resolving the problem are about 50-50 (resolution rate in the control group was 47% or 100% minus 53% who reported residual sleep problems). If she participates, however, it is most likely that her chances of resolving the problem increase to about 70% (100% minus 30% who reported residual sleep problems). One could frame it in the opposite but equivalent way: her likelihood of persisting sleep problems drops from 53% to 30% with the behavioral

Table 29-3 Comparison of Sleep Problems in Behavioral Sleep Intervention Trial

	Intervention Group n = 76	Control Group n = 76	Absolute Difference	95% CI Around Difference	Relative Risk	95% CI Around Relative Risk	Relative Risk Reduction	95% CI Around Relative Risk Reduction	P Value
Sleep problems	23 (30%)	40 (53%)	−23%	−8% to −38%	0.57	0.38 to 0.86	43%	14% to 62%	0.005

Data from Hiscock H, Wake M. Randomised controlled trial of behavioural infant sleep intervention to improve infant sleep and maternal mood. BMJ. 2002; 324:1062-1065.
CI, Confidence interval.

sleep intervention (and in framing the same information differently, one may make a different impression). Yet another way to express this would be that of every four families who participate, one child who would otherwise have continued to have sleep problems would be getting a good night's sleep (i.e., the number needed to treat [NNT] is 100%/23% [absolute difference], or approximately 4).

What if the mother were to ask: "But nurse, are you sure the sleep program is that good?" You would have to say that no, you are not. You can be confident, however, that the chances of resolving the sleep problem will increase from 47% without the sleep program to 55% with it (47% plus the 8% that represents the lower boundary of the confidence interval around the absolute difference between intervention and control groups). If this lower boundary represents the truth, then 12 families would have to participate for a single infant to benefit (NNT = 100%/8%). If, before recommending the behavioral sleep intervention, you were to require a greater reduction than 8% in the proportion of mothers who report resolved infant sleep problems, a larger trial (with correspondingly narrower confidence intervals) would be needed.

WAS THE TRIAL LARGE ENOUGH?

As implied in our previous discussion, confidence intervals provide a way of determining whether a trial was large enough. We illustrate the approach in Figure 29-1.[6] In this figure, each of the distribution curves represents the results of one hypothetical randomized trial of an experimental intervention to reduce mortality (trials A, B, C, and D). The solid *vertical line* at 0% represents an absolute risk reduction of zero, when the intervention and control groups have exactly the same mortality. Values to the *right of the vertical line* represent results in which the treated group had a lower mortality rate than the control group. Values to the *left of the vertical line* represent results in which the treated group fared worse and had a higher mortality rate than the control group.

The highest point of each distribution represents the result actually observed (the point estimate). In trials A and B, the investigators observed that mortality was 5% lower in the intervention group than in the control group. In trials C and D, they observed that mortality was 1% higher in the intervention group than in the control group.

The distributions of the likelihood of possible true results of each trial are based on the point estimate and the size of the sample. The point estimate is the single value that is most likely to represent the true effect. Values farther from the results observed are less likely than values closer to the point estimate to represent the true difference in mortality.

Suppose we assume that an absolute reduction in mortality greater than 1% warrants intervention (i.e., such a result is clinically important) and a reduction of less than 1% means that intervention is not warranted (i.e., the result is trivial). For instance, if the experimental intervention results in a true reduction in mortality from 5% to 4% or less, we would want to use the intervention. Conversely, if the true reduction in mortality was 5% to 4.5%, we would consider the benefit of the experimental intervention was not worth the associated side effects and expense. What implication does this have for the way in which we interpret the results of the four studies?

In trial *A* in Figure 29-1, the entire distribution and, hence, the entire 95% confidence interval lies above the threshold risk reduction of 1%. We could be confident that the true

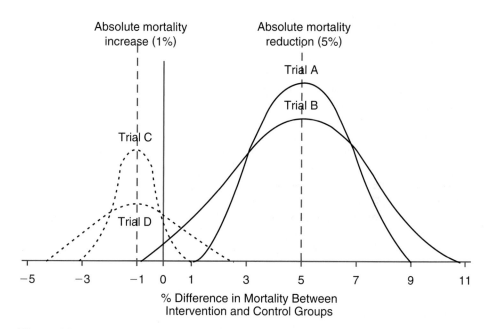

Figure 29-1. Deciding whether a trial is definitive: Distributions of the likelihood of the true results of four trials (A, B, C, and D). Trial *A* is a definitive positive trial, and Trial *B* is a nondefinitive positive trial. Trial *C* is a definitive negative trial, and Trial *D* is a nondefinitive negative trial. *(Modified and reproduced with permission of the Canadian Medical Association from Guyatt G, Jaeschke R, Heddle N, Cook D, Shannon H, Walter S. Basic statistics for clinicians. Interpreting study results: confidence intervals. Can Med Assoc J. 1995;152:169-173.)*

intervention effect was above our threshold, and that we had a definitive "positive" trial. In other words, we would be very confident that the true reduction in risk was greater than 1% (and most likely, appreciably greater), a finding suggesting that many patients would be interested in receiving the intervention. The sample size in this trial would be adequate to demonstrate that the intervention provides a clinically important benefit.

Trial *B* in Figure 29-1 has the same point estimate of intervention effect as trial A (5%) and is also "positive" ($P < 0.05$) but it includes fewer patients. In a hypothesis test, the null hypothesis (i.e., no difference between the intervention and control groups), would be rejected. However, more than 2.5% of the distribution is to the left of the 1% threshold. When the 95% confidence interval includes values less than 1%, the data are consistent with an absolute risk reduction less than 1%. We are left in doubt that the intervention effect is really greater than our threshold. This trial is still "positive," but its results would not be definitive. The sample size of this trial would be too small to establish definitively the appropriateness of administering the intervention.

Trial *C* in Figure 29-1 is "negative" in that its results would not exclude the null hypothesis of "no intervention effect." The investigators would observe a mortality rate that was 1% higher in the intervention group than in the control group. The entire distribution and, therefore, the 95% confidence interval lie to the left of our 1% threshold. The finding that the upper limit of the confidence interval is 1% would mean that we can be very confident that, if there is a benefit, it is very small and unlikely to be appreciably greater than the risks, costs, and inconvenience of the intervention. The trial would therefore exclude any patient-important benefit of the intervention, and it could be considered definitive. We would therefore dismiss the intervention, at least for this type of population.

The result of trial D in Figure 29-1 shows the same difference in absolute risk as that of trial C, in which the mortality rate is 1% higher in the intervention group than in the control group. Trial D, however, had a smaller sample size and, consequently, a much wider distribution of results. Because an appreciable portion of the confidence interval lies to the right of our 1% threshold, we would conclude that it remains plausible (although unlikely) that the true effect of the intervention is a reduction in mortality greater than 1%. Although we would still refrain from using this intervention (indeed, we would conclude it most likely kills people), we would not totally dismiss it. Trial D therefore would not be definitive, and we would require larger trials enrolling more patients to exclude a clinically important intervention effect.

CONCLUSION

Confidence intervals provide the plausible range within which the true difference in outcome between an intervention and control group falls. The smaller the sample size is, the wider the confidence interval will be. As the sample size becomes very large, the confidence interval narrows, and we become increasingly certain that the truth is not far from the point estimate. In addition, confidence intervals provide us with the information we need to help us determine the likelihood that, despite the lack of a statistically significant difference, a patient-important difference is still present.

In a negative trial, the confidence interval around the difference between groups helps to determine whether the trial was large enough to exclude a patient-important benefit. If the boundary of the confidence interval most in favor of the intervention excludes any important benefit of the intervention, you can indeed conclude that the trial is definitively negative. Conversely, if the confidence interval includes an important benefit, the trial has not ruled out the possibility that the intervention may still be worthwhile. In this case, further studies with larger sample sizes are required.

In a positive trial establishing that the effect of the intervention is greater than zero, look at the smallest plausible intervention effect compatible with the data. If this smallest intervention effect is greater than the smallest difference that you consider important, the sample size is adequate, and the trial is definitive. If it is less than this smallest important difference, the trial is nondefinitive, and further trials are required.

REFERENCES

1. Simon R. Confidence intervals for reporting results of clinical trials. *Ann Intern Med.* 1986;105:429-435.
2. Gardner MJ, Altman DG, eds. *Statistics With Confidence: Confidence Intervals and Statistical Guidelines.* London: BMJ Publishing Group; 1989.

3. Bulpitt CJ. Confidence intervals. *Lancet.* 1987;1:494-497.
4. Crichton N. Information point: confidence interval. *J Clin Nurs.* 1999;8:618.
5. Braitman LE. Confidence intervals assess both clinical significance and statistical significance. *Ann Intern Med.* 1991;114:515-517.
6. Guyatt G, Jaeschke R, Heddle N, Cook D, Shannon H, Walter S. Basic statistics for clinicians. 2. Interpreting study results: confidence intervals. *Can Med Assoc J.* 1995;152:169-173.
7. Mitchell-DiCenso A, Guyatt G, Marrin M, et al. A controlled trial of nurse practitioners in neonatal intensive care. *Pediatrics.* 1996;98:1143-1148.
8. Witlin AG, Friedman SA, Sibai BM. The effect of magnesium sulfate therapy on the duration of labor in women with mild preeclampsia at term: a randomized, double-blind, placebo-controlled trial. *Am J Obstet Gynecol.* 1997;76:623-627.
9. Moodley J, Moodley J. Prophylactic anticonvulsant therapy in hypertensive crises of pregnancy: the need for a large randomized trial. *Hypertens Preg.* 1994;13:245-252.
10. Anthony J, Rush R. A randomised controlled trial of intravenous magnesium sulphate versus placebo. *Br J Obstet Gynaecol.* 1998;105:809-810.
11. Chen FP, Chang SD, Chu KK. Expectant management in severe preeclampsia: does magnesium sulfate prevent the development of eclampsia? *Acta Obstet Gynecol Scand.* 1995;74:181-185.
12. Duley L, Gülmezoglu AM, Henderson-Smart DJ. Anticonvulsants for women with pre-eclampsia (Cochrane review: updated 7 October 1999). *Cochrane Database Syst Rev.* 2002;(2):CD000025.
13. Magpie Trial Collaborative Group. Do women with pre-eclampsia, and their babies, benefit from magnesium sulphate? The Magpie Trial: a randomised placebo-controlled trial. *Lancet.* 2002;359:1877-1890.
14. Duley L, Gülmezoglu AM, Henderson-Smart DJ. Magnesium sulphate and other anticonvulsants for women with pre-eclampsia (Cochrane review: updated 25 February 2003). *Cochrane Database Syst Rev.* 2003;(2):CD000025.
15. Hiscock H, Wake M. Randomised controlled trial of behavioural infant sleep intervention to improve infant sleep and maternal mood. *BMJ.* 2002;324:1062-1065.

30

Measuring Agreement
Beyond Chance

Andrew Jull, Alba DiCenso, and Gordon Guyatt

The following Editorial Board members also made substantive contributions to this chapter: Rien de Vos, Teresa Icart Isern, and Mary van Soeren.

We gratefully acknowledge the work of Thomas McGinn, Richard Cook, and Maureen Meade on the original chapter that appears in the Users' Guides to the Medical Literature, *edited by Guyatt and Rennie.*

In This Chapter

Clinicians Often Disagree

Chance Will Always Be Responsible for Some of the Apparent Agreement Between Observers

Alternatives for Dealing With the Problem of Agreement by Chance

One Solution to Agreement by Chance: Chance-Corrected Agreement or Kappa

Calculating Kappa

Kappa With Three or More Raters or Three or More Categories

A Limitation of Kappa

An Alternative to Kappa: Chance-Independent Agreement or Phi

Advantages of Phi Over Other Approaches

CLINICIANS OFTEN DISAGREE

Clinicians often disagree in their assessments of patients, be it in physical examinations or interpretation of diagnostic tests. Disagreement between two clinicians about the presence of a particular physical sign in a patient (e.g., elevated blood pressure) may be the result of different approaches to the examination or different interpretations of the findings. Similarly, disagreement among repeated examinations of the same patient by the same clinician may result from inconsistencies in the way the examination is conducted or different interpretations of the findings with each examination.

Researchers may also have difficulties agreeing on whether patients meet the eligibility requirements for a clinical trial (e.g., whether a patient has severe pain), whether patients in a randomized trial have experienced an outcome of interest (e.g., whether a patient has improved functional ability), or whether a study meets the eligibility criteria for a systematic review.

Agreement between two observers is often called *interobserver* (or *interrater*) *agreement,* and agreement within the same observer is referred to as *intraobserver* (or *intrarater*) *agreement.*

CHANCE WILL ALWAYS BE RESPONSIBLE FOR SOME OF THE APPARENT AGREEMENT BETWEEN OBSERVERS

Any two people judging the presence or absence of an attribute will agree some of the time by chance. This means that even if the people making the assessment are doing so by guessing in a completely random way, their random guesses will agree some of the time. When investigators present agreement as raw agreement—that is, by simply counting the number of times agreement has occurred—this chance agreement gives a misleading impression.

ALTERNATIVES FOR DEALING WITH THE PROBLEM OF AGREEMENT BY CHANCE

In this chapter, we describe approaches developed by statisticians to separate chance agreement from nonrandom agreement (or agreement over and above chance). When we are dealing with categorical data (i.e., placing patients in discrete categories such as mild or severe pain, a present or absent sign, or a positive or negative test), the most popular approach is *chance-corrected agreement.* Chance-corrected agreement is quantified as *kappa*. Kappa is a statistic used to measure nonrandom agreement among observers, investigators, or measurements.

ONE SOLUTION TO AGREEMENT BY CHANCE: CHANCE-CORRECTED AGREEMENT OR KAPPA

Conceptually, kappa removes agreement by chance and informs clinicians about the extent of possible agreement over and above chance. If raters agree on every judgment, the total possible agreement is 1.0 (also expressed as 100%). Figure 30-1 depicts a situation in which agreement by chance is 50%, leaving possible agreement above and beyond

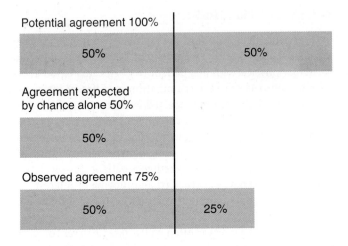

$$\text{Kappa} = \frac{\text{Observed agreement} - \text{Agreement expected by chance alone}}{\text{Total potential agreement} - \text{Agreement expected by chance alone}}$$

$$= \frac{75\% - 50\%}{100\% - 50\%}$$

$$= \frac{25\%}{50\%}$$

$$= 50\% \ \text{(moderate agreement)}$$

Figure 30-1. Kappa.

chance of 50%. As depicted in this figure, the raters have achieved an agreement of 75%. Of this 75%, 50% was achieved by chance alone. Of the remaining possible 50% agreement, the raters have achieved half, resulting in a kappa value of 0.25/0.50, or 0.50 (or 50%).

CALCULATING KAPPA

Kappa is calculated by following three steps: (1) calculating observed agreement, (2) calculating agreement expected by chance alone, and (3) calculating agreement beyond chance. Assume that two observers are assessing the presence of respiratory wheeze. However, they have no skill in auscultating the chest, and their evaluations are no better than blind guesses. Let us say that they are both guessing in a ratio of 50:50; they guess that wheezing is present in half of the patients and that it is absent in half of the patients. On average, if both raters were evaluating the same 100 patients, they would achieve the results presented in Figure 30-2. Referring to this figure, you observe that both raters detected a wheeze in 25 patients *(cell A)* and neither of the raters detected a wheeze in 25 patients *(cell D)*. By adding these two cells and dividing by the total number of patients (or observations) *(T)*, we calculate observed agreement to be (25 + 25)/100. This represents an agreement of 50% (i.e., they correctly guessed the presence or absence of a wheeze in 50 of 100 patients). Thus, simply by guessing (and thus by chance), the raters achieved 50% agreement.

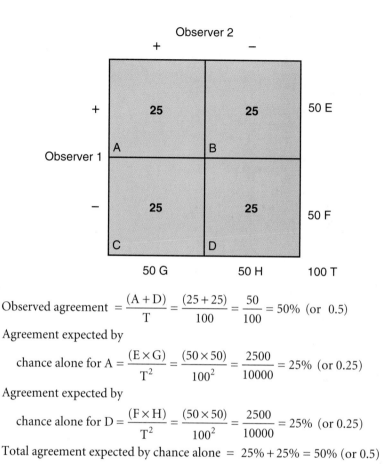

$$\text{Observed agreement} = \frac{(A+D)}{T} = \frac{(25+25)}{100} = \frac{50}{100} = 50\% \text{ (or } 0.5)$$

Agreement expected by

$$\text{chance alone for A} = \frac{(E \times G)}{T^2} = \frac{(50 \times 50)}{100^2} = \frac{2500}{10000} = 25\% \text{ (or } 0.25)$$

Agreement expected by

$$\text{chance alone for D} = \frac{(F \times H)}{T^2} = \frac{(50 \times 50)}{100^2} = \frac{2500}{10000} = 25\% \text{ (or } 0.25)$$

Total agreement expected by chance alone $= 25\% + 25\% = 50\%$ (or 0.5)

Figure 30-2. Agreement by chance when both reviewers are guessing in a ratio of 50% target positive and 50% target negative. **A,** Patients in whom both observers detect respiratory wheeze. **B,** Patients in whom observer 1 detects a respiratory wheeze, and observer 2 does not detect a wheeze. **C,** Patients in whom observer 1 does not detect a wheeze, and observer 2 detects a wheeze. **D,** Patients in whom both observers do not detect a wheeze. **E,** Patients in whom observer 1 detects a wheeze. **F,** Patients in whom observer 1 does not detect a wheeze. **G,** Patients in whom observer 2 detects a wheeze. **H,** Patients in whom observer 2 does not detect a wheeze. **T,** Total number of patients.

Having determined observed agreement, we go on to calculate agreement expected by chance alone, which involves calculating the number of observations we expect by chance to fall in cells A and D. We do this by multiplying the corresponding marginal totals (E, F, G, H) and dividing by the square of the total number of observations (T). To calculate how many observations we expect by chance to fall in *cell A*, we multiply E times G and divide this number by T^2: $(50 \times 50)/100^2 = 0.25$. Similarly, to calculate the number of observations we expect in *cell D*, we multiply F times H and divide by T^2: $(50 \times 50)/100^2 = 0.25$. Total chance agreement is therefore $0.25 + 0.25 = 0.50$ or 50%.

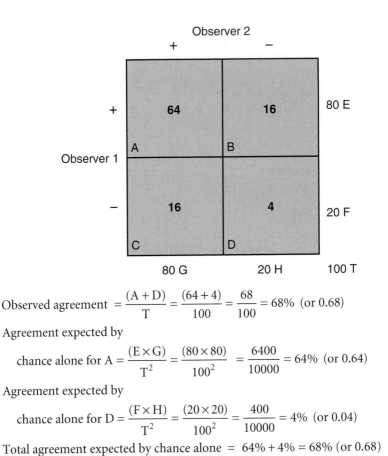

Observer 2

Observed agreement $= \dfrac{(A+D)}{T} = \dfrac{(64+4)}{100} = \dfrac{68}{100} = 68\%$ (or 0.68)

Agreement expected by

chance alone for A $= \dfrac{(E \times G)}{T^2} = \dfrac{(80 \times 80)}{100^2} = \dfrac{6400}{10000} = 64\%$ (or 0.64)

Agreement expected by

chance alone for D $= \dfrac{(F \times H)}{T^2} = \dfrac{(20 \times 20)}{100^2} = \dfrac{400}{10000} = 4\%$ (or 0.04)

Total agreement expected by chance alone $= 64\% + 4\% = 68\%$ (or 0.68)

Figure 30-3. Agreement by chance when both reviewers are guessing in a ratio of 80% target positive and 20% target negative. +, Target positive; –, target negative. In this case, + is respiratory wheeze present and – is respiratory wheeze absent.

What happens if the raters repeat the exercise of rating 100 patients, but this time each guesses in a ratio of 80% positive and 20% negative? Figure 30-3 depicts what, on average, will occur. The observed agreement (*cells A and D*) has increased to (64 + 4)/100 or 68% and total chance agreement has increased to 68%.

As two observers classify an increasing proportion of patients in one category or the other (e.g., positive or negative; sign present or absent), agreement by chance increases as shown in Table 30-1. Once we have determined observed agreement and agreement expected by chance alone, we are ready to calculate kappa (or agreement beyond chance).

Figure 30-4 illustrates the calculation of kappa with a hypothetical data set. First, we calculate the agreement observed. The two observers agreed that respiratory wheeze was present in 41 patients (*cell A*) and was absent in 80 patients (*cell D*). Thus, total agreement is (41 + 80)/200 = 0.605, or 60.5%. Next, we calculate agreement expected by chance in *cell A* by multiplying the marginal totals E and G and dividing by T^2

Table **30-1**   Relationship Between the Proportion Positive and the Expected Agreement by Chance

Proportion Positive (E/T = G/T)*	Agreement by Chance
0.5	0.5 (50%)
0.6	0.52 (52%)
0.7	0.58 (58%)
0.8	0.68 (68%)
0.9	0.82 (82%)

*E/T and G/T refer to letters in Figures 30-2 and 30-3; E/T, the proportion of patients observer 1 finds positive; G/T, the proportion of patients observer 2 finds positive.

$[(60 \times 101)/200^2 = 0.15]$, and we calculate agreement expected by chance in *cell D* by multiplying the marginal totals F and H and dividing by T^2 $[(140 \times 99)/200^2 = 0.35]$. Total chance agreement is $0.15 + 0.35 = 0.50$ or 50%. We can then calculate kappa using the principle illustrated in Figure 30-1:

$$\frac{\text{(observed agreement } - \text{ agreement by chance)}}{\text{(agreement possible [100\%]} - \text{ agreement by chance)}}$$

or, in this case:

$$\frac{(0.605 - 0.50)}{(1.0 - 0.50)} = 0.105 \div 0.50 = 0.21 \text{ or } 21\%$$

To summarize, observed agreement was 60.5%. Agreement of 50% would be expected to occur by chance, resulting in a kappa, or agreement over and above chance of 21%. Although there are numerous approaches to valuing the kappa levels achieved by raters, a widely accepted interpretation is the following: 0 = poor agreement; 0 to 0.2 = slight agreement; 0.2 to 0.4 = fair agreement; 0.4 to 0.6 = moderate agreement; 0.6 to 0.8 = substantial agreement; and 0.8 to 1.0 = almost perfect agreement[1]

Examples of chance-corrected agreement that investigators have calculated in clinical studies include exercise stress test cardiac T-wave changes, kappa = 0.25;[2] jugular venous distention, kappa = 0.50;[3] presence or absence of goiter, kappa = 0.82 to 0.95;[4,5] and straight-leg raising for diagnosis of low back pain, kappa = 0.82.[6]

KAPPA WITH THREE OR MORE RATERS OR THREE OR MORE CATEGORIES

Using similar principles, one can calculate chance-corrected agreement when there are more than two raters.[7] Furthermore, one can calculate kappa when raters place patients into more than two categories (e.g., patients with heart failure may be rated as New York Heart Association class I, II, III, or IV). In these situations, one may give partial credit for intermediate levels of agreement (e.g., one observer may classify a patient as class II, whereas another may observe the same patient as class III) by adopting a so-called

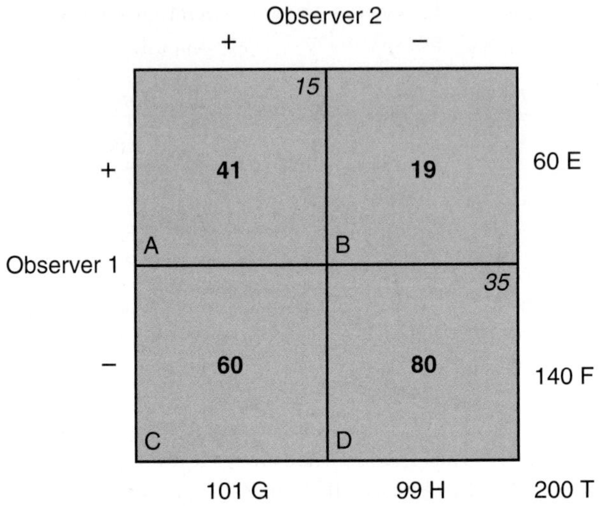

Observer 2

Observed agreement $= \dfrac{(A+D)}{T} = \dfrac{(41+80)}{200} = \dfrac{121}{200} = 60.5\%$ (or 0.605)

Agreement expected by chance alone for A $= \dfrac{(E \times G)}{T^2} = \dfrac{(60 \times 101)}{200^2} = \dfrac{6060}{40000}$

$= 15\%$ (or 0.15)

Agreement expected by chance alone for D $= \dfrac{(F \times H)}{T^2} = \dfrac{(140 \times 99)}{200^2} = \dfrac{13860}{40000}$

$= 35\%$ (or 0.35)

Total agreement expected by chance alone $= 15\% + 35\% = 50\%$ (or 0.5)

Kappa $(\kappa) = \dfrac{\text{observed agreement } - \text{ agreement expected by chance alone}}{\text{total potential agreement } - \text{ agreement expected by chance alone}}$

$= \dfrac{60.5\% - 50\%}{100\% - 50\%} = \dfrac{10.5\%}{50\%} = 21\%$ (or 0.21)

Figure 30-4. Observed and expected agreement. +, Target positive; − target negative. In this case, + is respiratory wheeze present and − is respiratory wheeze absent. Expected agreement by chance appears in italics in cells A and D.

weighted kappa statistic (weighted because full agreement receives full credit, and partial agreement receives partial credit).[8]

A LIMITATION OF KAPPA

Kappa provides an accurate measurement of agreement beyond chance when the marginal frequencies are similar to one another (e.g., 50% positive observations and 50% negative observations). When the distribution of results is extreme (e.g., 90% positive observations and 10% negative observations), kappa is invariably low, in the absence of perfect agreement. If two observers believe that the prevalence of a clinical entity of interest (e.g., respiratory wheeze) is high or low in a given population, and both make a high or low proportion of positive ratings, raw agreement or agreement by chance will be high, even if the raters are just guessing. For this reason, when the proportion of positive ratings is extreme (i.e., extreme differences in the marginal frequencies), possible agreement beyond chance agreement is small, and it is difficult to achieve even moderate values of kappa.[9–11]

AN ALTERNATIVE TO KAPPA: CHANCE-INDEPENDENT AGREEMENT OR PHI

One solution to this problem is chance-independent agreement using the *phi* statistic, which is a relatively new approach to assessing observer agreement.[12] One begins by estimating the odds ratio from a 2 × 2 table displaying the agreement between two observers. Figure 30-5 contrasts the formulas for raw agreement, kappa, and phi.

The *odds ratio* (OR = ad/bc in Figure 30-5) provides the basis for calculating phi. The odds ratio is simply the odds of a positive classification by observer 2 when observer 1 gives a positive classification, divided by the odds of a positive classification by observer 2 when observer 1 gives a negative classification (see Chapter 27, Measures of Association). The odds ratio would not change if we were to reverse the rows and columns. Thus, it does not matter which observer we identify as observer 1 and which we identify as observer 2. The odds ratio provides a natural measure of agreement. Interpretation of this agreement can be simplified by converting it to a form that takes values from −1.0 (representing extreme disagreement) to 1.0 (representing extreme agreement).

The phi statistic makes this conversion using the following formula:

$$\text{Phi} = \frac{\sqrt{OR} - 1}{\sqrt{OR} + 1} = \frac{\sqrt{ad} - \sqrt{bc}}{\sqrt{ad} + \sqrt{bc}}$$

$$\text{Raw agreement} = \frac{a + d}{a + b + c + d}$$

$$\text{Kappa} = \frac{\text{observed agreement} - \text{expected agreement}}{1 - \text{expected agreement}}$$

$$\text{where observed agreement} = \frac{a + d}{a + b + c + d}$$

$$\text{and expected agreement} = \frac{(a + b)(a + c)}{(a + b + c + d)^2} + \frac{(c + d)(b + d)}{(a + b + c + d)^2}$$

$$\text{Odds Ratio \{OR\}} = \frac{ad}{bc} \qquad \text{Phi} = \frac{\sqrt{OR} - 1}{\sqrt{OR} + 1} = \frac{\sqrt{ad} - \sqrt{bc}}{\sqrt{ad} + \sqrt{bc}}$$

Figure 30-5. Calculations of agreement. *a, b, c,* and *d,* the four cells of a 2 × 2 table.

When both margins are 0.5 (that is, when both raters conclude that 50% of the patients are positive and 50% are negative for the trait of interest), phi is equal to kappa.

ADVANTAGES OF PHI OVER OTHER APPROACHES

The use of phi has four important advantages over other approaches. First, it is independent of the level of chance agreement. Thus, investigators could expect to find similar levels of phi if the distribution of results is 50% positive and 50% negative or if it is 90% positive and 10% negative. This is not true for measures of the kappa statistic, a chance-corrected index of agreement.

Second, phi allows statistical modeling approaches that the kappa statistic does not. For instance, such flexibility allows investigators to take advantage of all ratings when observers assess patients on multiple occasions.[12] Third, phi allows testing of whether differences in agreement between pairings of raters are statistically significant, an option that is not available with kappa.[12] Fourth, because phi is based on the odds ratio, one can carry out exact analyses. This feature is particularly attractive when the sample is small or when there is a zero cell in the chart.[13]

Statisticians may disagree about the relative usefulness of kappa and phi. The key point for clinicians reading studies that report measures of agreement is that investigators not mislead readers by presenting only raw agreement.

REFERENCES

1. Maclure M, Willett WC. Misinterpretation and misuse of the kappa statistic. *Am J Epidemiol*. 1987;126: 161-169.
2. Blackburn H. The exercise electrocardiogram: differences in interpretation. *Am J Cardiol*. 1968;21:871.
3. Cook DJ. Clinical assessment of central venous pressure in the critically ill. *Am J Med Sci*. 1990;299: 175-178.
4. Kilpatrick R, Milne JS, Rushbrooke M, Wilson ESB. A survey of thyroid enlargement in two general practices in Great Britain. *BMJ*. 1963;1:29-34.
5. Trotter WR, Cochrane AL, Benjamin IT, Mial WE, Exley D. A goitre survey in the Vale of Glamorgan. *Br J Prev Soc Med*. 1962;16:16-21.
6. McCombe PF, Fairbank JC, Cockersole BC, Pynsent PB. 1989 Volvo Award in clinical sciences. Reproducibility of physical signs in low-back pain. *Spine*. 1989;14:908-918.
7. Cohen J. Weighted kappa: Nominal scale agreement with provision for scaled disagreement or partial credit. *Psychol Bull*. 1968;70:213-220.
8. Landis JR, Koch GG. The measurement of observer agreement for categorical data. *Biometrics*. 1977;33: 159-174.
9. Thompson WD, Walter SD. A reappraisal of the kappa coefficient. *J Clin Epidemiol*. 1988;41:949-958.
10. Feinstein AR, Cicchetti DV. High agreement but low kappa, I: the problems of two paradoxes. *J Clin Epidemiol*. 1990;43:543-549.
11. Cook RJ, Farewell VT. Conditional inference for subject-specific and marginal agreement: two families of agreement measures. *Can J Stat*. 1995;23:333-344.
12. Meade MO, Cook RJ, Guyatt GH, et al. Interobserver variation in interpreting chest radiographs for the diagnosis of acute respiratory distress syndrome. *Am J Respir Crit Care Med*. 2000;161:85-90.
13. Armitage P, Colton T, eds. *Encyclopedia of Biostatistics*. Chichester, UK: John Wiley & Sons; 1998.

Regression and Correlation

Alba DiCenso and Gordon Guyatt

The following Editorial Board members also made substantive contributions to this chapter: Andrew Jull and Jenny Ploeg.

We gratefully acknowledge the work of Stephen Walter, Deborah Cook, and Roman Jaeschke on the original chapter that appears in the Users' Guides to the Medical Literature, *edited by Guyatt and Rennie.*

In This Chapter

Correlation
An Example of Correlation: Relationship Between Walk Test Scores
and Conventional Measures of Exercise Capacity

Regression
An Example of Linear Regression: Predicting Walk Test Scores
An Example of Logistic Regression: Predicting Clinically Important Bleeding

Investigators are sometimes interested in the relationship between different measures, or variables. They pose questions related to the correlation between these variables. For example, they might ask: How strong is the relationship between patients' and relatives' perspectives on a clinical situation? How strong is the relationship between a patient's physical well-being and emotional function?

By contrast, other investigators are primarily interested in causal relationships between phenomena. For instance, they might ask: What determines the extent to which patients feel dyspneic when they exercise or if they have a cardiac or respiratory illness?

Clinicians may be interested in the answers to both of these types of questions. To the extent that the relationship between patients' and relatives' perspectives on a clinical situation is weak, clinicians must obtain both perspectives. If physical well-being and emotional function are related only weakly, then clinicians must probe both areas thoroughly. If clinicians know that hypoxemia is strongly related to dyspnea, they will be more inclined to administer oxygen to patients with dyspnea. If the demonstrated hypoxemia–dyspnea relationship is weak, they will be less inclined to administer oxygen to these patients.

Correlation refers to the magnitude of the relationship between different variables or phenomena. *Regression* is the statistical technique for predicting or making a causal inference. In this chapter, we provide examples to illustrate the use of correlation and regression in the health care literature.

CORRELATION

An Example of Correlation: Relationship Between Walk Test Scores and Conventional Measures of Exercise Capacity

Traditionally, we obtain laboratory measurements of exercise capacity in patients with cardiac and respiratory illnesses using a treadmill or cycle ergometer. About 25 years ago, investigators began to use a simpler test that is related more closely to day-to-day activity.[1] In this walk test, patients are asked to cover as much ground as they can in an enclosed corridor during a specified time period (typically 6 minutes). For several reasons, we may be interested in the strength of the relationship between the walk test and conventional laboratory measures of exercise capacity. If the tests relate strongly enough to one another, we might be able to substitute one test for the other. In addition, the strength of the relationship might inform us about the potential of laboratory tests of exercise capacity to predict patients' ability to undertake physically demanding activities of daily living.

What do we mean by the strength of the relationship between two variables? A relationship between two variables is strong when patients who obtain high scores on the first variable also obtain high scores on the second variable, when those who obtain intermediate scores on the first variable also obtain intermediate scores on the second variable, and when those who obtain low scores on the first variable obtain low scores on the second variable. If patients who score low on one measure are equally likely to score low or high on another measure, then the relationship between the two measures is poor, or weak.

We can gain a sense of the strength of the correlation by examining a visual plot that relates patients' scores on the two measures. Figure 31-1[5] presents such a plot relating the results of the walk test (on the *x*-axis) to the results of a cycle ergometer exercise test (on the *y*-axis). The data for this plot, and for subsequent analyses using walk test results, are from three studies of patients with chronic airflow limitation.[2–4] Each dot in Figure 31-1 represents an individual patient and provides two pieces of information: the patient's walk test score and cycle ergometer exercise score. Although the walk test results are truly continuous, the cycle ergometer results tend to take only certain values because patients usually stop the test at the end of a particular level, rather than part-way through a level. Examining Figure 31-1, you can see that, in general, patients who score well on the walk test also tend to score well on the cycle ergometer exercise test, and patients who score poorly on the cycle ergometer test tend to score poorly on the walk test. Nevertheless, there are exceptions, with some patients scoring better than most patients on one test and not as well on the other test.

These data therefore represent a moderate relationship between two variables: the walk test and the cycle ergometer exercise test. The strength of the relationship can be summarized in a single number, the *correlation coefficient*. The correlation coefficient, denoted by the letter *r*, can range from −1.0 (representing the strongest possible negative relationship, in which the person who scores the highest on one test scores the lowest on

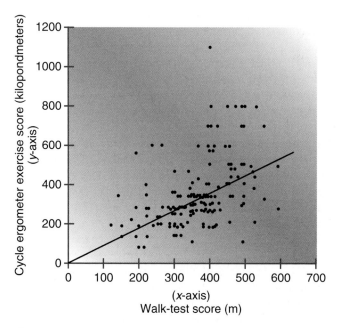

Figure 31-1. Relationship between walk test scores and cycle ergometer exercise scores. *(Modified and reproduced with permission of the Canadian Medical Association from Guyatt G, Walter S, Shannon H, Cook D, Jaeschke R, Heddle N. Basic statistics for clinicians: 4. Correlation and regression. CMAJ. 1995;152:497-504.)*

the other test) to 1.0 (representing the strongest possible positive relationship, in which the person who scores the highest on one test also scores the highest on the other test). A correlation coefficient of 0 denotes no relationship between the two variables (i.e., people with high scores on test A have the same range of values on test B as those with low scores on test A). The plot of data with a correlation of 0 looks like a starry sky.

The correlation coefficient assumes a linear relationship between the variables. There may be a relationship between the variables, but it may not take the form of a straight line when viewed visually. For example, even if scores on the variables increase together, one score may increase more slowly than the other for low values but may increase more quickly than the other for high values. The correlation coefficient may be misleading if a strong, but nonlinear, relationship exists between variables. In Figure 31-1, the relationship appears to approximate a straight line, and the r value for the correlation between the cycle ergometer and the walk test is 0.50.

Is this moderately strong correlation good or bad? It depends on how we wish to apply the information. If we wanted to use the walk test as a substitute for the cycle ergometer— after all, the walk test is much simpler to carry out—then we would be disappointed. A correlation of 0.8 or higher would be required for us to be confident in making that kind of substitution. If the correlation was less than 0.8, there would be too great a risk that a person who did poorly on the walk test would do well on the cycle ergometer test, or vice versa. On the other hand, if we assume that the walk test gives a good indication of exercise capacity in daily life, the moderate correlation suggests that the cycle ergometer result tells us something (less, but still something) about day-to-day exercise capacity.

You will often see a P value associated with a correlation coefficient (see Chapter 28, Hypothesis Testing). This P value is associated with the *null hypothesis* that the true correlation between the two measures is 0. Thus, the P value represents the probability that the correlation we observe occurred by chance if the true correlation were 0. The smaller the P value, the less likely it is that chance explains the apparent relationship between the two measures.

The P value depends not only on the strength of the relationship, but also on the sample size. In this case, we had data on both the walk test and the cycle ergometer for 179 patients; with a correlation of 0.50, the associated P value is < 0.0001. A relationship can be very weak, but if the sample size is sufficiently large, the P value may be small. For example, with a sample size of 500, we reach the conventional threshold P value of 0.05 at a correlation of only 0.10.

In evaluating intervention effects, the size of the effect and the confidence intervals around the effect tend to be much more informative than P values (see Chapter 29, Confidence Intervals). The same is true of correlations, in which the magnitude of the correlation and the confidence interval around the correlation are the key parameters. The 95% confidence interval around the correlation between the walk test and cycle ergometer test ranges from 0.38 to 0.60.

REGRESSION

As clinicians, we are often interested in prediction. We want to know which person will develop a disease and which person will not, which patient will do well and which patient will do poorly. Regression techniques are useful in addressing this type of question. We will once again use the walk test to illustrate the concepts involved in statistical regression.

An Example of Linear Regression: Predicting Walk Test Scores

Let us assume we are trying to predict patients' walk test scores using more easily measured variables: sex, height, and a measure of lung function—forced expiratory volume in 1 second (FEV_1). Alternately, we can think of the investigation as examining a causal hypothesis: to what extent are patients' walk test scores determined by sex, height, and pulmonary function? Either way, we have a target or response variable that we call the *dependent variable* (in this case, the walk test) because it is influenced or determined by other variables or factors. We also have the explanatory or predictor variables, called *independent variables*: sex, height, and FEV_1.

Figure 31-2[5], a bar graph of the walk test scores of 219 patients with chronic lung disease, shows that walk test scores vary widely among patients. If we had to predict an individual's walk test score without any other information, our best guess would be the mean score of all patients (394 m). For many patients, however, this prediction would be well off the mark.

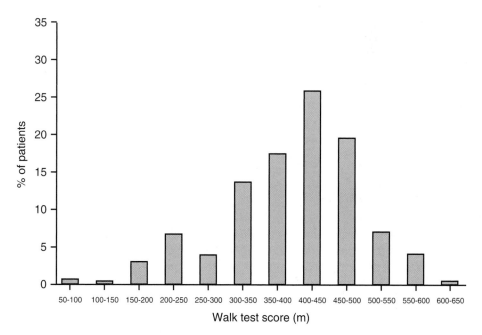

Figure 31-2. Distribution of walk test scores in the total sample of 219 patients. *(Modified and reproduced with permission of the Canadian Medical Association from Guyatt G, Walter S, Shannon H, Cook D, Jaeschke R, Heddle N. Basic statistics for clinicians: 4. Correlation and regression. CMAJ. 1995;152:497-504.)*

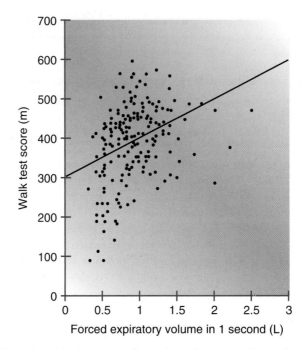

Figure 31-3. Relationship between forced expiratory volume in 1 second and walk test scores in 219 patients. *(Modified and reproduced with permission of the Canadian Medical Association from Guyatt G, Walter S, Shannon H, Cook D, Jaeschke R, Heddle N. Basic statistics for clinicians: 4. Correlation and regression. CMAJ. 1995;152: 497-504.)*

Figure 31-3[5] shows the relationship between FEV_1 and the walk test. Note that a relationship exists between the two variables, although it is not as strong as the relationship between the walk test and the exercise test depicted in Figure 31-1. Thus, some of the difference, or variation, in walk test scores seems to be explained by, or attributable to, the patient's FEV_1. We can construct an equation using FEV_1 to predict walk test scores. Because there is only one independent variable, we call this a *univariate or simple regression*.[6]

Generally, when we construct regression equations, we refer to the predictor (independent) variable as x and the target (dependent) variable as y. The regression equation assumes a linear fit between FEV_1 and walk test scores, and specifies the point at which the straight line meets the y-axis (the intercept) and the steepness of the line (the slope). In this case, the regression is expressed as follows:

$$y = 298 + 108x$$

where y is the value of the walk test, 298 is the intercept, 108 is the slope of the line, and x is the value of FEV_1. In this case, the intercept of 298 has little practical meaning; it predicts the walk test distance of a patient with an FEV_1 of 0. The slope of 108, however, does have some meaning: it predicts that for every increase in FEV_1 of 1 L, the patient will walk 108 m farther. The regression line corresponding to this formula is shown in Figure 31-3.

Having constructed the regression equation, we can examine the correlation between the two variables, and we can determine whether the correlation can be explained by chance. The correlation is 0.40, and the corresponding P value suggests that chance is a very unlikely explanation ($P = 0.0001$). Thus, we conclude that FEV_1 explains or accounts for a statistically significant proportion of the variability, or *variance*, in walk test scores.

We can also examine the relationship between walk test scores and patients' sex (Figure 31-4[5]). Although considerable variability exists within the sexes, men tend to have higher scores than women. If we had to predict a man's score, we would choose the mean score of the men (410 m); to predict a woman's score, we would choose the women's mean score (363 m).

Does the apparent relationship between sex and walk test score result from chance? One way of answering this question is to construct another simple regression equation with walk test as the dependent variable and patient's sex as the independent variable. As it turns out, chance is an unlikely explanation of the relationship between sex and the walk test ($P = 0.0005$). These two examples show that the independent variable can be an either/or variable—such as sex (male or female), which we call a *dichotomous variable*—or a variable that can theoretically take any value (such as FEV_1), which we call a *continuous variable*.

In Figure 31-5[5], we have separated the men from the women and divided each into groups with high and low FEV_1 results. Although there is a range of scores within each of these groups, the range is narrower than among all women or all men, and even more so than all patients. When we use the mean of a specific group as our best guess of the walk test score of any member of that group, we will on average be closer to the true value than if we had used the mean for all patients.

Figure 31-5[5] illustrates how we can take more than one independent variable into account at the same time in explaining or predicting the dependent variable. We can construct a mathematical model that explains or predicts the walk test score by simultaneously considering all the independent variables and thus creating a *multivariate regression equation.*

We can learn several things from such an equation. First, we can determine if the variables that were associated with the dependent variable in the univariate equations each make independent contributions to explaining the variation. In the current example, we have used an approach in which the independent variable with the strongest relationship to the dependent variable is considered first, followed by the variable with the next strongest relationship. FEV_1 and sex each make independent contributions to explaining walk test results ($P < 0.0001$ for FEV_1 and $P = 0.03$ for sex in the multiple regression analysis), but height (which was significant at the $P = 0.02$ level when considered in a univariate regression) does not make a comparable contribution to the explanation.

If we had chosen both FEV_1 and peak expiratory flow rates as independent variables, they would both show significant associations with the walk test score. However, because FEV_1 and peak expiratory flow rates are associated very strongly with one another, they are unlikely to provide independent contributions to explaining the

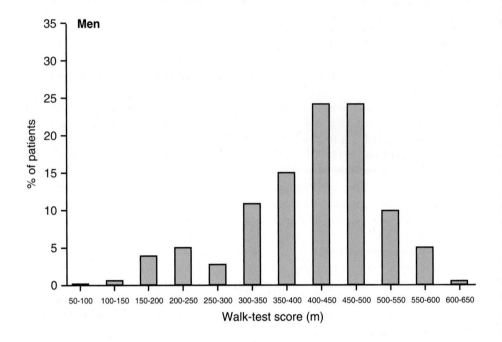

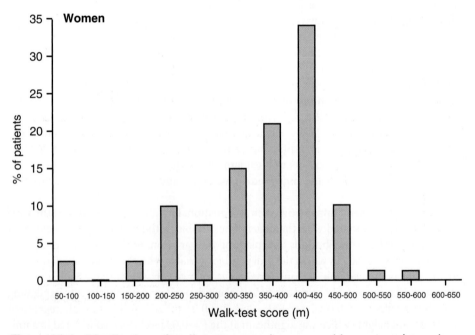

Figure 31-4. Distribution of walk test scores in men and in women (sample of 219 patients). *(Modified and reproduced with permission of the Canadian Medical Association from Guyatt G, Walter S, Shannon H, Cook D, Jaeschke R, Heddle N. Basic statistics for clinicians: 4. Correlation and regression. CMAJ. 1995;152:497-504.)*

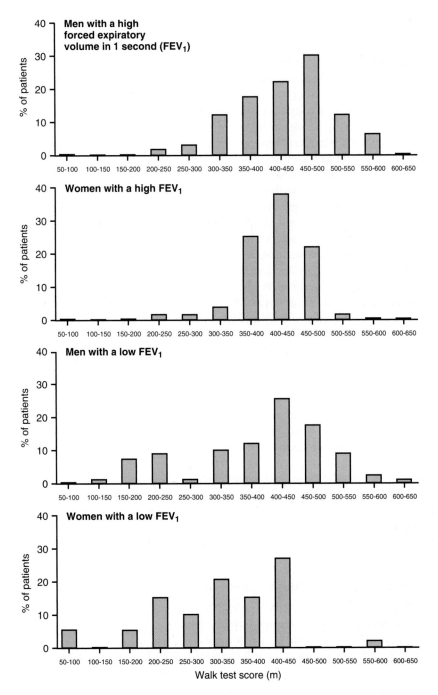

Figure 31-5. Distribution of walk test scores in men and women with high and low forced expiratory volume in 1 second (sample of 219 patients). *(Modified and reproduced with permission of the Canadian Medical Association from Guyatt G, Walter S, Shannon H, Cook D, Jaeschke R, Heddle N. Basic statistics for clinicians: 4. Correlation and regression. CMAJ. 1995;152:497-504.)*

variation in walk test scores. In other words, once we take FEV_1 into account, peak flow rates will not likely help to predict walk test scores, and if we first take peak flow rates into account, FEV_1 will not provide further explanatory power to our predictive model. Similarly, height was a significant predictor of the walk test score when considered alone but was no longer significant in the multivariate regression because of its correlation with sex and FEV_1. When exploring which variables should go into a predictive model, investigators should have considered which variables are likely to have an independent effect on the dependent variable.

We have emphasized how the P value associated with a correlation provides little information about the strength of the relation between two values; the correlation coefficient itself is required. Similarly, knowing that sex and FEV_1 independently explain some of the variation in walk test scores tells us little about the power of our predictive model. Figure 31-5 gives us some sense of the model's predictive power. Although the distributions of walk test scores in the four subgroups differ appreciably, considerable overlap remains. The regression equation can tell us the proportion of the variation in the dependent variable (i.e., the differences between people in walk test scores) that is associated with each of the independent variables (sex and FEV_1) and, therefore, the proportion explained by the entire model. In this case, FEV_1 explains 15% of the variation when it is the first variable entered into the model, sex explains an additional 2% of the variation conditional on FEV_1 being in the model already, and the total model explains 17% of the variation. We can therefore conclude that many other factors that have not been measured—and perhaps cannot be measured—determine how far people with chronic lung disease can walk in 6 minutes. Other investigations using regression techniques have found that patients' experience of the intensity of their exertion, as well as the perception of the severity of their illness, may be more powerful determinants of walk test distance than is their FEV_1.[7]

In our example, the dependent variable—the walk test—was a continuous variable. When the dependent variable is a continuous variable and the relationship between the variables is linear, we refer to the regression as *linear regression*. In our next example, the dependent variable is a dichotomous variable (e.g., present or absent; alive or dead). The term *logistic regression* refers to regression models in which the target (or dependent) variable is dichotomous.

An Example of Logistic Regression: Predicting Clinically Important Bleeding

Cook and colleagues addressed the question of predicting which critically ill patients are at risk for clinically important gastrointestinal bleeding.[8] In this case, the dependent variable was whether or not patients had a clinically important bleeding episode. When the dependent variable is a dichotomous variable, we use the term *logistic* (because it uses a model that relies on logarithms) to describe the regression analysis. The independent variables included whether patients were breathing independently or required ventilator support for respiratory failure, and the presence or absence of coagulopathy, hypotension, sepsis, hepatic failure, renal failure, enteral feeding, steroid administration, organ transplant, or anticoagulant therapy.

Table 31-1[5] shows some of the results from the study, in which the investigators followed up 2252 critically ill patients to determine who had a clinically important bleeding episode.[8] It shows that in univariate logistic regression equations, many independent variables (i.e., respiratory failure, coagulopathy, hypotension, sepsis, hepatic failure, renal failure, enteral feeding, steroid administration, organ transplantation, anticoagulant therapy) were significantly associated with clinically important bleeding. For several variables, the odds ratio (see Chapter 27, Measures of Association), which indicates the strength of the association, is quite large. However, when the investigators constructed a multiple logistic regression equation, only two of the independent variables, respiratory failure and coagulopathy, were significantly and independently associated with risk of bleeding. All of the other variables that predicted bleeding in the univariate analysis were correlated either with respiratory failure or with coagulopathy, and therefore did not reach conventional levels of statistical significance in the multiple regression. Among patients who were not ventilated, 3 of 1597 (0.2%) had a bleeding episode; among those who were ventilated, 30 of 655 (4.6%) had a bleeding episode; among patients with no coagulopathy, 10 of 1792 (0.6%) had a bleeding episode; among those with coagulopathy, 23 of 455 (5.1%) had a bleeding episode.

The primary clinical interest was to identify a subgroup with a sufficiently low risk that bleeding prophylaxis might be withheld. Separate from the regression analysis, they divided the patients into two groups—those who were neither ventilated nor had coagulopathy, of whom only 2 in 1405 (0.14%) had a bleeding episode, and those who were

Table 31-1 Odds Ratios and *P* Values According to Simple (Univariate) and Multiple (Multivariate) Logistic Regression Analysis for Risk Factors for Clinically Important Gastrointestinal Bleeding in Critically Ill Patients

	Simple Regression		Multiple Regression	
Risk Factors	*Odds Ratio*	*P Value*	*Odds Ratio*	*P Value*
Respiratory failure	25.5	<0.0001	15.6	<0.0001
Coagulopathy	9.5	<0.0001	4.3	0.0002
Hypotension	5.0	0.03	2.1	0.08
Sepsis	7.3	<0.0001	Not significant	
Hepatic failure	6.5	<0.0001	Not significant	
Renal failure	4.6	<0.0001	Not significant	
Enteral feeding	3.8	0.0002	Not significant	
Steroid administration	3.7	0.0004	Not significant	
Organ transplant	3.6	0.006	Not significant	
Anticoagulant therapy	3.3	0.004	Not significant	

Modified and reproduced with permission of the Canadian Medical Association from Guyatt G, Walter S, Shannon H, Cook D, Jaeschke R, Heddle N. Basic statistics for clinicians: 4. Correlation and regression. CMAJ. 1995;152:497-504.

either ventilated or had coagulopathy, of whom 31 of 847 (3.7%) had a bleeding episode. Prophylaxis may reasonably be withheld in the former group.

CONCLUSION

Correlation is a statistical tool that permits researchers to examine the strength of the relationship between two variables, when neither one is necessarily considered the target variable. Regression, by contrast, examines the strength of relationship between one or more predictor (or independent) variables and a target (or dependent) variable. Regression can be useful in formulating predictive models that purport to assess risks (e.g., the predictors of postpartum depression,[9] the predictors of motor urge urinary incontinence,[10] or the predictors of treatment-seeking delays for acute myocardial infarction symptoms[11]). Such predictive models can help us make better clinical decisions. Regardless of whether you are considering an issue of correlation or regression, you should consider whether the relationship between variables is statistically significant as well as the magnitude or strength of the relationship—either in terms of the proportion of variation explained or the extent to which groups with different risks of the target event can be specified.

References

1. McGavin CR, Gupta SP, McHardy GJ. Twelve-minute walking test for assessing disability in chronic bronchitis. *BMJ*. 1976;1:822-823.
2. Guyatt GH, Berman LB, Townsend M. Long-term outcome after respiratory rehabilitation. *CMAJ*. 1987;137:1089-1095.
3. Guyatt G, Keller J, Singer J, Halcrow S, Newhouse M. Controlled trial of respiratory muscle training in chronic airflow limitation. *Thorax*. 1992;47:598-602.
4. Goldstein RS, Gort EH, Stubbing D, Avendano MA, Guyatt GH. Randomised controlled trial of respiratory rehabilitation. *Lancet*. 1994;344:1394-1397.
5. Guyatt G, Walter S, Shannon H, Cook D, Jaeschke R, Heddle N. Basic statistics for clinicians: 4. Correlation and regression. *CMAJ*. 1995;152:497-504.
6. Godfrey K. Simple linear regression. *N Engl J Med*. 1985;313:1629-1636.
7. Morgan AD, Peck DF, Buchanan DR, McHardy GJ. Effect of attitudes and beliefs on exercise tolerance in chronic bronchitis. *BMJ*. 1983;286:171-173.
8. Cook DJ, Fuller HD, Guyatt GH, et al. Risk factors for gastrointestinal bleeding in critically ill patients. *N Engl J Med*. 1994;330:377-381.
9. Beck CT. Predictors of postpartum depression: an update. *Nurs Res*. 2001;50:275-285.
10. Gray M, McClain R, Peruggia M, Patrie J, Steers WD. A model for predicting motor urge urinary incontinence. *Nurs Res*. 2001;50:116-122.
11. Zerwic JJ, Ryan CJ, DeVon HA, Drell MJ. Treatment seeking for acute myocardial infarction symptoms: differences in delay across sex and race. *Nurs Res*. 2003;52:159-167.

Moving From Evidence to Action

Chapter **32** Number Needed to Treat

Chapter **33** Applying Results to Individual Patients

Chapter **34** Incorporating Patient Values

Chapter **35** Interpreting Levels of Evidence and Grades of Health Care Recommendations

Chapter **36** Recommendations About Screening

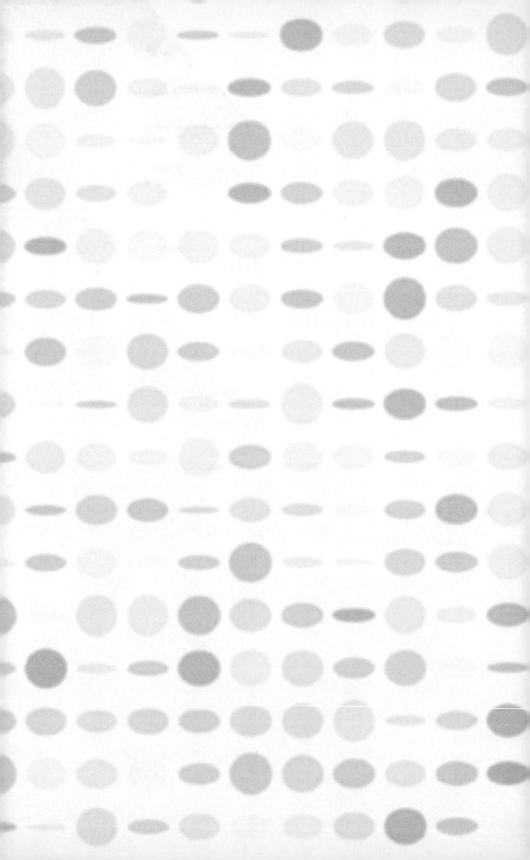

Number Needed to Treat

32

Alba DiCenso, Donna Ciliska, and Gordon Guyatt

The following Editorial Board members also made substantive contributions to this chapter: Rien de Vos, Andrew Jull, Cathy Kessenich, and Ania Willman.

We gratefully acknowledge the work of Christina Lacchetti and P. J. Devereaux on the original chapter that appears in the Users' Guides to the Medical Literature, *edited by Guyatt and Rennie.*

In This Chapter

How Can We Summarize Benefits and Risks?

Number Needed to Treat in Weighing Benefit and Harm
Number Needed to Treat and Dichotomous Outcomes
Number Needed to Treat Versus Relative Risk Reduction
Number Needed to Treat and Baseline Risk
Number Needed to Treat and Precision
Number Needed to Treat and Follow-up Time
Number Needed to Harm

HOW CAN WE SUMMARIZE BENEFITS AND RISKS?

Evidence-based practice requires that clinicians summarize the benefits and risks of health care interventions for patients. Furthermore, clinicians must incorporate patient values and benefit and risk data to judge which management strategies are in patients' best interests (see Chapter 34, Incorporating Patient Values).

These activities require clear and vivid summaries of the magnitude of intervention benefits. The *relative risk reduction* (RRR, the arithmetic difference between the control and intervention event rates, divided by the control event rate), the *absolute risk reduction* (ARR, the arithmetic difference between the control and intervention event rates), and the *number needed to treat* (NNT) represent alternative ways of summarizing the impact of an intervention (see Chapter 27, Measures of Association). In this chapter, we focus on NNTs.

NUMBER NEEDED TO TREAT IN WEIGHING BENEFIT AND HARM

The NNT, the number of patients a clinician must treat for a specific period of time to prevent one adverse outcome (e.g., pain) or produce one positive outcome (e.g., increased functional ability),[1,2] may be the most attractive single measure for summarizing the magnitude of an intervention effect. Knowing the NNT helps clinicians to determine whether the likely intervention benefits are worth the potential harm and costs. For example, we would be comfortable providing 10 patients with a safe, low-cost intervention to prevent one patient from experiencing a pressure ulcer (an NNT of 10), but we would be more reluctant to provide 10,000 patients with a risky, high-cost intervention to prevent one patient from experiencing a pressure ulcer (an NNT of 10,000).[3]

Arithmetically, the NNT is the inverse of the absolute difference (i.e., 1/ARR). A randomized controlled trial by Moller and colleagues[4] of a preoperative smoking intervention to reduce postoperative complications in patients having elective knee or hip replacement illustrates the usefulness of the NNT. At 6 to 8 weeks before surgery, the investigators allocated 60 patients to a smoking intervention involving weekly meetings with a nurse, who provided advice about smoking cessation or reduction and management of withdrawal symptoms and weight gain. The 60 patients allocated to usual care received little or no information or counseling on smoking. The risk of a postoperative complication (death or postoperative morbidity) was 18% in patients who received the smoking intervention and 52% in those who received usual care.

The relative risk (RR) of developing a postoperative complication with the smoking intervention is calculated by dividing the proportion of patients developing a postoperative complication in the intervention group by the proportion of patients developing a postoperative complication in the control group; in this case, the RR is 0.35 (0.18/0.52). The RRR is the proportional reduction in postoperative complication rates between the two groups and is calculated by dividing the absolute risk reduction by the absolute risk in the control group; in this case, the RRR is 65% [(0.52 − 0.18)/0.52 × 100]. One may also derive the RRR by subtracting the relative risk from 1.0 and multiplying by 100% [(1.0 − 0.35) × 100 = 65%)] or by subtracting the relative risk (expressed as a percentage) from 100% (100% − 35% = 65%).

The ARR, or the difference in the proportion of patients who experience postoperative complications in each group is 34% (52% − 18%), and the NNT, or the inverse of the ARR, is 3 (1/0.34 or 100%/34%). An NNT of 3 means that if we provide the preoperative smoking intervention to three patients who are daily smokers and are scheduled for elective knee or hip replacement, we could prevent one patient from developing a postoperative complication by the time of hospital discharge. Table 32-1 provides examples of NNTs for various nursing interventions. The remainder of this chapter addresses important points to consider when calculating and interpreting NNTs.

Number Needed to Treat and Dichotomous Outcomes

The only outcomes that lend themselves to calculation of NNTs are dichotomous outcomes, which are counts of the number of people who experience an outcome (e.g., alive or dead, recovered or not recovered, healed or not healed). One cannot calculate an NNT for an outcome expressed as a mean value such as mean blood pressure or mean length of stay. However, some trials dichotomize continuous outcomes by reporting the percentage of patients who attain a threshold value (e.g., the percentage of patients who attain a glycosylated hemoglobin concentration of less than 7.0%). In the preoperative smoking intervention trial, the outcome (i.e., development of a postoperative complication—yes or no) was a dichotomous event, which allowed calculation of an NNT.

Number Needed to Treat Versus Relative Risk Reduction

Why not confine our description of the clinical significance of a result to the RRR? The reason is that the RRR fails to discriminate huge absolute intervention effects from those that are trivial. For example, if the postoperative complication rate in the earlier example had been 10 times less than that observed in the trial (i.e., 1.8% of preoperative smoking intervention patients and 5.2% of control group patients), the RRR would still be 65%. This is because the RRR ignores how frequently the outcome occurs.[10] The effect of providing the smoking intervention to preoperative patients with a low risk of postoperative complications will differ from the effect of providing it to patients with a higher risk of complications.

In contrast to the nondiscriminating RRR, the absolute difference in postoperative complication rates between intervention and control group patients clearly *does* discriminate between these extremes. Contrast an ARR of 34% (52% − 18%) with the ARR of 3.4% (5.2% − 1.8%) in the hypothetical example provided earlier, in which 5.2% of control group patients and 1.8% of intervention group patients had postoperative complications. The ARR takes into account the baseline risk of patients and provides more detailed information than the RRR. By dividing the ARR into 1, we generate the NNT. Thus, if the postoperative complication rates had been 10 times less than those observed in the trial, the NNT would have been 30 (1/0.034 or 100%/3.4%), rather than 3 (1/0.34 or 100%/34%).

Number Needed to Treat and Baseline Risk

When considering the NNT associated with treating a particular patient, we must consider the patient's level of risk relative to the average control patient in the trial.

Table **32-1** Examples of Numbers Needed to Treat

Condition or Disorder	Intervention Versus Control	Outcome	Control Group Rate	RRR (CI) (%)	ARR (%)	NNT (CI)
Patients who had coronary angiography[5]	Pressure bandage versus no pressure bandage	Bleeding 6 to 12 hr after coronary angiography	6.7%	48 (10 to 70)	3.2	32 (17 to 175)
Patients who had coronary angiography[5]	Pressure bandage versus no pressure bandage	Groin pain 6 to 12 hr after coronary angiography	4.7%	Relative risk increase = 275 (148 to 469)	Absolute risk increase = 12.8	NNH = 8 (6 to 11)
Critically ill neonates[6]	Chlorhexidine versus 10% povidone-iodine	Central venous catheter tip colonization until catheter removal and culture	24%	40 (10 to 50)	9	11 (9 to 42)
Pregnant women with no health insurance or on Medicaid[7]	Nurse home-visits versus no visits	Children with emotional vulnerability at 6 mo of age	25%	36 (8 to 55)	9	12 (7 to 58)
Patients admitted to hospital with heart failure[8]	Nurse-led transitional care versus usual discharge planning	Emergency department visits over 12 wk after hospital discharge	46%	38 (6 to 59)	17	6 (3 to 48)
High-risk older adults[9]	Outpatient geriatric evaluation and management versus usual care	Loss of functional ability over 18 mo	52%	24 (9 to 37)	12	9 (5 to 24)

ARR, *absolute risk reduction;* CI, *confidence interval;* NNH, *number needed to harm;* NNT, *number needed to treat;* RRR, *relative risk reduction.*

NNTs vary with baseline risk: the lower the baseline risk is, the higher the NNT will be. For example, applying the RRR (31%) of pravastatin therapy over conventional therapy for patients without diagnosed cardiovascular disease[12] (first row of Table 32-2), we find that we must treat approximately 161 patients in the low-risk group with pravastatin therapy to prevent a single cardiovascular event over 5 years. In contrast, we must treat approximately nine patients in the very high-risk group with pravastatin therapy to prevent a single cardiovascular event over 5 years. Clinicians may make different decisions about recommending this therapy to these low-risk and very high-risk patients.

Our patient's expected event rate can be estimated in several ways. First, we can assign our patient the same event rate as that of the control group in the trial. Although this approach is simple, it is sensible only if our patient is very similar to the average control group patient. Second, if the study presents data for subgroups of patients, and our patient has similar characteristics to one of these subgroups, we can assign our patient the control group rate for that subgroup. Third, we can look for a prospective study that examined the prognosis of patients similar to ours and use its results to assign a baseline risk rate to our patient.[10]

For patients at very high risk of the target event, the NNT will tend to be low, and intervention is likely to be justified. For patients at very low risk of the target event, the NNT is likely to be high enough to raise doubts about whether the intervention is warranted, even if the outcome being prevented is serious.[3] Chatellier and colleagues[29] described a systematic review[30] of coronary artery bypass graft surgery in patients with stable coronary heart disease that illustrates the importance of establishing a patient's baseline risk when determining the NNT. Five-year mortality in patients with the lowest, middle, and highest risk was 6.3%, 13.9%, and 25.2%, respectively. Assuming that the same 39% relative risk reduction in 5-year mortality risk existed in each subgroup, the NNT to avoid a single death in the groups with the lowest, middle, and highest risk would be 40, 19, and 10, respectively (Table 32-3). Some may argue against using resources for coronary artery bypass graft surgery in 40 low-risk patients to prevent a single death. In Table 32-2, we apply the RRRs associated with various interventions to groups of patients at varying levels of risk and calculate the associated NNTs. After considering the adverse events associated with an intervention and its additional cost, clinicians may make different decisions about whether to administer an intervention to low-risk and high-risk patients.

Number Needed to Treat and Precision

Because NNTs are only estimates of truth, they should be accompanied by 95% confidence intervals (CIs)—the limits within which the true NNT lies 95% of the time. Because estimates of precision are directly dependent on sample size, the smaller the number of patients in a study, the wider the CI around the NNT will be. In the preoperative smoking intervention trial by Moller and colleagues,[4] the 95% CI around the NNT of 3 ranged from 2 to 6,[31] a finding indicating that the true NNT may be as low as 2 and as high as 6. Given that the true NNT could fall anywhere within the CI, the decision to implement the preoperative smoking intervention should consider the outer limits of the CI.

Table 32-2 Numbers Needed to Treat Associated With Varying Levels of Risk

Condition or Disorder	Intervention Versus Control	Outcome	Risk Groups	RRR (CI) (%)	ARR (%)	NNT
Persons without diagnosed cardiovascular disease[a]	Pravastatin therapy versus conventional therapy	Cardiovascular event[b] over 5 yr	Low[c] = < 2.5% Moderate = 12.5% High = 17.5% Very high = > 30%	31 (17 to 43)[12]	0.62 3.88 5.43 10.85	161 26 18 9
Persons without diagnosed cardiovascular disease	Aspirin versus placebo	Cardiovascular event[b] over 5 yr	Low[c] = < 2.5% Moderate = 12.5% High = 17.5% Very high = > 30%	15 (1 to 27)[13]	0.30 1.88 2.63 5.25	333 53 38 19
Persons without diagnosed cardiovascular disease	Aspirin versus placebo	Major bleeding episodes (fatal and nonfatal) over an average of 3.8 yr	NA	Relative risk increase = 74 (31 to 130)[13]	0.62	Number needed to harm = 161
Congestive heart failure	Spironolactone versus placebo	Total mortality over 1 yr	Low[d] = 8% Medium = 21% High = 33%	30 (18 to 40)[15]	2.40 6.30 9.90	42 16 10
Congestive heart failure	Angiotensin-converting enzyme inhibitor versus placebo	Total mortality over 1 yr	Low[d] = 8% Medium = 21% High = 33%	23 (12 to 33)[16]	1.84 4.83 7.59	54 21 13
Congestive heart failure	Beta-blocker therapy versus placebo	Total mortality over 1 yr	Low[d] = 8% Medium = 21% High = 33%	32 (12 to 47)[17]	2.56 6.72 10.56	39 15 9

Condition	Treatment	Outcome	Baseline risk	NNT (95% CI)		
Acute myocardial infarction	Angiotensin-converting enzyme inhibitor versus placebo	Mortality over 6 mo	Low[e] = 1.8% Medium = 2.0% High = 9.9% Very high = 14.4%	6.3 (1 to 10)[19]	0.11 0.13 0.62 0.91	882 794 160 110
Postmyocardial infarction	Beta-blocker therapy versus placebo	Total mortality over 6 mo	Low[e] = 1.8% Medium = 2.0% High = 9.9% Very high = 14.4%	23 (15 to 31)[20]	0.4 0.5 2.3 3.3	242 217 44 30
Hypertension	Antihypertensive treatment (primarily beta-blockers or diuretics) versus placebo/usual care	Cardiovascular event (includes fatal/nonfatal myocardial infarction, stroke, or coronary death) over 5 yr	Low[f] = 2% Medium = 5% High = 10%	25 (14 to 29)[22,23]	0.5 1.25 2.5	200 80 40
Hypertension	Antihypertensive treatment (primarily beta-blockers or diuretics) versus placebo/usual care	Cardiovascular event (includes fatal/nonfatal myocardial infarction, stroke, or coronary death) over 20 yr	Low[f] = 15% Medium = 30% High = 50%	25 (14 to 29)[22,23]	3.75 7.5 12.5	27 13 8
Nonvalvular atrial fibrillation	Warfarin versus placebo	Stroke over 1 yr	Very low[g] = ≤ 1% Low = 4.9% Medium = 5.7% High = 8.1%	62 (48 to 72)[25]	0.62 3.04 3.53 5.02	161 33 28 20

Continued

Table 32-2   Numbers Needed to Treat Associated With Varying Levels of Risk—cont'd

Condition or Disorder	Intervention Versus Control	Outcome	Risk Groups	RRR (CI) (%)	ARR (%)	NNT
Rheumatoid arthritis treated with nonsteroidal anti-inflammatory drugs	Concurrent misoprostol versus placebo	Development of serious upper gastrointestinal complications over 6 mo	Low[h] = 0.4% Medium = 1.0% High = 9.0%	40 (1.8 to 64)[26]	0.16 0.40 3.60	625 250 28
HIV infection	Ritonavir versus placebo	AIDS-defining illness at 6 yr[i]	Low = 2.4% Medium = 4.3% High = 7.5% Very high = 12.8%	42 (29 to 52)[28]	1.01 1.81 3.15 5.38	99 85 32 19

[a] >90% of patients studied did not have diagnosed cardiovascular disease.

[b] Cardiovascular event is defined as death related to coronary artery disease, nonfatal myocardial infarction, new angina, fatal or nonfatal stroke or transient ischemic attack, development of congestive heart failure, or peripheral vascular disease.

[c] Risk varies according to a patient's sex, diabetic status, smoking status, and age. For example, low risk = patients aged 40-49 yr with blood pressure 120-140 mm Hg systolic or 75-85 mm Hg diastolic, who do not have diabetes and do not smoke; moderate risk = patients aged 50 yr and older with blood pressure 140-160 mm Hg systolic or 85-95 mm Hg diastolic, who may have diabetes and do not smoke; high risk = patients aged 60 yr and older with blood pressure 160-180 mm Hg systolic or 95-105 mm Hg diastolic, who may have diabetes and do not smoke; very high risk = patients aged 70 yr and older with blood pressure = 180 mm Hg systolic or 105 mm Hg diastolic, who may have diabetes and do not smoke. Refer to Jackson[11] to identify the various combinations of factors that determine a patient's risk category.

[d] Low risk = New York Heart Association (NYHA) functional class II; medium risk = NYHA functional class III; high risk = NYHA functional class IV.[14]

[e] Low risk = no premature ventricular beats (PVBs) and no clinical heart failure (CHF); medium = 1-10 PVBs and no CHF; high = 1-10 PVBs and CHF; very high = >10 PVBs and CHF.[18]

[f] Low risk = diastolic blood pressure 90 mm Hg; medium = diastolic blood pressure 95 mm Hg; high = diastolic blood pressure 100 mm Hg.[21]

[g] Very low risk = age < 65 yr with no risk factors; low risk = age < 65 yr with ≥ 1 risk factors (history of hypertension, diabetes, and prior stroke or transient ischemic attack); medium risk = age 65-75 yr with ≥ 1 risk factors; high risk = age > 75 yr with ≥ 1 risk factors.[24]

[h] Low risk = patients with none of the following risk factors: age ≥ 75 yr; history of peptic ulcer; history of gastrointestinal bleeding; or history of cardiovascular disease; medium risk = patients with any single factor; high risk = patients with all four factors.[26]

[i] Baseline HIV-1 RNA level (copies/mL): low = 501-3000; medium = 3001-10,000; high = 10,001-30,000; very high = > 30,000.[27]

ARR, Absolute risk reduction; CI, confidence interval; NA, not applicable; NNT, number needed to treat; RRR, relative risk reduction.

Table 32-3   Relationship Between Baseline Risk of Mortality and Number Needed to Treat in Patients With Stable Coronary Heart Disease

	CER (5 Year Mortality)	RRR	ARR = CER × RRR	NNT = 1/ARR
Low risk	6.3%	39%	2.5%*	40
Middle risk	13.9%	39%	5.4%	19
High risk	25.2%	39%	9.8%	10

ARR, *Absolute risk reduction;* CER, *control event rate;* NNT, *number needed to treat;* RRR, *relative risk reduction.*
Data from Yusuf S, Zucker D, Peduzzi P, et al. Effect of coronary bypass graft surgery on survival: overview of 10-year results from randomised trials by the Coronary Artery Bypass Graft Surgery Trialists Collaboration. Lancet. 1994;344:563–570.
*[(0.063 × 0.39) × 100] = 2.45% (rounded to 2.5%)

Number Needed to Treat and Follow-up Time

Because the number of reported events in a study is determined by following up the study patients for a specified period, this must be reflected in the interpretation of NNTs. For example, in the preoperative smoking intervention study, patients were followed up to hospital discharge. The NNT for postoperative complications at hospital discharge was 3 (95% CI, 2 to 6). In other words, three patients who were scheduled for elective hip or knee replacement and were daily smokers would need to receive the intervention to prevent one additional patient from having a postoperative complication by the time of hospital discharge, and the true NNT could be as low as 2 and as high as 6.

Number Needed to Harm

Interventions often have adverse effects as well as benefits. To determine the impact of adverse effects, we calculate the *number needed to harm* (NNH), which is the number of patients who, if they received the experimental intervention, would lead to a single additional patient being harmed compared with patients who receive the control intervention.[32] Like the NNT, the NNH is calculated as 1/absolute difference (or 100%/absolute difference expressed as a percentage) and is accompanied by a CI.

A study that evaluated the effectiveness and safety of pressure bandages applied immediately after coronary angiography illustrates the need to consider both the benefits and adverse effects of an intervention (see the first row of Table 32-1).[5] Within 6 to 12 hours after coronary angiography, only 3.5% of patients assigned to the pressure bandage group had bleeding compared with 6.7% of patients assigned to the no-bandage control group. The RRR is 48% [(6.7% − 3.5%)/6.7%], meaning that pressure bandages decreased the relative risk of bleeding after coronary angiography by 48%. The ARR is 3.2% (6.7% − 3.5%). The NNT is 32 (1/0.032), which means that we would need to treat 32 people with pressure bandages for 6 to 12 hours after coronary angiography to prevent one additional person from bleeding.

Although this appears to be an important beneficial effect, it must be considered in conjunction with the adverse effects. Patients in the bandage group had a higher incidence of nausea, back pain, groin pain, leg pain, and urinary difficulties. Looking more closely at groin pain (see the second row of Table 32-1), 17.5% of patients in the bandage group and 4.7% of patients in the control group had groin pain during the 6- to 12-hour period. This absolute risk increase of 12.8% (17.5% − 4.7%) generates an NNH over 6 to 12 hours of 8, meaning that treating eight patients with pressure bandages for 6 to 12 hours would cause a single additional patient to have groin pain.

Clinicians and patients must decide when adverse effects are large enough to more than offset the positive effects of an intervention. The Women's Health Initiative trial of estrogen plus progestin[33] illustrates the usefulness of NNHs and NNTs in helping clinicians to judge the degree of harm and the degree of benefit patients can expect from an intervention. The Women's Health Initiative study was stopped early (at a mean of 5.2 years instead of the expected 8.5 years) because the investigators found that women who received combination hormone replacement therapy had a greater incidence of coronary heart disease (NNH = 1152; 95% CI, 531 to 16,693), stroke (NNH = 1164; 95% CI, 562 to 6811), and venous thromboembolism (NNH = 565; 95% CI, 345 to 1079) than women who received placebo.[33] At the same time, women in the study had a reduced incidence of vertebral fractures (NNT = 1962; 95% CI, 1191 to 33,358), hip fractures (NNT = 1962; 95% CI, 1213 to 33,358), and colorectal cancer (NNT = 1691; 95% CI, 1097 to 7819).[33]

The example in the second row of Table 32-2 further illustrates this point. As a result of taking aspirin, patients with hypertension without known coronary artery disease can expect a reduction of approximately 15% in their relative risk of cardiovascular-related events.[13] For an otherwise low-risk woman with hypertension and a *baseline risk* of cardiovascular-related events of less than 2.5%, this translates into an NNT of approximately 333 during a 5-year period. However, as presented in the third row of the table, for every 161 patients treated with aspirin (NNH), 1 patient would experience a major hemorrhage. Thus, in 1000 patients, aspirin would be responsible for preventing three cardiovascular events, but it would also be responsible for causing approximately six serious bleeding episodes. Recommending aspirin to such low-risk patients would be questionable at best. For a patient at very high risk of cardiovascular events (e.g., a man with hypertension and diabetes who is more than 70 years old), the NNT of approximately 20 (in 1000 patients, 50 cardiovascular events prevented by aspirin and six bleeding episodes caused by aspirin) suggests that recommending aspirin may be much more appropriate.

Finally, another example from Table 32-2 emphasizes the importance of considering the time frame in evaluating the NNT. During a 5-year period, the NNT for prevention of major cardiovascular events with antihypertensive treatment in low-risk, medium-risk, and high-risk patients is 200, 80, and 40, respectively (ninth row of Table 32-2). Over 20 years, the corresponding numbers are 27, 13, and 8 (tenth row of Table 32-2). This reduction in the NNT with longer time frames is due to the increased number of events that occur over this time and the resulting increase in the absolute difference between event rates. These figures help to demonstrate how different presentations of NNT data can determine the impact of the information on clinicians and patients.

Clinicians can use NNTs in making intervention decisions with patients. However, when using NNTs, it is important to consider an individual patient's baseline risk, the RRR, and the NNH associated with the intervention before advising patients about the optimal management of their health problems.

REFERENCES

1. Laupacis A, Sackett DL, Roberts RS. An assessment of clinically useful measures of the consequences of treatment. *N Engl J Med.* 1988;318:1728-1733.

2. DiCenso A. Clinically useful measures of the effects of treatment [editorial]. *Evid Based Nurs.* 2001;4:36-39.

3. Sinclair JC, Cook RJ, Guyatt GH, Pauker SG, Cook DJ. When should an effective treatment be used? Derivation of the threshold number needed to treat and the minimum event rate for treatment. *J Clin Epidemiol.* 2001;54:253-262.

4. Moller AM, Villebro N, Pedersen T, et al. Effect of preoperative smoking intervention on postoperative complications: a randomised clinical trial. *Lancet.* 2002;359:114-117.

5. Botti M, Williamson B, Steen K, et al. The effect of pressure bandaging on complications and comfort in patients undergoing coronary angiography: a multicenter randomized trial. *Heart Lung.* 1998;27:360-373.

6. Garland JS, Alex CP, Mueller CD, et al. A randomized trial comparing povidone-iodine to a chlorhexidine gluconate–impregnated dressing for prevention of central venous catheter infections in neonates. *Pediatrics.* 2001;107:1431-1437.

7. Olds DL, Robinson J, O'Brien R, et al. Home visiting by paraprofessionals and by nurses: a randomized, controlled trial. *Pediatrics.* 2002;110:486-496.

8. Harrison, MB, Browne GB, Roberts J, et al. Quality of life of individuals with heart failure: a randomised trial of the effectiveness of two models of hospital-to-home transition. *Med Care.* 2002;40:271-282.

9. Boult C, Boult LB, Morishital L, et al. A randomized clinical trial of outpatient geriatric evaluation and management. *J Am Geriatr Soc.* 2001;49:351-359.

10. Sackett DL. On some clinically useful measures of the effects of treatment [editorial]. *Evid Based Med.* 1996;1:37-38.

11. Jackson R. Updated New Zealand cardiovascular disease risk-benefit prediction guide. *BMJ.* 2000;320:709-710.

12. Shepherd J, Cobbe SM, Ford I, et al. Prevention of coronary heart disease with pravastatin in men with hypercholesterolemia. *N Engl J Med.* 1995;333:1301-1307.

13. Hansson L, Zanchetti A, Carruthers SG, et al. Effects of intensive blood-pressure lowering and low-dose aspirin in patients with hypertension: principal results of the Hypertension Optimal Treatment (HOT) randomised trial. *Lancet.* 1998;351:1755-1762.

14. Matoba M, Matsui S, Hirakawa T, et al. Long-term prognosis of patients with congestive heart failure. *Jpn Circ J.* 1990;54:57-61.

15. Pitt B, Zannad F, Remme WJ, et al. The effect of spironolactone on morbidity and mortality in patients with severe heart failure. *N Engl J Med.* 1999;341:709-717.

16. Garg R, Yusuf S. Overview of randomized trials of angiotensin-converting enzyme inhibitors on mortality and morbidity in patients with heart failure: Collaborative Group on ACE Inhibitor Trials. *JAMA.* 1995;273:1450-1456.

17. Lechat P, Packer M, Chalon S, Cucherat M, Arab T, Boissel JP. Clinical effects of beta-adrenergic blockade in chronic heart failure: a meta-analysis of double-blind, placebo-controlled, randomized trials. *Circulation.* 1998;98:1184-1191.

18. Maggioni AP, Zuanetti G, Franzosi MG, et al. Prevalence and prognostic significance of ventricular arrhythmias after acute myocardial infarction in the fibrinolytic era: GISSI-2 results. *Circulation.* 1993;87:312-322.

19. ACE inhibitor Myocardial Infarction Collaborative Group. Indications for ACE inhibitors in early treatment of acute myocardial infarction: systematic overview of individual data from 100,000 patients in randomized trials. *Circulation.* 1998;97:2202-2212.

20. Freemantle N, Cleland J, Young P, Mason J, Harrison J. Beta blockade after myocardial infarction: systematic review and meta regression analysis. *BMJ*. 1999;318:1730-1737.

21. McAlister FA, O'Connor AM, Wells G, Grover SA, Laupacis A. When should hypertension be treated? The different perspectives of Canadian family physicians and patients. *Can Med Assoc J*. 2000;163:403-408.

22. Collins R, Peto R, MacMahon S, et al. Blood pressure, stroke, and coronary heart disease. Part 2. Short-term reductions in blood pressure: overview of randomised drug trials in their epidemiological context. *Lancet*. 1990;335:827-838.

23. Gueyffier F, Boutitie F, Boissel JP, et al. Effect of antihypertensive drug treatment on cardiovascular outcomes in women and men: a meta-analysis of individual patient data from randomized, controlled trials. *Ann Intern Med*.1997;126:761-767.

24. Atrial Fibrillation Investigators. Risk factors for stroke and efficacy of antithrombotic therapy in atrial fibrillation: analysis of pooled data from five randomized controlled trials. *Arch Intern Med*. 1994;154:1449-1457.

25. Hart RG, Benavente O, McBride R, Pearce LA. Antithrombotic therapy to prevent stroke in patients with atrial fibrillation: a meta-analysis. *Ann Intern Med*. 1999;131:492-501.

26. Silverstein FE, Graham DY, Senior JR, et al. Misoprostol reduces serious gastrointestinal complications in patients with rheumatoid arthritis receiving nonsteroidal anti-inflammatory drugs: a randomized, double-blind, placebo-controlled trial. *Ann Intern Med*. 1995;123:241-249.

27. Mellors JW, Munoz A, Giorgi JV, et al. Plasma viral load and $CD4^+$ lymphocytes as prognostic markers of HIV-1 infection. *Ann Intern Med*. 1997;126:946-954.

28. Cameron DW, Heath-Chiozzi M, Danner S, et al. Randomised placebo-controlled trial of ritonavir in advanced HIV-1 disease: the Advanced HIV Disease Ritonavir Study Group. *Lancet*. 1998;351:543-549.

29. Chatellier G, Zapletal E, Lemaitre D, et al. The number needed to treat: a clinically useful nomogram in its proper context. *BMJ*. 1996;312:426-429.

30. Yusuf S, Zucker D, Peduzzi P, et al. Effect of coronary bypass graft surgery on survival: overview of 10-year results from randomised trials by the Coronary Artery Bypass Graft Surgery Trialists Collaboration. *Lancet*. 1994;344:563-570.

31. A preoperative smoking intervention decreased postoperative complications in elective knee or hip replacement. *Evid Based Nurs*. 2002;5:84. Abstract of: Moller AM, Villebro N, Pedersen T, et al. Effect of preoperative smoking intervention on postoperative complications: a randomised clinical trial. *Lancet*. 2002;359:114-117.

32. Sackett DL, Straus SE, Richardson WS, et al. *Evidence-Based Medicine: How to Practice and Teach EBM*. Edinburgh, UK: Churchill Livingstone; 2000.

33. Rossouw JE, Anderson GL, Prentice RL, et al. Risks and benefits of estrogen plus progestin in healthy postmenopausal women: principal results from the Women's Health Initiative randomized controlled trial. *JAMA*. 2002;288:321-333.

33

Applying Results to Individual Patients

Alba DiCenso and Gordon Guyatt

The following Editorial Board members also made substantive contributions to this chapter: Rien de Vos, Marie Driever, Kate Flemming, Linda Johnston, Dorothy McCaughan, Mark Newman, and Ania Willman.

We gratefully acknowledge the work of Antonio Dans, Finlay McAlister, Leonilla Dans, Scott Richardson, and Sharon Straus on the original chapter that appears in the Users' Guides to the Medical Literature, *edited by Guyatt and Rennie.*

In This Chapter

How Can I Apply the Results to Patient Care?
Biologic Issues
Socioeconomic Issues
Epidemiologic Issues

Are the Likely Benefits Worth the Potential Risks?
What Is the Patient's Risk of Sustaining Adverse Events?

Having found a high-quality study related to the health problem or situation facing a patient in your clinical setting, the challenge is to determine whether the study results apply to that patient. For example, for many years, research on heart disease was conducted primarily on men, and results were then applied to women, sometimes inappropriately. As clinicians look to randomized controlled trials (RCTs) to guide their clinical care, they must decide how to apply the results to individual patients in their practice settings. Chapter 4, Health Care Interventions, suggested three criteria for deciding on applicability: (1) Is the patient before you similar to those included in the study? (2) Did the investigators measure all important outcomes? and (3) What is the balance between the benefits and risks of intervening?

With regard to the first of these three questions, we suggested that clinicians could apply the results to patients in their settings unless there was a compelling reason to believe that the results would differ substantially as a function of the particular characteristics of those patients. Empirical support for this position comes from several sources. In general, meta-analyses of therapeutic interventions have suggested that effects of interventions are usually similar across subgroups of patients.[1] For example, a systematic review of interventions aimed at improving immunization rates found that reminders were effective for both childhood and adult vaccinations and for patients in various settings, including academic settings, private practice settings, and public health clinics.[2]

Nevertheless, the underlying biologic characteristics of a group of patients may differ from those of most participants in a clinical trial to such an extent that we must question the applicability of the study findings. Clinicians managing patients who differ economically, racially, or culturally from those recruited in typical clinical trials face particular challenges in deciding whether patient groups are sufficiently different that applicability of results is threatened.

In this chapter, we expand on the criteria related to applying results to individual patients and achieving a balance of benefits and risks. Table 33-1 summarizes the guides, categorizing them into biologic and socioeconomic issues (to help us decide if an intervention can work) and epidemiologic issues (to help us decide on the magnitude of the likely benefits and risks).

HOW CAN I APPLY THE RESULTS TO PATIENT CARE?

Biologic Issues

Are There Pathophysiologic Differences in the Health Problem Under Study That May Lead to a Diminished Response to the Intervention?

A specific disease, such as hypertension, may actually represent conditions with important pathophysiologic differences. These differences can sometimes lead to diminished treatment responses because of divergence in pathogenetic mechanisms among patients or biologic differences in causative agents. For example, hypertension in African Americans or black non-Americans is relatively responsive to diuretics but unresponsive to beta-blockers.[3] This selective response reflects a state of relative volume excess that

Table 33-1   Users' Guides for Applying Study Results to Individual Patients

How Can I Apply the Results to Patient Care?

Biologic issues

- Are there pathophysiologic differences in the health problem under study that may lead to a diminished response to the intervention?
- Are there patient differences that may diminish the response to the intervention?

Socioeconomic issues

- Are there important differences in patient adherence that may diminish the response to the intervention?
- Are there important differences in provider adherence that may diminish the safety and efficacy of the intervention?

Epidemiologic issues

- Do patients in my setting have comorbid conditions that significantly alter the potential benefits and risks of the intervention?

Are the Likely Benefits Worth the Potential Risks?

- What is the patient's risk of sustaining adverse events?

investigators now theorize may have served a protective function in hot and arid ancestral environments.[4]

Malaria is an example of a condition that may vary because of biologic differences in the causative agent. Malaria treatment protocols vary depending on drug-resistance patterns.[5] In such instances, clinicians should anticipate variations in response to treatment and temper hasty conclusions about the applicability of trial results.

Are There Patient Differences That May Diminish the Response to the Intervention?

Between-population differences in response to an intervention may arise from differences in drug metabolism, immune response, or environmental factors. For example, women with heart disease may respond differently to interventions that have been shown to work in men. Differences in drug metabolism may directly influence the efficacy of a treatment regimen. If these differences are not identified, patients in whom drugs are metabolized slowly may be at risk of greater toxicity, whereas those in whom drugs are metabolized rapidly might experience decreases in efficacy. Such differences are usually based on genetic polymorphism in the activity of metabolizing enzymes. A well-known example is hepatic N-acetyltransferase, an enzyme with increased activity in persons of Asian descent.[6] For this reason, clinicians prescribe higher dosages of drugs such as isoniazid and hydralazine for such patients.

Differences in patients' immune response may also modulate the effect of an intervention. *Haemophilus influenzae* vaccine, for example, has a lower efficacy rate in indigenous Alaskan populations than in nonindigenous populations.[7] Finally, environmental factors may affect patients' response to an intervention. For instance, children with asthma who live in homes in which their mothers smoke are less responsive to treatment.[8]

Socioeconomic Issues

When clinicians are satisfied that biologic differences do not compromise treatment applicability, they must consider constraints related to the social environment that may diminish the effectiveness of an intervention.

Are There Important Differences in Patient Adherence That May Diminish the Response to the Intervention?

To the extent that groups of people exhibit different levels of adherence to an intervention, clinicians can expect variations in the effectiveness of an intervention. Variability in adherence between populations may stem from obvious resource limitations in particular settings or from less obvious attitudinal or behavioral characteristics. Examples of resource limitations include low income, illiteracy, and lack of access to health insurance and drug benefits, all of which may influence patient adherence to interventions. For example, in an observational study evaluating a smoke alarm–giveaway program, visits to a random sample of homes at 12 months revealed that the alarms were properly installed and functioning in more than 50% of homes.[9] In contrast, in an RCT evaluating the effect of providing free smoke alarms in a deprived, multiethnic, urban community, home visits revealed that few alarms had been installed or maintained.[10] Injuries from residential fires were significantly reduced in the observational study but not in the RCT.

One explanation for the differences in study results may relate to the study designs. Because an observational study does not incorporate random allocation of participants to comparison groups, those responsible for determining who will and will not receive the intervention may be influenced, consciously or unconsciously, by known prognostic factors. Therefore, prognostic factors will likely be unbalanced between groups, and the study will yield biased, misleading results (in this case, overestimation of the intervention's effect) (see Chapter 14, Surprising Results of Randomized Controlled Trials). Although the benefit found in the observational study may have been related to the study design, the authors of the RCT suggest that the differential results may have been related to population differences that could have affected the likelihood of alarms being installed and maintained. Participants in the RCT may not have understood installation instructions or brochures about the benefits of alarms because of illiteracy or poor comprehension of the English language. Tenants may have lacked installation skills or tools or may have worried about landlords objecting to installation. Because of the small size of some apartments, incorrect installation near sources of steam or cooking smoke may have increased the incidence of false or nuisance alarms, leading to removal of the battery or disconnection.[10] These studies illustrate how we cannot always expect the same adherence to an intervention among different populations and how differences in adherence can have a powerful impact on the intended benefit of the intervention.

Although clinicians are often unable to predict patient adherence, a systematic examination of adherence in individual patients—or groups of patients—is likely to aid in identifying varying adherence patterns. Clinicians may also refer to more general sources of evidence, such as sociologic descriptions of attitudes of specific groups of people (see Chapter 8, Qualitative Research).

Are There Important Differences in Provider Adherence That May Diminish the Safety and Efficacy of the Intervention?

In this section, the term *provider adherence* refers to a host of diagnostic tests, monitoring equipment, interventional requirements, and other technical specifications that clinicians must use or satisfy to administer an intervention safely and effectively. Financial conditions in a health care center, access to equipment, technologic expertise, and the availability and skill of health care personnel may influence the effectiveness of an intervention. For example, in hospitals with high patient-to-nurse ratios, surgical patients have higher risk-adjusted 30-day mortality and failure-to-rescue rates.[11]

Epidemiologic Issues

When clinicians are satisfied that biologic and socioeconomic differences do not compromise applicability, they should then consider patient characteristics that could influence the magnitude of the benefits or risks of an intervention (and, thus, the trade-off between the two).[12]

Do Patients in My Setting Have Comorbid Conditions That Significantly Alter the Potential Benefits and Risks of the Intervention?

The presence of other conditions in a particular locality may affect treatment efficiency in two ways: as competing diagnostic possibilities or as competing etiologies of outcome. The management of pneumonia in developing countries provides an example of a competing diagnostic possibility. The acute respiratory infection management protocol includes a symptom-driven *algorithm* for differentiating pneumonia from nonpneumonia. This protocol identifies children who need antibiotics and has proved effective in reducing mortality from pneumonia in children younger than 5 years of age.[13] However, similarities exist in the clinical presentation of pneumonia and malaria. In malaria-endemic areas, clinicians may expect an increase in *false-positive* diagnoses of pneumonia. Patients with results that mimic pneumonia when malaria is actually present will not respond to antibiotics for pneumonia, and a delay in antimalarial treatment may result. If the drop in accuracy is large enough, the balance between harm and benefit will change.

In addition to reducing benefits, other morbidity may affect the magnitude of risk. For example, surgical mortality may increase in malnourished patients, shifting the balance between benefit and risk.

ARE THE LIKELY BENEFITS WORTH THE POTENTIAL RISKS?

What Is the Patient's Risk of Sustaining Adverse Events?

In applying this guide, there are two issues to consider: (1) Does the patient in your clinical setting have a baseline risk that is similar to that of the patients in the study? and

(2) What is the relationship between a patient's risk of an adverse event and the magnitude of the intervention effect?

An individual patient's baseline risk is the key issue in determining the impact of an intervention on that patient. Clinicians can derive estimates of a patient's baseline risk from various sources. First, they can use their intuition, which may sometimes be accurate—at least in terms of the extent to which risk is increased or decreased relative to a typical patient. Second, if randomized trials report risks for patient subgroups, clinicians can choose the risk that best applies to the patient in their setting.[14] However, most trials are not large enough to allow the generation of precise estimates of baseline risk in patient subgroups and those that are large enough often do not provide the required information. Systematic reviews that pool data from multiple trials can provide more precise estimates. For example, Yusuf and colleagues[15] pooled individual patient data from randomized trials comparing coronary artery bypass graft surgery with medical therapy in patients with stable coronary heart disease and were able to provide estimates of prognosis for patients in clinically important subgroups.

Clinicians are most likely to find information about risks in easily identifiable subgroups of patients from studies of prognosis (see Chapter 7, Prognosis). For example, analysis of the Malmo Stroke Registry showed that during the 3 years after a stroke, patients have a 6% risk of recurrent nonfatal stroke and a 43% risk of death.[16] When contemplating stroke-prevention interventions in individual patients, clinicians can take into account that these risks are even higher in older patients and those with diabetes mellitus or cardiac disease.[16] Investigators sometimes use data from prognostic studies to construct models that incorporate several variables to create clinically helpful risk strata (see Chapter 22, Clinical Prediction Rules). When prospectively validated in new populations, these risk-stratification systems can provide accurate patient-specific estimates of prognosis.

We discuss the relationship between a patient's risk of an adverse event and the magnitude of the intervention effect elsewhere in this book (see Chapter 4, Health Care Interventions; Chapter 27, Measures of Association; and Chapter 32, Number Needed to Treat). Because this issue is so important when assessing applicability of study results, we review it here as well. We assume that readers have achieved a basic understanding of the statistical tools known as relative risk reduction (RRR), absolute risk reduction (ARR), number needed to treat (NNT), and number needed to harm (NNH).

Consider, for example, the decision about whether to recommend enteral nutrition for malnourished patients having elective surgery for gastrointestinal cancer. A study by Bozzetti and colleagues[17] found that 34% of patients in the enteral nutrition group had postoperative complications by the time of hospital discharge compared with 49% of patients in the parenteral nutrition group (control group). The RRR is [(49% − 34%)/49%] = 31%, meaning that enteral nutrition decreased the relative risk of postoperative complications after surgery for gastrointestinal cancer by 31%. The ARR is (49% − 34%) = 15%. The NNT is (100%/15%) or (1.0/0.15) = 7, which means that we would need to give enteral nutrition to seven malnourished patients with gastrointestinal cancer to prevent one additional patient from experiencing postoperative complications by the time of hospital discharge. For those who prefer to avoid arithmetic altogether, a nomogram allows determination of the NNT using only a ruler or straight edge and information about the patient's baseline risk and the RRR[18] (see Figure 27-2 in Chapter 27, Measures of Association).

One can consider a patient's risk of harm from an intervention in the same way. In the enteral nutrition trial,[17] 35% of patients in the enteral nutrition group and 14% of patients in the parenteral nutrition group experienced adverse events such as abdominal cramping and distention, diarrhea, and vomiting, resulting in an ARR of (35% − 14%) = 21% and an NNH of (100%/21%) = 5. This means that for every five malnourished patients given enteral nutrition, one patient will have adverse events. If one considers benefits and risks to be equivalent (in this instance, prevention of postoperative complications is equivalent to adverse events such as abdominal cramping and distention), one can construct a ratio of NNT to NNH to provide an index of the relative likelihood of benefit versus harm.[19] For the typical patient for whom we are considering enteral nutrition after surgery for gastrointestinal cancer, the likelihood of harm (the absolute increase in risk of adverse events with treatment, or 21%) is higher than the likelihood of benefit (the absolute decrease in risk of postoperative complications, or 15%). However, one would want to know more about how severe the adverse effects were; if they were mild, one might consider that the benefit of reduced complications would outweigh the risk of mild adverse effects.

NNTs vary with baseline risk: the lower the baseline risk is, the higher the NNT will be. To illustrate, we will examine a study in which patients' baseline risks varied by country of origin and residence. Keys compared the 20-year incidence of death from coronary heart disease in the United States, five European countries, and Japan.[20] He found an extremely low incidence of death from coronary heart disease in the Japanese cohort, despite adjustment for baseline differences in recognized risk factors. Similar results have been observed in reports of the Multinational Monitoring of Cardiovascular Disease and Their Determinants (MONICA) project.[21] This study involving 39 centers from 26 countries found a much lower incidence of death from coronary heart disease in East Asians than their Western counterparts. Age-standardized mortality rates for coronary heart disease were lowest in Japan (40 of 100,000) and highest in North Ireland (414 of 100,000). If we consider the NNT, this 10-fold reduction in incidence among the Japanese would translate to a 10-fold increase in the NNT for an intervention preventing coronary deaths. This decrease in efficiency may warrant reconsideration of applying the results of a trial to low-risk patients.

CONCLUSION

This chapter addresses the task of applying the results of clinical trials of restricted populations to other groups. The guides are relevant to all situations in which clinicians must make decisions about applicability. By breaking down the problem into specific questions, we have provided guides for clinicians in their daily attempts to strike a balance between making unjustifiably broad generalizations and being too conservative in their conclusions.

What can clinicians do when they suspect limited applicability? The answer depends on whether the anticipated differences are important, and if they are important, whether they are remediable. For example, differences in disease pathophysiology do not always mean that applicability is limited. Management of cataracts, for example, will probably be the same regardless of the cause. Differences in response to an intervention can sometimes be accommodated by altering the way in which an intervention is administered (e.g., adjusting insulin dosage). Education, training, provision of necessary equipment, and other attempts to optimize adherence may address problems of patient and provider adherence.

For differences in comorbid conditions or expected target event rates, a clinician's response will depend on the difference observed. If an increase in efficiency is anticipated (e.g., disease prognosis is worse or incidence of an adverse outcome is greater), a recommendation to intervene can be accepted more easily. A decrease in efficiency, on the other hand, should lead clinicians to be more cautious in accepting a recommendation to intervene. When differences in patient populations are important and not easily remediable, clinicians should not assume that the trial results can be readily applied. In such instances, an additional RCT may be warranted.

The patient in your clinical setting will often not be entirely similar to the patients included in clinical studies. The challenge is to determine whether differences between patients are important enough that the patient in your clinical setting will not benefit from the intervention in the same way that study participants did. This chapter has provided a series of guides to consider when you wish to apply study findings to patients in your clinical setting who differ biologically or socioeconomically from those in the study. Having considered the guides, you may decide the results are applicable as they are, applicable with some modification, or not at all applicable.

REFERENCES

1. Schmid CH, Lau J, McIntosh MW, Cappelleri JC. An empirical study of the effect of the control rate as a predictor of treatment efficacy in meta-analysis of clinical trials. *Stat Med.* 1998;17:1923-1942.
2. Szilagyi P, Vann J, Bordley C, et al. Interventions aimed at improving immunization rates. *Cochrane Database Syst Rev.* 2002;(4):CD003941.
3. Falkner B, Kushner H. Effect of chronic sodium loading on cardiovascular response in young blacks and whites. *Hypertension.* 1990;15:36-43.
4. Wilson TW. History of salt supplies in West Africa and blood pressure today. *Lancet.* 1986;1:784-786.
5. World Health Organization. World malaria situation in 1992. Part 1. *Wkly Epidemiol Rec.* 1994;69: 309-314.
6. Horai Y, Ishizaki T. Pharmacogenetics and its clinical implication: N-acetylation polymorphism. *Ration Drug Ther.* 1987;21:1-7.
7. Ward J, Brenneman G, Letson GW, Heyward WL. Limited efficacy of a *Haemophilus influenzae* type b conjugate vaccine in Alaska Native infants. The Alaska *H. influenza* Vaccine Study Group. *N Engl J Med.* 1990;323:1393-1401.
8. Soussan D, Liard R, Zureik M, Touron D, Rogeaux Y, Neukirch F. Treatment compliance, passive smoking, and asthma control: a three year cohort study. *Arch Dis Child.* 2003;88:229-233.
9. Mallonee S, Istre GR, Rosenberg M, et al. Surveillance and prevention of residential-fire injuries. *N Engl J Med.* 1996;335:27-31.
10. DiGuiseppi C, Roberts I, Wade A, et al. Incidence of fires and related injuries after giving out free smoke alarms: cluster randomised controlled trial. *BMJ.* 2002;325:995-997.
11. Aiken LH, Clarke SP, Sloane DM, Sochalski J, Silber JH. Hospital nurse staffing and patient mortality, nurse burnout, and job dissatisfaction. *JAMA.* 2002;288:1987-1993.

12. Glasziou PP, Irwig LM. An evidence based approach to individualising treatment. *BMJ.* 1995;311:1356-1359.
13. Sazawal S, Black RE. Meta-analysis of intervention trials on case management of pneumonia in community settings. *Lancet.* 1992;340:528-533.
14. DiCenso A. Clinically useful measures of the effects of treatment [editorial]. *Evid Based Nurs.* 2001;4:36-39.
15. Yusuf S, Zucker D, Peduzzi P, et al. Effect of coronary artery bypass graft surgery on survival: overview of 10-year results from randomised trials by the Coronary Artery Bypass Graft Surgery Trialists Collaboration. *Lancet.* 1994;344:563-570.
16. Elneihoum AM, Goransson M, Falke P, Janzon L. Three-year survival and recurrence after stroke in Malmo, Sweden: an analysis of stroke registry data. *Stroke.* 1998;29:2114-2117.
17. Bozzetti F, Braga M, Gianotti L, et al. Postoperative enteral versus parenteral nutrition in malnourished patients with gastrointestinal cancer: a randomized multicentre trial. *Lancet.* 2001;358:1487-1492.
18. Chatellier G, Zapletal E, Lemaitre D, Menard J, Degoulet P. The number needed to treat: a clinically useful nomogram in its proper context. *BMJ.* 1996;312:426-429.
19. Straus SE. Individualizing treatment decisions: the likelihood of being helped versus harmed. *Evaluation and the Health Professions.* 2002;25:210-224.
20. Keys A. *Seven Countries: A Multivariate Analysis of Death and Coronary Heart Disease.* Cambridge, MA: Harvard University Press; 1980.
21. Tuomilehto J, Kuulasmaa K. WHO MONICA Project: assessing CHD mortality and morbidity. *Int J Epidemiol.* 1989;18:S38-45.

34

Incorporating Patient Values

Annette O'Connor, Dawn Stacey, Peter Tugwell, and Gordon Guyatt

The following Editorial Board members also made substantive contributions to this chapter: Maureen Dobbins, Andrew Jull, and Andrea Nelson.

We gratefully acknowledge the work of Sharon Straus, Finlay McAlister, Brian Haynes, Jack Sinclair, P.J. Devereaux, and Christina Lacchetti on the original chapter that appears in the Users' Guides to the Medical Literature, *edited by Guyatt and Rennie.*

In This Chapter

Finding the Evidence
Search for Evidence on Infliximab for Rheumatoid Arthritis
Search for Evidence on Associated Patient Decision Aids

Strategies for Incorporating Patient Values
Implicit Values Elicitation
Explicit Values Elicitation
Levels of Patient Participation in Decision Making

Patient Decision Aids
The Ottawa Decision Support Framework
Advantages of Patient Decision Aids
Do Patient Decision Aids Work?

Identification of Patient Values
Balance Scales
Formal Utility Assessments
Threshold Techniques
Analytic Hierarchy Process

Would This Patient With Refractory Rheumatoid Arthritis Choose To Add Infliximab To Current Treatment To Control Persistent Joint Pain and Swelling?

A 51-year-old woman was diagnosed with rheumatoid arthritis 6 years ago. Her primary care practitioner treated her with nonsteroidal anti-inflammatory drugs (NSAIDs) for several years, but about 6 months ago, her condition worsened, and she was referred to a rheumatologist. At her first visit with the rheumatologist, she described increasing joint pain and swelling that had become so uncomfortable that she had to reduce her employment status from full time to part time. An x-ray showed erosions in four metacarpophalangeal joints, and she was started on oral methotrexate. At her 6-month follow-up appointment, it is clear that the oral methotrexate has helped slightly but has not controlled her symptoms or disease activity.

The rheumatologist suggests two possible options: (1) continue taking methotrexate alone; or (2) add infliximab to the methotrexate treatment. The patient has read a bit about infliximab because she has been searching the Internet for information on treatments for rheumatoid arthritis. The rheumatologist explains that infliximab is an immune-suppressing drug administered through intravenous infusion that has been shown to be effective in combination with methotrexate. After some discussion about the potential benefits and harms of adding infliximab to her current treatment, the patient remains uncertain about what to do, stating "I'm not sure about taking a stronger drug. I worry about the unknown risks. It has not been studied for very long, and I understand it might be linked to infections including tuberculosis. On the other hand, I can't function the way I am, and I would like to prevent further damage to my joints. It's hard to know if the good outweighs the bad."

The patient requests more time to think this over. You are a nurse who provides patient education at the clinic and are asked to meet with the patient to help her consider the treatment plan options in preparation for her return appointment. You realize that your role is to prepare the patient for informed, values-based decision making, which involves (1) finding evidence-based information on the options and their related benefits and harms; and (2) finding workable methods for incorporating the patient's values into decision making.

FINDING THE EVIDENCE

You decide to conduct two searches, one on infliximab for treatment of rheumatoid arthritis and the second on associated decision aids.

Search for Evidence on Infliximab for Rheumatoid Arthritis

You frame the question as follows: Does the addition of infliximab to methotrexate decrease pain and swelling in patients with rheumatoid arthritis compared with methotrexate alone? To search for studies that address this question, you decide to use a hierarchy that you learned at a recent workshop provided by the hospital librarian. The hierarchy, which progresses from the most to the least evolved preprocessed evidence-based information sources, begins with *systems* as the highest level resource, followed by *synopses of syntheses* (systematic reviews), *syntheses, synopses of single studies,* and finally *single studies* (see Chapter 2, Finding the Evidence, for details about this hierarchy). Using this framework, you begin by searching *Clinical Evidence,* a systems-level, regularly updated, Web-based and print publication that integrates evidence-based information about specific clinical problems. You type in "infliximab," which results in a few hits. You learn that infliximab is a tumor necrosis factor antagonist, the effectiveness of which is summarized in *Clinical Evidence.* The authors of this section found three placebo-controlled randomized trials, one of which included people with active disease not responsive to methotrexate.[1,2] Although these authors do not mention a systematic review on the topic, you also check *Evidence-Based Nursing* for synopses of syntheses (systematic reviews) and the *Cochrane Library* for a synthesis. You type in the keyword "infliximab." Although you get no hits in *Evidence-Based Nursing,* you do get one hit in the *Cochrane Database of Systematic Reviews,* entitled "Infliximab for the treatment of rheumatoid arthritis."[3]

The systematic review identifies the same randomized controlled trial that was summarized in *Clinical Evidence,* with results reported at 30 weeks[1] and 54 weeks.[2] In this trial, 428 patients who had active rheumatoid arthritis despite methotrexate therapy were randomized to methotrexate (same dose they had been receiving before the study) plus infusions of infliximab, 3 mg/kg every 4 weeks, or methotrexate plus placebo. Patients were unaware of whether they were receiving infliximab or placebo. An independent assessor, who had no knowledge of the patient's treatment assignment, evaluated the number of tender and swollen joints in each group. Other outcomes included quality of life and effect on joint damage assessed radiographically. The investigators conducted an intention-to-treat analysis and, at 54 weeks, found that patients who received methotrexate plus infliximab had a sustained reduction in number of swollen joints (50% reduction with methotrexate plus infliximab vs. 13% with methotrexate alone; $P < 0.001$) and number of tender joints (55% reduction vs. 23%; $P < 0.001$) compared with patients who received methotrexate alone. Quality of life was also significantly better with methotrexate plus infliximab than with methotrexate alone. Radiographic evidence of joint damage increased in patients who received methotrexate alone, but not in those who received methotrexate plus infliximab (mean change in radiographic score, 7.0 vs. 0.6; $P < 0.001$).[2]

Despite these impressive findings about the clinical benefits of infliximab and its ability to halt the progression of joint damage, you appreciate the difficult decision the patient has to make. Although *Clinical Evidence* categorizes tumor necrosis factor antagonists such as infliximab as "likely to be beneficial" in the treatment of rheumatoid arthritis, it also states that short-term toxicity is relatively low, but the long-term safety is unclear. Common side effects include upper respiratory infections (cold), headache, diarrhea, and stomach pain. Other side effects, such as headache, nausea, and hives, can occur during or immediately after the injection of infliximab. Larger and longer-term studies of this drug are required because it has been associated with tuberculosis and other life-threatening infections.[4]

Search for Evidence on Associated Patient Decision Aids

The rheumatology clinic has just purchased *Evidence-based Rheumatology,* a reference book available in both print[5] and electronic *(www.evidbasedrheum.com)* form that reviews and updates the best evidence for treatments of rheumatologic disorders and also provides decision aids. You click on the chapter on Decision Aids and then click on infliximab. You find a decision aid, "Should I take infliximab?"[4]

The decision aid is based on evidence from the Cochrane systematic review described previously and can be used either by patients alone in preparation for discussions with their practitioner or by patients together with their practitioners. It guides patients to verify the decision, clarify their values about the benefits and harms of infliximab, determine their preferred role in decision making, identify remaining decisional needs, plan the next steps, and share their thinking with their practitioners.

Armed with the evidence and the decision aid, you prepare to meet with the patient. You are aware that the treatment decision will depend on the relative value the patient places on reduction of disability coupled with improved quality of life and prevention of progressive joint damage, compared with avoiding the risk of tuberculosis and other life-threatening infections. The patient's values are crucial in making the decision.

STRATEGIES FOR INCORPORATING PATIENT VALUES

In other chapters of this book (Chapter 1, Introduction to Evidence-Based Nursing; Chapter 4, Health Care Interventions; Chapter 10, Moving from Evidence to Action Using Clinical Practice Guidelines; and Chapter 33, Applying Results to Individual Patients), we have proposed that clinical decision making should begin by using the best evidence to estimate the benefits, harms, and costs associated with alternative courses of action. We have pointed out that because interventions always have advantages and disadvantages, evidence alone cannot determine the best course of action. Most would agree that clinicians must use the values and preferences of the patient to balance harms and benefits. Not surprisingly, patients vary greatly in the value they place on different outcomes. Given this variability in patient's values, clinicians should proceed with great care. It is easy to assume that a patient's values are similar to one's own, but this may be an incorrect assumption. The challenge, then, is to integrate the evidence with the patient's values.

For many clinical decisions, the trade-off is sufficiently clear that clinicians do not need to be concerned about variability in patient values. Previously healthy patients will all want antibiotics to treat their pneumonia and anticoagulation to treat their pulmonary embolus; bedridden patients will want regular skin care and turning to prevent decubiti. Under such circumstances, a brief explanation of the rationale for treatment and the expected benefits and side effects will suffice. However, not all decisions are so straightforward. When benefits and risks are balanced more precariously and the best choice may differ across patients, clinicians must attend to the variability in patients' values.

Implicit Values Elicitation

An *implicit* strategy for integrating evidence with preferences and values involves communicating the benefits and harms to patients, thus permitting them to incorporate their own values into the decision. The clinician typically shares the evidence, in some form, with the patient, while attempting to understand the patient's values. One advantage of this approach is that it avoids the problem of measuring patients' values. Unfortunately, communicating evidence about benefits and harms to patients in a way that allows them to understand their choices and incorporate their preferences and values may be as difficult as directly measuring patient values.

Explicit Values Elicitation

An *explicit* strategy is to directly elicit patient values using formal measurement techniques, such as standard gambles or balance scales. These explicit approaches have the advantage of facilitating communication of values between patients and clinicians. Moreover, the more formal techniques provide values or utilities that can be incorporated into decision trees using decision analysis to determine which option has the highest expected value for the patient. The disadvantages of formal techniques include their complexity, impracticality in most practice settings, and potential for measurement errors.

Levels of Patient Participation in Decision Making

Patients often have preferences not only about the outcomes, but also about the decision-making process. These preferences can vary, and the patient's desired level of involvement should determine which approach the clinician takes.[6-8] At one end of the spectrum, the clinician acts as a technician, providing the patient with information and taking no active part in the decision-making process. At the opposite extreme, the clinician ascertains the patient's values and then makes a recommendation in light of the likely advantages and disadvantages of alternative management approaches. In this paternalistic approach, the clinician decides what is best in light of the patient's preferences.

Intermediate approaches of shared decision making are generally more popular than those at either extreme. Shared decision making uses both fundamental approaches to decision making: The clinician typically shares the evidence, in some form, with the patient, while attempting to understand the patient's values. Evidence that more active patient involvement in the process of health care delivery can improve outcomes and reported quality of life—and possibly reduce health care expenditures[9-13]—provides support for secular trends toward patient autonomy and movement away from paternalistic approaches.

PATIENT DECISION AIDS

To support patient decision making, researchers and clinicians have developed patient decision aids as adjuncts to counseling.[14] *Decision aids* are shared decision-making interventions that describe options in sufficient detail for patients to judge their value. They often include (1) information on the condition, options, benefits, and harms; (2) probabilities of benefits and harms, which may be tailored to a patient's risk profile; (3) information about the level of scientific uncertainty regarding the probabilities of benefits and harms; (4) values clarification strategies to help patients consider the value or personal importance of benefits versus harms; (5) balanced stories of others' experiences with decision making; and (6) guidance or coaching in the steps of decision making and communication, using strategies such as personal worksheets.

The Ottawa Decision Support Framework

Although the developers of decision aids have different conceptual frameworks of decision support,[15–21] most are based on decision theories from economics and cognitive psychology [22–24] that structure decisions according to options, outcomes, and probabilities of outcomes so that patients can better judge the value of the benefits versus the harms. Many frameworks broaden this cognitive perspective by including emotional, social, and environmental dimensions.[25–29]

We developed the Ottawa Decision Support Framework,[15] based on expectancy value, decisional conflict, and social support theories.[22–30] The purpose of the framework is to guide clinicians in the process of decision support for health decisions that (1) are stimulated by a new circumstance, diagnosis, or developmental transition; (2) require careful deliberation because of the uncertain and/or value-sensitive nature of the benefits and harms; and (3) need relatively more effort during the deliberation phase than the implementation phase.

The framework (Table 34-1) includes three process elements: (1) assessment of needs or determinants of decisions that are suboptimal; (2) provision of decision support interventions that address the suboptimal determinants; and (3) evaluation of the effects of decision support on the quality of decision making and outcomes of decisions. The variables in the framework apply to both clinicians and patients, but discussion in this chapter is focussed on the patient.

Determinants of Decisions

Essential inputs into decisions include the patients' demographic, clinical, and practice characteristics, perceptions of the decision, perceptions of important others involved in the decision, and personal and external resources to make and implement a choice. The selection of one option over another depends not only on patient characteristics, but also on whether patients are knowledgeable about the issues, expect that the preferred option will likely lead to the outcomes they value most, are reasonably certain this is the best option, perceive that important others agree with and support the option, and have the necessary personal and external resources to make and implement the choice.

Decision Support

Decision support involves preparing patients for decision making and structuring follow-up counseling. The goal is to improve the quality of decision making by addressing the modifiable determinants of decisions that are suboptimal: inadequate knowledge, unrealistic expectations of outcomes, unclear values, unclear norms, unwanted pressure, inadequate support, and inadequate personal and external resources to make the decision. These factors also contribute to decisional conflict.[31] High decisional conflict or uncertainty results in poor decision quality, decision delay, regret, discontinuance, dissatisfaction, and overuse of health services that patients do not value.

Decision support includes providing tailored information, realigning outcome expectations, clarifying values, and augmenting skills in decision making and communication. Decision aids use these strategies in preparing patients for follow-up counseling. They include information about the problem, options, and benefits and harms to

Table **34-1** Ottawa Decision Support Framework

Assess Needs (Determinants of Decisions)	Provide Decision Support	Evaluate Effects of Decision Support
Characteristics **Client:** Age, sex, marital status, education, occupation, culture, locale, medical diagnosis and duration, health status **Practitioner:** Age, sex, education, specialty, culture, practice locale, experience, counseling style	**Provide Access to Information** • Health situation • Options • Outcomes • Other's opinions and choices	**Decision Making** • Reduced decisional conflict • Improved knowledge • Realistic outcome expectations and norms • Clear values • Agreement between values and choice • Implementation of chosen option • Satisfaction with decision making
Perceptions of Decision • Knowledge • Expectations • Values • Decisional conflict • Stage of decision making • Predisposition toward options	**Realign Expectations of Outcomes** **Clarify Personal Values for Outcomes** **Augment Skills by Providing Guidance/ Coaching in:** • Steps in decision making • Communicating with others • Handling pressure • Accessing support and resources	**Outcomes of Decision** • Persistence with choice • Improved values-linked quality of life • Reduced distres • Reduced regret • Informed use of resources
Perceptions of Others • Perceptions of others' opinions and practices • Support • Pressures • Roles in decision making		
Resources to Make Decision **Personal:** • Previous experience • Self-confidence • Motivation • Skill in decision making **External:** • Support (information, advice, emotional, instrumental, financial, professional help) from social networks and agencies		

improve knowledge of the decision. Probabilities tailored to a patient's clinical risk are included to create more realistic expectations or subjective judgments of the likelihood of benefits and harms. Decision aids may also clarify personal values by either implicitly or explicitly asking individuals to consider the personal importance they place on each benefit and harm and to identify the trade-offs they will need to make in choosing one option. As a result, there is likely to be better congruence between patients' values and their choices.

Evaluating Decision Support

The framework distinguishes between quality decision making and quality outcomes, because good decisions can still result in bad outcomes as a result of the probabilistic nature of clinical events. Because decisions that depend on patients' values cannot be judged as right or wrong, the framework defines a high-quality decision as one that reduces decisional conflict, improves knowledge, incorporates realistic outcome expectations, is consistent with personal values, is enacted, and results in decision maker satisfaction.[31] Improving decision making may impact favorably on behavioral, clinical, and health services outcomes of decisions, such as adherence to the chosen option, improved values-linked quality of life, reduced distress about the expected consequences of options, reduced regret, and appropriate use of resources.

Advantages of Patient Decision Aids

A well-constructed decision aid has two advantages over implicit values elicitation. One advantage is that someone has reviewed the literature and produced a rigorous summary of the probabilities. Clinicians who doubt the rigor of the summary of probabilities can go back to the original literature on which those probabilities are based and, using the principles of this book, determine their accuracy. A second advantage of a well-constructed decision aid is that it will offer a pretested and effective way of communicating the information to patients, who may have little background in quantitative decision making. Most commonly, decision aids use visual props to present outcome data in terms of the percentage of people with a certain condition who do well without an intervention compared with the percentage who do well with an intervention. Decision aids will summarize the data regarding all outcomes of importance to patients; however, many decision aids fail to address the scientific uncertainty about related benefits and harms.

Do Patient Decision Aids Work?

Theoretically, decision aids present an attractive strategy for ensuring that patient values guide clinical decision making. However, what impact do decision aids actually have on clinical practice? O'Connor and colleagues conducted a systematic review and identified 34 randomized trials that used 29 unique decision aids.[32] In the trials comparing decision aids with usual care, the decision aid group had higher knowledge scores (weighted mean difference [WMD], 19 on a 100-point scale; 95% confidence interval [CI], 13 to 24), more realistic expectations (relative risk [RR], 1.4; 95% CI, 1.1 to 1.9), and lower decisional conflict related to feeling informed (WMD, −9.1; of 100; 95% CI, −12 to −6). A higher proportion of the decision aid group was active in decision making (RR, 1.4;

95% CI, 1.0 to 2.3), and a smaller proportion of this group remained undecided after the intervention (RR, 0.43; 95% CI, 0.3 to 0.7).

Decision aids with detailed information resulted in only marginally higher knowledge scores when compared with decision aids with briefer information (WMD, 4 out of 100; 95% CI, 3 to 6). Decision aids that included probabilities of outcomes produced more realistic expectations (perceived probabilities of benefits and harms) than decision aids without information on probabilities (RR, 1.5; 95% CI, 1.3 to 1.7), and those that included explicit values clarification exercises had greater agreement between values and choices than those that did not include these exercises.

Exposure to decision aids reduced rates of elective invasive surgery in favor of conservative options (RR, 0.77; 95% CI, 0.7 to 0.9), with variable effects on other decisions. Generally, decision aids were no better than comparators in affecting satisfaction with decision making or anxiety. Most trials showed no improvements in health outcomes. However, the health outcomes measured were not linked to personal values (e.g., did the decision aid increase the health outcomes patients valued most and decrease the outcomes patients valued least?).

As part of the systematic review to evaluate the impact of decision aids on patient decision making, O'Connor and colleagues also created a global inventory of existing patient decision aids and evaluated the quality of these aids using CREDIBLE criteria (C: competently developed; R: recently updated; E: evidence-based; DI: disclosure of conflicts of interest; BL: balanced presentation of options, benefits, and harms; and E: efficacious in improving decision making). The decision aids and more information about the CREDIBLE criteria can be found at *http://decisionaid.ohri.ca/*.

The medium for delivery of decision aids varies (e.g., print, boards, videos, audioguided workbooks), and many developers are now producing Web-based applications. Nurses can provide coaching in the use of decision aids. One randomized trial[33] focusing on treatment decisions for menorrhagia, compared usual care, a video decision aid, and a video decision aid with nurse coaching that included values clarification. The video plus nurse coaching was superior to the other interventions in terms of patient satisfaction and cost-effectiveness. Moreover, hysterectomy rates were significantly lower.

In summary, decision aids increase patient participation in decision making without affecting anxiety. They improve decision quality by increasing the chances that choices are based on better knowledge, more realistic outcome expectations, and personal values. They may have a role in preventing the overuse of aggressive surgical options that informed patients do not value, without adversely affecting health outcomes. Simple decision aids that clinicians can integrate into usual patient care could increase the extent to which patient values truly determine health care decisions.

IDENTIFICATION OF PATIENT VALUES

A key objective of decision aids is to help patients clarify and communicate the value they place on the outcomes associated with each option. Doing so requires that the patient understands the nature of those options and outcomes and improves the match between what is personally most desirable and the option the patient chooses. There are several ways to help patients consider the value they attach to various options. The relative efficacy of different approaches is still under investigation.

Virtually all decision aids describe what it is like to undergo the related procedures and to live with the physical, emotional, and social consequences. Patients are better able to judge the value of consequences when the consequences are familiar, simple, and directly experienced.[24]

Some decision aids use *social matching strategies*. They begin by showing examples of how others value the features of an option to illustrate how different values may lead to different choices. Then they ask the patient to indicate which examples most closely match their own and which do not. This strategy may be more helpful for those who are not quantitatively oriented.

Some decision aids guide patients to compare, rate, or trade off different features of options using more quantitative methods. These engaging processes may increase awareness of personal values and provide insight into the trade-offs that need to be made in choosing one option over another. Some specific quantitative techniques for clarifying values in decision aids include balance scales, formal utility assessments, threshold techniques, and an analytic hierarchy process.

Balance Scales

In balance scale values clarification,[15,34] standard features of an option are visually displayed on a "weighing scale" in which the benefits (pros) of an option are listed on the left and the harms (cons) on the right. Patients review the standard features and add others that are important in their situation. They then rate the desirability of each feature by shading or assigning stars (0 stars = not at all important to me; 5 stars = very important to me). Next, they make an overall value judgment using a "leaning scale" anchored by "Willing to consider treatment: pros are more important to me than the cons" and "Not willing to consider treatment: cons are more important to me than the pros," with "unsure" situated in the middle. This technique is simple to administer, can be self-administered, and promotes communication of values at a glance. It has been used successfully in decision aids, and direct comparisons with more formal methods are under investigation.[34]

Formal Utility Assessments

Formal utility assessment techniques are based on expected utility theory and elicit the desirability of the outcomes of each option.[21,35–37] These are more complex strategies and include the visual analog scale, standard gamble, and time trade-off. They are usually administered by a clinician or data collector rather than self-administered, although investigators have developed computer-based applications that may lend themselves to self-administration. Two randomized trials have successfully used the computer-based application.[35,38]

When using a *visual analogue scale*, the clinician asks the patient to place a mark on a 100-point scale or "feeling thermometer" (Figure 34-1). The mark signifies how the patient feels about the health state in question and can be placed anywhere between 0

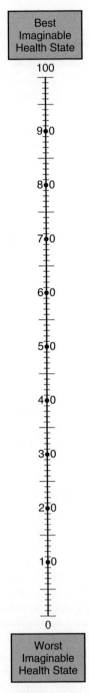

Figure 34-1. Visual analogue scale as a "Feeling Thermometer."

(the worst imaginable health state) and 100 (the best imaginable health state). The value of the health state or outcome is the point where the patient places the mark. For example, if the patient places the mark on 90, the value of the health state is $90/100 = 0.90$. Because some health states, such as an infection, are temporary, whereas others, such as a stroke, are permanent, clinicians must ensure that patients incorporate the duration of the health state in their rating. Schünemann and colleagues validated a self-administered approach to the feeling thermometer.[39]

In the *standard gamble*, patients are asked to choose between living in a state of impaired health and taking a gamble in which they may return to full health or die immediately (see Chapter 12, Quality of Life). In a series of paired choices, patients indicate the probability at which they are indifferent between (1) the certainty of living the rest of their lives in an intermediate health state/outcome; or (2) a gamble in which there is a probability (p) of being restored to perfect health but a corresponding probability ($1 - p$) of immediate death. The utility for the health state/outcome is the probability (p) at which the patient is indifferent (e.g., 0.90 chance of perfect health).

In *time trade-off*, patients choose between a longer period in a state of impaired health (such as recovery from severe stroke) and a shorter period in a state of full health. Patients are given a series of paired choices through which they indicate the length of time in perfect health that is equivalent to a lifetime in an intermediate health state/outcome. The patient's value for the outcome is calculated as the proportion that is indicated (e.g., 9/10 years' life expectancy = 0.90).

Threshold Techniques

The simplest form of threshold technique involves evaluating whether to choose option A or option B.[40] Standard features of both options (their procedures, consequences, and chances) are visually displayed in parallel columns. After considering this information, patients indicate their initially preferred option. The relative strength of the preference for the initially preferred option is gauged by hypothetically altering the level of one of the features (e.g., probability of a positive or a negative outcome) in either the preferred or the rejected option, until the patient gives up the initially preferred option and switches to other option.

Analytic Hierarchy Process

The analytic hierarchy process begins with explicit definitions of the decision goal, the alternative options, and the criteria used to compare the options' abilities to meet the goal.[41] These elements are then organized into a hierarchical decision model, with the goal at the top, the alternatives at the bottom, and the criteria in the middle. The elements at each level are then compared relative to the element(s) at the next higher level to derive a ratio-level scale: for the criteria, the ratio-level scale indicates their importance relative to the decision goal; for the options, the ratio-level scale indicates how well they can be expected to meet the criteria. Finally, information about the relationships among the elements on each horizontal level of the hierarchy is combined vertically to determine the relative abilities of the alternative options to meet the decision goal. This technique has been used successfully in a randomized trial of a decision aid.[41]

CLINICAL RESOLUTION

You meet with the patient and show her the decision aid you found in *Evidence-based Rheumatology:* Should I take Infliximab?[4] (Figure 34-2). You were also able to find this same decision aid in the inventory of patient decision aids created by O'Connor and colleagues (*http://decisionaid.ohri.ca/*). The patient is clear from her visit with the rheumatologist that the decision she needs to make is whether or not she should start taking infliximab along with methotrexate to control the joint pain and swelling related to her rheumatoid arthritis. You move on to Step 2 and describe the 30-week and 54-week results of the randomized trial of infliximab.[1,2] You then ask her to review the balance scale summarizing the pros and cons of taking infliximab and clarify her values by circling the appropriate number of stars in each box. She then needs to indicate whether she is willing to consider infliximab given the relative importance she places on the pros and cons. After identifying the role she wants to have in choosing her treatment (Step 3), you move on to Step 4, in which you assess her current decision making needs using a Decisional Conflict Scale.[31] This scale allows her to consider what she knows, what's important, how others help, and how sure she feels. From her responses to the decisional conflict scale, you feel that the patient is reassured that the information you have provided confirms what her rheumatologist explained to her. Through scoring the pros and cons in Step 2, she realizes that the personal importance of controlling her symptoms and slowing disease progression outweighs her concerns about harms and the use of powerful drugs. She feels reasonably sure that this is the best choice for her, and her next step is to take the aid to her rheumatologist to share her values associated with her preference for starting infliximab.

Nurses who coach patients in preparation for shared decision making with their practitioners need to know the evidence about patients' options and tailor their support to patients' decisional needs. For example, they must address knowledge deficits by providing evidence-based information, resolve unclear values with values clarification exercises, help patients manage support deficits, and provide guidance in the steps of decision making. Evidence-based decision aids may streamline this process and help in follow-up discussions with the practitioner.

Furthermore, patients can carry over these basic skills in decision making to subsequent decisions in the chronic disease trajectory. For each choice, patients need to be involved in clearly articulating the decision, the timing of the decision, their role in decision making, their understanding of outcomes related to the options, and balancing the benefits and harms in relation to personal values. Evidence-based patient decision making continues to evolve, with an emphasis on identifying simple, effective ways to support patients in the process.

Decision Aid: Should I Take Infliximab?

This guide can help you make decisions about the treatment your doctor is asking you to consider.

It will help you to:
1. Clarify what you need to decide.
2. Consider the pros and cons of different choices.
3. Decide what role you want to have in choosing your treatment.
4. Identify what you need to help you make the decision.
5. Plan the next steps.
6. Share your thinking with your doctor.

Step 1. Clarify what you need to decide.

What is the decision?

Should I start taking infliximab when methotrexate alone is not working to control rheumatoid arthritis?

Infliximab is an intravenous (IV) injection given at set times every few weeks.

When does this decision have to be made? *Check ✓ one*
- ☐ *within days*
- ☑ *within weeks*
- ☐ *within months*

How far along are you with this decision? *Check ✓ one*
- ☐ *I have not thought about it yet*
- ☑ *I am considering the choices*
- ☐ *I am close to making a choice*
- ☐ *I have already made a choice*

Continued

Figure 34-2. Decision aid to assist patients in making treament decisions.
(Modified and reproduced with permission of BMJ Books from Tugwell P, Shea B, Boers M, et al., eds. Evidence-based Rheumatology. *London: BMJ Publishing Group; 2003.)*

Step 2. Consider the pros and cons of different choices.

What does the research show?

Infliximab is classified as: "Trade off between benefits and harms"

There is 'gold' level evidence from two studies of 428 people with rheumatoid arthritis. The studies tested infliximab and lasted 6 months to 1 year. (See chart for pros and cons.)

What do I think of the pros and cons of infliximab?
1. Review the common pros and cons.
2. Add any other pros and cons that are important to you.
3. Show how important each pro and con is to you by circling from one (∗) star if it is a little important to you to up to five stars (∗∗∗∗∗) if it is very important to you.

Pros and Cons of Infliximab Treatment				
PROS (? number of people affected)	How important is this to you?		**CONS** (? number of people affected)	How important is this to you?
Improves pain and function 41 out of 100 people are helped at least a little 31 out of 100 are helped a lot	⟨∗ ∗ ∗ ∗ ∗⟩		**Side effects: colds, headache, diarrhea, abdominal pain** 5 out of 100 people stopped taking infliximab because of the side effects 7 out of 100 people stopped taking methotrexate/placebo because of side effects	⊙∗ ∗ ∗ ∗
Slows progress of disease X-rays are better in 47 out of 100 people	⟨∗ ∗ ∗⟩∗		**Reactions during or immediately after the injection** Headache, nausea, and hives	⊙∗ ∗ ∗ ∗
Works within weeks rather than months	⟨∗ ∗⟩∗ ∗		**Serious harms: tuberculosis and other serious infections** (some have caused death)	⟨∗ ∗ ∗⟩∗ ∗
Other pros:	∗ ∗ ∗ ∗ ∗		Unsure if can travel with this medicine	∗ ∗ ∗ ∗ ∗
			Extra clinic visits and blood tests needed	∗ ∗ ∗ ∗ ∗
			Cost of medicine My drug plan covers this	∗ ∗ ∗ ∗ ∗
			Other cons: Unknown long term effects	⟨∗ ∗⟩∗ ∗ ∗

What do you think about taking infliximab? *Check ✓ one*

☑   ☐   ☐

Willing to consider this treatment   Unsure   Not willing to consider this treatment
Pros are more important   Cons are more important
to me than the Cons   to me than the Pros

Figure 34-2—cont'd.

Step 3. Decide the role you want to have in choosing your treatment. *Check ✓ one*

☐ *I prefer to decide on my own after listening to the opinions of others*
☑ *I prefer to share the decision with:* <u>my rheumatologist</u>
☐ *I prefer someone else to decide for me, namely:*_____

Step 4. Identify what you need to help you make the decision.

Please circle your answers to these questions.

What I know	Do you know enough about your condition to make a choice?	(Yes)	No	Unsure
	Do you know which options are available to you?	(Yes)	No	Unsure
	Do you know the good points (pros) of each option?	(Yes)	No	Unsure
	Do you know the bad points (cons) of each option?	(Yes)	No	Unsure
What's important	Are you clear about which **pros** are most important to you?	(Yes)	No	Unsure
	Are you clear about which **cons** are most important to you?	(Yes)	No	Unsure
How others help	Do you have enough support from others to make a choice?	(Yes)	No	Unsure
	Are you choosing without pressure from others?	(Yes)	No	Unsure
	Do you have enough advice to make a choice?	Yes	(No)	Unsure
How sure I feel	Are you clear about the best choice for you?	(Yes)	No	Unsure
	Do you feel sure about what to choose?	Yes	(No)	Unsure

Decisional Conflict Scale © A. O'Connor 1993, Revised 1999

If you answered No or Unsure to many of these questions, you should talk to your doctor.

Step 5. Plan the next steps.

What do you need to do before you make this decision?

For example, I need to discuss the treatment plan with my rheumatologist

Step 6. Share the information on this form with your doctor.

It will help your doctor understand what you think about this treatment.

Figure 34-2.—cont'd.

REFERENCES

1. Maini R, St Clair EW, Breedveld F, et al. Infliximab (chimeric anti-tumour necrosis factor alpha mono-clonal antibody) versus placebo in rheumatoid arthritis patients receiving concomitant methotrexate: a randomised phase III trial. ATTRACT Study Group. *Lancet*. 1999;354:1932-1939.

2. Lipsky PE, van der Heijde DM, St. Clair EW, et al. Infliximab and methotrexate in the treatment of rheumatoid arthritis. *N Engl J Med*. 2000;343:1594-1602.

3. Blumenauer B, Judd M, Wells G, et al. Infliximab for the treatment of rheumatoid arthritis. *Cochrane Database Syst Rev*. 2002;(3):CD003785.

4. Suarez-Almazor M, Osiri M, Emery P, Ottawa Methods Group. Rheumatoid Arthritis. In: Tugwell P, Shea B, Boers M, et al., eds. *Evidence-based Rheumatology*. London: BMJ Publishing Group; 2003:306-314. Available at: http://www.evidbasedrheum.com. Accessed January 16, 2004.

5. Tugwell P, Shea B, Boers M, et al., eds. *Evidence-based Rheumatology*. London: BMJ Publishing Group; 2003. Available at: http://www.evidbasedrheum.com. Accessed January 16, 2004.

6. Strull WM, Lo B, Charles G. Do patients want to participate in medical decision making? *JAMA*. 1984;252:2990-2994.

7. Degner LF, Kristjanson LJ, Bowman D, et al. Information needs and decisional preferences in women with breast cancer. *JAMA*. 1997;277:1485-1492.

8. Stiggelbout AM, Kiebert GM. A role for the sick role: patient preferences regarding information and participation in clinical decision-making. *CMAJ*. 1997;157:383-389.

9. Szabo E, Moody H, Hamilton T, Ang C, Kovithavongs C, Kjellstrand C. Choice of treatment improves quality of life: a study of patients undergoing dialysis. *Arch Intern Med*. 1997;157:1352-1356.

10. Greenfield S, Kaplan SH, Ware JE Jr, Yano EM, Frank HJL. Patients' participation in medical care: effects on blood sugar control and quality of life in diabetes. *J Gen Intern Med*. 1988;3:448-457.

11. Kaplan SH, Greenfield S, Ware JE Jr. Assessing the effects of physician-patient interactions on the outcomes of chronic disease. *Med Care*. 1989;27:S110-S127.

12. Schulman BA. Active patient orientation and outcomes in hypertension treatment: application of a socio-organizational perspective. *Med Care*. 1979;17:267-280.

13. Stewart MA. Effective physician-patient communication and health outcomes: a review. *CMAJ*. 1995;152:1423-1433.

14. Entwistle VA, Sowden AJ, Watt IS. Evaluating interventions to promote patient involvement in decision making: by what criteria should effectiveness be judged? *J Health Serv Res Policy*. 1998;3:100-107.

15. O'Connor AM, Tugwell P, Wells GA, et al. A decision aid for women considering hormone therapy after menopause: decision support framework and evaluation. *Patient Educ Couns*. 1998;33:267-279.

16. Charles C, Gafni A, Whelan, T. Shared decision-making in the medical encounter: what does it mean? *Soc Sci Med*. 1997;44:681-692.

17. Llewellyn-Thomas HA. Patients' health-care decision making: a framework for descriptive and experimental investigations. *Med Decis Making*. 1995;15:101-106.

18. Hersey J, Matheson J, Lohr K. *Consumer Health Informatics and Patient Decision-Making*. (AHCPR Pub. No. 98-N001). Washington, DC: Agency for Health Care Policy and Research; 1997.

19. Mulley A. Outcomes research: implications for policy and practice. In: Smith R, Delamothe T, eds. *Outcomes in Clinical Practice*. London: BMJ Publishing Group; 1995:13-27.

20. Rothert M, Talarcyzk GJ. Patient compliance and the decision making process of clinicians and patients. *J Compliance Health Care*. 1987;2:55-71.

21. Pauker SP, Pauker SG. The amniocentesis decision: ten years of decision analytic experience. *Birth Defects*. 1987;23:151-169.

22. Keeney RL, Raiffa H. *Decisions with Multiple Objectives: Preferences and Value Tradeoffs*. New York: John Wiley & Sons; 1976.

23. Tversky A, Kahneman D. The framing of decisions and the psychology of choice. *Science*. 1981;211:453-458.

24. Fischhoff B, Slovic P, Lichtenstein S. Knowing what you want: measuring labile values. In: Wallsten TS, ed. *Cognitive Processes in Choice and Decision Behavior*. Hillsdale, NJ: Lawrence Erlbaum; 1980:117-141.

25. Janis IL, Mann L. *Decision Making*. New York: The Free Press; 1977.

26. Orem DE. *Nursing: Concepts of Practice*. Toronto: Mosby; 1995.

27. Norbeck JS. Social support. *Annu Rev Nur Res.* 1988;6:85-109.

28. Ajzen I, Fishbein M. *Understanding Attitudes and Predicting Social Behavior.* Englewood Cliffs, NJ: Prentice Hall; 1980.

29. Bandura A. Self-efficacy mechanism in human agency. *Am Psych.* 1982;37:122-147.

30. Feather NT. *Expectations and Actions: Expectancy-Value Models in Psychology.* Hillsdale, NJ: Lawrence Erlbaum; 1982.

31. O'Connor AM. Validation of a decisional conflict scale. *Med Decis Making.* 1995;15:25-30.

32. O'Connor AM, Stacey D, Entwistle V, et al. Decision aids for people facing health treatment or screening decisions. *Cochrane Database Syst Rev.* 2003;(2):CD001431.

33. Kennedy AD, Sculpher MJ, Coulter A, et al. Effects of decision aids for menorrhagia on treatment choices, health outcomes, and costs: a randomized controlled trial. *JAMA.* 2002;288:2701-2708.

34. Araki SS, Tosteson ANA, Kuntz KM, et al. Decision support in endometriosis: Do patients prefer a particular method of preference elicitation [abstract]? *Med Decis Making.* 2003:23:559.

35. Montgomery AA, Fahey T, Peters TJ. A factorial randomized controlled trial of decision analysis and information video plus leaflet for newly diagnosed hypertensive patients. *Br J Gen Pract.* 2003;53:446-453.

36. Torrance GW. Utility approach to measuring health-related quality of life. *J Chronic Dis.* 1987;40:593-603.

37. Froberg DG, Kane RL. Methodology for measuring health-state preferences. II: scaling methods. *J Clin Epidemiol.* 1989;42:459-471.

38. Kupperman M, Learman LA, Gates E, Gildengorin V, Washington AE, Nease RF. The effect of utility assessment on decisional conflict regarding prenatal testing: findings from a randomized controlled trial [abstract]. *Med Decis Making.* 2003:23:550.

39. Schünemann HJ, Armstrong D, Degl'innocenti A, et al. A randomized multi-center trial to evaluate simple utility elicitation techniques in patients with gastroesophageal reflux disease. *Med Care.* 2004;42:1132-1142.

40. Palda VA, Llewellyn-Thomas HA, Mackenzie RG, Pritchard KI, Naylor CD. Breast cancer patients' attitudes about rationing postlumpectomy radiation therapy: applicability of trade-off methods to policy-making. *J Clin Oncol.* 1997;15:3192-3200.

41. Dolan JG, Frisina S. Randomized controlled trial of a patient decision aid for colorectal cancer screening. *Med Decis Making.* 2002;22:125-139.

35 Interpreting Levels of Evidence and Grades of Health Care Recommendations

Alba DiCenso and Gordon Guyatt

The following Editorial Board members also made substantive contributions to this chapter: Lazelle Benefield and Mariko Koyama.

We gratefully acknowledge the work of Robert Hayward, Scott Richardson, Lee Green, Mark Wilson, Jack Sinclair, Deborah Cook, Paul Glasziou, Alan Detsky, and Eric Bass on the original chapter that appears in the Users' Guides to the Medical Literature, *edited by Guyatt and Rennie.*

In This Chapter

Health Care Recommendations

Developing Health Care Recommendations
  Health Care Recommendations and Clinical Practice Guidelines

Assessing Health Care Recommendations
  Do the Recommendations Consider All Relevant Patient Groups, Management Options, and Possible Outcomes?
  Is There a Systematic Review of Evidence Linking Options to Outcomes for Each Relevant Question?
  Is There an Appropriate Specification of Values or Preferences Associated With Outcomes?
  Do the Authors Indicate the Strength of Their Recommendations?

Relationship Between Levels of Evidence and Grades of Health Care Recommendations

Problems with Existing Systems for Grading Evidence and Health Care Recommendations

A New Grading System
  Levels of Evidence
  Grading of Recommendations

Evaluating the Trade-off Between Benefits and Risks

HEALTH CARE RECOMMENDATIONS

Each day, clinicians make dozens of patient management decisions. Some are relatively inconsequential, whereas others are important. Each one involves weighing benefits and risks, gains and losses, and recommending or instituting a course of action judged to be in the patient's best interest. Implicit in each decision is a consideration of the relevant evidence, an intuitive integration of that evidence, and a weighing of the likely benefits and risks in light of the patient's preferences. When making choices, nurses may benefit from structured summaries of options and outcomes, systematic reviews of the evidence on the relationship between options and outcomes, and recommendations about the best choices. This chapter outlines the process for developing recommendations, summarizes criteria for critically evaluating the methodological quality of recommendations, and introduces a taxonomy for grading evidence and recommendations that facilitates consideration of the trade-off between benefits and risks.

Traditionally, authors of original research on health care interventions include recommendations about the use of these interventions in clinical practice in the discussion sections of their papers. Authors of systematic reviews also tend to provide their impressions of the management implications derived from the summarization of evidence. Typically, however, authors of individual trials or systematic reviews do not consider all possible management options, but instead focus on comparisons of two or three alternatives. They may also fail to identify subpopulations in which the impact of the intervention may vary considerably. In addition, they may not consider some of the important outcomes associated with alternative management options. Finally, when the authors of systematic reviews provide recommendations, they typically are not grounded in an explicit presentation of societal or patient preferences.

Failure to consider these issues may lead to variability in recommendations based on the same data. For example, various recommendations emerged from different systematic reviews of adolescent pregnancy prevention interventions despite similar results.[1,2] The recommendations varied from suggesting to rejecting implementation of interventions such as sex education. Varying recommendations reflect the fact that investigators reporting primary studies and systematic reviews often make their recommendations without benefit of an explicit standardized process or set of rules.

When benefits or risks are dramatic and essentially homogeneous across an entire population, intuition may provide an adequate guide to making treatment recommendations. However, such situations are unusual. In most instances, intuitive recommendations risk misleading clinicians and patients because of their susceptibility to both bias and random error. These considerations suggest that nurses should critically evaluate the methodological quality of health care recommendations before implementing them.

DEVELOPING HEALTH CARE RECOMMENDATIONS

Figure 35-1 presents the steps involved in developing a recommendation, along with the formal strategies for doing so. The first step in clinical decision making is to define the decision. This involves specifying the alternative courses of action and the possible outcomes. Interventions are often designed to delay or prevent adverse outcomes, such as

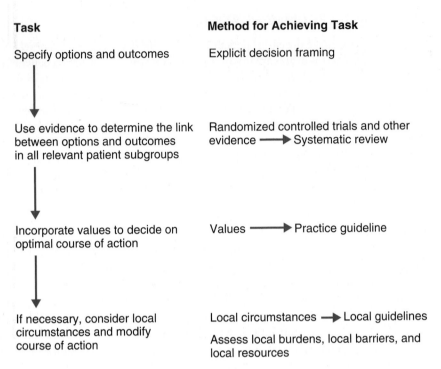

Task	Method for Achieving Task
Specify options and outcomes	Explicit decision framing
Use evidence to determine the link between options and outcomes in all relevant patient subgroups	Randomized controlled trials and other evidence ⟶ Systematic review
Incorporate values to decide on optimal course of action	Values ⟶ Practice guideline
If necessary, consider local circumstances and modify course of action	Local circumstances ⟶ Local guidelines. Assess local burdens, local barriers, and local resources

Figure 35-1. A schematic view of the process of developing a health care recommendation.

falls, pressure ulcers, urinary incontinence, or death. As usual, we refer to the outcomes that an intervention is designed to prevent as *target outcomes.* Interventions are associated with their own adverse outcomes: pain, worry, inconvenience, and side effects. In addition, new interventions may markedly increase—or decrease—costs. Ideally, the definition of the decision will be comprehensive: developers of health care recommendations should consider all reasonable alternatives and identify all possible beneficial and adverse outcomes. For example, in considering recommendations for prevention of falls in the elderly, options include doing nothing, performing individualized assessments, or offering an exercise program to everyone or only those who are at particularly high risk. Major outcomes include falls and fractures, the inconvenience associated with participating in the assessment or exercise program, and costs to participants, the health care system, and society.

Having identified the options and outcomes, developers of recommendations must evaluate the links between the two. What will the alternative management strategies yield in terms of benefits and harms?[3,4] How are potential benefits and risks likely to vary in different groups of patients?[4,5] Once these questions are answered, making recommendations about interventions involves value judgments about the relative desirability or undesirability of possible outcomes. We use the term *preferences* synonymously with *values* or *value judgments* in referring to the process of trading off positive and negative consequences of alternative management strategies.

Health Care Recommendations and Clinical Practice Guidelines

Health care recommendations are found in clinical practice guidelines. *Practice guidelines*, or "systematically developed statements to assist practitioner and patient decisions about appropriate health care for specific clinical circumstances,"[6] represent an attempt to distill a large body of health care knowledge into a convenient, readily usable format.[7–11] Similar to systematic reviews, they gather, appraise, and combine evidence. Guidelines, however, go beyond systematic reviews in attempting to address all of the issues relevant to a clinical decision and all of the values that might sway a clinical recommendation. Guidelines balance trade-offs between benefits and risks and make explicit recommendations, often on behalf of health organizations, with a definite intent to influence what clinicians do. Practice guideline methodology relies on the consensus of a group of decision makers, ideally including (or reflecting the views of) content experts, front-line clinicians, and patients, who carefully consider the evidence and decide on its implications. The mandate of guideline developers may focus on recommendations for a country, region, city, hospital, or clinic. Guidelines based on the same evidence may differ depending on the country (e.g., China or the United States), regional characteristics (urban or rural), size of the institution (e.g., a large teaching hospital or a small community hospital), and the population served (e.g., a poor community or an affluent one). For a detailed description of practice guidelines, see Chapter 10, Moving from Evidence to Action Using Clinical Practice Guidelines.

ASSESSING HEALTH CARE RECOMMENDATIONS

In Table 35-1, we offer four guidelines to assess the validity of a health care recommendation.

Do the Recommendations Consider All Relevant Patient Groups, Management Options, and Possible Outcomes?

Recommendations pertain to decisions, and decisions involve particular groups of patients, choices for those patients, and the consequences of the choices. Regardless of whether recommendations apply to diagnosis, prevention, treatment, or rehabilitation, they should specify all relevant patient groups, the interventions of interest, and sensible alternative options. Health care recommendations often vary for different subgroups of patients. In particular, patients at lower risk of the *target outcomes* that an intervention is designed to prevent are less likely to benefit from the intervention than are those at higher risk (see Chapter 33, Applying Results to Individual Patients). For instance, in a guideline on colorectal cancer screening for asymptomatic people, the Canadian Task Force on Preventive Health Care provided separate recommendations for people at normal risk and those at above-average risk because of a family history of colorectal cancer.[12]

Guideline developers who formulate recommendations must consider not only all relevant patient groups and management options, but all important consequences of the options as well. Evidence about the effects on morbidity, mortality, and quality of life are all relevant to patients, and efficient use of resources dictates attention to costs.

Table **35-1**   Users' Guides for the Validity of Health Care
             Recommendations

- Do the recommendations consider all relevant patient groups, management options, and possible outcomes?
- Is there a systematic review of evidence linking options to outcomes for each relevant question?
- Is there an appropriate specification of values or preferences associated with outcomes?
- Do the authors indicate the strength of their recommendations?

Costs, regardless of whether they are based on the perspective of patients, insurers, or the health care system—or whether they consider broader issues, such as the consequences of time lost from work—can affect the recommendations (see Chapter 18, Economic Evaluation).

Making recommendations about screening requires particular attention to identifying all potential outcomes. Attempting to identify disease in asymptomatic individuals may result in several negative outcomes that clinicians do not face when diagnosing and treating symptomatic patients. Asymptomatic individuals who screen positive for a disease must live for a longer time with awareness of their illness and the associated negative psychologic consequences. This is particularly problematic if patients remain asymptomatic for long periods. For example, consider a man who screened positive for prostate cancer, but who was destined to die of heart disease before the prostate cancer became clinically manifest. Those who screen positive but ultimately are found not to have the disease, such as with false positives in breast cancer screening, may find the experience traumatic, whereas people who screen negative but ultimately are found to have the target condition may feel betrayed (see Chapter 36, Recommendations About Screening).

Is There a Systematic Review of Evidence Linking Options to Outcomes for Each Relevant Question?

Having specified options and outcomes, the next task for guideline developers is to estimate the likelihood that each outcome will occur. In effect, they have a series of specific questions. For hormone replacement therapy, the initial question may be, "What is the effect of alternative approaches on the incidence of hip fracture, breast cancer, endometrial cancer, myocardial infarction, and sudden coronary death?"

Recommendations must consolidate and combine all of the relevant evidence in an appropriate manner. In formulating recommendations, guideline developers must avoid bias that will distort the results. This requires access to, or conduct of, a systematic review of the evidence bearing on each question. Chapter 9, Summarizing the Evidence Through Systematic Reviews, provides guidelines for assessing the likelihood that collection and summarization of the evidence are free from bias.

The best recommendations define admissible evidence, report how it was selected and combined, make key data available for review, and report randomized trials that link interventions with outcomes. However, such randomized trials may be unavailable, and the authors of systematic reviews may reasonably abandon their project if there are no high-quality studies to summarize. Those making recommendations, however, must do so even in the absence of high-quality studies. For important but ethically, technically, or economically difficult questions, strong scientific evidence may never become available. Because recommendations must deal with the best (often inadequate) evidence available, guideline developers may need to consider a variety of studies (published and unpublished) and reports of expert and consumer experience. This means that the strength of the evidence in support of recommendations can vary widely, and poor-quality evidence may yield weak recommendations.

Is There an Appropriate Specification of Values or Preferences Associated With Outcomes?

Linking treatment options with outcomes is largely based on fact and science. Assigning preferences to outcomes, by contrast, is a matter of values. Consider, for example, a guideline panel examining just two of the outcomes associated with using, or not using, hormone replacement therapy (HRT). First, the panel must consider the risk of breast cancer in women using, and not using, HRT. Second, they must consider the risk of osteoporotic fracture with and without HRT. These are matters of fact and science. In making a decision, however, the panel must also trade off the increased risk of breast cancer with HRT against the decreased risk of osteoporotic fracture. This judgment is a matter of values and preferences. Because they need to make such judgments, it is important that guideline developers report the values and preferences that lie behind their decisions.

Clinicians should look for information about who was involved in assigning values to outcomes or who, by influencing recommendations, was implicitly involved in assigning values. Expert panels and consensus groups often determine what a guideline will say. You need to know who the "experts" are, bearing in mind that panels dominated by members of specialty groups may be subject to intellectual, territorial, and financial biases. Panels that include a balance of experts in research methodology, practicing clinicians, and public representatives are more likely to have considered diverse views in their deliberations than panels restricted to content area experts.

Even with broad representation, the actual process of deliberation can influence recommendations. Therefore, clinicians should look for a report of methods used to synthesize preferences from multiple sources. Informal and unstructured processes may be vulnerable to undue influence by individual panel members, particularly that of the panel chair. Explicit strategies for describing and dealing with dissent among judges, or frank reports of the degree of consensus strengthen the credibility of recommendations.

Knowing the extent to which panelists considered *patient preferences* is particularly important. Many guideline reports, by their silence on the matter of patient preferences, assume that guideline developers adequately represent patients' interests. Although they are reported rarely, it also would be valuable to know which principles—such as patient autonomy, nonmaleficence, or distributive justice—were given priority in guiding decisions about the value of alternative interventions. Excellent guidelines will state whether a guideline is intended to optimize values for individual patients, reimbursement agencies, or society as a whole. Ideally, guidelines will state the underlying value judgments on which they are based.

Do the Authors Indicate the Strength of Their Recommendations?

Multiple considerations should inform the strength or grade of recommendations: (1) quality of the sources contributing to the systematic review or reviews that bring together the relevant evidence, (2) magnitude and consistency of the intervention effects in different studies, (3) magnitude of adverse effects, (4) burden to patients and the health care system, (5) costs, and (6) relative value placed on different outcomes. Thus recommendations may vary from those that rely on evidence from a systematic review of randomized controlled trials that show large effects of the intervention on patient-important outcomes with minimal side effects, inconvenience, and costs (yielding a very strong recommendation) to those that rely on evidence from observational studies showing a small magnitude of treatment effect with appreciable side effects and costs (yielding a very weak recommendation).

RELATIONSHIP BETWEEN LEVELS OF EVIDENCE AND GRADES OF HEALTH CARE RECOMMENDATIONS

Groups developing recommendations should make sequential judgments about the quality of evidence (i.e., the extent to which one can be confident that an estimate of effect is correct) and the strength of the recommendation (i.e., the extent to which one can be confident that adherence to a recommendation will do more good than harm).[13] These judgments are typically indicated through formal grading systems, one categorizing levels of evidence and one categorizing levels of recommendations.

However, many current grading systems do not adequately distinguish between evidence and recommendations. Although the quality of evidence serves as the principal basis for clinical practice recommendations, the review of the evidence is a conceptually distinct process from the setting of clinical policy. Because of the health, economic, and social implications of clinical practice guidelines, the scientific evidence must be viewed within the context of the clinical practice and health care settings to which the recommendations apply.[14] Examples of factors other than evidence that can affect the grade of a recommendation include questionable transfer of study results to other countries or practice settings, limited availability of a particular technology, demonstrated poor adherence with a procedure, potential for harm, overwhelming burden of suffering, large numbers needed to treat, costly procedures or technology, and the values and preferences that determine decisions about the balance between benefits and harms.[14] For this reason, two rating scales are required: one for levels of evidence and one for grades of recommendations.

Appreciation of the need for these rating scales has led to a proliferation of hierarchies that use various systems of codes to communicate grades of evidence and recommendations, with the most common falling into three categories: letters (e.g., A, B, C, etc.), numbers (e.g., I, II, III, etc.), and a combination of letters and numbers (e.g., Ia,

Ib, IIa, etc.).[13] The existence of multiple classifications for evaluating and structuring evidence and the differing interpretations of grades of recommendations on the basis of this evidence pose potential problems for clinicians. Table 35-2 illustrates four evidence hierarchies.[14-17] Considerable differences exist among them with respect to what counts as the highest-quality evidence and what constitutes the strongest possible recommendation.[18]

Scientists develop evidence hierarchies and grades of recommendations to promote the use of evidence-based approaches in health care and provide clinicians with a guide to reliable knowledge. However, the large number of systems threatens to create confusion for clinicians. The various hierarchies are differentially restrictive with respect to what counts as best evidence.[18] They give differential weight to consensus of expert opinion and evidence. To address this problem of multiple hierarchies, the GRADE Working Group has developed yet another system for grading evidence and recommendations.[19] The GRADE Working Group consists of more than 25 scientists from around the world with extensive experience in conducting systematic reviews and developing guidelines. They have developed their system through a critical appraisal of six prominent systems, review of other systems, iterative discussions, and a pilot study.[19] Their system has one key difference from all other systems: it includes detailed guides for working through a recommendation to arrive at a grade of methodological quality and strength of recommendation. Before describing this system, we illustrate some of the problems with existing systems.

PROBLEMS WITH EXISTING SYSTEMS FOR GRADING EVIDENCE AND HEALTH CARE RECOMMENDATIONS

The American Diabetes Association has published recommendations to prevent foot ulcers in people with diabetes.[20] The guideline developers used a rating scheme for levels of evidence, which ranged from randomized controlled trials (RCTs), representing the strongest level of evidence, to expert and consensus opinion, representing the lowest level of evidence (I-A: RCT, crossover trials; I-B: controlled trial, nonrandomized; II-A: cohort, case-control; II-B: time-series, pre-post studies, repeated panel; II-C: cross-sectional population-based data; III: descriptive studies, case series, case reports; IV: expert opinion and consensus opinion).[21] Three issues arise in review of the recommendations.

First is the use of expert opinion as level IV evidence. The concept of evidence supported by expert opinion is often ill defined. What do we mean by evidence? In the broadest definition, we mean experiences in the world. When those experiences are reported to others, they become evidence that we can all consider. Consider the following statement: I am an expert in condition x, and I know that treatment y is extremely effective and provides much more benefit than harm. This statement provides no evidence. It is an opinion. Consider an alternative statement: I have administered treatment y to 1000 patients with condition x. They all improved markedly with minimal side effects, and treatment y was associated with little cost and inconvenience. This statement provides evidence. It may be anecdotal and subject to a several biases, but it constitutes evidence.

Table 35-2 Highest Level of Evidence and Strongest Grade of Recommendation in Four Evidence Hierarchies

Source of Evidence Hierarchy	Highest Level of Evidence for a Treatment or Intervention	Conditions for Strongest Recommendation
Canadian Task Force on Preventive Health Care[14]	1 = at least one RCT	A study (including meta-analysis or systematic review) that meets all design-specific criteria well
Scientific Advisory Council of the Osteoporosis Society of Canada[15]	1+ = systematic review or meta-analysis of RCTs 1 = one randomized trial with adequate power	Supportive level 1 or 1+ evidence plus consensus
Centre for Evidence-Based Medicine[16]	1a = systematic review with homogeneity of RCTs 1b = one RCT with narrow confidence interval 1c = all or none*	Consistent level 1 studies
Scottish Intercollegiate Guidelines Network[17]	1++ = high-quality meta-analyses, systematic reviews of RCTs, or RCTs with very low risk of bias 1+ = well-conducted meta-analyses, systematic reviews of RCTs, or RCTs with low risk of bias 1− = meta-analyses, systematic reviews of RCTs, or RCTs with high risk of bias	At least one meta-analysis, systematic review, or RCT rated as 1++ and directly applicable to the target population; or a systematic review of RCTs or a body of evidence consisting principally of studies rated as 1+ directly applicable to the target population and demonstrating overall consistency

RCT, *Randomized controlled trial.*
The Center for Evidence-Based Medicine explains "all or none" as follows: "met when all patients died before the treatment became available but some now survive on it; or when some patients died before the treatment became available but none now die on it."
Modified and reproduced with permission of the Canadian Medical Association from Upshur RE. Are all evidence-based practices alike? Problems in the ranking of evidence. CMAJ. 2003;169:672-673.

Systems of grading recommendations that specify "expert opinion" as a level of evidence ignore the distinction between opinion and evidence. Perhaps such systems are implicitly suggesting that expert members of the panel bring their individual clinical experience to bear on the decision and are therefore providing evidence. If so, an explicit and clear statement of that assumption would be helpful. Moreover, if that is what they are saying, such systems need to confront the fact that many experts become increasingly distant from clinical practice with increasing years of widely acknowledged expertise and that evidence available only within the panel (in contrast to, for example, published case series) lacks transparency. Clearly specifying that evidence, and not opinion, bears on grading the strength of evidence represents a superior approach to this issue.

Second, although the guideline developers outlined the rating scheme for the strength of evidence, they did not link the strength of evidence to each recommendation. Readers are left with an undifferentiated list of recommendations with no accompanying information about the strength of evidence for each recommendation.

Finally, the guideline developers did not provide information about the strength of the recommendations. With the absence of grades of recommendations, readers have no information about the balance between benefits and harm, adherence problems, and cost implications of implementing the recommendations.

The New Zealand Guidelines Group (NZGG) developed an evidence-based best practice guideline for health professionals working in cardiac rehabilitation in hospitals and communities in New Zealand.[22] The group rated the evidence using an adapted version of the Scottish Intercollegiate Guidelines Network (SIGN) grading system for recommendations in evidence-based guidelines.[17] Table 35-3 outlines the levels of evidence and grades of recommendations. The highest level of evidence (1++) is derived from high-quality meta-analyses, systematic reviews of RCTs, or RCTs with a very low risk of bias, and the lowest level of evidence (4) is derived from expert opinion. A recommendation is assigned the highest grade of A if it is substantiated by at least one meta-analysis, systematic review, or RCT rated as 1++, and if it is directly applicable to the target population; or if it is substantiated by a body of evidence consisting principally of studies rated as 1+, and if it is directly applicable to the target population and demonstrates overall consistency of results. A recommendation is assigned the lowest grade of D if it is based on level 3 or 4 evidence or is extrapolated from studies rated as 2+, or expert opinion.

These guideline developers created separate levels of evidence and grades of recommendation, but only the grades of recommendation (which incorporate the levels of evidence) accompany the recommendation statements. As with the guideline on foot ulcers described previously, they included expert opinion as the weakest level of evidence. The grades of recommendation are based largely on the levels of evidence, although the guideline developers also stipulate direct applicability to the target population for levels A, B, and C.

The biggest problem with this approach is that it ignores the fact that one can have very high-quality evidence accompanying a weak recommendation. Consider a series of large, well-planned, and brilliantly executed randomized trials of the highest methodological quality summarized in a rigorous systematic review and meta-analysis. All of us

Table **35-3** Grading System Used by New Zealand Guidelines Group in Cardiac Rehabilitation Guideline

Levels of Evidence

1++	High-quality meta-analyses, systematic reviews of RCTs, or RCTs with a very low risk of bias
1+	Well-conducted meta-analyses, systematic reviews of RCTs, or RCTs with a low risk of bias
1−	Well-conducted meta-analyses, systematic reviews of RCTs, or RCTs with a high risk of bias
2++	High-quality systematic reviews of case-control or cohort studies with a very low risk of confounding or bias and a high probability that the relationship is causal
2+	Well-conducted case-control or cohort studies with a low risk of confounding or bias and a moderate probability that the relationship is causal
2−	Case-control or cohort studies with a high risk of confounding or bias and a significant risk that the relationship is not casual
3	Nonanalytic studies (case reports, case series)
4	Expert opinion

Grades of Recommendation

A	At least one meta-analysis, systematic review, or RCT rated as 1++, and directly applicable to the target population, OR a body of evidence consisting principally of studies rated as 1+, directly applicable to the target population, and demonstrating overall consistency of results
B	A body of evidence including studies rated as 2++, directly applicable to the target population, and demonstrating overall consistency of results, OR extrapolated evidence from studies rated as 1++ or 1+
C	A body of evidence including studies rated as 2+, directly applicable to the target population, and demonstrating overall consistency of results, OR extrapolated evidence from studies rated as 2++
D	Evidence levels 3 or 4, OR extrapolated evidence from studies rated as 2+, or expert opinion

RCTs, *Randomized controlled trials.*
Modified and reproduced with permission from the New Zealand Guidelines Group. Best practice evidence-based guideline: cardiac rehabilitation. *Available at:*
http:// www.nzgg.org.nz/guidelines/0001/cardiac_rehabilitation.pdf

would classify this as highest-quality evidence. Now, what would we recommend if the intervention was administered to 1000 people and prevented a single premature death. All 1000 people, however, became moderately to severely nauseated for 6 months, and 100 of these people lost all their hair. Would we recommend this intervention? Some of us might, whereas others would not. But whatever our decision, none of us would claim that our recommendation is a strong one. Thus, systems such as SIGN that assume that high-quality evidence leads to strong recommendations are problematic.

The Canadian Task Force on Preventive Health Care developed recommendations on the effectiveness of specific screening techniques for colorectal cancer in asymptomatic patients.[12,23] Table 35-4 outlines the levels of evidence and grades of recommendations used by the Task Force.[23] The strongest level of evidence (I) is derived from at least one well-designed randomized controlled trial, and the weakest level of evidence (III) is derived from opinions of respected authorities, clinical experience, or descriptive

Table 35-4 Canadian Task Force on Preventive Health Care Levels of Evidence and Grades of Recommendations*

Levels of Evidence

I	Evidence from at least one well-designed randomized controlled trial
II-1	Evidence from well-designed controlled trials without randomization
II-2	Evidence from well-designed cohort or case-control analytic studies, preferably from more than one center or research group
II-3	Evidence from comparisons between times or places with or without the intervention: dramatic results from uncontrolled studies could be included here
III	Opinions of respected authorities, based on clinical experience; descriptive studies or reports of expert committees

Grades of Recommendations

A	Good evidence to support the recommendation that the condition or maneuver be specifically considered in a periodic health examination (PHE)
B	Fair evidence to support the recommendation that the condition or maneuver be specifically considered in a PHE
C	Insufficient evidence regarding inclusion or exclusion of the condition or maneuver in a PHE, but recommendations may be made on other grounds
D	Fair evidence to support the recommendation that the condition or maneuver be specifically excluded from a PHE
E	Good evidence to support the recommendation that the condition or maneuver be specifically excluded from a PHE

*Since this systematic review was published, the Canadian Task Force on Preventive Health Care (CTFPHC) has made revisions to their grades of recommendations. Grade C now means the following: "Existing evidence is conflicting and does not allow making a recommendation for or against use of the clinical preventive action." They have also added a Grade I recommendation indicating "insufficient evidence (in quantity and/or quality) to make a recommendation." For more detailed information about the most recent levels of evidence and grades of recommendations, please refer to the CTFPHC History/Methodology section on their Web site at www.ctfphc.org.[24,25]

Modified and reproduced with permission of the Canadian Task Force on Preventive Health Care from McLeod R, with the Canadian Task Force on Preventive Health Care. Screening Strategies for Colorectal Cancer: Systematic Review & Recommendations. CTFPHC Technical Report #01-2. February 2001. London, Ontario: Canadian Task Force. Available at: http://www.ctfphc.org

studies or reports of expert committees. With respect to this weakest level of evidence, parts of it constitute evidence (clinical experience and descriptive studies), but parts of it do not (opinions of respected authorities and reports of expert committees).

A recommendation is assigned the highest grade of A if good evidence suggests that the condition or maneuver should be specifically considered in a periodic health examination; a grade of C if there is insufficient evidence; and a grade of E if good evidence suggests that the condition or maneuver should be specifically excluded from the periodic health examination.

In this system, Grade C is not a recommendation at all. For example, a man asks a nurse practitioner if he should be tested with prostate-specific antigen (PSA). The NP refers to a guideline for information about what to advise the patient. Using the Canadian Task Force system, a guideline tells the NP that there is insufficient evidence to decide (which is, at the time of this writing, the case for PSA screening). The NP is no further ahead in knowing what to advise the patient because there is no recommendation. For clinicians seeking guidance about how to proceed in the absence of adequate evidence (and, after all, the patient and NP must proceed one way or the other, screen or not screen), the guideline has not been helpful.

Unlike the previous two examples, each recommendation statement has both a level of evidence and a grade of recommendation. This is useful because it is possible, as noted previously, for any one recommendation statement to have strong evidence and a weak recommendation. For example, although administration of anticoagulant therapy in atrial fibrillation is supported by strong evidence, it might warrant only a weak recommendation for implementation in rural settings, where travel distances are large and anticoagulant intensity monitoring is difficult, or in more severely resource-constrained settings where there is a direct inverse relationship between the resources available for purchase of antibiotic drugs and those allocated to monitoring levels of anticoagulation.

It is also possible to have weak evidence and a strong recommendation. Evidence for the long-term health benefits of exercising in one's youth comes from weak observational studies. We may nevertheless provide a strong recommendation for exercise on the basis that costs and side effects are negligible.

These three examples of health care recommendations illustrate the diversity in the presence and nature of hierarchies that rank levels of evidence and grades of recommendations. Given the existence of numerous and varied systems, readers must look for and review the specific hierarchy for levels of evidence and grades of recommendations so that the strength of the recommendations can be accurately interpreted.

A NEW GRADING SYSTEM

The Grades of Recommendation Assessment, Development, and Evaluation (GRADE) Working Group has developed a new system for evaluating evidence and recommendations.[19] We propose consideration and adoption of this system because it has been developed by many experienced scientists from around the world based on critical appraisal of other systems, iterative discussions, and a pilot study.[19] This system facilitates consideration of the trade-off between benefits and risks and includes detailed guides for working through a recommendation to arrive at a grade of methodological quality and strength of recommendation.

Levels of Evidence

With respect to quality of evidence, the group suggests that systematic reviews guide judgments. Reviewers should consider four key elements of quality: study design, study quality, consistency, and directness. *Study designs* are broadly categorized as randomized controlled trials, quasi-randomized trials (trials using nonrandom allocation such as alternation), and observational studies. Some study designs are more subject to bias than others, and therefore provide weaker justification for clinical decisions.[18] As a result, observational studies do not always predict the findings of subsequent randomized trials, and they frequently overestimate treatment effects.[19] A dramatic example of such a discrepancy occurred when the results of observational studies that suggested HRT decreased the risk of coronary heart disease were contradicted by subsequent randomized trials that found no such reduction in risk and the possibility of an increased risk.[26,27]

Study quality refers to the detailed study design and execution. Reviewers should use appropriate criteria to assess quality for each important outcome.[19] For randomized trials, for example, reviewers might use criteria such as the adequacy of allocation concealment, blinding, and follow-up (see Chapter 4, Health Care Interventions). Reviewers should make explicit their reasons for downgrading a quality rating. For example, they may state that failure to blind patients and clinicians reduced the quality of evidence for an intervention's impact on pain severity and that they considered this to be a serious flaw.[19]

Consistency refers to the similarity of estimates of effect across studies. Differences in the direction of effect, the size of differences, and the statistical significance of differences decrease our confidence in the estimate of effect for a particular outcome.[19] *Directness* refers to the extent to which the people, interventions, and outcome measures are similar to those of interest. For example, there may be uncertainty about the directness of the evidence if the patients of interest are older, sicker, or have more comorbidity than those included in the studies (see Chapter 33, Applying Results to Individual Patients).[19] To determine whether important uncertainty exists, one can ask whether there is a compelling reason to expect important differences in effect sizes. Use of surrogate outcomes for outcomes that are important to patients (e.g., bone density as a surrogate for fractures) often results in appropriately increased uncertainty (see Chapter 13, Surrogate Outcomes).[19]

To grade levels of evidence, the Working Group suggests first categorizing the evidence based on study design (Table 35-5) and subsequently considering whether the studies have serious flaws, important inconsistencies in the results, or whether uncertainty about the directness of the evidence is warranted. They suggest the following definitions in grading the quality of evidence[19]:

High: Further research is very unlikely to change our confidence in the estimate of effect.
Moderate: Further research is likely to have an important impact on our confidence in the estimate of effect and may change the estimate.

Table 35-5 Criteria for Assigning Grade of Evidence

Type of Evidence

Randomized trial = high
Observational study = low
Any other evidence = very low

Decrease Grade if:

- Serious (–1) or very serious (–2) limitation to study quality
- Important inconsistency (–1)
- Some (–1) or major (–2) uncertainty about directness
- Imprecise or sparse data (–1)
- High probability of reporting bias (–1)

Increase Grade if:

- Strong evidence of association—significant relative risk of > 2 (< 0.5) based on consistent evidence from two or more observational studies, with no plausible confounders (+ 1)
- Very strong evidence of association—significant relative risk of > 5 (< 0.2) based on direct evidence with no major threats to validity (+2)
- Evidence of a dose-response gradient (+1)
- All plausible confounders would have reduced the effect (+1)

Modified and reproduced with permission of BMJ Publishing Group from GRADE Working Group. Grading quality of evidence and strength of recommendations. BMJ. *2004;328:1490-1498.*

Low: Further research is very likely to have an important impact on our confidence in the estimate of effect and is likely to change the estimate.

Very low: Any estimate of effect is very uncertain.

Limitations in study quality, important inconsistency of results, or uncertainty about the directness of evidence can lower the grade of evidence. For instance, if all available studies have serious flaws, the grade will drop by one level, and if all studies have very serious flaws, the grade will drop by two levels. Fatally flawed studies may be excluded from consideration.[19] Limitations act cumulatively. For example, if randomized trials have both serious flaws and uncertainty exists about the directness of the evidence, the grade of evidence drops from high to low.

Grading of Recommendations

Recommendations involve a trade-off between benefits and harms. Making that trade-off involves placing a value on each outcome. Different people will have different values and, therefore, it is difficult to judge how much weight to give to different outcomes. Grading recommendations entails making explicit judgments about the balance between the main health benefits and harms. Recommendations must apply to specific settings and groups of patients whenever the benefits and harms differ across settings or patient groups.[19] The Working Group suggests a simple scheme to, in effect, categorize recommendations as strong (the trade-offs are clear) or weak (benefits and downsides are closely balanced). The final grade of recommendation becomes very explicit[19]:

"Do it" or **"Don't do it"**: Indicating a judgment that most well-informed people will make the same choice.

"Probably do it" or **"Probably don't do it"**: Indicating a judgment that most well-informed people will make the same choice, but a substantial minority will not.

In some instances, it may not be appropriate to make a recommendation because of unclear trade-offs or lack of agreement (although, as pointed out earlier, this is unhelpful for clinicians looking for guidance).

EVALUATING THE TRADE-OFF BETWEEN BENEFITS AND RISKS

Depending on the balance between benefits and risks, methodologically strong studies that suggest a benefit of one intervention over another intervention may lead to varying recommendations. When side effects are minimal, risk reductions are large, or a patient's risk of the target event that the intervention will prevent is very high, guideline developers may make a strong recommendation to administer the more effective intervention to patients with compatible values and preferences. When benefits and risks are closely balanced, we may see conflicting recommendations and practice. When risk reductions are small and toxicity is high, guideline developers may even recommend the less effective intervention or recommend not to treat at all. As the magnitude of benefits and risks become more closely balanced, decisions about administration of effective interventions also become more cost sensitive.

The categories for recommendations suggested by the GRADE Working Group reflect the balance between benefits and risks of health care interventions. If the benefits clearly outweigh the risks (or vice versa) and virtually all patients would make the same choice, the recommendation is designated as "do it" or "don't do it." An example is the prophylaxis of deep venous thrombosis after hip fracture surgery, in which heparin reduces the risk of deep venous thrombosis by approximately 40%.[28] Here, because sample sizes of the studies are relatively large and confidence intervals are narrow, and because prophylaxis is associated with low costs and complications, benefits clearly outweigh the downsides of treatment, and the recommendation is strong. If they understand the benefits and risks, virtually all patients will comply with prophylaxis to reduce thromboembolism after hip fracture. Thus, one way of thinking about a "do it" or "don't do it" recommendation is that variability in patient values or individual clinician values is unlikely to influence treatment choice in typical patients.

When the balance is less certain and different patients may make different choices, they designate the recommendation as "probably do it" or "probably don't do it." Several factors may create uncertainty in the balance between benefits and risks, including marked variation in patient values, a wide range of confidence intervals around estimates of benefits and risks, high costs, or small effect sizes (see Chapter 10, Moving From Evidence to Action Using Clinical Practice Guidelines).

If the balance between benefits and risks is uncertain, we may have methodologically rigorous studies but recommendations may still be weak ("probably do it" or "probably don't do it"). The more balanced the trade-off between benefits and risks, the greater is the influence of individual patient values in decision making. When the trade-off between benefits and risks is less clear, clinicians will want to ensure that individual patient values bear strongly on the final decision (see Chapter 34, Incorporating Patient Values). In considering the duration of anticoagulation after an episode of idiopathic deep venous thrombosis, patients may make different choices depending on the relative value they place on avoiding a fatal pulmonary embolus, avoiding bleeding, and the inconvenience and worry associated with repeated testing to determine the intensity of anticoagulation. "Probably do it" or "probably don't do it" recommendations are those in which variation in patient values or individual clinician values will often mandate different treatment choices, even among typical patients.

CONCLUSION

In this chapter, we outlined the process of developing recommendations, summarized criteria for critically evaluating the methodological quality of recommendations, and introduced a taxonomy for grading evidence and recommendations that facilitates consideration of the trade-off between benefits and risks. We have illustrated the importance and added value of having information on both the level of evidence and the grade of recommendation and how the two are not always entirely dependent on one another.

REFERENCES

1. DiCenso A, Guyatt G, Willan A, Griffith L. Interventions to reduce unintended pregnancies among adolescents: systematic review of randomised controlled trials. *BMJ*. 2002;324:1426.
2. NHS Centre for Reviews and Dissemination. *Preventing and Reducing the Adverse Effects of Unintended Teenage Pregnancies*. York, England: NHS Centre for Reviews and Dissemination; 1997.
3. Glasziou PP, Irwig LM. An evidence based approach to individualising treatment. *BMJ*. 1995;311:1356-1358.
4. Sinclair JC, Cook R, Guyatt GH, Pauker SG, Cook DJ. When should an effective treatment be used? Derivation of the threshold number needed to treat and the minimum event rate for treatment. *J Clin Epidemiol*. 2001;54:253-262.
5. Smith GD, Egger M. Who benefits from medical interventions? *BMJ*. 1994;308:72-74.
6. Field MJ, Lohr KN (eds.). *Clinical Practice Guidelines: Directions for a New Program*. Washington, DC: National Academy Press; 1990.
7. Hayward RS, Laupacis A. Initiating, conducting and maintaining guidelines development programs. *CMAJ*. 1993;148:507-512.
8. Grimshaw J, Eccles M, Russell I. Developing clinically valid practice guidelines. *J Eval Clin Pract*. 1995;1:37-48.
9. Field MJ, Lohr KN (eds.). *Guidelines for Clinical Practice: From Development to Use*. Washington, DC: National Academy Press; 1992.
10. Browman GP, Levine MN, Mohide EA, et al. The practice guidelines development cycle: a conceptual tool for practice guidelines development and implementation. *J Clin Oncol*. 1995;13:502-512.
11. Grinspun D, Virani T, Bajnok I. Nursing best practice guidelines. The RNAO project. *Hosp Q*. 2002;5:56-60.
12. Canadian Task Force on Preventive Health Care. Colorectal cancer screening. *CMAJ*. 2001;165:206-208.
13. Schunemann HJ, Best D, Vist G, Oxman AD, for the GRADE Working Group. Letters, numbers, symbols and words: how to communicate grades of evidence and recommendations. *CMAJ*. 2003;169:677-680.

14. Canadian Task Force on Preventive Health Care. "History and methods." Available at: *http://www.ctfphc.org/*. Accessed December 21, 2003.

15. Brown JP, Josse RG, for the Scientific Advisory Council of the Osteoporosis Society of Canada. 2002 clinical practice guidelines for the diagnosis and management of osteoporosis in Canada. *CMAJ*. 2002;167(10 Suppl):S1-S34.

16. Centre for Evidence-Based Medicine. Levels of evidence and grades of recommendation. Available at: *http://www.cebm.net/levels_of_evidence.asp*. Accessed December 21, 2003.

17. Scottish Intercollegiate Guidelines Network (SIGN). SIGN 50: A guideline developers' handbook, Section 6: forming guideline recommendations. Available at: *http://www.sign.ac.uk/guidelines/fulltext/50/section6.html*. Accessed December 21, 2003.

18. Upshur RE. Are all evidence-based practices alike? Problems in the ranking of evidence. *CMAJ*. 2003;169:672-673.

19. GRADE Working Group. Grading quality of evidence and strength of recommendations. *BMJ*. 2004;328:1490-1498.

20. American Diabetes Association. Preventive foot care in diabetes. *Diabetes Care*. 2004;27:S63-S64.

21. Mayfield JA, Reiber GE, Sanders LJ, Janisse D, Pogach LM. American Diabetes Association. Preventive foot care in people with diabetes. *Diabetes Care*. 2003;26:S78-S79.

22. New Zealand Guidelines Group. Best practice evidence-based guideline: cardiac rehabilitation. Available at: *http://www.nzgg.org.nz/guidelines/0001/cardiac_rehabilitation.pdf*. Accessed June 30, 2004.

23. McLeod R, with the Canadian Task Force on Preventive Health Care. *Screening Strategies for Colorectal Cancer: Systematic Review & Recommendations*. CTFPHC Technical Report #01-2. February 2001. London, Ontario: Canadian Task Force. Available at: *http://www.ctfphc.org*. Accessed December 21, 2003.

24. Woolf SH, Battista RN, Anderson GM, Logan AG, Wang E, and other members of the Canadian Task Force on the Periodic Health Examination. Assessing the clinical effectiveness of preventive maneuvers: analytic principles and systematic methods in reviewing evidence and developing clinical practice recommendations. *J Clin Epidemiol*. 1990;43:891-905.

25. Canadian Task Force on Preventive Health Care. New grades for recommendations from the Canadian Task Force on Preventive Health Care. *CMAJ*. 2003;169:207-208.

26. Grodstein F, Manson JE, Colditz GA, Willett WC, Speizer FE, Stampfer MJ. A prospective, observational study of postmenopausal hormone therapy and primary prevention of cardiovascular disease. *Ann Intern Med*. 2000;133:933-941.

27. Writing Group for the Women's Health Initiative Investigators. Risks and benefits of estrogen plus progestin in healthy postmenopausal women: principal results from the Women's Health Initiative randomized controlled trial. *JAMA*. 2002;288:321-333.

28. Handoll HH, Farrar MJ, McBirnie J, Tytherleigh-Strong G, Milne AA, Gillespie WJ. Heparin, low molecular weight heparin and physical methods for preventing deep vein thrombosis and pulmonary embolism following surgery for hip fractures. *Cochrane Database Syst Rev*. 2002;(4):CD000305.

36

Recommendations About Screening

Alba DiCenso and Gordon Guyatt

The following Editorial Board members also made substantive contributions to this chapter: Susan Marks, Andrea Nelson, and Mark Newman.

We gratefully acknowledge the work of Alexandra Barratt, Les Irwig, Paul Glasziou, Robert Cumming, Angela Raffle, Nicholas Hicks, and Muir Gray on the original chapter that appears in the Users' Guides to the Medical Literature, *edited by Guyatt and Rennie.*

In This Chapter

Finding the Evidence

Consequences of Screening

Are the Recommendations Valid?
  Is There Randomized Trial Evidence That Earlier Intervention Works?
  Were the Data Identified, Selected, and Combined in an Unbiased Fashion?

What Are the Recommendations?
  What Are the Benefits?
  What Are the Risks?

Can I Apply the Recommendations to Patient Care?
  How Do Benefits and Risks Compare in Different People and With Different
    Screening Strategies?
  What Is the Impact of Individuals' Values and Preferences?
  What Is the Impact of Uncertainty Associated With the Evidence?
  What Is the Cost-effectiveness?

Should a 47-Year-Old Couple Undergo Colon Cancer Screening?

You are a primary care nurse practitioner seeing a 47-year-old woman and her husband of the same age. They are concerned because a friend recently was diagnosed with colon cancer, and she has urged them both to undergo screening with the fecal occult blood test (FOBT).

Both of these patients have no family history of colon cancer and no change in bowel habit. They ask whether you agree that they should be screened. You know that trials of FOBT screening have shown that screening can reduce mortality from colorectal cancer, but you also recall that FOBTs can have a high false-positive rate, which then necessitates investigation by colonoscopy. You are unsure whether screening these relatively young, asymptomatic people at average risk of colon cancer is likely to do more good than harm. You decide to check the literature to see whether there are any guidelines or recommendations about screening for colorectal cancer that could help you respond to their question.

FINDING THE EVIDENCE

Because you know that more than one randomized trial exists on this topic, you first look for a *systematic review*. You search the Cochrane Database of Systematic Reviews using the terms "fecal occult blood test" and "colon cancer." Your search identifies a systematic review by Towler and colleagues.[1] However, because there may be additional evidence that might influence your decision to recommend screening to this couple (e.g., the *false-positive* rate of the test, side effects of subsequent investigation and treatment, and associated costs), you also check for a clinical practice guideline. You go to the National Guideline Clearinghouse Web site (*http://www.guideline.gov/*), enter the same keywords, and find eight guidelines, the most recent of which is by the American Gastroenterological Association (AGA), "Colorectal Cancer Screening and Surveillance: Clinical Guidelines and Rationale—Update Based on New Evidence."[2] The guideline is based on the same trials as the systematic review and also provides the additional information you were hoping to find. The full text is provided, so you print a copy to review.

CONSEQUENCES OF SCREENING

The best way to think about *screening* is as a therapeutic intervention. This clarifies the methodology required to support a policy of screening: randomized trials examining the effect of screening on patient-important outcomes.[3-6] Screening can be used to identify the presence of disease or the presence of risk factors for disease (e.g., cholesterol screening).

Table 36-1 presents the possible consequences of screening. Some people will have *true-positive* results (a) with clinically significant disease (a^0); a proportion of this group

Table **36-1**　Summary of Benefits and Risks of Screening by
Underlying Disease State

	Reference Standard Results		
	Disease or Risk Factor Present		Disease or Risk Factor Absent
Screening test positive	a^0—true positives (significant disease)	or　a^1—true positives (inconsequential disease)	b—false positives
Screening test negative	c^0—false negatives (significant disease)	or　c^1—false negatives (inconsequential disease)	d—true negatives

a^0, disease or risk factor that will cause symptoms in the future (significant disease); a^1, disease or risk factor asymptomatic until death (inconsequential disease); b, false-positive results; c^0, missed disease that will be significant in the future; c^1, missed disease that will be inconsequential in the future; d, true-negative results.
Note: sensitivity = $a/(a+c)$ and specificity = $d/b+d$.
Modified and reproduced with permission of the American Medical Association from Barratt A, Irwig L, Glasziou P, et al. Users' guides to the medical literature. XVII. How to use guidelines and recommendations about screening. JAMA. 1999;281:2029–2034.

will benefit depending on the effectiveness of treatment and the severity of the detected disease. For example, children found to have phenylketonuria will experience large, long-lasting benefits of screening. Other people will have true-positive results with inconsequential disease (a^1); they may experience the consequences of labeling, investigation, and treatment for a disease or risk factor that otherwise never would have affected their lives. Consider, for instance, a man in whom screening reveals low-grade prostate cancer. This man will most likely die of coronary artery disease before his prostate cancer becomes clinically manifest. Thus, he may be advised to undergo unnecessary treatment and experience associated adverse effects.

People with *false-positive* results (b) may be adversely affected by the risks associated with investigation of the screen-detected condition. People with *false-negative* results of clinically important disease (c^0) may experience harm if false reassurance results in delayed presentation or investigation of symptoms; some patients may be angry when they discover they have disease despite having negative screening test results. By contrast, patients with false-negative results with inconsequential disease (c^1) are not harmed by their "disease" being missed because it was never destined to affect them. Patients with *true-negative* results (d) may experience the benefits associated with an accurate reassurance of being disease free, but they may also experience the inconvenience, cost, and anxiety associated with screening.

The longer the gap is between possible detection and clinically important consequences, the greater will be the number of people in the inconsequential disease category (a^1). When screening for risk factors, very large numbers of people need to be screened and treated to prevent one adverse event years later.[7] Thus, most people found to have a risk factor at screening will be treated for inconsequential disease. Table 36-2 summarizes the criteria for evaluating a study about screening.

ARE THE RECOMMENDATIONS VALID?

Is There Randomized Trial Evidence that Earlier Intervention Works?

Guidelines recommending screening are on strong ground if they are based on randomized controlled trials that compare screening with conventional care. In the past, many screening programs, some of them effective (e.g., screening for cervical cancer and for phenylketonuria), were implemented on the basis of observational data. When the benefits are enormous and the disadvantages are minimal, randomized trials are not needed. More often, however, the benefits and risks of screening are balanced more evenly. In these situations, observational studies of screening may be misleading. Survival, as measured from the time of diagnosis, may be increased not because patients live longer, but because screening lengthens the time that they know they have a disease *(lead-time bias)*. Patients whose disease is discovered by screening also may appear to live longer because screening tends to detect slowly progressing disease, yet it often misses rapidly progressive disease that becomes symptomatic between screening rounds *(length-time bias)*. Therefore, unless the evidence of benefit is overwhelming, randomized trial assessment is required.

Investigators may choose one of two study designs to test the impact of a screening process. Trials may assess the entire screening process (early detection and early intervention; Figure 36-1A), in which case people are randomized to be screened and treated if early abnormality is detected or not screened (and treated only if symptomatic disease occurs). Trials of mammographic screening have used this design.[8–10] Alternatively, all participants may undergo screening, and those with positive results can be randomized to be treated or not treated (Figure 36-1B). If those who receive treatment do better than those who do not, then one can conclude that early treatment has provided some benefit. Investigators usually

Table 36-2　Users' Guides for an Article About Screening

Are the Recommendations Valid?

- Is there randomized trial evidence that earlier intervention works?
- Were the data identified, selected, and combined in an unbiased fashion?

What Are the Recommendations?

- What are the benefits?
- What are the risks?

Can I Apply the Recommendations to Patient Care?

- How do benefits and risks compare in different people and with different screening strategies?
- What is the impact of individuals' values and preferences?
- What is the impact of uncertainty associated with the evidence?
- What is the cost-effectiveness?

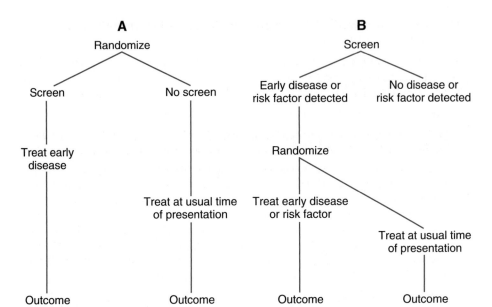

Figure 36-1. Designs for randomized controlled trials of screening.
A, Randomized controlled trial can assess the entire screening process,
in which case participants are randomized to be screened (and treated)
or not screened. **B,** Alternatively, everyone can participate in the
screening, and those with positive results are randomized to be treated or
not treated. *(Modified and reproduced with permission of the American Medical
Association from Barratt A, Irwig L, Glasziou P, et al. Users' guides to the medical
literature. XVII. How to use guidelines and recommendations about screening. JAMA.
1999;281:2029–2034.)*

use this study design when screening detects factors that increase the risk of disease rather
than the disease itself. Tests of screening programs for hypertension and high cholesterol
have used this design.[11,12] The principles outlined in this chapter apply to both of these
study designs (see Figure 36-1) when used to address screening issues.

Regardless of which design is used (see Figure 36-1), a successful outcome of
screening depends on optimal, or at least appropriate, application of testing and treatment after a positive screening test. One way that investigators can deal with this issue is
to include recommendations for the investigative tests and interventions to be delivered
if the target condition is detected. The limitation of this approach is that it may not
simulate usual clinical practice and thus may limit the applicability of the results.
An alternative is to allow clinicians to manage patients as they ordinarily would and document the investigative tests and interventions they use. Without such monitoring, the
clinical community may be unaware that the reason screening failed to improve outcome
was because of suboptimal management of patients with positive screening results.

Were the Data Identified, Selected, and Combined in an Unbiased Fashion?

As is true for all systematic reviews and guidelines, developers must specify the inclusion and exclusion criteria for the studies they choose to consider, conduct a comprehensive search, and assess the methodological quality of the studies they include.

USING THE GUIDE

In their systematic review, Towler and colleagues[1] identified four randomized controlled trials that evaluated the effectiveness of screening with the FOBT Hemoccult.[13–16] Three trials[14–16] randomly allocated individuals or households identified from general practitioner records or population registers to invitation to screening with Hemoccult or control groups, and one trial[13] allocated volunteers to screening or control groups. Meta-analysis of the results of the four randomized controlled trials showed that those allocated to screening had a 16% reduction in the relative risk of dying of colorectal cancer (relative risk, 0.84; 95% confidence interval, 0.77 to 0.93).

The AGA guideline[2] states that three randomized controlled trials[13–15] (all included in the systematic review) showed that testing of two samples from each of three consecutive stools for the presence of occult blood using a guaiac-impregnated slide test reduced the risk of death from colorectal cancer. One of the trials included in the systematic review[16] was not cited in the AGA guideline, possibly because the authors had not yet published mortality data but had provided these data for the meta-analysis via personal communication. After completion of the systematic review, investigators of one of the trials[13] reported an 18-year follow-up of study participants in which they found that FOBT screening every other year reduced colorectal cancer mortality by 21%.[17]

Towler and colleagues[1] searched for published and unpublished trials and assessed the quality of individual trials using criteria recommended by the Cochrane Collaboration.[18] The investigators abstracted data from the trials and combined them in a meta-analysis on an intention-to-screen basis.

For the AGA guideline,[2] panel members updated the original guideline[19] by conducting literature searches, preparing evidence tables to summarize scientifically strong studies that were relevant to colorectal cancer screening and surveillance, and circulating the tables to the entire panel for comments. The panel then met to critique the new evidence and used a consensus process to draft guidelines.

WHAT ARE THE RECOMMENDATIONS?

A good guideline should summarize the trial evidence about the benefits and risks of a screening program, for example, in a balance sheet.[20] The guideline should also provide information about how the benefits and risks might vary in population subgroups and with different screening strategies.

What Are the Benefits?

Which *outcomes* need to be measured to estimate the benefits of a screening program? Some of the people who test positive will experience a reduction in mortality or an increase in quality of life. The benefit can be estimated as an absolute risk reduction (ARR) or a relative risk reduction (RRR) in adverse outcomes such as mortality (or an absolute benefit increase [ABI] or a relative benefit increase [RBI] in positive outcomes such as improved quality of life) (see Chapter 27, Measures of Association). Briefly, the ARR depends on the baseline risk of disease and thus presents a more realistic estimate of the size of the mortality benefit. By contrast, the RRR is independent of baseline risk and may provide a misleading impression of benefit (Table 36-3). The number of people needed to screen to prevent an adverse outcome is another way of representing the benefit of screening (see Chapter 27, Measures of Association, and Chapter 32, Number Needed to Treat).

When the benefit is a reduction in mortality, we would like to see a reduction in both disease-specific mortality and total mortality. However, because the target condition is typically only one of many causes of death, even important reductions in disease-specific mortality are unlikely to result in statistically significant reductions in total mortality (i.e., mortality from any and all possible causes). In some conditions with high mortality rates, it may be reasonable to expect reductions in both total and disease-specific mortality. An example is screening and treatment for high cholesterol in people who already have symptomatic heart disease. In this instance, the risk of death from heart disease is high and is the most likely cause of death. Meta-analyses have shown significant effects of screening and treatment on both disease-specific and total mortality.[21] For the most part, we will have to be satisfied with demonstrated reductions in disease-specific mortality, although it is reassuring if data show no increase in total mortality.

In addition to prevention of adverse outcomes, people may also regard knowledge of the presence of an abnormality as a benefit, as in antenatal screening for Down syndrome. Another potential benefit of screening comes from the reassurance afforded by

Table 36-3   Comparison of Data Presented as Relative and Absolute Risk Reductions and Number Needed to Screen With Varying Baseline Risks of Disease and Constant Relative Risk

Baseline Risk (Risk in Unscreened Group)	Risk in Screened Group	Relative Risk Reduction	Absolute Risk Reduction	Number Needed to Screen
4%	2%	50%	2%	50
2%	1%	50%	1%	100
1%	0.5%	50%	0.5%	200
0.1%	0.05%	50%	0.05%	2000

Modified and reproduced with permission of the American Medical Association from Barratt A, Irwig L, Glasziou P, et al. Users' guides to the medical literature. XVII. How to use guidelines and recommendations about screening. JAMA. 1999;281:2029–2034.

a negative test, particularly in people who feel anxious because a family member or friend has developed the target condition or because of discussion in the popular media. However, a person's self-perception of being "at risk" can be enhanced rather than reduced by testing. When people experience anxiety as a result of publicity surrounding the screening program itself, we would not view anxiety reduction as a benefit. For example, assume that women are not anxious about breast cancer. However, extensive publicity about a new screening program for breast cancer causes them to become anxious. The screening program should not be credited with achieving a benefit if women's anxiety—generated by the publicity of the screening test—decreases after negative screening test results.

Testing for fecal occult blood can be done using guaiac-based or immunochemical tests, both of which can detect blood in the stool. The sensitivity of guaiac-based tests is increased if the test slide is rehydrated with a few drops of water before adding the hydrogen peroxide reagent. However, although rehydration increases sensitivity, the readability of the test is unpredictable, and rehydration substantially increases the false-positive rate. Because elements of an ordinary diet can cause false-positive reactions of guaiac-based tests, the person being tested may be asked to restrict intake of red meat and certain vegetables. The AGA guideline[2] reports that offering yearly FOBT with rehydration reduced colorectal cancer deaths by 33% after 13 years; biennial testing reduced colorectal cancer deaths by 15% and 18% after 7.8 and 10 years, respectively, without rehydration[14,15] and 21% at 18 years with rehydration.[17] The guideline recommends against the use of rehydration for the reasons cited earlier. An estimate of the uncertainty associated with these RRRs (e.g., the 95% confidence interval around a pooled RRR) would help readers to appreciate the range within which the true RRR plausibly lies. Based on a computer simulation using data from the original AGA guideline for annual screening with FOBT,[19] and assuming 100% participation, screening of 100,000 people beginning at age 50 years and continuing until age 85 or death would result in a reduction of 1330 deaths (13.3 per 1000) from colon cancer (Table 36-4).[22]

What Are the Risks?

Among those who test positive, adverse consequences may include the following:
1. Complications arising from investigation
2. Side effects of treatment
3. Unnecessary treatment of persons with true-positive results but inconsequential disease
4. Adverse effects of labeling or early diagnosis
5. Anxiety generated by investigations and treatment
6. Costs and inconvenience incurred during investigations and treatment

The AGA guideline[2] reports that most people who test positive do not have colorectal neoplasia (i.e., have *false-positive* test results) and thus undergo the discomfort, cost, and risk of colonoscopy without benefit. In the trials, only 2% to 6% of those who tested positive actually had colon cancer. Thus, for every 100 participants who have a positive test result, only 2 to 6 will have cancer, but all 100 will be exposed to colonoscopy and its attendant risks (see Table 36-4). Although colonoscopies will reveal few cancers, they will show many polyps (25% of people aged 50 years or older have polyps, some of which will be judged to need removal, depending on their size). Part of the benefit of screening will come from removal of the small proportion of polyps that would have

Table **36-4** Clinical Consequences for 1000 People Entering a Program of Annual Fecal Occult Blood Test Screening for Colorectal Cancer at Age 50 Years and Remaining in it Until Age 85 or Death

Clinical Consequences	Number of Events in 1000 People
Risks	
Screening tests	27,030
Diagnostic evaluations (by colonoscopy)	2263
False-positive screening tests	2158
Deaths from colonoscopy complications	0.5
Bowel perforations from colonoscopy	3
Major bleeding episodes from colonoscopy	7.4
Minor complications from colonoscopy	7.7
Benefits	
Deaths averted	13.3
Years of life saved	123.3
Years of life gained per person whose cancer death was prevented	9.3

(Data from Winawer S, Fletcher R, Rex D, et al. Colorectal cancer screening and surveillance: clinical guidelines and rationale—update based on new evidence.Gastroenterology. 2003;124:544-560.)
(Modified and reproduced with permission of the American Medical Association from Barratt A, Irwig L, Glasziou P, et al. Users' guides to the medical literature. XVII. How to use guidelines and recommendations about screening. JAMA. 1999;281:2029–2034.)

progressed to invasive cancer. Part of the risk of screening will come from regular colonoscopies that are recommended for people who have had benign or inconsequential polyps removed. The AGA guideline[2] includes certain recommendations to reduce the false-positive rate, including avoiding rehydration when examining stools and restricting diet for the more sensitive guaiac-based tests.

Among those who test negative, adverse consequences may include the following:

1. Anxiety generated by the screening test (waiting for result)
2. False reassurance (and delayed presentation of symptomatic disease later)
3. Costs and inconvenience incurred during the screening test

According to the AGA guideline,[2] the sensitivity of a single FOBT is low, ranging from 30% to 50%. Patients who present with symptoms after a *false-negative* result may experience a sense of anger and betrayal that they would not suffer in the absence of a screening program.

Using computer simulation, the original AGA guideline[19] presents data on the frequency of some of these risks. Table 36-4 summarizes data for 1000 people, 50 to 85 years of age, who participate in annual screening by FOBT. The model assumes that those who test positive undergo colonoscopy.

We now know the magnitude of both benefits and risks (as presented in Table 36-4). This balance sheet tells us that screening 1000 people annually with FOBT from age

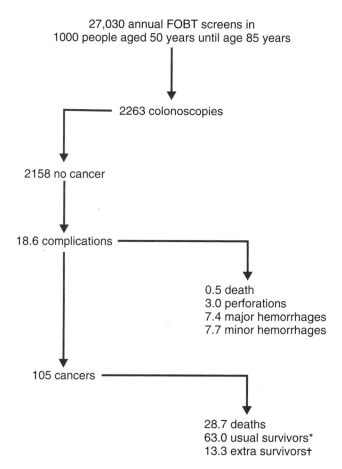

Figure 36-2. Clinical consequences for 1000 people in a program of annual fecal occult blood test screening for colorectal cancer. FOBT, Fecal occult blood test *Usual survivors are those who would have survived with or without screening †Extra survivors are those in whom the earlier detection of cancer averts death. *(Data from Winawer S, Fletcher R, Rex D, et al. Colorectal cancer screening and surveillance: clinical guidelines and rationale—update based on new evidence. Gastroenterology. 2003;124:544-560. Modified and reproduced with permission of the American Medical Association from Barratt A, Irwig L, Glasziou P, et al. Users' guides to the medical literature. XVII. How to use guidelines and recommendations about screening. Evidence-Based Medicine Working Group. JAMA. 1999;281:2029–2034.)*

50 years will prevent 13.3 deaths from colorectal cancer but will cause 0.5 deaths from complications of investigation and surgery. There will also be 10.4 major complications (perforations and major bleeding episodes) and 7.7 minor complications. The authors provide no data on anxiety, but we can assume that some people will feel anxious before colonoscopy. Figure 36-2[22] presents these data as a flow diagram.

These data assume that the screening programs will deliver the same magnitude of benefits and risks as found in randomized controlled trials, but this will be true only if the programs are delivered to the same standard of quality as those in the trials. Otherwise, the benefits will be smaller, and the risks will be greater.

CAN I APPLY THE RECOMMENDATIONS TO PATIENT CARE?

How Do Benefits and Risks Compare in Different People and With Different Screening Strategies?

The AGA guideline[2] recommends that clinicians offer screening for colorectal cancer to men and women at average risk beginning at age 50 years. The authors of the guideline recommend any one of several screening strategies, including FOBT, sigmoidoscopy, combined FOBT and flexible sigmoidoscopy, colonoscopy, and double-contrast barium enema, because no single test is unequivocally superior and giving patients a choice allows them to apply personal preferences. In relation to FOBT, the authors of the guideline recommend annual screening. The magnitude of benefits and adverse consequences will vary in different patients and with different screening strategies, as the following discussion reveals.

Risk for Disease

Assuming that the RRR is constant over a broad range of disease risk, benefits will be greater for people at higher risk for disease. For example, mortality from colorectal cancer increases with age, and the mortality benefit achieved by screening increases accordingly (Figure 36-3, top).[22] However, life-years lost to colorectal cancer are related to both the age at which mortality is highest and the length of life still available. Thus, the number of life-years that can be saved by colorectal cancer screening increases with age to about 75 years and then decreases again as life expectancy declines (Figure 36-3, bottom).[22] The number of deaths averted by screening over 10 years for those aged 40, 50, and 60 years at first screening (0.2, 1.0, and 2.4 per 1000 people, respectively[1]) reflects these differences. Because of greater benefits, it may be rational for a person aged 60 years to decide that screening is worthwhile, whereas a person aged 40 years (or 80 years) with smaller potential benefits could decide that it is not worthwhile.

Risk for disease—and therefore the benefits of screening—may be increased by other factors, such as family history of disease. The AGA guideline[2] reports that people with a first-degree relative (parent, sibling, or child) or two second-degree relatives (grandparents, aunts, and uncles) with colorectal cancer should be advised to begin having colonoscopies at age 40 years. This recommendation is based on their estimate that the incidence of colorectal cancer in people aged 40 years who have a first-degree relative with colorectal cancer is comparable to that of people aged 50 years who do not have a family history of disease.

Screening Interval

As the screening interval is shortened, the effectiveness of a screening program will tend to improve, although there is a limit to the amount of improvement that is possible. For example, screening twice as often could theoretically double the relative mortality reduction obtained by screening, but in practice, the effect is usually much less. Cervical

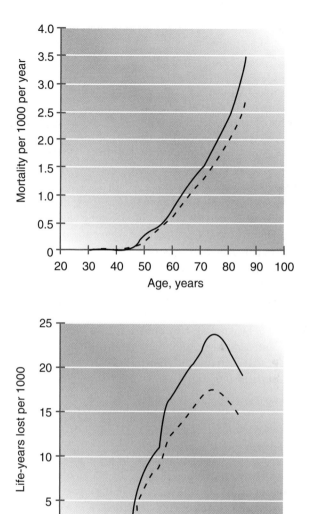

Figure 36-3. Mortality from colorectal cancer and years of life lost due to colorectal cancer with and without screening. **Top,** Mortality from colorectal cancer. **Bottom,** Life-years lost due to colorectal cancer. Broken lines indicate with screening, solid lines without screening. *(Data from Towler BP, Irwig L, Glasziou P, Weller D, Kewenter J. Screening for colorectal cancer using the faecal occult blood test, Hemoccult.* Cochrane Database Syst Rev. *2000;(2):CD001216.) (Modified and reproduced with permission of the American Medical Association from Barratt A, Irwig L, Glasziou P, et al. Users' guides to the medical literature. XVII. How to use guidelines and recommendations about screening.* JAMA. *1999;281: 2029–2034.)*

cancer screening, for instance, may reduce the incidence of invasive cervical cancer by 64%, 84%, and 94% if screening is conducted at 10-year, 5-year, and 1-year intervals, respectively.[23]

The frequency of risks also will increase with more frequent screening, potentially in direct proportion to the frequency of screening. Thus, we will see diminishing marginal return as the screening interval is shortened. Ultimately, the marginal risks will outweigh the marginal benefits of further reductions in the screening interval. The AGA guideline recommends yearly screening with FOBT using a guaiac-based test with dietary restriction or an immunochemical test without dietary restriction.

Test Characteristics

If the sensitivity of a new test is greater than that of the test used in the trials and if it detects significant disease earlier, the benefit of screening will increase. However, it may be that the new, apparently more sensitive, test is detecting more cases of inconsequential disease (e.g., more low-grade prostate cancers or more low-grade cervical epithelial abnormalities[24]), which will increase the potential for risk. Conversely, if specificity is improved and testing produces fewer false-positive results, net benefit will increase, and the new test may be useful in groups in which the old test was not as useful.

Ideally, clinicians should look to randomized trials of the new test compared with the old test (see Chapter 6, Diagnosis). However, new tests often appear in profusion, and randomized trials are expensive and often require long follow-up periods. Being pragmatic, we accept that if trials have shown that earlier detection reduces the risk of adverse effects, a comparison of a new and an old test only needs to examine test characteristics.

In the case of colorectal cancer screening, randomized trials have shown reduced mortality after early detection by FOBT, and thus, we may assume that early detection works in principle. It seems reasonable to assume that early detection using other methods, such as flexible sigmoidoscopy, will also reduce mortality from colorectal cancer even though there are no published reports of randomized trials of the effects of screening with flexible sigmoidoscopy on mortality. This theoretical approach is supported by the available observational data, which indicate benefits from other methods of screening for colorectal cancer.[2]

What Is the Impact of Individuals' Values and Preferences?

The ways and extent to which people value the benefits and risk of screening can vary. For example, pregnant women who are considering fetal screening for Down syndrome may make different choices depending on the value they place on having a child with Down syndrome, as opposed to the risk of iatrogenic abortion from amniocentesis.[25]

Perception plays a large role. Persons who choose to participate in screening programs are benefiting (in their view) from screening, and others are benefiting (in their view) from not participating. Individuals can make the right choice for themselves only if they have access to high-quality information about the benefits and risks of screening and if they are able to weigh that information. This probably will require better educational and decision-support materials than traditionally have been provided, although some examples of such materials are already available.[26,27]

What Is the Impact of Uncertainty Associated With the Evidence?

Uncertainty about the benefits and risks of screening will always exist. The 95% confidence intervals around the estimates of each benefit and adverse consequence provide an indication of the amount of uncertainty for each estimate. Studies with small sample sizes will have wider confidence intervals, and nurses should explain to potential screening participants that the magnitude of benefits or risks could be considerably smaller or greater than the *point estimate.*

What Is the Cost-effectiveness?

Although clinicians will be most interested in the balance of benefits and risks for individual patients, policy makers must consider issues of cost-effectiveness and local resources in their decisions (see Chapter 18, Economic Evaluation).

The AGA guideline[2] reports that cost-effectiveness analyses have shown that each of the screening strategies recommended (FOBT, flexible sigmoidoscopy, colonoscopy, and double-contrast barium enema) costs less than US$25,000 per year of life saved.[28-31] This cost per year of life saved is within the range of what is currently paid in some countries for the benefits of other screening programs, such as mammographic screening for women aged 50 to 69 years (estimated at US$21,400 per life-year saved[32]), ultrasound screening for patients with carotid stenosis (estimated incremental cost per quality-adjusted life-year gained of US$39,495[33]), and ultrasound screening for abdominal aortic aneurysm in men aged 60 to 80 years (estimated US$41,550 per life-year gained[34]). Costs increase out of proportion to benefits with shorter intervals between screening examinations.

CLINICAL RESOLUTION

A clinical practice guideline should quantify the benefits of screening according to age so that accurate information can be provided to individual patients about the potential benefits of screening. The AGA guideline does not provide age-specific mortality reductions attributable to screening, and therefore, you cannot easily quantify the benefits for the couple in your practice. Based on the AGA guideline, you can say with confidence that screening a group of 1000 people with FOBT beginning at age 50 years and continuing annually to age 85 will avert about 13 deaths from colorectal cancer. We know from the systematic review by Towler and colleagues[1] that the mortality benefit for people 40 to 50 years of age is about 0.2 to 1.0 deaths averted over 10 years per 1000 people screened. The AGA guideline cites a study of screening colonoscopy[35] in people 40 to 49 years of age that confirms that colorectal cancers are uncommon in this age group and estimates that at least 250 persons, and perhaps 1000 or more, would need to be screened to detect a single case of cancer in this age group.

Based on these data and given the couple's age, negative family history, and lack of symptoms, you explain that the absolute benefit of screening with FOBT at their age is extremely small. Next, you outline the potential risks of screening. According to the computer simulation based on the original AGA guideline,[19] for every 1000 people screened annually with FOBT, there will be 0.5 deaths, 3.0 bowel perforations, 7.4 major bleeding episodes, and 7.7 minor complications related to colonoscopy. In addition, issues of cost, inconvenience, and anxiety should be considered.

Continued

CLINICAL RESOLUTION—CONT'D

The couple must determine whether the benefit of reduced risk of death from colorectal cancer is worth the potential adverse consequences such as the inconvenience and potential complications of colonoscopy, the adverse effects of early treatment for colon cancer, side effects of treatment, and the anxiety generated by the investigations and treatment.

If the couple feels that they are unable to weigh the benefits and risks, you could help them to clarify their values about the possible outcomes. For example, if they are not bothered by the prospect of colonoscopy, they would probably choose to be screened. However, if either of them places a high value on avoiding colonoscopy now, he or she may prefer to reconsider screening in a few years, when the benefits will be greater than they are at the present time.

REFERENCES

1. Towler BP, Irwig L, Glasziou P, Weller D, Kewenter J. Screening for colorectal cancer using the faecal occult blood test, Hemoccult. *Cochrane Database Syst Rev.* 2000;(2):CD001216.
2. Winawer S, Fletcher R, Rex D, et al. Colorectal cancer screening and surveillance: clinical guidelines and rationale—update based on new evidence. *Gastroenterology.* 2003;124:544-560.
3. Wilson JMG, Jungner G. *Principles and Practice of Screening for Disease.* Geneva: World Health Organization; 1968.
4. Gray JA. *Evidence-Based Healthcare.* London: Churchill Livingstone; 1997.
5. Sackett DL, Haynes RB, Tugwell P. *Clinical Epidemiology: A Basic Science for Clinical Medicine.* 2nd ed. Boston: Little, Brown; 1991.
6. Welch HG, Black WC. Evaluating randomized trials of screening. *J Gen Intern Med.* 1997;12:118-124.
7. Khaw KT, Rose G. Cholesterol screening programmes: how much potential benefit? *BMJ.* 1989;299:606-607.
8. Andersson I, Aspegren K, Janzon L, et al. Mammographic screening and mortality from breast cancer: the Malmo mammographic screening trial. *BMJ.* 1988;297:943-948.
9. Tabar L, Fagerberg G, Duffy SW, Day NE. The Swedish two county trial of mammographic screening for breast cancer: recent results and calculation of benefit. *J Epidemiol Community Health.* 1989;43:107-114.
10. Roberts MM, Alexander FE, Anderson TJ, et al. Edinburgh trial of screening for breast cancer: mortality at seven years. *Lancet.* 1990;335:241-246.
11. Multiple Risk Factor Intervention Trial Research Group. Multiple risk factor intervention trial: risk factor changes and mortality results. *JAMA.* 1982;248:1465-1477.
12. Frick MH, Elo O, Haapa K, et al. Helsinki Heart Study: primary-prevention trial with gemfibrozil in middle-aged men with dyslipidemia. Safety of treatment, changes in risk factors, and incidence of coronary heart disease. *N Engl J Med.* 1987;317:1237-1245.
13. Mandel JS, Bond JH, Church TR, et al. Reducing mortality from colorectal cancer by screening for fecal occult blood. *N Engl J Med.* 1993;328:1365-1371.
14. Hardcastle JD, Chamberlain JO, Robinson MHE, et al. Randomised controlled trial of faecal-occult-blood screening for colorectal cancer. *Lancet.* 1996;348:1472-1477.
15. Kronborg O, Fenger C, Olsen J, Jorgensen OD, Sondergaard O. Randomised study of screening for colorectal cancer with faecal-occult-blood test. *Lancet.* 1996;348:1467-1471.
16. Kewenter J, Brevinge H, Engaras B, Haglind E, Ahren C. Results of screening, rescreening, and follow-up in a prospective randomized study for detection of colorectal cancer by fecal occult blood testing. Results for 68,308 subjects. *Scand J Gastroenterol.* 1994;29:468-473.
17. Mandel JS, Church TR, Ederer F, Bond JH. Colorectal cancer mortality: effectiveness of biennial screening for fecal occult blood. *J Natl Cancer Inst.* 1999;91:434-437.

18. Mulrow CD, Oxman AD, eds. Critical Appraisal of Studies. Cochrane Collaboration Handbook (updated September 1997); section 4. In: *The Cochrane Library* (database on disk and CD-ROM). Cochrane Collaboration. Oxford: Update Software; 1997, issue 4.

19. Winawer SJ, Fletcher RH, Millar L, et al. Colorectal cancer screening: clinical guidelines and rationale. *Gastroenterology*. 1997;112:594-642.

20. Eddy DM. Comparing benefits and harms: the balance sheet. *JAMA*. 1990;263:2493, 2498, 2501.

21. Barratt A, Irwig L. Is cholesterol testing/treatment really beneficial? *Med J Aust*. 1993;159:644-647.

22. Barratt A, Irwig L, Glasziou P, et al. Users' guides to the medical literature. XVII. How to use guidelines and recommendations about screening. *JAMA*. 1999;281:2029-2034.

23. IARC Working Group on Evaluation of Cervical Cancer Screening Programmes. Screening for squamous cervical cancer: duration of low risk after negative results of cervical cytology and its implication for screening policies. *Br Med J Clin Res Ed*. 1986;293:659-664.

24. Raffle AE. New tests in cervical screening. *Lancet*. 1998;351:297.

25. Fletcher J, Hicks NR, Kay JD, Boyd PA. Using decision analysis to compare policies for antenatal screening for Down's syndrome. *BMJ*. 1995;311:351-356.

26. Wolf AM, Nasser JF, Wolf AM, Schorling JB. The impact of informed consent on patient interest in prostate-specific antigen screening. *Arch Intern Med*. 1996;156:1333-1336.

27. Flood AB, Wennberg JE, Nease RF Jr, Fowler FJ Jr, Ding J, Hynes LM, for the Prostate Patient Outcomes Research Team. The importance of patient preference in the decision to screen for prostate cancer. *J Gen Intern Med*. 1996;11:342-349.

28. Wagner JL, Tunis S, Brown M, Ching A, Almeida R. Cost-effectiveness of colorectal cancer screening in average-risk adults. In: Young G, Rozen P, Levin B, eds. *Prevention and Early Detection of Colorectal Cancer*. London: WB Saunders; 1996:321-356.

29. Frazier AL, Colditz GA, Fuchs CS, Kuntz KM. Cost-effectiveness of screening for colorectal cancer in the general population. *JAMA*. 2000;284:1954-1961.

30. Loeve F, Brown ML, Boer R, van Ballegooijen M, van Oortmarssen GJ, Habbema JD. Endoscopic colorectal cancer screening: a cost-saving analysis. *J Natl Cancer Inst*. 2000;92:557-563.

31. Sonnenberg A, Delco F, Inadomi JM. Cost-effectiveness of colonoscopy in screening for colorectal cancer. *Ann Intern Med*. 2000;133:573-584.

32. Salzmann P, Kerlikowske K, Phillips K. Cost-effectiveness of extending screening mammography guidelines to include women 40 to 49 years of age. *Ann Intern Med*. 1997;127:955-965.

33. Yin D, Carpenter JP. Cost-effectiveness of screening for asymptomatic carotid stenosis. *J Vasc Surg*. 1998;27:245-255.

34. Frame PS, Fryback DG, Patterson C. Screening for abdominal aortic aneurysm in men ages 60 to 80 years: a cost-effectiveness analysis. *Ann Intern Med*. 1993;119:411-416.

35. Imperiale TF, Wagner DR, Lin CY, Larkin GN, Rogge JD, Ransohoff DF. Results of screening colonoscopy among persons 40 to 49 years of age. *N Engl J Med*. 2002;346:1781-1785.

Appendix

Calculations

Raymond Leung

In the Appendix

Measures of Association

Diagnostic Tests

Chance-Corrected Agreement: Kappa

Confidence Intervals

MEASURES OF ASSOCIATION

(See Chapter 4, Health Care Interventions; Chapter 5, Harm; and Chapter 27, Measures of Association.)

		Outcome	
		Present	Absent
Exposure/Intervention	Present	a	b
	Absent	c	d

Control Event Rate (CER)
$$= \frac{c}{c+d}$$

Experimental Event Rate (EER)
$$= \frac{a}{a+b}$$

Relative Risk (RR)
$$= \frac{a/(a+b)}{c/(c+d)}$$

Relative Risk Reduction (RRR)
$$= \frac{c/(c+d) - a/(a+b)}{c/(c+d)} \quad \text{or} \quad 1 - RR$$

Absolute Risk Reduction (ARR)
$$= \frac{c}{c+d} - \frac{a}{a+b}$$

Absolute Risk Increase (ARI)
$$= \frac{c}{c+d} - \frac{a}{a+b}$$

Number Needed to Treat (NNT)
$$= \frac{1}{ARR}$$

Number Needed to Harm (NNH)
$$= \frac{1}{ARI}$$

Odds Ratio (OR)
$$= \frac{a/b}{c/d} = \frac{ad}{bc}$$

Deriving number needed to treat from control event rate and odds ratio:

$$NNT = \frac{1 - [CER(1 - OR)]}{CER(1 - CER)(1 - OR)}$$

Deriving number needed to harm from control event rate and odds ratio:

$$NNH = \frac{1 + [CER(OR - 1)]}{CER(1 - CER)(OR - 1)}$$

DIAGNOSTIC TESTS

(See Chapter 6, Diagnosis.)

		Reference Standard	
		Positive	Negative
Test Result	Positive	a	b
	Negative	c	d

True Positive $\qquad = a$

True Negative $\qquad = d$

False Positive $\qquad = b$

False Negative $\qquad = c$

Sensitivity $\qquad = \dfrac{a}{a+c}$

Specificity $\qquad = \dfrac{d}{b+d}$

Likelihood Ratio for Positive Test (LR+) $\qquad = \dfrac{sensitivity}{1-specificity} = \dfrac{a/(a+c)}{b/(b+d)}$

Likelihood Ratio for Negative Test (LR−) $\qquad = \dfrac{1-sensitivity}{specificity} = \dfrac{c/(a+c)}{d/(b+d)}$

Positive Predictive Value (PPV) $\qquad = \dfrac{a}{a+b}$

Negative Predictive Value (NPV) $\qquad = \dfrac{d}{c+d}$

Diagnostic Accuracy $\qquad = \dfrac{a+d}{a+b+c+d}$

Pretest Probability (Prevalence) $\qquad = \dfrac{a+c}{a+b+c+d}$

Pretest Odds $\qquad = \dfrac{prevalence}{1-prevalence} = \dfrac{a+c}{b+d}$

Posttest Odds $\qquad = $ pretest odds × likelihood ratio

Posttest Probability $\qquad = $ posttest odds/(1 + posttest odds)

CHANCE-CORRECTED AGREEMENT: KAPPA

(See Chapter 30, Measuring Agreement Beyond Chance.)

		Rater B's Observation	
		Present	Absent
Rater A's Observation	Present	a	b
	Absent	c	d

Raw agreement $= \dfrac{a+d}{a+b+c+d}$

Kappa $= \dfrac{observed\ agreement - expected\ agreement}{1 - expected\ agreement}$

where observed agreement $= \dfrac{a+d}{a+b+c+d}$

and expected agreement $= \dfrac{(a+b)(a+c)}{(a+b+c+d)^2} + \dfrac{(c+d)(b+d)}{(a+b+c+d)^2}$

Odds Ratio (OR) $= \dfrac{ad}{bc}$

Phi $= \dfrac{\sqrt{OR}-1}{\sqrt{OR}+1} = \dfrac{\sqrt{ad}-\sqrt{bc}}{\sqrt{ad}+\sqrt{bc}}$

CONFIDENCE INTERVALS

(See Chapter 29, Confidence Intervals.)

The following is a 2 × 2 sample set:

	Column 1	Column 2	Total
Row 1	a	b	n
Row 2	c	d	m

Using the 2 × 2 sample set, the following confidence intervals can be calculated:[1]

	Point Estimate	Confidence Intervals	Examples
Binomial Proportion	$\dfrac{a}{n}$	$\dfrac{a}{n} \pm z\sqrt{\dfrac{a(n-a)}{n^3}}$	CER EER Sensitivity Specificity PPV NPV
Difference between 2 Proportions	$\dfrac{a}{n} - \dfrac{c}{m}$	$\left(\dfrac{a}{n} - \dfrac{c}{m}\right) \pm z\sqrt{\dfrac{a(n-a)}{n^3} + \dfrac{c(m-c)}{m^3}}$	ARR
Ratio between 2 Proportions	$\dfrac{a/n}{c/m}$	$\dfrac{a/n}{c/m}\, e^{\pm z\sqrt{\frac{1}{a}-\frac{1}{n}+\frac{1}{c}-\frac{1}{m}}}$	RR LR+ LR−
Ratio between 2 Ratios	$\dfrac{a/b}{c/d}$	$\dfrac{a/b}{c/d}\, e^{\pm z\sqrt{\frac{1}{a}+\frac{1}{b}+\frac{1}{c}+\frac{1}{d}}}$	OR

where z = 1.96 for 95% confidence interval and e = exponential constant = 2.718281828......

REFERENCE

1. SAS Institute Inc, SAS OnlineDoc, Version 8. Cary, NC: SAS Institute Inc; 1999. Available at: http://v8doc.sas.com/sashtml/. Accessed June 25, 2004.

Glossary

Absolute Benefit Increase (ABI)   The absolute arithmetic difference in rates of good outcomes between experimental (EER) and control groups (CER), calculated as rate of good outcome in experimental group minus rate of good outcome in control group (EER–CER).

Absolute Difference   The absolute arithmetic difference in rates of good or harmful outcomes between experimental (EER) and control groups (CER), calculated as event rate in experimental group minus event rate in control group (EER–CER).

Absolute Risk   The proportion of study participants who experience the harmful outcome in each comparison group.

Absolute Risk Increase (ARI)   The absolute arithmetic difference in rates of harmful outcomes between experimental (EER) and control groups (CER), calculated as rate of harmful outcome in experimental group minus rate of harmful outcome in control group (EER–CER). Typically used with a harmful exposure.

Absolute Risk Reduction (ARR)   The absolute arithmetic difference in rates of harmful outcomes between experimental (EER) and control groups (CER), calculated as rate of harmful outcome in experimental group minus rate of harmful outcome in control group (EER–CER). Use restricted to a beneficial exposure or intervention.

Academic Detailing (or Educational Outreach Visits)   A strategy for changing clinician behavior. Use of a trained person who meets with professionals in their practice settings to provide information with the intent of changing their practice.

Adjusted Analysis   An adjusted analysis takes into account differences in prognostic factors (or baseline characteristics) between groups that may influence the outcome. For instance, in a comparison between an experimental intervention and control, if the experimental group is on average older, and thus at higher risk of an adverse outcome than the control group, the adjusted analysis will show a larger intervention effect than the unadjusted analysis.

Alerting System   A type of computer decision support system that alerts the clinician to a circumstance that might require clinical action (e.g., a system that highlights patients' out-of-range laboratory values).

Allocation Concealment (or Concealment)   Randomization is concealed if the person who is making the decision about enrolling a patient is unaware of whether the next patient enrolled will be entered in the intervention or control group (using techniques such as central randomization or sequentially numbered opaque, sealed envelopes). If randomization is not concealed, patients with better prognoses may tend to be preferentially enrolled in the active intervention arm resulting in exaggeration of the apparent benefit of the intervention (or even falsely concluding that the intervention is efficacious).

Alpha Level The probability of erroneously concluding there is a difference between comparison groups when there is in fact no difference (type I error). Typically, investigators decide on the chance of a false-positive result they are willing to accept when they plan the sample size for a study (e.g., investigators often set alpha level at 0.05).

Artificial Neural Networks The application of nonlinear statistics to pattern recognition problems that can be used to develop clinical prediction rules. The technique identifies those predictors most strongly associated with the outcome of interest that belong in a clinical prediction rule and those that can be omitted from the rule without loss of predictive power.

Asymmetry Distribution of values is skewed (i.e., two halves that are not mirror images of each other). In a systematic review, asymmetry in a funnel plot may indicate publication bias.

Audit and Feedback A strategy for changing clinician behavior. Any written or verbal summary of clinician performance (e.g., based on chart review or observation of clinical practice) over a period of time. The summary may also include recommendations for clinical action.

Autocorrelation Occurs when the likelihood of an observation is not independent of its relationship with other observations. For example, autocorrelation occurs when a good day for a patient with chronic disease is more likely to follow a "good day" than a "bad day".

Axial Coding Second level of coding in a grounded theory study that involves categorizing, recategorizing, and condensing first level codes by connecting categories and subcategories.

Baseline Characteristics Factors that describe study participants at the beginning of the study (e.g., sex, age, disease severity); in comparison studies, it is important that these characteristics are initially similar in each group; if not balanced or if the imbalance is not statistically adjusted, these characteristics can cause confounding and can bias study results.

Baseline Risk The risk of an adverse outcome in the control group.

Bayesian Analysis An analysis that starts with a particular probability of an event (the prior probability) and incorporates new information to generate a revised probability (a posterior probability).

Before-After Design (or One-Group Pretest-Posttest Design) Study in which the investigators compare the status of study participants before and after the introduction of an intervention.

Bias A systematic error in the design, conduct or interpretation of a study that may cause a systematic deviation from the underlying truth.

   1. Channeling effect or Channeling bias Tendency for clinicians to prescribe treatment based on a patient's prognosis. As a result, in observational studies, treated patients are more likely to be high-risk patients than untreated patients, leading to a biased estimate of treatment effect.

2. Data completeness bias Using a computer decision support system (CDSS) to log episodes in the intervention group and using a manual system in the non-CDSS control group can create variation in the completeness of data.

3. Detection bias Tendency to look more carefully for an outcome in one of the comparison groups.

4. Expectation bias In data collection, an interviewer has information that influences her expectation of finding the exposure or outcome. In clinical practice, a clinician's assessment may be influenced by prior knowledge of the presence or absence of a disorder.

5. Incorporation bias Occurs when investigators study a diagnostic test that incorporates features of the target outcome.

6. Interviewer bias Greater probing by an interviewer in one of the groups being compared.

7. Publication bias Occurs when the publication of research depends on the direction of the study results and whether they are statistically significant.

8. Recall bias Occurs when patients who experience an adverse outcome have a different likelihood of recalling an exposure than patients who do not experience the adverse outcome independent of the true extent of exposure.

9. Social desirability bias Study participants misrepresent their responses in the direction of answers consistent with prevailing social norms or socially desirable behavior.

10. Surveillance bias Synonymous with detection bias, the tendency to look more carefully for an outcome in one of the comparison groups.

11. Verification bias Results of a diagnostic test influence whether patients are assigned to intervention group (sometimes called Work-up bias).

Blind (or Blinded or Masked) Patients, clinicians, those monitoring outcomes, judicial assessors of outcomes, data analysts, and/or those writing the paper are unaware of which patients have been assigned to the experimental or control group.

Boolean Operators (or Logical Operators) Words used when searching electronic databases. These operators are AND, OR, and NOT and are used to combine terms (AND/OR) or exclude terms (NOT) from the search strategy.

Bootstrap Technique A statistical technique for estimating parameters such as standard errors and confidence intervals based upon resampling from an observed data set with replacement from the original sample.

Case-Control Study A study designed to determine the association between an exposure and outcome in which study participants are sampled by outcome. Those with the outcome (cases) are compared to those without the outcome (controls) with respect to exposure to the suspected harmful agent.

Case Reports Descriptions of individual patients.

Case Series A study reporting on a consecutive collection of patients treated in a similar manner, without a control group. For example, a clinician might describe the outcome for 25 consecutive patients with diabetes who received education for prevention of foot ulcers.

Case Study An exploration of a "bounded system" or contemporary phenomenon within its real-life context, especially when the boundaries between phenomenon and context are not clearly evident.

Categorical Variable (or Nominal Variable) A variable with discrete values rather than values incrementally placed along a continuum (e.g., marital status, gender, race).

Chance-Corrected Agreement The proportion of possible agreement achieved beyond what one would expect by chance alone (kappa statistic).

Channeling Bias (or Channeling Effect) Tendency for clinicians to prescribe treatment based on a patient's prognosis. As a result, in observational studies, treated patients are more likely to be high-risk patients than untreated patients, leading to a biased estimate of treatment effect.

Chi-Square Test A nonparametric test of statistical significance used to compare the distribution of categorical outcomes in two or more groups, the null hypothesis of which is that the underlying distributions are identical.

Clinical Decision Rules (or Decision Rules), Clinical Prediction Rules (or Prediction Rules) A guide for practice that is generated by initially examining, and ultimately combining, a number of variables to predict the likelihood of a current diagnosis or a future event. Sometimes, if the likelihood is sufficiently high or low, the rule generates a suggested course of action.

Clinical Practice Guidelines (or Practice Guidelines) Systematically developed statements or recommendations to assist practitioner and patient decisions about appropriate health care for specific clinical circumstances. They present indications for performing a test, procedure, or intervention, or the proper management for specific clinical problems. Guidelines may be developed by government agencies, institutions, organizations such as professional societies or governing boards, or by convening expert panels.

Clinical Prediction Rules (or Prediction Rules), Clinical Decision Rules (or Decision Rules) A guide for practice that is generated by initially examining, and ultimately combining, a number of variables to predict the likelihood of a current diagnosis or a future event. Sometimes, if the likelihood is sufficiently high or low, the rule generates a suggested course of action.

Cluster Analysis A statistical procedure in which the unit of analysis is the cluster (e.g., school, clinic) rather than individual study participants.

Cluster Assignment The assignment of groups (e.g., schools, clinics) rather than individuals to comparison groups. This approach is often used in cases where assignment by individuals is likely to result in contamination (e.g., if adolescents within a school are assigned to receive or not receive a new sex education program, it is likely that they will share the information they learn with one another (contamination); instead, schools (clusters) form the unit of assignment meaning that entire schools are assigned to receive or not receive the new sex education program).

Cohort A group of persons with a common characteristic or set of characteristics. Typically, the group is followed for a specified period of time to determine the incidence of a disorder or complications of an established disorder (prognosis).

Cohort Study (or Longitudinal Study or Prospective Study) When used to study potential causes of a disorder, it is a prospective investigation in which a cohort of individuals who do not have evidence of an outcome of interest but who are exposed to the putative cause are compared with a concurrent cohort who are also free of the outcome but not exposed to the putative cause. Both cohorts are then followed forward in time to compare the incidence of the outcome of interest. When used to study the effectiveness of an intervention, it is a prospective investigation in which a cohort of individuals who receive the intervention are compared with a concurrent cohort who do not receive the intervention. Both cohorts are then followed forward in time to compare the incidence of the outcome of interest.

Cointervention Intervention other than intervention under study that may be differentially applied to intervention and control groups and, thus, potentially bias the results of a study.

Comorbidity Disease(s) that coexist(s) in study participants in addition to the index condition that is the subject of the study.

Complete Follow-Up The investigators are aware of the outcome in every patient who participated in a study.

Computer Decision Support System (CDSS) Computer software designed to aid in clinical decision-making about individual patients.

Concealment (or Allocation Concealment) Randomization is concealed if the person who is making the decision about enrolling a patient is unaware of whether the next patient enrolled will be entered in the intervention or control group (using techniques such as central randomization or sequentially numbered opaque, sealed envelopes). If randomization is not concealed, patients with better prognoses may tend to be preferentially enrolled in the active intervention arm resulting in exaggeration of the apparent benefit of intervention (or even falsely concluding that the intervention is efficacious).

Conceptual Framework An organization of interrelated ideas or concepts that provides a system of relationships between those ideas or concepts.

Conditional Probability The probability of a particular state, given another state (i.e., the probability of A, given B).

Confidence Interval (CI) Range between two values within which it is probable that the true value lies for the whole population of patients from which the study patients were selected.

Confounder (or Confounding Variable) A factor that distorts the true relationship of the study variable of interest by virtue of also being related to the outcome of interest. Confounders are often unequally distributed among the groups being compared. Randomized studies are less likely to have their results distorted by confounders than are observational studies.

Consecutive Sample (or Sequential Sample) A sample in which all potentially eligible patients seen over a period of time are enrolled.

Consequentialist (or Utilitarian) A consequentialist or utilitarian view of distributive justice would contend that even in individual decision making, the clinician should take a broad social view in which the action that would provide the greatest good to the greatest number is favored. In this broader view, the effect on others of allocating resources to a particular patient's care would bear on the decision. An alternative to the deontological view.

Consistency A key element to consider when grading the quality of evidence for a health care recommendation. Refers to the similarity of estimates of effect across studies; higher scores are given if the direction of the effect, the size of the differences, and the statistical significance of differences are similar across studies.

Constant Comparison A procedure used in qualitative research wherein newly collected data are compared in an ongoing fashion with data obtained earlier, to refine theoretically relevant categories.

Construct Validity A construct is a theoretically derived notion of the domain(s) we wish to measure. An understanding of the construct will lead to expectations about how an instrument should behave if it is valid. Construct validity therefore involves comparisons between measures, and examination of the logical relationships, which should exist between a measure and characteristics of patients and patient groups.

Contamination Occurs when participants in either the experimental or control group receive the intervention intended for the other arm of the study.

Continuous Variable A variable that can theoretically take any value and in practice can take a large number of values with small differences between them (e.g., height).

Control Event Rate (CER) Proportion of study participants in the control group in whom an event is observed.

Control Group A group that does not receive the experimental intervention. In many studies, the control group receives either usual care or a placebo.

Controlled Before-and-After Study A design in which the investigator identifies a control group or setting that has similar characteristics to the intervention group but is not exposed to the intervention, and collects data from both groups before and after the intervention.

Controlled Interrupted Time–Series Design This design incorporates a control group into an interrupted time–series study. Data are collected at several times both before and after the intervention in the intervention group and at the same times in a control group that does not receive the intervention. Data collected before the intervention allow the underlying trend and cyclical (seasonal) effects to be estimated. Data collected after the intervention allow the intervention effect to be estimated while accounting for underlying secular trends. The incorporation of a control group addresses the greatest threat to the validity of a time-series design: the occurrence of another event at the same time as the intervention, both of which may be associated with the outcome.

Controlled Trial (or Randomized Trial or Randomized Controlled Trial) Experiment in which individuals are randomly allocated to receive or not receive an experimental preventive, therapeutic, or diagnostic procedure and then followed to determine the effect of the intervention.

Convenience Sample Individuals or groups selected at the convenience of the investigator or primarily because they were available at a convenient time or place.

Correlation The magnitude of the relationship between two different variables or phenomena.

Correlation Coefficient A numerical expression of the magnitude and direction of the relationship between two variables, which can take values from –1.0 (perfect negative relationship) to 0 (no relationship) to 1.0 (perfect positive relationship).

Cost Analysis   An economic analysis in which only costs of various alternatives are compared. This comparison informs only the resource-use half of the decision (the other half being the expected outcomes).

Cost-Benefit Analysis   An economic analysis in which both the costs and the consequences (including increases in the length and quality of life) are expressed in monetary terms.

Cost-Effectiveness Analysis   An economic analysis in which the consequences are expressed in natural units. Examples include cost per life saved or cost per unit of blood pressure lowered.

Cost-Minimization Analysis   An economic analysis conducted in situations where the consequences of the alternatives are identical, and the only issue is their relative costs.

Cost-to-Charge Ratio   Where there is a systematic deviation between costs and charges, an economic analysis may adjust charges using a cost-to-charge ratio to approximate real costs.

Cost-Utility Analysis   A type of cost-effectiveness analysis in which the consequences are expressed in terms of life-years adjusted by peoples' preferences. Typically, one considers the incremental cost per incremental gain in quality-adjusted life-years (QALYs).

Cox Regression Model   A regression technique that allows adjustment for known differences in baseline characteristics between intervention and control groups applied to survival data.

Criterion Standard (or Gold Standard or Reference Standard)   A method having established or widely accepted accuracy for determining a diagnosis that provides a standard to which a new screening or diagnostic test can be compared. The method need not be a single or simple procedure but could include follow-up of patients to observe the evolution of their conditions or the consensus of an expert panel of clinicians.

Critiquing   A decision support approach in which the computer evaluates a clinician's decision and generates an appropriateness rating or an alternative suggestion.

Crossover Study   A study design in which all patients are switched, in a specified or random order, to the alternate intervention after a specified period of time.

Cross-Product Ratio (or Odds Ratio or Relative Odds)   A ratio of the odds of an event in an exposed group to the odds of the same event in a group that is not exposed.

Cross-Sectional Study   The observation of a defined population at a single point in time or during a specific time interval. Exposure and outcome are determined simultaneously.

Data Completeness Bias   Using a computer decision support system (CDSS) to log episodes in the intervention group and using a manual system in the non-CDSS control group can create variation in the completeness of data.

Data-Dredging   Searching a data set for differences between groups on particular outcomes, or in subgroups of patients, without explicit a priori hypotheses.

Data Saturation   A process of collecting data in qualitative research to the point where new data yield only redundant information.

Decision Aid   A tool that endeavors to present patients with the benefits and harms of alternative courses of action in a manner that is quantitative, comprehensive, and understandable.

Decision Analysis   A systematic approach to decision making under conditions of uncertainty. It involves identifying all available alternatives and estimating the probabilities of potential outcomes associated with each alternative, valuing each outcome, and, on the basis of the probabilities and values, arriving at a quantitative estimate of the relative merit of the alternatives.

Degrees of Freedom   A technical term in a statistical analysis that has to do with the power of the analysis. The more degrees of freedom, the more powerful the analysis.

Deontological   A deontological approach to distributive justice holds that the clinician's only responsibility should be to best meet the needs of the individual under her care. An alternative to the consequentialist or utilitarian view.

Dependent Variable (or Outcome)   The target variable of interest. The variable that is hypothesized to depend on or be caused by another variable, the *independent variable.*

Detection Bias (or Surveillance Bias)   The tendency to look more carefully for an outcome in one of the comparison groups.

Determinants of Outcome   The causal factors that determine whether or not a target event will occur.

Dichotomous Outcomes   "Yes" or "no" outcomes that either happen, or do not happen such as pregnancy, pressure ulcer, and death.

Dichotomous Variable   A variable that can take one of two discrete values rather than values incrementally placed along a continuum (e.g., male or female, pregnant or not pregnant, dead or alive).

Differential Diagnosis   The set of diagnoses that can plausibly explain a patient's presentation.

Directness   A key element to consider when grading the quality of evidence for a health care recommendation. Refers to the extent to which the people, interventions, and outcome measures in the various studies substantiating the recommendation are similar to those of interest.

Disability-Adjusted Life-Years (DALYs)   The number of years of life after downward adjustment for disabilities that patients experience.

Discriminant Analysis   A statistical technique, similar to logistic regression analysis, that identifies variables that are associated with the presence or absence of a particular categorical (nominal) outcome.

Document Analysis   Review of written material usually with intent to code and analyze.

Dose-Response Gradient (or Dose-Dependence)   Risk of an outcome increases as the quantity or the duration of exposure to the putative harmful agent increases.

Downstream Costs   Costs due to resources consumed in the future and associated with clinical events that are attributable to the intervention.

Economic Evaluation   Comparative analysis of alternative courses of action in terms of both their costs and consequences.

Educational Meetings (or Interactive Workshops)   A strategy for changing clinician behavior. Participation of professionals in workshops that include interaction and discussion.

Educational Outreach Visits (or Academic Detailing)   A strategy for changing clinician behavior. Use of a trained person who meets with professionals in their practice settings to provide information with the intent of changing their practice.

Effect Size   The difference in outcomes between the intervention and control groups divided by some measure of variability, typically the standard deviation.

Efficiency   Technical efficiency is the relationship between inputs (costs) and outputs (in health, quality-adjusted life-years [QALYs]). Interventions that provide more QALYs for the same or fewer resources are more efficient. Technical efficiency is assessed using cost minimization, cost-effectiveness, and cost-utility analysis. Allocative efficiency recognizes that health is not the only goal that society wishes to pursue, so competing goals must be weighted and then related to costs. This is typically done through cost-benefit analysis.

End Point   Health event or outcome that leads to completion or termination of follow-up of an individual in a trial or cohort study, for example, death or major morbidity.

Equivalence Studies (or Equivalence Trials)   Studies designed to determine if an intervention that is cheaper, less toxic, or simpler to administer is equivalent to the current standard in terms of benefit.

Ethnography (or Ethnographic Study)   An approach to inquiry that focuses on the culture or subculture of a group of people, with an effort to understand the world view of those under study.

Event Rate   Proportion of study participants in a group in which an event is observed. Control event rate (CER) and experimental event rate (EER) are used to refer to event rates in control and experimental groups of study participants, respectively.

Evidence-Based Nursing (EBN) (or Evidence-Based Health Care or Evidence-Based Clinical Practice or Evidence-Based Practice)   The conscientious, explicit, and judicious use of current best evidence in making decisions about the care of individual patients. Evidence-based clinical practice requires integration of individual clinical expertise and patient preferences with the best available external clinical evidence from systematic research, and consideration of available resources.

Exclusion Criteria   The characteristics that render potential subjects ineligible to participate in a particular study or that render studies ineligible for inclusion in a systematic review.

Expectation Bias   In data collection, an interviewer has information that influences her expectation of finding the exposure or outcome. In clinical practice, a clinician's assessment may be influenced by prior knowledge of the presence or absence of a disorder.

Experimental Event Rate (EER)   Proportion of study participants in the experimental or intervention group in whom an event is observed.

Exposure   A condition to which patients are exposed (either a potentially harmful agent or a potentially beneficial one) that may impact on their health.

External Validity (or Generalizability)   The degree to which the results of a study can be generalized to settings or samples other than the ones studied.

Face Validity   The extent to which a measuring instrument looks as though it can measure what it is intended to measure.

Fail-Safe N The minimum number of undetected negative studies that would be needed to change the conclusions of a meta-analysis. A small fail-safe N suggests that the conclusion of the meta-analysis may be susceptible to publication bias.

False Negative Those who have the target disorder but the test incorrectly identifies them as not having it.

False Positive Those who do not have the target disorder, but the test incorrectly identifies them as having it.

Field Observation The witnessing and recording of events as they occur.

Fixed-Effects Model A model used to give a summary estimate of the magnitude of effect in a meta-analysis that restricts inferences to the set of studies included in the meta-analysis, and assumes that a single true value underlies all of the primary study results. The assumption is that if all studies were infinitely large, they would yield identical estimates of effect; thus, observed estimates of effect differ from each other only because of random error. This model only takes within-study variation into account and not between-study variation, and therefore, is usually not used if there is significant heterogeneity between individual study results.

Focus Group A small group of individuals (typically gatherings of four to eight people with similar background or experience) who meet together and are asked questions by a moderator about a given topic.

Follow-Up (Complete) The investigators are aware of the outcome in every patient who participated in a study.

Funnel Plot A graphic technique for assessing the possibility of publication bias in a systematic review. The effect measure is plotted on the horizontal axis and the sample size on the vertical axis. In the absence of publication bias, because of sampling variability, the graph should have the shape of a funnel that is viewed sideways, with the large opening down and the tip pointed up and centered on the true effect size. If there is bias against the publication of null results or results showing an adverse effect of the intervention, the left corner of the pyramidal part of the funnel will be distorted or missing.

Generalizability (or External Validity) The degree to which the results of a study can be generalized to settings or samples other than the ones studied.

Gold Standard (or Reference or Criterion Standard) A method having established or widely accepted accuracy for determining a diagnosis that provides a standard to which a new screening or diagnostic test can be compared. The method need not be a single or simple procedure but could include follow-up of patients to observe the evolution of their conditions or the consensus of an expert panel of clinicians.

Grounded Theory An approach to collecting and analyzing qualitative data with the aim of developing a theory grounded in real-world observations.

Harm Adverse consequences of exposure to a stimulus.

Hawthorne Effect Human performance that is improved when participants are aware that their behavior is being observed.

Hazard Ratio The weighted relative risk of an outcome (e.g., death) over the entire study period; often reported in the context of survival analysis.

Health Outcomes All possible changes in health status that may occur for a defined population or that may be associated with exposure to an intervention. These include changes in the length and quality of life as a result of detecting or treating disease when it is present, the false security associated with failing to detect disease when it is present, and the mislabeling associated with detecting disease when it is really absent.

Health Profile　A type of data collection tool, intended for use in the entire population (including the healthy, the very sick, and patients with any sort of health problem) that attempts to measure all important aspects of health-related quality of life (HRQL).

Health-Related Quality of Life (HRQL)　Measurements of how people are feeling, or the value they place on their health state.

Heterogeneity　Differences in results of individual studies included in a systematic review.

Historical Cohort Design (or Nonrandomized Historical Control Study)　Cohort studies can be historical when the outcomes of individuals or organizations exposed and not exposed to the intervention at some time in the past are compared. The practical advantage of a historical cohort study is that information on the long-term effect of the intervention (e.g., 10 or 20 years) can be assessed without having to wait the full time for the outcome to manifest itself. The disadvantages are that detailed information about the intervention and potential confounding factors may be lacking (unless there are good historical records), and the investigator has no control over what information was collected on the individuals in the past or how it was collected.

Inception Cohort　A designated group of persons assembled at a common time early in the development of a specific clinical disorder (for example, at the time of first exposure to the putative cause or the time of initial diagnosis) and who are followed thereafter.

Incidence　Number of new cases of disease occurring during a specified period of time; expressed as a percentage of the number of people at risk during that time.

Inclusion Criteria　The characteristics that define the population who will be eligible for a study or that define the studies that will be eligible for inclusion in a systematic review.

Incorporation Bias　Occurs when investigators study a diagnostic test that incorporates features of the target outcome.

Incremental Cost-Effectiveness Ratio　The price at which additional units of benefit can be obtained.

Independent Association　When a variable is associated with an outcome after adjusting for multiple other potential prognostic factors, the association is an independent association.

Independent Variable　The variable that is believed to cause or influence the *dependent variable;* in experimental research, the manipulated (intervention) variable.

Index Date　The date of an important event that marks the beginning of monitoring patients for the occurrence of the outcome of interest.

Indicator Condition　A clinical situation (e.g., disease, symptom, injury, or health state) that occurs reasonably frequently and for which there is sound evidence that high-quality care is beneficial. Indicator conditions can be used to evaluate quality of care by comparing the care provided (as assessed through chart review or observation of clinical practice) to that which is recommended.

Indirect Costs and Benefits   The impact of alternative patient management strategies on the productivity of the patient and others involved in the patient's care.

Informational Redundancy (or Theoretical Saturation)   The point at which iterations among data collection, analysis, and theory development yield a well-developed concept and further observations yield minimal or no new information to further challenge or elaborate the concept.

Informed Consent   A potential participant's expression of willingness, after full disclosure of the implications, to participate in a study.

Intention to Treat Analysis (or Intention to Treat Principle)   Analyzing study participant outcomes based on the group to which they were randomized, even if they dropped out of the study or for other reasons did not actually receive the planned intervention. This analysis preserves the power of randomization, thus maintaining that important unknown factors that influence outcome are likely equally distributed across comparison groups.

Interactive Workshops (or Educational Meetings)   A strategy for changing clinician behavior. Participation of professionals in workshops that include interaction and discussion.

Internal Validity   Whether a study provides valid results depends on whether it was designed and conducted well enough that the study findings accurately represent the direction and magnitude of the underlying true effect.

Interobserver Agreement (or Interrater Agreement)   The degree to which two or more independent observers or raters assign the same ratings or values to an attribute being measured or observed.

Interrupted Time-Series (or Time-Series Design)   In this study design, data are collected at several times both before and after the intervention; data collected before the intervention allow the underlying trend and cyclical (seasonal) effects to be estimated. Data collected after the intervention allow the intervention effect to be estimated, while accounting for underlying secular trends. The time-series design monitors the occurrence of outcomes or end points over a number of cycles and determines if the pattern changes coincident with the intervention.

Intervention Effect (or Treatment Effect)   The results of comparative clinical studies can be expressed using various intervention effect measures. Examples are absolute risk reduction (ARR), relative risk reduction (RRR), odds ratio (OR), number needed to treat (NNT), and effect size. The appropriateness of using these to express an intervention effect, and whether probabilities, means, or medians are used to calculate them, depend upon the type of outcome variable used to measure health outcomes. For example, ARR, RRR and NNT are used for dichotomous variables and effect sizes are normally used for continuous variables.

Interview   A method of data collection in which one person (an interviewer) asks questions of another person, either face-to-face or by telephone.

Interviewer Bias   Greater probing by an interviewer in one of the groups being compared.

Intraobserver Agreement (or Intrarater Agreement)   The degree to which the same observer or rater assigns the same ratings or values when measuring or observing the same attribute repeatedly.

Investigator Triangulation   More than one investigator collects and analyzes the raw data, such that the findings emerge through consensus among investigators.

Judgmental Sampling (or Purposive or Purposeful Sampling)   A type of nonprobability sampling in which theory or personal judgment guide the selection of study participants who will be most representative of the population. Examples include (1) maximum variation sampling, to document range or diversity; (2) extreme or deviant case sampling, where one selects cases that are opposite in some way; (3) typical or representative case sampling, to describe and illustrate what is typical and common in terms of the phenomenon of interest; (4) critical sampling, to make a point dramatically; and, (5) criterion sampling, where all cases that meet some predetermined criteria of importance are studied.

Kaplan-Meier Curve (or Survival Curve)   A curve that starts at 100% of the study population and shows the percentage of the population still surviving (or free of disease or some other outcome) at successive times for as long as information is available.

Kappa Statistic (or Weighted Kappa)   A measure of the extent to which observers achieve agreement beyond the level expected to occur by chance alone. Kappa can take values from 0 (poor agreement) to 1.0 (perfect agreement).

Leading Hypothesis (or Working Diagnosis)   The clinician's single best explanation for the patient's clinical problem(s).

Levels of Evidence   A hierarchy of research evidence, usually ranging from strongest to weakest.

Likelihood Ratio   For a screening or diagnostic test (including clinical signs or symptoms), the relative likelihood that a given test result is expected in a patient with (as opposed to one without) the target disorder.

Likert Scales   Scales, typically with three to nine possible values, that include extremes of attitudes or feelings (such as from totally disagree to totally agree) which respondents mark to indicate their rating.

Linear Regression   The term used for a regression analysis when the dependent or target variable is a continuous variable and the relationship between the dependent and independent variables is thought to be linear.

Local Consensus Process   A strategy for changing clinician behavior. Inclusion of participating clinicians in discussions to ensure they agree with suggested approach to change provider practice.

Local Opinion Leaders (or Opinion Leaders)   A strategy for changing clinician behavior using respected academic and clinician peers who are recognized by their colleagues as "educationally influential".

Logical Operators (or Boolean Operators)   Words used when searching electronic databases. These operators are AND, OR, and NOT and are used to combine terms (AND/OR) or exclude terms (NOT) from the search strategy.

Logistic Regression   A multivariate regression analysis that analyzes relationships between multiple independent variables and categorical dependent variables.

Longitudinal Study (or Cohort Study or Prospective Study)   When used to study potential causes of a disorder, it is a prospective investigation in which a cohort of individuals who do not have evidence of an outcome of interest but who are exposed to the putative cause are compared with a concurrent cohort who are also free of the outcome but not exposed to the putative cause. Both cohorts are then followed forward in time to compare the incidence of the outcome of interest. When used to study the effectiveness of an intervention, it is a prospective investigation in which a cohort of individuals who receive the intervention are compared with a concurrent cohort who do not receive the intervention. Both cohorts are then followed forward in time to compare the incidence of the outcome of interest.

Lost to Follow-Up   Patients whose status on the outcome or end point of interest is unknown.

Marginal Utility   The change in a person's utility (preference or relative value) for an outcome as the outcome increases in magnitude.

Masked (or Blind or Blinded)   Patients, clinicians, those monitoring outcomes, judicial assessors of outcomes, data analysts, and/or those writing the paper are unaware of which patients have been assigned to the experimental or control group.

Matching   A deliberate process to make the study group and comparison group comparable with respect to factors (or confounders) that are extraneous to the purpose of the investigation but that might interfere with the interpretation of the study's findings. For example, in case control studies, individual cases may be matched with controls on the basis of comparable age, gender, and/or other clinical features.

Member Checking   Involves sharing draft study findings with the participants to inquire whether their viewpoints were faithfully interpreted, to determine whether there are gross errors of fact, and to ascertain whether the account makes sense to participants with different perspectives.

Meta-Analysis   A statistical technique for quantitatively combining the results of multiple studies, that measure the same outcome, into a single pooled or summary estimate.

Meta-Synthesis   A procedure for combining qualitative research on a specific topic in which researchers compare and analyze the texts of individual studies and develop new interpretations.

Mixed-Methods Study   A study that combines data collection approaches, sometimes both qualitative and quantitative, into the study methodology and is commonly used in the study of service delivery and organization. Some mixed-methods studies combine study designs (e.g., investigators may embed qualitative or quantitative process evaluations alongside quantitative evaluative designs to increase understanding of causal mechanisms, modifying factors, and findings). Some mixed-methods studies include a single overarching research design but use mixed-methods for data collection (e.g., surveys, interviews, observation, and analysis of documentary material).

Multifaceted Interventions   Use of multiple strategies to change clinician behavior. Multiple strategies may include a combination that includes two or more of: audit and feedback, reminders, local consensus processes, patient-mediated interventions.

Multiple Regression (or Multivariate Regression Equation)   A type of regression that provides a mathematical model that explains or predicts the dependent or target variable by simultaneously considering all of the independent or predictor variables.

Multivariate Analysis   An analysis that simultaneously considers a number of independent variables.

N of 1 Trial   An experiment designed to determine the effect of an intervention or exposure on a single study participant. The patient undergoes pairs of treatment periods organized so that one period involves the use of the experimental treatment and one period involves the use of an alternate treatment or placebo. The patient and clinician are blinded if possible and outcomes are monitored. Treatment periods are replicated until the clinician and patient are convinced that the treatments are definitely different or definitely not different.

Negative Predictive Value (NPV)   Proportion of people with a negative test who are free of disease.

Negative Studies   Studies in which the authors have concluded that the comparison groups do not differ statistically in the variables of interest. Research results that fail to support the researchers' hypotheses.

No Test-Test Threshold (or Test Threshold)   The probability below which the clinician decides a diagnosis warrants no further consideration.

Nominal Variable (or Categorical Variable)   A variable with discrete values rather than values incrementally placed along a continuum (e.g., marital status, gender, race).

Nomogram   Graphic scale facilitating calculation of a probability.

Nonrandomized Controlled Trial   Experiment in which assignment of patients to the intervention groups is at the convenience of the investigator or according to a preset plan that does not conform to the definition of random.

Nonrandomized Historical Control Study (or Historical Cohort Design)   Cohort studies can be historical when the outcomes of individuals or organizations exposed and not exposed to the intervention at some time in the past are compared. The practical advantage of a historical cohort study is that information on the long-term effect of the intervention (e.g., 10 or 20 years) can be assessed without having to wait the full time for the outcome to manifest itself. The disadvantages are that detailed information about the intervention and potential confounding factors may be lacking (unless there are good historical records), and the investigator has no control over what information was collected on the individuals in the past or how it was collected.

Null Hypothesis   In the hypothesis-testing framework, the starting hypothesis the statistical test is designed to consider and possibly reject, is that there is no relationship between the variables under study.

Null Result   A nonsignificant result; no statistically significant difference between groups.

Number Needed to Harm (NNH)   The number of patients who, if they received the experimental intervention, would lead to one additional patient being harmed over a specific period of time. It is the inverse of the absolute risk increase (1/ARI).

Number Needed to Treat (NNT)   The number of patients who need to be treated over a specific period of time to achieve one additional good outcome. When discussing NNT, it is important to specify the intervention, its duration, and the good outcome. It is the inverse of the absolute risk reduction (1/ARR).

Observational Studies (or Observational Study Design)   Studies in which participant or clinician preference determines whether a participant is assigned to the intervention or control group.

Odds   The ratio of events to non-events; the ratio of the number of study participants experiencing the outcome of interest to the number of study participants not experiencing the outcome of interest.

Odds Ratio (or Cross-Product Ratio or Relative Odds)   A ratio of the odds of an event in an exposed group to the odds of the same event in a group that is not exposed.

One-Group Pretest-Posttest Design (or Before-After Design)   Study in which the investigators compare the status of study participants before and after the introduction of an intervention.

Open Coding   First level of coding in a grounded theory study, consisting of basic descriptive coding of narrative content.

Open-Ended Questions   Questions that offer no specific structure for the respondent's answers and allow the respondents to answer in their own words.

Opinion Leaders (or Local Opinion Leaders)   A strategy for changing clinician behavior using respected academic and clinician peers who are recognized by their colleagues as "educationally influential".

Opportunistic Sampling   Availability of participants guides on-the-spot sampling decisions.

Opportunity Costs   The value of (health or other) benefits forgone in alternative uses when a resource is used.

Outcome (or Dependent Variable)   The target variable of interest. The variable that is hypothesized to depend on or be caused by another variable, the *independent variable*.

Outcome Evaluation   Assesses the impact of an intervention. It examines the changes that occurred as a result of the intervention and if the intervention is having the intended effect. It answers the question: "What is the impact of this intervention?" It may also answer the question: "Are the benefits of the intervention worth the costs?"

Overview   A type of review in which primary research relevant to a question is examined and summarized, and an effort is made to identify all available literature (published or unpublished) that pertains to that question.

Patient Expected Event Rate (PEER)   The probability of the occurrence of the end point or outcome of interest in the patient group of which the individual under consideration is representative.

Patient-Mediated Interventions   A strategy for changing clinician behavior. Any intervention aimed at changing the performance of professionals through interactions with, or information provided to, patients.

Patient Preferences   The relative value that patients place on varying health states.

Phase I Studies   Studies that investigate a drug's physiological effect or ensure that it does not manifest unacceptable early toxicity, often conducted in normal volunteers.

Phase II Studies   Initial studies on patients, which provide preliminary evidence of possible drug effectiveness.

Phase III Studies   Randomized controlled trials designed to definitively establish the magnitude of drug benefit.

Phase IV Studies (or Postmarketing Surveillance Studies)   Studies conducted after the effectiveness of a drug has been established and the drug marketed, typically to establish the frequency of unusual toxic effects.

Phenomenology   An approach to inquiry that emphasizes the complexity of human experience and the need to understand the experience holistically as it is actually lived.

Phi (or Phi Statistic)   A measure of chance-independent agreement calculated by the following formula: $\sqrt{OR} - 1 / \sqrt{OR} + 1$.

Placebo   A biologically inert substance (typically a pill or capsule) that is as similar as possible to the active intervention. Placebos are sometimes given to participants in the control arm of a trial to help conceal their group assignment.

Placebo Effect   The impact of an intervention independent of its biological effect.

Point Estimate   The single value that best represents the value of the population parameter.

Positive Predictive Value (PPV)   The proportion of people with a positive test who have the disease.

Positive Study (or Positive Trial)   A study with results that are consistent with the researchers' hypotheses.

Postmarketing Surveillance Studies (or Phase IV Studies)   Studies conducted after the effectiveness of a drug has been established and the drug marketed, typically to establish the frequency of unusual toxic effects.

Postpublication Bias   A result of conducting a systematic review that fails to seek published studies from more obscure sources, such as non-English journals; if, for example, non-English–language authors publish positive studies in English–language journals and negative studies (of equivalent methodological quality) in local non-English–language journals that are less likely to be indexed in MEDLINE, and these studies are not included in the review, the estimate of the intervention effect will be exaggerated.

Posttest Odds   The odds of the target condition being present after the results of a diagnostic test are available.

Posttest Probability   The probability of the target condition being present after the results of a diagnostic test are available.

Power   The ability of a study to reject a null hypothesis when it is false (and should be rejected). It is linked to the adequacy of the sample size; if a sample size is too small, the study will have insufficient power to detect differences between groups, if differences exist.

Practice Guidelines (or Clinical Practice Guidelines)   Systematically developed statements or recommendations to assist practitioner and patient decisions about appropriate health care for specific clinical circumstances. They present indications for performing a test, procedure, or intervention or the proper management for specific clinical problems. Guidelines may be developed by government agencies, institutions, organizations such as professional societies or governing boards, or by convening expert panels.

Predictive Value   Two categories: Positive Predictive Value — the proportion of people with a positive test who have the disease; Negative Predictive Value — proportion of people with a negative test and who are free of disease.

Preprocessed (or Prefiltered)   A process whereby someone has reviewed the literature, and chosen only the methodologically strongest studies.

Pretest Odds   The odds of the target condition being present before the results of a diagnostic test are available.

Pretest Probability   The probability of the target condition being present before the results of a diagnostic test are available.

Prevalence   Proportion of persons affected with a particular disease at a specified time. Prevalence rates obtained from high-quality studies can inform pretest probabilities.

Primary Studies   Studies that collect original data. Primary studies are differentiated from systematic reviews that summarize the results of primary studies.

Probability   Quantitative estimate of the likelihood of a condition existing (as in diagnosis) or of subsequent events (such as in an intervention study).

Process Evaluation   Evaluates how a program or intervention is implemented and used in practice. It focuses on what the intervention does and for whom. It answers the question: "Is implementation consistent with the way the intervention was planned?" and "How can the intervention be improved?".

Prognosis   The possible outcomes of a disease and the frequency with which they can be expected to occur.

Prognostic Factors   Patient or study participant characteristics that confer increased or decreased risk of a positive or adverse outcome.

Prognostic Study   A study that enrolls patients at a point in time and follows them forward to determine the frequency and timing of subsequent events.

Prospective Study (or Cohort Study or Longitudinal Study)   When used to study potential causes of a disorder, it is a prospective investigation in which a cohort of individuals who do not have evidence of an outcome of interest but who are exposed to the putative cause are compared with a concurrent cohort who are also free of the outcome but not exposed to the putative cause. Both cohorts are then followed forward in time to compare the incidence of the outcome of interest. When used to study the effectiveness of an intervention, it is a prospective investigation in which a cohort of individuals who receive the intervention are compared with a concurrent cohort who do not receive the intervention. Both cohorts are then followed forward in time to compare the incidence of the outcome of interest.

Provider Adherence (or Provider Compliance)   Extent that health care providers carry out the host of diagnostic tests, monitoring equipment, interventional requirements, and other technical specifications that define optimal patient management.

Publication Bias   Occurs when the publication of research depends on the direction of the study results and whether they are statistically significant.

Purposeful Sampling (or Purposive Sampling or Judgmental Sampling)   A type of nonprobability sampling in which theory or personal judgment guide the selection of study participants who will be most representative of the population. Examples include (1) maximum variation sampling, to document range or diversity; (2) extreme or deviant case sampling, where one selects cases that are opposite in some way; (3) typical or representative case sampling, to describe and illustrate what is typical and common in terms of the phenomenon of interest; (4) critical sampling, to make a point dramatically; and (5) criterion sampling, where all cases that meet some predetermined criteria of importance are studied.

P **Value**   The probability that results as or more extreme than those observed would occur if the null hypothesis were true and the experiment were repeated over and over. A *P* value < 0.05 means that there is a less than 1 in 20 probability of the result occurring by chance alone if the null hypothesis were true.

Qualitative Research   The investigation of phenomena in a non-quantitative, in-depth and holistic fashion, through the collection of rich narrative materials. Examples of data collection include observation, interviews, and document analysis.

Quality-Adjusted Life Expectancy   The number of years of expected life corrected for the quality of life that patients are expected to experience in those years.

Quality-Adjusted Life-Year (QALY)   A unit of measure for survival that accounts for the effects of suboptimal health status and the resulting limitations in quality of life. For example, if a patient lives for 10 years and her quality of life is decreased by 50% because of chronic lung disease, her survival would be equivalent to 5 quality-adjusted life-years.

Quality Assurance   Any procedure, method, or philosophy for collecting, processing, or analyzing data that is aimed at maintaining or improving the appropriateness of health care services.

Quality of Care   The extent to which health care meets technical and humanistic standards of optimal care.

Quantitative Research   The investigation of phenomena that lend themselves to test well-specified hypotheses through precise measurement and quantification of pre-determined variables that yield numbers suitable for statistical analysis.

Quasi-Randomized Controlled Trial   Experiment in which individuals are allocated by investigators to receive or not receive an experimental preventive, therapeutic or diagnostic procedure and then followed to determine the effect of the intervention. Allocation is not random but systematic (e.g., on even and odd days of the week or on even and odd days of birth).

Random   Governed by a formal chance process in which the occurrence of previous events is of no value in predicting future events. The probability of assignment of, for example, a given participant to a specified study group is fixed and constant (typically 0.5) but the participant's actual assignment cannot be known until it occurs.

Random Allocation (or Randomization)   Allocation of individuals to groups by chance, usually done with the aid of a table of random numbers. Not to be confused with systematic allocation (e.g., on even and odd days of the month) or allocation at the convenience or discretion of the investigator.

Random-Effects Model   A model used to give a summary estimate of the magnitude of effect in a meta-analysis that assumes that the studies included are a random sample of a population of studies addressing the question posed in the meta-analysis. Each study estimates a different underlying true effect, and the distribution of these effects is assumed to be normal around a mean value. Because a random-effects model takes into account both within-study and between-study variability, the confidence interval around the point estimate is wider than it would be if a fixed-effects model were used. This method is usually used instead of the fixed-effects model if there is significant heterogeneity between individual study results.

Random Error   We can never know with certainty the true value of an intervention effect because of random error. It is inherent in all measurement. The observations that are made in a study are only a sample of all possible observations that could be made from the population of relevant patients. Thus, the average value of any sample observations is subject to some variation from the true value for that entire population. When the level of random error associated with a measurement is high, the measurement is less precise and we are less certain about the value of that measurement.

Random Sample   A sample derived by selecting sampling units (e.g., individual patients) such that each unit has an independent and fixed (generally equal) chance of selection. Whether or not a given unit is selected is determined by chance, for example, by a table of randomly ordered numbers.

Randomization (or Random Allocation)   Allocation of individuals to groups by chance, usually done with the aid of a table of random numbers. Not to be confused with systematic allocation (e.g., on even and odd days of the month) or allocation at the convenience or discretion of the investigator.

Randomized Controlled Trial (or Randomized Trial or Controlled Trial)   Experiment in which individuals are randomly allocated to receive or not receive an experimental preventive, therapeutic, or diagnostic procedure and then followed to determine the effect of the intervention.

Recall Bias   Occurs when patients who experience an adverse outcome have a different likelihood of recalling an exposure than patients who do not experience the adverse outcome, independent of the true extent of exposure.

Reference Standard (or Gold Standard or Criterion Standard)   A method having established or widely accepted accuracy for determining a diagnosis that provides a standard to which a new screening or diagnostic test can be compared. The method need not be a single or simple procedure but could include follow-up of patients to observe the evolution of their conditions or the consensus of an expert panel of clinicians.

Regression   A technique that uses predictor or independent variables to build a statistical model that predicts an individual patient's status with respect to a dependent or target variable.

Relative Benefit Increase (RBI)   The proportional increase in rates of good outcomes between experimental and control participants. It is calculated by dividing the rate of good outcome in the experimental group (EER) minus the rate of good outcome in the control group (CER) by the rate of good outcome in the the control group [(EER – CER)/CER].

Relative Odds (or Cross-Product Ratio or Odds Ratio)   A ratio of the odds of an event in an exposed group to the odds of the same event in a group that is not exposed.

Relative Risk (or Risk Ratio)   Ratio of the risk of an event among an exposed population to the risk among the unexposed.

Relative Risk Increase (RRI)   The proportional increase in rates of harmful outcomes between experimental and control participants. It is calculated by dividing the rate of harmful outcome in the experimental group (EER) minus the rate of harmful outcome in the control group (CER) by the rate of harmful outcome in the control group [(EER – CER)/CER]. Typically used with a harmful exposure.

Relative Risk Reduction (RRR)   The proportional reduction in rates of harmful outcomes between experimental and control participants. It is calculated by dividing the rate of harmful outcome in the experimental group (EER) minus the rate of harmful outcome in the control group (CER) by the rate of harmful outcome in the control group [(EER – CER)/CER]. Used with a beneficial exposure or intervention.

Reliability (or Reproducibility)   The degree of consistency with which an instrument measures the attribute it is designed to measure.

Reminder Systems (or Reminders)   A strategy for changing clinician behavior. Manual or computerized reminders to prompt behavior change.

Reproducibility (or Reliability)   The degree of consistency with which an instrument measures the attribute it is designed to measure.

Responsiveness   The ability of an instrument to detect change over time.

Review   A general term for all attempts to obtain and synthesize the results and conclusions of two or more publications on a given topic.

Risk   Measure of the association between exposure and outcome (including incidence, side effects, toxicity).

Risk Aversion   People are said to be risk averse if they would accept a fixed outcome with certainty rather than a lottery with a higher expected value. For example, they would choose $10 for sure rather than a 50/50 chance of $0 or $30.

Risk Factors   Authors often distinguish between prognostic factors and risk factors. Risk factors are patient characteristics associated with the development of a disease in the first place. Prognostic factors are patient characteristics that confer increased or decreased risk of a positive or adverse outcome from a given disease.

Risk Ratio (or Relative Risk)   Ratio of the risk of an event among an exposed population to the risk among the unexposed.

ROC Curve (Receiver Operating Characteristic Curve)   A figure depicting the power of a diagnostic test. The ROC curve presents the test's true-positive rate (i.e., sensitivity) on the horizontal axis and the false-positive rate (i.e., 1 – specificity) on the vertical axis for different cut-points dividing a positive from a negative test. An ROC curve for a perfect test has an area under the curve = 1.0 while a test that performs no better than chance has an area under the curve of only 0.5.

Screening Services, designed to detect people at high risk of suffering from a condition associated with a modifiable adverse outcome, offered to persons who have neither symptoms of, nor risk factors (other than age or gender) for, a target condition.

Secondary Journals A secondary journal does not publish original research but rather includes synopses of published research studies that meet pre-specified criteria of both clinical relevance and methodological quality.

Secular Trends Changes in the probability of events with time, independent of known predictors of outcome.

Selective Coding The third level of coding in a grounded theory study that involves the process of selecting the core category, systematically integrating relationships between the core category and other categories, and validating those relationships.

Selective Screening Services to be offered to asymptomatic persons with one or more risk factors for a target condition, such as family history of the disease, certain personal behaviors, or membership in a population with increased prevalence of the disease.

Semi-Structured Interview Interviewer asks a number of specific questions, but additional questions or probes are used at the discretion of the interviewer.

Sensitivity The proportion of people who truly have a designated disorder who are so identified by the test. The test may consist of, or include, clinical observations.

Sensitivity Analysis Any test of the stability of the conclusions of a health care evaluation over a range of probability estimates, value judgments, and assumptions about the structure of the decisions to be made. This may involve the repeated evaluation of a decision model in which one or more of the parameters of interest are varied.

Sentinal Effect Human performance may improve when participants are aware that their behavior is being evaluated.

Sequential Sample (or Consecutive Sample) A sample in which all potentially eligible patients seen over a period of time are enrolled.

Sign Test A nonparametric test for comparing two paired groups based on the relative ranking of values between the pairs.

Signal-to-Noise Ratio Signal is based on the observed difference between groups and noise is the variability between individuals within the group. Nearly all statistical tests are based on a signal-to-noise ratio, where the signal is the important relationship and the noise is a measure of individual variation.

When trying to discriminate among people at a single point in time, the signal comes from differences in scores among patients. The noise comes from variability within patients. The greater the noise, the more difficult it is to detect the signal.

When trying to evaluate change over time in the same patients, the signal comes from the difference in scores in patients whose status has improved or deteriorated. The noise comes from the variability in scores in patients whose status has not changed.

Silo Effect One of the main reasons for considering narrower viewpoints in conducting an economic analysis is to assess the impact of change on the main budget holders, as budgets may need to be adjusted before a new intervention can be adopted.

Simple Regression (or Univariate Regression)   Regression where there is only one independent variable.

SnNout   When a test with a high **Sen**sitivity is **N**egative, it effectively rules **out** the diagnosis of disease.

Snowball Sampling   Study participants nominate or refer other potential study participants who meet the study inclusion criteria.

Social Desirability Bias   Study participants misrepresent their responses in the direction of answers consistent with prevailing social norms or socially desirable behavior.

Specificity   The proportion of people who are truly free of a designated disorder who are so identified by the test. The test may consist of, or include, clinical observations.

SpPin   When a test is highly **Sp**ecific, a **P**ositive result can rule **in** the diagnosis.

Stakeholder   An individual, group and/or organization with a vested interest in the clinical question or decision.

Stakeholder Analysis   A strategy that seeks to increase understanding of stakeholder behavior, plans, relationships and interests and seeks to generate information about stakeholders' levels of influence, support and resources.

Standard Error   The standard deviation of an estimate of a population parameter. The standard error of the mean is the standard deviation of the estimate of the population mean value.

Standard Gamble   A direct preference or utility measure that effectively asks respondents to rate their quality of life on a scale from 0 to 1.0, where 0 is death and 1.0 is full health. Respondents choose between a specified time x in their current health state and a gamble in which they have probability P (anywhere from 0 to 0.99) of full health for time x, and a probability $1 - P$ of immediate death.

Statistical Inference   Statistical methodologies to make deductions about underlying truth. There are two principle functions: (1) To predict or estimate a population parameter from a sample statistic, and (2) to test statistically based hypotheses.

Statistical Significance   A term indicating that the results obtained in an analysis of study data are unlikely to have occurred by chance and the null hypothesis is rejected. When statistically significant, the probability of the observed results, given the null hypothesis, falls below a specified level of probability (most often $P < 0.05$).

Structure Evaluation   Assesses settings and instruments available and used for the provision of care. This covers facilities, supplies, and equipment and may also include organizational structure and numbers and qualifications of the health agency staff. It signifies the properties and resources used to provide care and the manner in which they are organized.

Study Quality   A key element to consider when grading the quality of evidence for a health care recommendation. Refers to the detailed assessment of study design and execution to determine whether the study was conducted so that it avoided, or minimized bias and yielded valid results.

Subgroup Analysis   The separate analysis of data for subgroups of patients, such as those at different stages of their illness, those with different comorbid conditions, or those of different ages.

Surrogate Outcomes or End Points (or Substitute Outcomes or End Points)   Outcomes that are not in themselves important to patients, but are associated with outcomes that are important to patients, (e.g., bone density for fracture, cholesterol for myocardial infarction, and blood pressure for stroke).

Surveillance Bias (or Detection Bias)   The tendency to look more carefully for an outcome in one of the comparison groups.

Survey Research   Observational or descriptive non-experimental study that focuses on obtaining information about activities, beliefs, preferences or attitudes through self-report by study participants.

Survival Analysis   A statistical procedure used to compare the proportion of patients in each group who experience an outcome or end point at various time intervals over the duration of the study (e.g., death).

Survival Curve (or Kaplan-Meier Curve)   A curve that starts at 100% of the study population and shows the percentage of the population still surviving (or free of disease or some other outcome) at successive times for as long as information is available.

Symbolic Interactionism   A qualitative research method that focuses on the way in which people make sense of social interactions and the meanings they attach to social symbols such as language.

Synopses   Brief summaries that encapsulate the key methodological details and results of a single study or systematic review.

Syntheses   Systematic reviews of all the evidence addressing focused clinical questions.

Systematic Review   The consolidation of research evidence that incorporates a critical assessment and evaluation of the research (not simply a summary) and addresses a focused clinical question using methods designed to reduce the likelihood of bias.

Systems   Systems include practice guidelines, clinical pathways, or evidence-based textbook summaries that integrate evidence-based information about specific clinical problems and provide regular updating.

Target Condition   In diagnostic test studies, the condition the investigators or clinicians are particularly interested in identifying (such as tuberculosis, lung cancer, or iron-deficiency anemia).

Target End Points (or Target Outcomes or Target Events)   In intervention studies, the condition the investigators or clinicians are particularly interested in identifying and which it is anticipated the intervention will decrease (such as myocardial infarction, stroke, or death) or increase (such as ulcer healing).

Target-Negative   In diagnostic test studies, patients who do not have the target condition.

Target-Positive   In diagnostic test studies, patients who do have the target condition.

Test Threshold (or No Test–Test Threshold)   The probability below which the clinician decides a diagnosis warrants no further consideration.

Theoretical Sampling   In qualitative studies, selection of study participants based on emerging findings to ensure adequate representation of important themes.

Theoretical Saturation (or Informational Redundancy)   The point at which iterations among data collection, analysis, and theory development yield a well-developed concept and further observations yield minimal or no new information to further challenge or elaborate the concept.

Theory-Based Operational Construct Sampling Where incidents, time periods, people, or other data sources are sampled on the basis of their potential manifestation or representation of important theoretical constructs.

Theory Triangulation Theory triangulation is a process whereby emergent findings are corroborated with existing social science theories.

Time-Series Design (or Interrupted Time-Series) In this study design, data are collected at several times both before and after the intervention; data collected before the intervention allow the underlying trend and cyclical (seasonal) effects to be estimated. Data collected after the intervention allow the intervention effect to be estimated, while accounting for underlying secular trends. The time-series design monitors the occurrence of outcomes or end points over a number of cycles, and determines if the pattern changes coincident with the intervention.

Time Trade-off A formal utility assessment. In time trade-off, patients choose between a longer period in a state of impaired health (such as recovery from severe stroke) and a shorter period in a state of full health. Patients are given a series of paired choices through which they indicate the length of time in perfect health that is equivalent to a lifetime in an intermediate health state/outcome. The patient's value for the outcome is calculated as the proportion that is indicated (e.g., 9/10 years' life expectancy = 0.90).

Treatment Effect (or Intervention Effect) The results of comparative clinical studies can be expressed using various intervention effect measures. Examples are absolute risk reduction (ARR), relative risk reduction (RRR), odds ratio (OR), number needed to treat (NNT), and effect size. The appropriateness of using these to express an intervention effect, and whether probabilities, means, or medians are used to calculate them, depend upon the type of outcome variable used to measure health outcomes. For example, ARR, RRR and NNT are used for dichotomous variables and effect sizes are normally used for continuous variables.

Treatment Threshold Probability above which a clinician would consider a diagnosis confirmed and would stop testing and initiate treatment.

Triangulation In the course of qualitative analysis, key findings are corroborated using multiple sources of information.

Trigger Orders Orders in response to which the computer decision support system (CDSS) would initiate action.

Trim-and-Fill Method When publication bias is suspected in a systematic review, investigators may attempt to estimate the true intervention effect by removing, or trimming, small positive studies that do not have a negative study counterpart and then calculating a supposed true effect from the resulting symmetric funnel plot. The investigators then replace the positive studies they have removed and add hypothetical studies that mirror these positive studies to create a symmetric funnel plot that retains the new pooled effect estimate. This method allows the calculation of an adjusted confidence interval and an estimate of the number of missing trials.

True Negative Those who the test correctly identifies as not having the target disorder.

True Positive Those who the test correctly identifies as having the target disorder.

T-Test A parametric statistical test that examines the difference between the means of two groups of values.

Type I Error An error created by rejecting the null hypothesis when it is true (i.e., investigators conclude that a relationship exists between variables when it does not).

Type II Error An error created by accepting the null hypothesis when it is false (i.e., investigators conclude that no relationship exists between variables when, in fact, a relationship does exist).

Unblinded (or Unmasked) Patients, clinicians, those monitoring outcomes, judicial assessors of outcomes, data analysts, and those writing the paper are aware of whether patients have been assigned to the experimental or control group.

Unit of Allocation The basic unit or focus used for assignment to comparison groups (e.g., individuals or clusters such as schools, health care teams, hospital wards, or outpatient practices).

Unit of Analysis The basic unit or focus of the analysis; while it is most often the individual study participant, in a study that uses cluster allocation, the unit of analysis is the cluster (e.g., school, clinic).

Univariate Regression (or Simple Regression) Regression where there is only one independent variable.

Unmasked (or Unblinded) Patients, clinicians, those monitoring outcomes, judicial assessors of outcomes, data analysts, and those writing the paper are aware of whether patients have been assigned to the experimental or control group.

Utilitarian (or Consequentialist) A consequentialist or utilitarian view of distributive justice would contend that even in individual decision making, the clinician should take a broad social view in which the action that would provide the greatest good to the greatest number is favored. In this broader view, the effect on others of allocating resources to a particular patient's care would bear on the decision. An alternative to the deontological view.

Utility Patient preferences that are measured with techniques consistent with modern utility theory. Patient preferences refer to the degrees of subjective satisfaction, distress, or desirability that patients or potential patients associate with a particular health outcome. Utility theory is based on specific axioms that describe how a rational decision maker ought to make a decision when the outcomes of that decision are uncertain. Commonly used measures of utility include the "standard gamble" or "time trade-off" techniques.

Utility Measures Measures that provide a single number that summarizes all of health-related quality of life (HRQL) and are preference- or value-weighted; these have the preferences or values anchored to death and full health and are called utility measures.

Utilization Review An organized procedure carried out through committees to review admissions, duration of stay, and professional services provided, and to evaluate the necessity of those services and promote their most efficient use.

Validity The extent to which an instrument measures what it is intended to measure.

Values (or Value Judgments) The basis for individual personal preferences.

Variance The technical term for the statistical estimate of the variability in results.

Verification Bias (or Work-Up Bias)   Results of a diagnostic test influence whether patients are assigned to an intervention group.

Visual Analogue Scale   A scaling procedure consisting of a straight line anchored on each end with words or phrases that represent the extremes of some phenomenon (e.g., "worst pain I have ever had" to "absolutely no pain"). Respondents are asked to make a mark on the line at the point that corresponds to their experience of the phenomenon.

Washout Period   In a crossover or N of 1 trial, the period required for the treatment to cease to act once it has been discontinued.

Weighted Kappa (or Kappa Statistic)   A measure of the extent to which observers achieve agreement beyond the level expected to occur by chance alone. Kappa can take values from 0 (poor agreement) to 1.0 (perfect agreement).

Working Diagnosis (or Leading Hypothesis)   The clinician's single best explanation for the patient's clinical problem(s).

Work-Up Bias (or Verification Bias)   Results of a diagnostic test influence whether patients are assigned to an intervention group.

Index

A

A priori analyses, 255
ABI (absolute benefit increase), 60, 532
Absolute differences, 60
Absolute risk, 409-410
Absolute risk reduction, 60, 253-254, 409-410, 413-414, 470-479, 532, 532t
Academic detailing, 175f, 189, 191t
Academy Health, 268
Acceptance-related issues, 330-331
ACP Journal Club, 23, 37
Action plans, 177b, 178f-179f, 189b, 187b-190b
Adjusted analyses, 428-429
Administration (differential), 400-401
Administrative databases use, 281-282, 282t, 287
Adult Asthma Care Guidelines for Nurses, 173, 176b-177b, 185b
Advanced concepts (education- and application-related principles). *See also under individual topics.*
  diagnoses-related topics, 370
  health care intervention topics, 203-262
  health services research topics, 263-336
  practice applications topics, 467-541
  results-related topics, 395-466
  systematic review and summarization topics, 371-394
Adverse effects risks, 487
AGA (American Gastroenterological Association) guidelines, 527-536
Agency for Health Care Policy and Research, 14-15
Agency for Healthcare Research and Quality, 14-15, 155
Agreement beyond chance measures, 446-454
  vs. agreement by chance, 447-448
  future perspectives of, 454
  interobservers/interraters and, 447
  kappa, 447-454
    calculations for, 448-451, 449f, 451t, 545
    limitations of, 452-453
    ORs and, 453-454, 453f
    overviews and summaries of, 447-448, 448f
    vs. phi, 453-454, 453f
    with three or more raters/categories, 451-452, 452f

Agreement beyond chance measures *(Continued)*
  weighted statistics for, 452
  overviews and summaries of, 447
  reference resources for, 454
Agreement by chance, 447-448
AHCPR (Agency for Health Care Policy and Research), 14-15
AHRQ (Agency for Healthcare Research and Quality), 14-15, 155
Aids (decision), 494-498
Alerting systems, 320-322, 321t
Allocation concealment, 52-54
Alpha levels, 425
American Gastroenterological Association guidelines, 527-536
Analogue scales (visual), 499-501, 500f
Analyses. *See also under individual topics.*
  adjusted, 428-429
  cost, 300-309
  decision, 300
  decision trees for, 300
  differences, adjustments for, 279-280, 280t
  document, 126-128, 126f
  economic, 298-317
  impact, 361-362, 367-369
    accuracy rates of, 368
    meta-analyses and, 367-368
    overviews and summaries of, 361-362, 367-368
    steps of, 361-362
  intention-to-treat, 249-250
  meta-analyses, 12, 139-140, 145-149, 148f, 367, 382-385, 383f-384f
  multivariate, 280
  post hoc, 255
  a priori, 255
  sensitivity, 146-147, 310-311
  subgroup, 251-262
  survival analyses, 60
  unit/cluster assignment, 287-288
Antibiotic Assistant, 322
Apparent trials, 438-442
  negative, 438-440
  positive, 440-442, 441t
Applicability-related issues, 103-104

Note: Entries followed by "b" indicate boxes, "f" indicate figures, and "t" indicate tables.

Application-related topics. *See also* Practice-related topics.
  evidence level interpretations and health care grade recommendations, 508-525
  NNT factors, 469-480
  patient care applications, 481-489. *See also* Patient care applications.
  patient values incorporation topics, 490-507
  screening recommendations, 526-541
Appropriateness, 123-124, 125-126
ARIMA (autoregressive integrated moving average) models, 291
ARR (absolute risk reduction), 60, 253-254, 409-410, 413-414, 470-479, 532, 532t
Arthur, Heather, 108, 397
Aspect omissions, 212-213
Assessments and evaluations. *See* Evaluation-related topics.
Assignment analyses, 287-288
Assisting systems, 321t
Association measures, 407-422
  2 × 2 tables for, 409, 410t, 416
  absolute risk and, 409-410
  ARR, 409-411, 413-414
  calculations for, 543
  case-control studies for, 420-421, 421t
  CIs for, 418
  control event rates for, 410
  Cox regression models for, 419-420
  dichotomous *vs.* continuous outcomes for, 409
  future perspectives of, 421
  NNH and, 409, 416
  NNT and, 409, 414-415, 415f
  ORs for, 409-413
  overviews and summaries of, 407-409, 408f
  RDs for, 408-410
  reference resources for, 422
  relative risks and, 410-411, 413-414
  RRR and, 408, 411
  selection of, 421
  survival data for, 418-420, 419f
Association of Registered Nurses, 6
Associations (independent), 226
Asymmetry, 377
Atheoretical aspects, 9-10
Attia, John, 407
Audit and feedback, 189
Author revisions and resubmissions, 375t
Autocorrelation, 291
Autoregressive integrated moving average models, 291

B

Background *vs.* foreground questions, 21-23, 22f
Balance scales, 499
Bandolier, 42
Barratt, Alexandra, 407, 526
Barrier-related issues, 15-17, 16t

Baselines, 306-307, 428-429, 471-473, 477t
  differences of, 428-429
  risks and, 306-307, 471-473, 477t
Basic concepts (nursing literature use principles). *See also under individual topics.*
  clinical practice guidelines-related topics, 154-171
  diagnoses-related topics, 87-107
  evidence discovery, 20-43
  fundamental topics, 3-19
  harm-related topics, 44-47, 71-86
  health care intervention topics, 48-70
  organizational practice change topics, 172-200
  prognoses-related topics, 108-119
  qualitative research topics, 120-136
  systematic review and summarization topics, 137-153
Bass, Eric, 154, 508
Before-and-after studies (controlled), 271-272
Benefield, Lazelle, 20, 71, 508
Benefit-harm factors. *See also* Harm-related topics.
  ARR, 470-479, 532, 532t
  baseline risks, 306-307, 471-473, 477t
  CIs, 473-478
  dichotomous outcomes, 471
  NNH, 477-479
  overviews and summaries of, 470-479
  precision, 473-477
  ratios for, 105-106
  risk levels, 474t-476t
  RRR, 470-479
  RRs, 470-479
Benefit-risk ratios, 523-524
  ABI and, 531-536
  NNH and, 486-487
  NNT and, 486-487
  RBI and, 531-536
  RRR and, 486-487
  screening recommendations and, 528t
Best Practice Guidelines Project, 34-39, 34f, 35t-36t, 42
Best research evidence, 4
Between-study *vs.* within-study differences, 254-255
Bias-related topics. *See also under individual topics.*
  channeling bias, 76, 78
  cointervention, 400-401
  degrees (bias *vs.* random error), 401-403, 402f
  detection bias, 79
  differential administration, 400-401
  differential measures, 401
  expectation bias, 94
  follow-up loss, 401
  future perspectives of, 406
  harm and, 404-406, 404t
  incorporation bias, 342
  interviewer bias, 79
  outcomes determinants, 399-400
  overviews and summaries of, 397-399
  placebo effect, 400

Bias-related topics (Continued)
   prognostic factors, 111, 399-400
   publication bias, 373-380
   random error and, 397-399
   reduction strategies, 404-406, 404t
   reference resources for, 406
   surveillance bias, 79, 286
   target outcomes, 399-400, 401
   verification bias, 94-95
   work-up bias, 94-95
Biologic issues, 482-485
Blinding, 52-54
Bootstrap techniques, 364
Braden Scale for Predicting Pressure Sore Risk,
   210-211
Brenner, Phyllis, 20, 265, 432
Bucher, Heiner, 108, 222
Budgetary viewpoints, 305

C
CAGE (Cut down, Annoyed, Guilty, Eye-opener)
   scores, 367
Calculations, 542-546
   association measures, 543
   for CIs, 546
   for diagnostic tests, 544
   for kappa, 448-451, 449f, 451t, 545
   multivariate regression equations, 461, 464
   overviews and summaries of, 542
Canadian Task Force on Preventive Health Care,
   516t, 519-520, 519t
CANDI (Computer Aided Nursing Diagnosis and
   Intervention), 322
Care grade recommendations, 515-523, 526-541.
   See also Evidence level interpretations
   and health care grade recommendations.
Care organizations (economic issues), 301-302
CAREPLAN, 322
Case-control studies, 47, 75t, 77-78, 274-275,
   420-421, 421t. See also Observational designs.
   overviews and summaries of, 274-275
   surprising results of, 236-243, 238t-242t
Case series and case reports, 78
Cautious detachment, 131
CDSS (computer decision support systems),
   318-335
   clinical acceptance of, 330-331
   clinical scenarios and resolutions for, 319b, 333b
   computer-aided diagnostic systems, 321t, 322
      Antibiotic Assistant, 322
      CANDI, 322
      CAREPLAN, 322
      COMMES, 322
      FLORENCE, 322
      UNIS, 322
   conditional probabilities and, 320
   evidence discovery for, 319-322
   evidence sources, 319-322

CDSS (computer decision support systems)
   (Continued)
   future perspectives of, 333
   identification factors (results), 328-329
   overviews and summaries of, 318
   patient care applications for, 329-333
   portability of, 330
   reference resources for, 334-335
   reliability of, 331
   types of, 320-322, 321t
      alerting systems, 320-322, 321t
      assisting systems, 321t
      computer-aided diagnostic systems, 321t, 322
      critiquing systems, 321-322, 321t
      facilitating systems, 321t
      interpreting systems, 321t
      predicting systems, 321t
      reminder systems, 320-322, 321t
      suggesting systems, 321t
   users' guides for, 323t, 326b-329b
   validity factors (results), 322-328, 323t
Centre for Evidence-Based Medicine (Oxford), 36t
Centre for Evidence-Based Medicine (Toronto), 36t
Centre for Evidence-Based Nursing, 36t
Chance-related topics. See also under individual
   topics.
   agreement beyond chance measures, 446-454
      agreement vs. disagreement, 447
      future perspectives of, 454
      kappa (chance-corrected agreement),
         447-454, 545
      overviews and summaries of, 446
      reference resources for, 454
   agreement by, 447-448
   calculations, 545
   hypotheses and, 423-431. See also Hypotheses
      and hypotheses testing topics.
Channeling bias, 76, 78
Checklist effects, 329-330
Chronic Heart Failure Questionnaire, 304
Ciliska, Donna. See also under individual topics.
   advanced concepts (education- and application-
      related principles) and, 388-394
      differences evaluations (results), 381-387
      fixed-effects vs. random-effects models,
         388-394
      HRQL topics, 205-221
      NNT factors, 469-480
      publication bias, 373-380
      subgroup analyses topics, 251-262
   basic concepts (nursing literature use principles)
      and, 3-19
CINAHL (Cumulative Index to Nursing and Allied
   Health Literature), 33, 35t, 39-40, 142
CIs (confidence intervals), 432-445. See also under
   individual topics.
   association measures and, 418
   calculations for, 546

CIs (confidence intervals) *(Continued)*
clinical prediction rules and, 366-367
definitions for, 433-435
differential diagnoses and, 355-356
future perspectives of, 444
interpretation factors for, 366-367, 435-444
of apparent negative trials, 438-440
of apparent positive trials, 440-442, 441t
of clinical trials, 435-438, 436t
ORs, 438
overviews and summaries of, 366-367
trial magnitudes and, 442-444, 443f
NNT and, 473-477
overviews and summaries of, 432-435
prognoses and, 115-116
reference resources for, 444-445
Classifications (manifestation), 343
Clinical acceptance issues, 330-331
Clinical diagnoses, 361. *See also* Diagnoses-related
topics.
Clinical Evidence, 16-17, 34-39, 34f, 35t, 39, 157
Clinical manifestations of disease topics, 339-348.
See also Diagnoses-related topics.
clinical scenarios and resolutions
for, 340b, 347b
definitions for, 341-342
future perspectives of, 347
identification factors (results), 344-346
estimates precision, 345
manifestation frequencies, 344-345
symptom temporal sequences (presenting,
concurring, eventual), 345-346
incorporation bias, 342
overviews and summaries of, 339-340
patient care applications, 346-347
differential diagnoses generation, 347
manifestation changes over time, 346-347
study patient-clinical setting patient
similarities, 346
reference resources for, 348
reference standard tests, 342
representative samples, 341
syndrome diagnoses, 342
users' guides for, 341t, 343b-344b, 346b
validity factors (results), 340-344
definitive diagnostic standard appropriateness,
342
diagnoses verification criteria credibility and
independence, 342
manifestation classifications, 343
representative patient samples, 340-342
target population mirroring, 340-342
Clinical practice guidelines-related topics, 154-171.
See also Users' guides.
AGA guidelines, 526-536
clinical scenarios and resolutions for, 155b, 169b
development processes and cycles, 155-159,
156f, 159f

Clinical practice guidelines-related topics
(Continued)
evidence discovery, 155-159, 156f, 159f
evidence sources, 155-159
future perspectives of, 170
identification factors (results), 164-167
GRADE Working Group and, 165
overviews and summaries of, 164
practical and clinically important
recommendations, 164
recommendation strengths, 164-166, 167t
implementation processes, 170
interpretation, 254-260, 254t
National Guideline Clearinghouse, 527
patient care applications, 167-169
primary objectives consistency, 167
recommendation applicability, 167-169
reference resources for, 170-171
users' guides, 158t, 163b-164b, 167b-168b
validity factors (results), 159-164
evidence identification, selection, and
combination, 160-161
inclusiveness, 159-160
patient values and preferences specification, 161
peer review and testing, 162
preferences, 158
recent developments inclusion, 162
target outcomes, 158-160
Clinical prediction rules, 359-370
clinical scenarios and resolutions for, 360b, 369b
creation and derivation of, 361-362
definitions for, 360-362, 361f-362f
development of, 362-363, 363t
evidence hierarchies for, 362-363, 363t
overviews and summaries of, 359-360
future perspectives of, 369
impact analyses for, 361-362, 367-369
accuracy rates of, 368
meta-analyses and, 367-368
overviews and summaries of, 360-362, 367-368
steps of, 361-362
interpretation factors of, 366-367
CAGE scores, 367
CIs, 367
Ottawa ankle rules, 360b, 361f, 367-369
overviews and summaries of, 366-367
overviews and summaries of, 359-362, 362f
reference resources for, 369-370
STRATIFY (risk assessment tool), 360
validation processes for, 361-366, 362f, 363t
bootstrap techniques, 364
derivation methodological standards, 364t
overviews and summaries of, 361-362
Clinical records reviews, 283-285, 283t
Clinical scenarios and resolutions. *See also under
individual topics.*
for advanced concepts (education- and
application-related principles)

Clinical scenarios and resolutions *(Continued)*
  CDSS, 319b, 333b
  clinical manifestations of disease topics,
    340b, 347b
  clinical prediction rules, 360b, 369b
  differential diagnoses topics, 350b, 357b
  health services interventions, 266b-267b, 294b
  HRQL topics, 206, 231b
  patient values incorporation topics, 491b, 502b
  screening recommendations, 527b, 539b-540b
  surrogate outcomes topics, 223b, 231b
  for basic concepts (nursing literature use
    principles)
    clinical practice guidelines-related topics,
      155b, 169b
    diagnoses-related topics, 91b, 106b
    fundamental topics, 4b
    harm-related topics, 72b, 84b-85b
    health care intervention topics, 49b, 69b
    organizational practice change topics, 173b
    prognoses-related topics, 109b, 118b
    qualitative research topics, 121b, 134b
    systematic review and summarization topics,
      138b, 151b-152b
Clinical setting-study patients similarities, 65-66,
  82, 117, 346, 356
Clinical states, 4
Clinically important recommendations, 164
Cluster assignment analyses, 287-288
Cluster randomization, 271
CMA Infobase, 223
Cochrane Central Register of Controlled Trials,
  142-143
Cochrane Database of Systematic Reviews, 39, 138,
  223, 527
Cochrane Library, 16-17, 34-39, 34f, 35, 49-50, 138,
  223-224
Coefficients (correlation), 457
Cohen, Marlene, 120
Cohort studies, 46, 52, 75-76, 75t, 273-274. *See also*
  Observational designs.
  historical *vs.* nonrandomized, 273-274
  overviews and summaries of, 273-274
  surprising results of, 236-243, 238t-242t
Cointerventions, 57, 400-401
Collins, Seana, 20-43
COMMES (Creighton Online Multiple Modular
  Expert System), 322
Compatibility characteristics, 180
Completions (reports and studies), 375t
Complexity characteristics, 180
Computer-aided diagnostic systems, 321t, 322. *See
  also* CDSS (computer decision
  support systems).
  Antibiotic Assistant, 322
  CANDI, 322
  CAREPLAN, 322
  COMMES, 322

FLORENCE, 322
  UNIS, 322
Computer Aided Nursing Diagnosis and
  Intervention, 322
Computer decision support systems, 318-335. *See also*
  CDSS (computer decision support systems).
Concealed randomization, 52-54, 276-277
Conditional probabilities, 320
Confirmation components, 190-198, 191t-192t
Confounding variables, 75-76
Consequentialist approaches, 302-303
Consistency issues, 259-260, 521
Constant comparative methods, 124
Constructs, 125-126, 211-212
  sampling of, 125-126
  validity of, 211-212
Continuous outcomes, 409
Continuous quality improvement processes, 272
Continuous variables, 428, 461
Control event rates, 410
Controlled before-and-after studies, 271-272.
  See also Observational designs.
Convenience samples, 124
Cook, Deborah, 48, 120, 137, 154, 205, 222, 318,
  349, 388, 407, 423, 432, 455, 508
Cook, Richard, 446
Correlation topics, 455-466. *See also* Regression and
  correlation topics.
Cortes, Olga, 20
Cost-benefit analyses, 303-304
Cost-benefit ratios, 151
Cost-effectiveness analyses, 303-304
Cost expectation transferability, 314-315
Cost-risk ratios, 151
Cost-to-charge ratios, 307
Cost-utility analyses, 303
Costs as outcomes, 299-304. *See also* Economic
  evaluations.
Cox regression models, 419-420
CQI (continuous quality improvement)
  processes, 272
Craig, Jonathan, 20
CREDIBLE criteria, 498
Creighton Online Multiple Modular Expert
  System, 322
Criteria, 47, 342
  applications of, 47
  credibility and independence of, 342
Critical question explicitness and sensibility, 141-142
Critiquing systems, 321-322, 321t
CTFPHC (Canadian Task Force on Preventive
  Health Care), 516t, 519-520, 519t
Cullum, Nicky, 44-47, 71-86
Cumming, Robert, 71, 526
Cumulative Index to Nursing and Allied Health
  Literature, 33, 35t, 39-40, 142
Cut down, Annoyed, Guilty, Eye-opener (CAGE)
  scores, 367

D

DALYs (disability-adjusted life-years), 214-215, 310
Dans, Antonio, 481
Dans, Leonilla, 481
Database indexing, 375t
de Vos, Rien, 20, 48, 87, 339, 349, 359, 423, 446, 469, 481
Decision aids, 494-498
  advantages of, 497
  CREDIBLE criteria, 498
  Ottawa Decision Support Framework, 495-497, 496t
  overviews and summaries of, 494
  success of, 497-498
Decisions, 186-188, 292-294, 300-302, 375t, 494
  analyses for, 300-302
  components of, 186-188
  decision-maker retrieval, 375t
  decision-making processes, 292-294, 303-304, 494
  decision trees, 300
  models for, 300-302
Definitions. *See also under individual topics.*
  for advanced concepts (education- and application-related principles)
    CIs, 433-435
    clinical manifestations of disease topics, 341-342
    clinical prediction rules, 360-362, 361f-362f
    differential diagnoses topics, 350
    economic evaluations, 299-300
    health services interventions, 269-270
    subgroup analyses topics, 252-253
  for basic concepts (nursing literature use principles)
    fundamental topics, 4-9
    harm-related topics, 45
    systematic review and summarization topics, 138-141
Degrees (bias vs. random error), 401-403, 402f
Demers, Catherine, 298-317
Deontologic approaches, 302-303
Dependent vs. independent variables, 459-466
Derivation methodological standards, 364t
Designs (research), 269-276. *See also under individual topics.*
  mixed method studies, 275
  negative vs. positive studies, 374
  observational designs, 236-243, 271-275
    before-and-after studies (controlled), 271-272
    case-control studies, 236-243, 238t-242t, 274-275, 420-421, 421t
    cohort studies (historical vs. nonrandomized), 236-243, 238t-242t, 273-274
    CQI processes and, 272
    overviews and summaries of, 271
    time-series studies (interrupted), 272-273
  overviews and summaries of, 269-270
  RCTs, 236-243, 238t-242t, 270-271

Designs (research) *(Continued)*
  cluster randomization and, 271
  overviews and summaries of, 270-271
  systematic reviews, 137-153, 275-276
    clinical scenarios and resolutions for, 138b, 151b-152b
    definitions for, 138-141, 140t
    evidence discovery for, 138
    evidence sources for, 138
    future perspectives of, 151
    identification factors (results) for, 141-150, 148f
    overviews and summaries of, 138-141, 140t, 137-138
    patient care applications of, 150-151
    reference resources for, 152-153
    users' guides, 141t-142t, 144b-145b
    validity factors (results) for, 141-145, 141t-142t
Detachment (cautious), 131
Detailing (academic), 189, 191t
Detection bias, 79
Determinants (outcomes), 399-400
Detsky, Alan, 154, 508
Development processes and cycles, 155-159, 156f, 159f
Devereaux, P.J., 48, 245, 469, 490
Diabetes Life Satisfaction Scale, 216b-217b
Diabetes Quality of Life for Youth Measure, 209b-213b
Diagnoses-related topics. *See also under individual topics.*
  advanced concepts (education- and application-related principles), 337-370
    clinical manifestations of disease topics, 339-348
    clinical prediction rules, 359-370
    differential diagnoses topics, 349-358
  basic concepts (nursing literature use principles), 87-107
    calculations (diagnostic tests), 89, 544
    clinical scenarios and resolution for, 91b, 106b
    computer-aided diagnostic systems, 321t, 322. *See also* CDSS (computer decision support systems).
    diagnostic processes, 88-91, 89f
      active alternatives, 89
      choices of, 88-89
      diagnoses probabilities, 89f
      diagnostic and therapeutic thresholds, 89-90, 89f
      diagnostic tests, 91
      false-positive diagnoses, 90
      DSM-IV and, 94
      evidence discovery, 92
      evidence sources, 92
      future perspectives of, 105-106
      identification factors (results), 95-102, 96t, 98t-102t
      likelihood ratios, 95-102, 96t, 98t, 99t-102t
      LR+, 97

Diagnoses-related topics *(Continued)*
  LR–, 97
  nomograms, 97-99, 98f
  sensitivity, 99-102
  specificity, 99-102
  leading hypotheses, 89
  no-test *vs.* test thresholds, 90
  overviews and summaries of, 87-88, 88
  patient care applications, 102-106
    applicability, 103-104
    benefit-harm ratios, 105-106
    diagnostic test reproducibility, 102-103
    management strategy changes, 104-105
  pretest *vs.* posttest probabilities, 88
  reference resources for, 106-107
  systematic research and, 90-91
  users' guides, 92t, 95b, 101b, 103b-105b
  validity factors (results), 93-95
    evaluation and assessments, 93
    expectation bias, 94
    test gold standards, 94-95
    verification bias, 94-95
    work-up bias, 94-95
  verification criteria credibility and
    independence, 342
  working diagnoses, 89
DiCenso, Alba. *See also under individual topics.*
  advanced concepts (education- and application-
    related principles) and, 205-541
  agreement beyond chance measures,
    446-454
  association measures, 407-422
  bias and random error topics, 397-406
  CIs, 432-445
  clinical manifestations of disease topics,
    339-348
  clinical prediction rules, 359-370
  evidence level interpretation and health care
    grades recommendations, 508-525
  health services intervention topics, 265-297
  HRQL topics, 205-221
  hypothesis testing topics, 423-431
  individual patient care applications, 481-489
  intention to treat principle, 245-250
  NNT factors, 469-480
  regression and correlation topics, 455-466
  screening recommendations, 526-541
  surprising results-related topics, 235-244
  surrogate outcomes topics, 222-234
  basic concepts (nursing literature use principles)
    and, 3-153
  clinical practice guidelines-related topics,
    154-171
  evidence discovery factors, 20-43
  fundamental topics, 3-19
  health care intervention topics, 48-70
  prognosis-related topics, 108-119
  qualitative research topics, 120-136

DiCenso, Alba *(Continued)*
  systematic review and summarization topics,
    137-153
Dichotomous outcomes, 60, 409, 471
Dichotomous variables, 461
Differences evaluations (results), 381-387
  future perspectives of, 387
  heterogeneity and, 382, 385
  meta-analyses and, 382-385, 383f-384f
  overviews and summaries of, 381
  pooling and, 382-387
  reference resources for, 387
  systematic reviews and, 382
  variability, 383-385, 383f-384f
Differential administration, 400-401
Differential diagnoses topics, 349-358. *See also*
  Diagnoses-related topics.
  clinical manifestations and, 347
  clinical scenarios and resolutions for, 350b, 357b
  definitions for, 350
  evidence discovery, 350-351, 351t
    assessment of, 351t
    overviews of, 350
  evidence sources, 350
  future perspectives of, 357
  generation of, 347
  identification factors (results), 355-356
    CIs, 355-356
    diagnoses identification and probability
      estimates, 355
    disease probability estimate precision, 355-356
    precision formulae, 355
  patient care applications, 347, 356-357
    disease probability changes over
      time, 356-357
    overviews and summaries of, 347
    study patient-clinical setting patient
      similarities, 356
  reference resources for, 357-358
  users' guides for, 351t, 354b-357b
  validity factors (results), 351-355
    diagnoses reproducibility, 352-353
    follow-up durations and completeness,
      354-355
    patient enrollments, 351-352
    representative patient samples, 351-352
    standards appropriateness, explicitness, and
      credibility, 352-353
    target population mirroring, 351-352
    underdiagnosed patients, 354-355
Differential measures, 401
Diffusion Innovations theory, 174
DiGiulio, Paola, 48, 71, 235
Disability-adjusted life-years, 214-215, 310
Disagreement *vs.* agreement (chance), 447
Discovery-related factors, 20-43. *See also* Evidence
  discovery.
Disease Impact Scale, 216b

Disease manifestations topics, 339-348. *See also* Clinical manifestations of disease topics.

Disease-Related Worries Scale, 216b

Dissertation Abstracts Online, 143

Dobbins, Maureen, 154-171, 172-200, 490

Document analyses, 126-128, 126f

Dose response gradients, 81

Dowding, Dawn, 318-336

Down-stream costs, 309

Driever, Marie, 265, 318, 481

Drug evaluations, 224-225

Drummond, Michael, 298

DSM-IV (Diagnostic and Statistical Manual of Mental Disorders, fourth edition), 94

E

EBN (evidence-based nursing) concepts. *See also under individual topics.*
  advanced concepts (education- and application-related principles), 201-541
    diagnoses-related topics, 337-370
    health care intervention topics, 203-262
    health services research topics, 263-336
    practice applications topics, 467-541
    results-related topics, 395-466
    systematic review and summarization topics, 371-394
  basic concepts (nursing literature use principles), 1-200
    clinical practice guidelines-related topics, 154-171
    diagnoses-related topics, 87-107
    evidence discovery factors, 20-43
    fundamental topics, 3-19
    harm-related topics, 44-47, 71-86
    health care intervention topics, 44-70
    organizational practice change topics, 172-200
    prognoses-related topics, 108-119
    qualitative research topics, 120-136
    systematic review and summarization topics, 137-153
  calculations, 542-546
  overviews and summaries of, 3-19
  reference resources for. *See* Reference resources.

Economic analyses, 303-304

Economic evaluations, 298-317
  costs as outcomes, 299-304
    care organizations and, 301-302
    challenges of, 303-304
    Chronic Heart Failure Questionnaire and, 304
    consequentialist approaches and, 302-303
    controversies about, 302-303
    cost analyses and, 300-301, 308
    cost-benefit analyses and, 303-304
    cost-effectiveness analyses and, 303-304
    cost-utility analyses and, 303
    DALYs, 310
    decision analyses and models, 300-302

Economic evaluations *(Continued)*
    decision trees for, 300-301
    deontologic approaches, 302-303
    economic analyses and, 303-304
    health care policy decision-making and, 303-304
    overviews and summaries of, 299-301
    QALYs and, 303
    resource-intensive approaches and, 303
    strategies and models for, 300-301
    utilitarian approaches and, 302-303
    variability levels (costs *vs.* other outcomes), 301-302
  definitions for, 299-300
  evidence sources for, 299
  future perspectives of, 315
  hierarchies for, 299
  identification factors (results), 308-311
    down-stream costs, 309
    effects differences, 310
    Global Burden of Disease Study and, 310
    Health Utilities Index and, 310
    incremental costs, 308-310, 309t
    sensitivity analyses, 310-311
    statistical significance tests, 311
    strategy effects, 308-310, 309t
    subgroup differences, 310
    up-front costs, 309
  overviews and summaries of, 298-299
  patient care applications, 311-315, 312f
    cost expectation transferability, 314-315
    opportunity costs, 313
    outcomes matrices for, 311-313, 312f
    overviews and summaries of, 311
    treatment benefits *vs.* risks and costs, 311-313, 312f
  quality of, 299
  reference resources for, 315-317
  users' guides for, 304t
  validity factors (results), 304-308
    baseline risk reporting differences, 306-307
    cost measurements accuracy, 307-308
    cost timing consequences, 308
    cost-to-charge ratios, 307
    incremental cost differences, 310
    methodological factors and, 305-306, 306t
    narrow budgetary viewpoints, 305
    silo effects, 305
    societal viewpoints, 305-306
    United States Panel on Cost-Effectiveness in Health and Medicine and, 308
    viewpoint broadness, 304-306

Editorial considerations, 375t

Education- and application-related principles (advanced topics). *See also under individual topics.*
  diagnoses-related topics, 337-370
  health care intervention topics, 203-262

Education- and application-related principles
    (advanced topics) *(Continued)*
  health services research topics, 263-336
  interactive education, 192t
  practice applications topics, 467-541
  results-related topics, 395-466
  systematic review and summarization topics,
    371-394
Education outreach visits, 189, 191t
Edwards, Nancy, 154, 265-297
Effects. *See also under individual topics.*
  adverse effects risks, 485-487
  checklist, 329-330
  differences of, 310
  hypothesized, 255-260
    consistency of, 259-260
    magnitudes of, 256-257
    statistical significance of, 257-259, 258f
  measures of, 253-254, 254t
  models for, 147
    fixed-effects, 147
    random-effects, 147
  strategy, 308-310, 309t
Electronic database indexing, 375t
EMBASE, 35t, 41, 142
End points (surrogate), 229, 236-243, 238t-242t
Enrollments (patients), 351-352
Environmental characteristics, 180, 185b
Epidemiologic issues, 485
Equations (multivariate regression), 461-464
Equivalence studies, 428
ERIC, 142
Estabrooks, Carole, 3, 137, 172
Estimates precision, 61-64, 63f, 115-116, 345
Ethics/institutional review board approval, 375t
Ethnographies, 123
Evaluation components, 194t-197t
Evaluation-related topics. *See also under individual
    topics.*
  differences evaluations (results), 381-387
  drug evaluations, 224-225
  economic evaluations, 298-317
  formal utility assessments, 499-501
  health care recommendations, 511-514, 512t
  patient-derived assessments, 209-210
  process evaluations, 190
  STRATIFY (risk assessment tool), 360
  structure evaluations, 190
Evidence-Based Cardiovascular Medicine, 23
Evidence-Based Mental Health, 23
Evidence-Based Nursing, 16-17, 23, 37, 49-50,
    56, 121
Evidence-based nursing concepts. *See* EBN
    (evidence-based nursing concepts).
Evidence discovery, 20-43. *See also under individual
    topics.*
  for advanced concepts (education- and
    application-related principles), 337-370

Evidence discovery *(Continued)*
  CDSS, 319-322
  differential diagnoses topics, 350-352, 351t
  patient values incorporation topics, 491-507
  screening recommendations, 525-541
  surrogate outcomes topics, 222-234
  assessment of, 351t
  for basic concepts (nursing literature use
    principles)
    clinical practice guidelines-related topics,
      155-159, 156f, 159f
    diagnoses-related topics, 92
    harm-related topics, 72
    health care intervention topics, 49-50
    prognoses-related topics, 109-111
    qualitative research topics, 121-122
    systematic review and summarization
      topics, 138
  evidence sources for. *See* Evidence sources.
  future perspectives of, 42
  literature use methods for, 21-23, 22f
    background *vs.* foreground questions,
      21-23, 22f
    for informed decision-making, 23
    novice *vs.* expert questions, 21-23, 22f
    overviews and summaries of, 21
    research currency, 23
  overviews and summaries of, 20-21, 42
  question framing methods for, 23-27
  reference resources for, 42-43
  search methods for, 28-32, 28f-31f
    overviews and summaries of, 28
    for qualitative studies, 32
    for quantitative studies, 28-32, 28f-31f
    question type determinations, 28
    for systematic reviews, 32, 138
Evidence hierarchies, 12-14, 13t, 16t, 362-363, 363t
Evidence level interpretations and health care grade
    recommendations, 508-525
  benefit-risk ratios and, 523-524
  future perspectives of, 524
  health care grade recommendations, 515-523
    Centre for Evidence-Based Medicine, 516t
    consistency and, 521
    criteria for, 522-523, 522t
    CTFPHC, 516t, 519-520, 519t
    directness and, 521
    vs. evidence levels, 514-515
    examples of, 516t, 518t-519t
    GRADE Working Group, 520-523, 522t
    NZCG, 517, 518t
    problems of, 515-520
    Scientific Advisory Council of the
      Osteoporosis Society of Canada, 516t
    Scottish Intercollegiate Guidelines Network,
      516t
  health care recommendations, 509-515
    vs. clinical practice guidelines, 511

Evidence level interpretations and health care grade recommendations *(Continued)*
  development of, 509-511, 510f
  evaluations of, 511-514, 512t
  vs. health care grade recommendations, 514-515
  overviews and summaries of, 509
  overviews and summaries of, 508, 524
  reference resources for, 524-525
  users' guides for, 512t
Evidence sources, 21-42, 34f, 35t-36t. *See also under individual topics.*
  ACP Journal Club, 23
  Adult Asthma Care Guidelines, 173, 176b-177b, 184b-190b, 193b
  for advanced concepts (education- and application-related principles)
    CDSS, 319-322
    differential diagnoses topics, 350
    economic evaluations, 299
    screening recommendations, 526
    surrogate outcomes topics, 224-225
  AGA guidelines, 527-536
  AHRQ, 42, 155
  Bandolier, 42
  for basic concepts (nursing literature use principles)
    clinical practice guidelines-related topics, 155-159
    diagnoses-related topics, 92
    harm-related topics, 72
    health care intervention topics, 49-50, 56
    prognoses-related topics, 109-111
    qualitative research topics, 121-122
    systematic reviews, 138-141
  Centre for Evidence-Based Medicine (Oxford), 36t
  Centre for Evidence-Based Medicine (Toronto), 36t
  Centre for Evidence-Based Nursing, 36t
  CINAHL, 33, 35t, 39-40, 142
  Clinical Evidence, 16-17, 34-37, 34f, 35t, 157
  clinical practice guidelines, 34, 36t
  CMA Infobase, 223
  Cochrane Central Register of Controlled Trials, 142
  Cochrane Database of Systematic Reviews, 39, 138, 223
  Cochrane Library, 16-17, 34-39, 34f, 35t 49-50, 138, 223-224
  Dissertation Abstracts Online, 143
  EBM Toolkit, 36t
  EMBASE, 35t, 41, 142, 439
  ERIC, 142
  Evidence-Based Cardiovascular Medicine, 23
  Evidence-Based Mental Health, 23
  Evidence-Based Nursing, 16-17, 23, 37, 49-50, 56, 121
  German Centre for Evidence-Based Nursing, 36t
  Google.com, 155
  Joanna Briggs Institute, 36t

Evidence sources *(Continued)*
  journal selections, 375t
  Knowledge Finder, 40
  MEDLINE, 35t, 38-41, 92, 142
  National Guidelines Clearinghouse, 36t, 42
  overviews and summaries of, 33
  OVID, 40
  PreMEDLINE, 40-41
  preprocessed sources, 34-39, 34f, 35t
  PsycINFO, 142
  PubMed, 34-39, 34f, 35t, 92, 109, 319, 350
  RNAO Best Practice Guidelines Project, 34-39, 34f, 36t, 42
  Sarah Cole Hirsh Institute, 36t
  ScHARR Netting the Evidence, 36t
  selection criteria for, 33
  Silver Platter, 40
  TRIP Database, 42
  Ulrich's Periodicals Directory, 21
  United Kingdom National Health Service Economic Evaluation Database, 299
  unprocessed sources, 35t, 39-42
Expectation bias, 94
Expert *vs.* novice questions, 21-23, 22f
Explicit strategies, 494
Exposed patient identification, 79
Exposure stoppages, 83-84
Externals *vs.* internal validity, 269-270

F
Face *vs.* construct validity, 211-212
Facilitating systems, 321t
False-negative risks, 427-428
False-positive diagnoses, 90
False-positive *vs.* false-negative results, 528-529
Feedback, 189, 329-330
Feeling thermometers, 499-501, 500f
Field observations, 126-127, 126f
Fineout-Overholt, Ellen, 3
Fixed-effects *vs.* random-effects models, 388-394
  data pooling models and, 389
  definitions for, 389
  differences evaluations (results) for, 389-392, 390f, 392f
  future perspectives of, 392
  overviews and summaries of, 388
  reference resources for, 392-393
Flanagin, Annette, 3, 318, 397
Flemming, Kate, 3, 20, 48, 235, 481
FLORENCE, 322
Follow-ups, 57-59, 113-118, 354-355, 401
  completeness of, 57-59, 58t, 113, 354-355
  durations of, 117, 354
  loss, 401
Foreground *vs.* background questions, 21-23, 22f
Formal utility assessments, 499-501
Frameworks (organizational), 173-198
  confirmation components of, 190-198, 191t-192t

Frameworks (organizational) *(Continued)*
  decision components of, 186-188
  evaluation components of, 194t-197t
  implementation components of, 188-190,
      194t-197t
  knowledge components, 174-177, 175t
  overviews and summaries of, 173-174
  persuasion components of, 177-186, 178f-179f,
      181t-183t
Fundamental topics, 3-19
  barrier-related issues, 15-17, 16t
  clinical scenarios and resolutions for, 4b
  clinical skills, 6-7
  definitions for, 4-9
  evidence hierarchies, 12-14, 13t, 16t
  future perspectives of, 17
  humanism, 6-7
  misconceptions, 8-12, 11t
    about atheoretical aspects, 9-10
    about meta-analyses, 12
    about patient preference and values, 8-9
    about quantitative *vs.* qualitative research,
        10-11, 11t
    about RCT overemphasis, 12
    about systematic reviews overemphasis, 12
  overviews and summaries of, 3, 17
  reference resources for, 17-19
  relevancy-related issues, 11t
  social responsibility, 6-7
Funding-related issues, 375t-376t
Funnel plots (magnitude *vs.* precision), 377-379,
      378f-379f
Future perspectives. *See also under individual topics.*
  of advanced concepts (education- and
      application-related principles)
    agreement beyond chance measures, 454
    association measures, 421
    bias- and random error-related topics, 406
    CDSS, 333
    CIs, 444
    clinical manifestations of disease topics, 347
    clinical prediction rules, 369
    differences evaluations (results), 387
    differential diagnoses topics, 357
    economic evaluations, 315
    evidence level interpretations and health care
        grade recommendations, 524
    hypotheses and hypotheses testing topics, 431
    intention to treat principle, 250
    NNT factors, 478-479
    patient care applications, 488
    publication bias, 379
    regression and correlation topics, 465-466
    subgroup analyses topics, 260-261
    surprising results-related topics, 243
    surrogate outcomes topics, 230-231
  of basic concepts (nursing literature use
      principles)

Future perspectives *(Continued)*
    clinical practice guidelines-related topics, 170
    diagnoses-related topics, 105-106
    evidence discovery, 42
    fundamental topics, 17
    harm-related topics, 47
    health care intervention topics, 68
    prognoses-related topics, 118

G

Gambles (standard), 214-215, 214f, 501
German Centre for Evidence-Based Nursing, 36t
Giacomini, Mita, 120
Glasziou, Paul, 154, 508, 526
Global Burden of Disease Study, 310
Gold standards, 94-95
Google.com, 155
GRADE (Grades of Recommendation Assessment,
      Development, and Evaluation) Working
      Group, 165, 520-523, 522t
Grading recommendations, 515-541. *See also*
      Evidence level interpretations and health care
      grade recommendations.
Gray, Muir, 526
Green, Lee, 154, 508
Gregory, David, 120-136
Grimshaw, Jeremy, 265-297
Grounded theories, 123-124
Guides and guidelines. *See* Clinical practice
      guidelines-related topics; Users' guides.
Guyatt, Gordon. *See also under individual topics.*
    advanced concepts (education- and application-
        related principles) and, 205-541
    agreement beyond chance measures and,
        446-454
    association measures, 407-422
    bias and random error topics, 397-406
    CDSS, 318-336
    CIs, 432-445
    clinical manifestations of disease topics,
        339-348
    clinical prediction rules, 359-370
    differences evaluations (results), 381-387
    differential diagnoses topics, 349-358
    economic evaluations, 298-317
    evidence levels interpretations and health care
        grades recommendations, 508-525
    fixed effects *vs.* random effects models, 388-393
    health services intervention topics, 265-297
    HRQL topics, 205-221
    hypothesis testing topics, 423-431
    individual patient care applications, 481-489
    intention to treat principle, 245-250
    NNT factors, 469-480
    patient values incorporation topics, 490-507
    publication bias, 373-380
    regression and correlation topics, 455-466
    screening recommendations, 526-541

Guyatt, Gordon *(Continued)*
   subgroup analyses topics, 251-262
   surprising results-related topics, 235-244
   surrogate outcomes topics, 222-234
   basic concepts (nursing literature use principles) and, 3-171
     clinical practice guidelines-related topics, 154-171
     fundamental topics, 3-19
     harm-related topics, 44-47, 71-86
     health care intervention topics, 48-70
     prognoses-related topics, 108-119
     qualitative research topics, 120-136
     systematic review and summarization topics, 137-153
   users' guides and, 20, 48, 71, 87, 108, 120, 137, 154, 205, 235, 251, 265, 298, 318, 339, 349, 373, 381, 397, 407, 423, 432, 446, 455, 469, 481, 508, 526

H

Haines, Ted, 71
Harm-related topics, 44-46, 71-86
   benefit-harm ratios, 105-106
   bias and, 404-406, 404t
   clinical scenarios and resolutions for, 72b, 84-85
   criteria applications, 47
   definitions for, 44
   evidence discovery, 72
   evidence sources, 72
   future perspectives of, 47
   harm-benefit factors, 470-479
     ARR, 470-479
     baseline risks, 471-473, 477t
     CIs, 473-478
     dichotomous outcomes, 471
     NNH, 477-478
     overviews and summaries of, 470-471
     precision, 473-477
     risk levels, 474t-476t
     RRR, 470-479
     RRs, 470-479
   health care interventions and, 44-47
   identification factors (results), 45, 81-82
     CIs, 81-82
     dose response gradients, 81
     exposure-outcome association strengths, 81
     overviews and summaries of, 45
     relative risks, 81
     risk estimate precision, 81-82
   NNH, 409, 486-487
   overviews and summaries of, 44, 71
   patient care applications, 45-46, 82-84
     absolute risk increases, 83
     exposure stoppages, 83-84
     follow-up durations, 82
     overviews and summaries of, 45-46
     risk magnitudes, 82-83

Harm-related topics *(Continued)*
     study patient-clinical setting patient similarities, 82
   reference resources for, 47, 85-86
   study designs, 46-47, 75-79, 75t
     case-control studies, 47, 75t, 77-78
     case series and case reports, 78
     cohort studies, 46, 75-76, 75t
     observational studies, 46-47
     overviews and summaries of, 46, 75t, 78
     RCTs, 46, 72-80
   users' guides, 73t, 79b-80b
   validity factors (results), 45, 72-80
     channeling bias, 76
     confounding variables, 75-76
     controls, 77-78
     detection bias, 79
     exposed patient identification, 79
     follow-up completeness, 79
     inquiry directions for, 75t
     interviewer bias, 79
     ORs, 77-78, 81
     outcomes assessments uniformity, 79
     overviews and summaries of, 45, 72-74, 75t
     surveillance bias, 79
Haslam, David, 71
Hatala, Rose, 381
Hawthorne effects, 332
Haynes, Brian, 20, 318, 490
Hayward, Robert, 20, 154, 508
Hayward, Sarah, 3, 137, 172
Hazard ratios, 60
Health care grade recommendations, 515-523, 526-641. *See also* Evidence level interpretations and health care grade recommendations.
Health care intervention topics, 44-86, 203-262. *See also under individual topics.*
   advanced concepts (education- and application-related principles), 203-297
     health services interventions, 265-297
     HRQL topics, 205-221
     intention to treat principle, 245-250
     subgroup analyses topics, 251-262
     surprising results-related topics, 235-244
     surrogate outcomes topics, 222-234
   basic concepts (nursing literature use principles), 44-86
     harm-related topics, 44-86
     health care interventions, 48-70
   clinical scenarios and resolutions, 49b, 69b
   evidence discovery, 49-50
   evidence sources, 49-50, 56
   future perspectives of, 68
   identification factors (results), 60-65
     ABI, 60
     absolute differences, 60
     ARR, 60

Health care intervention topics *(Continued)*
CIs, 64
dichotomous outcomes, 60
effects magnitudes, 60-61, 61t
estimates precision, 61-64, 63f
hazard ratios, 60
relative benefit increases, 60
relative differences, 60
RRR, 60-64, 63f
survival analyses, 60
overviews and summaries, 48
patient care applications, 65-69
cost-benefit ratios, 67-69, 67t
economic analyses, 67
harm-benefit ratios, 67-69, 67t
inclusion *vs.* exclusion criteria, 65
NNT factors, 67-68, 67t
outcomes inclusivity, 66-67
study patient-clinical setting patient
similarities, 65-66
reference resources for, 69-70
study designs, 52-59
cohort studies, 52
observational studies, 52
RCTs, 52-59
users' guides for, 51t
validity factors (results), 50-59
allocation concealment, 52-54
blinding, 56-59
cointerventions, 57
concealed randomization, 52-54
event rates, 59
follow-up completeness, 57-59, 58t
group allocation awareness, 52-54, 56-57
intention-to-treat principle, 54
lost to follow-up concept, 57-59, 58t
masking, 56
non-adherent patients, 54
outcome assessor awareness, 56-57
overviews and summaries of, 50-51
patient-group exclusions, 54
patient randomization, 51-52
placebo effects, 55-56
Health care personnel influences, 485
Health care policy decision-making, 303-304
Health care recommendations, 509-515
vs. clinical practice guidelines, 511
development of, 509-511, 510f
evaluations of, 511-514, 512t
overviews and summaries of, 509
Health profiles, 213
Health services interventions, 265-297
clinical scenarios and resolutions for, 266b-267b,
294b
decision-making factors for, 292-293
outcomes inclusivity, 293-294
overviews and summaries of, 292
processes inclusivity, 293-294

Health services interventions *(Continued)*
definitions for, 269-270
identification factors (results), 290-292
ARIMA models and, 291
autocorrelation and, 291
effects magnitudes, 290-291
effects precision, 291
time-series regression techniques and, 291
overviews and summaries of, 265, 267-268
patient care applications, 292-293
reference resources for, 294-297
research designs for, 269-276. *See also* Designs
(research).
mixed-method studies, 275
observational designs, 271-275
overviews and summaries of, 269-270
RCTs, 270-271
systematic reviews, 275-276
users' guides for, 277t, 289b-292b
validity factors (results), 276-290, 278t, 280t,
282t-283t
administrative databases use, 281-282, 282t
analyses differences adjustments, 279-280, 280t
assessments for, 278t
clinical records reviews, 283-285, 283t
comparison group data collection measures
and, 285
concealed randomization, 276-277
for determinants, 280-285
determinants similarities, 279-280, 280t
exposures and outcomes assessment
uniformity and bias, 285-286
exposures and outcomes completeness,
286-287
group allocation blinding, 286
independent outcomes and, 288
intention-to-treat principle, 279
internal *vs.* external validity, 288-289
multivariate analyses and, 288
nonrandomized studies and, 288-289
for outcomes measures, 280-285
overviews and summaries of, 276, 277t
for processes, 280-285
vs. reliability factors, 281
rival plausible explanations and, 288-289
self-reported data reviews, 285
study patient groups analyses, 276-277
study patient randomization, 276-277, 279
surveillance bias and, 286
unit/cluster assignment analyses adjustments,
287-288
Health services research topics, 263-335. *See also*
under individual topics.
CDSS, 318-335
economic evaluations, 298-317
health services interventions, 265-297
Health Utilities Index, 310
Heterogeneity, 382, 385

Heterogeneity tests, 145-146
Heyland, Daren, 205, 298
Hicks, Nicholas, 526
Hierarchies (evidence), 12-14, 13t, 16t, 299,
    362-363, 363t, 501-502
Historical *vs.* nonrandomized cohort studies,
    273-274
Holbrook, Anne, 71, 222
Homogeneity, 112-113
HRQL (health-related quality of life) topics,
    205-221
  clinical scenarios and resolutions for, 206b, 219b
  HRQL-specific factors, 207-208, 207t
  measurement instruments, 209-217
    Braden Scale for Predicting Pressure Sore Risk,
        210-211
    Diabetes Life Satisfaction Scale, 216b
    Diabetes Quality of Life for Youth Measure,
        209b-213b
    Disease Impact Scale, 216b
    Disease-Related Worries Scale, 216b-217b
    Medical Outcomes Study, 213
    New York Heart Association functional
        classification, 216
    Owestry Back-Disability Index, 215-216
    Sickness Impact Profile, 213
  NNT factors, 216-217, 217t. *See also* NNT
      (number needed to treat) factors.
  overviews and summaries of, 205-207
  patient care applications, 217-219
  reference resources for, 219-221
  result description and analysis factors, 215-216
  users' guides for, 207t, 208b-213b, 215b-219b
  validity factors (results), 209-215, 214f
    aspect omissions, 212-213
    face *vs.* construct validity, 211-212
    health profiles, 213
    measurement properties, 210-212
    patient-derived assessments, 209-210
    QALYs *vs.* DALYs, 214-215
    quantity-quality of life trade-offs, 213-215, 214f
    responsiveness, 211
    signal-noise relationships, 210-211
    standard gambles, 214-215, 214f
    utility measures, 214-215
Humanism, 6-7
Hunt, Dereck, 20
Hutchison, Brian, 265-297
Hypotheses and hypotheses testing topics, 423-431
  baseline differences, 428-429
    adjusted analyses, 428-429
    randomization, 428-429
  chance, 424-425. *See also* Chance-related topics.
  continuous variables, 428
  effects, 255-260
    consistency of, 259-260
    magnitudes of, 256-257
    statistical significance of, 257-259, 258f

Hypotheses and hypotheses testing topics
    (Continued)
  examples for, 428
  false-negative risks, 427-428
    equivalence studies and, 428
    power and, 427-428
    type II errors, 427-428
  future perspectives of, 431
  leading hypotheses, 89
  limitations of, 431
  multiple tests, 429-430
  null hypotheses, 374, 433, 458
  overviews and summaries of, 423-424
  P values, 425-427
    alpha levels, 425
    statistical significance, 426-427
    type I errors, 425
  reference resources for, 431

I
Icart Isern, Teresa, 87, 235, 339, 446
Identification factors (results). *See also under*
    individual topics.
  ABI, 60
  absolute differences, 60
  for advanced concepts (education- and
      application-related principles)
    CDSS, 328-329
    clinical manifestations of disease topics,
        344-346
    differential diagnoses topics, 355-356
    economic evaluations, 308-311
    health services interventions, 290-292
    HRQL topics, 215-217
    surrogate outcomes topics, 229-231
  autocorrelation, 291
  for basic concepts (nursing literature use principles)
    clinical practice guidelines-related topics,
        164-167
    diagnoses-related topics, 95-102, 96t, 98f,
        99t-102t
    harm-related topics, 45, 81-82
    health care intervention topics, 60-65
    prognoses-related topics, 115-117
    qualitative research topics, 131-132
    systematic review and summarization topics,
        145-150, 148f
  cautious detachment, 131
  CIs, 115-116, 355-356
  diagnoses identification and probability
      estimates, 355
  dichotomous outcomes, 60
  down-stream costs, 309
  effects, 60-61, 61t, 310
    differences of, 310
    magnitudes of, 60-61, 61t
  estimates precision, 61-64, 63f, 115-116, 345
  fixed-effects models, 147

Identification factors (results) *(Continued)*
  Global Burden of Disease Study and, 310
  hazard ratios, 60
  Health Utilities Index and, 310
  heterogeneity tests, 145-146
  incremental costs, 308-310, 309t
  intervention magnitudes, precision, and
      duration, 229-230
  likelihood ratios, 95-102, 96t, 98f, 99t, 102t
    LR+, 97
    LR−, 97
  manifestation frequencies, 344-345
  meta-analyses, 145-149, 148f
  nomograms, 97-99, 98f
  outcomes occurrences over time, 115
  overall results, 146-149
  practical and clinically important
      recommendations, 164
  precision, 149, 355
  probability estimates, 355
  random-effects models, 147
  recommendation strengths, 164-167, 167t
  results similarities, 145-146
  sensitivity, 99-102, 146, 310-311
  specificity, 99-102
  statistical significance tests, 311
  strategy effects, 308-310, 309t
  subgroup differences, 310
  surrogate end points, 229
  survival analyses, 60, 115-116, 116f
  symptom temporal sequences (presenting,
      concurring, eventual), 345
  thoroughness, 131
  time-series regression techniques and, 291
  up-front costs, 309
Identification (publication bias), 377-379,
    378f-379f
  asymmetry and, 377
  funnel plots (magnitude *vs.* precision) for,
      377-378, 378f-379f
  overviews and summaries of, 377-378
  trim-and-fill methods and, 378
Identification (screening recommendations),
    531-536
Identification (values), 498-505. *See also* Patient
    values incorporation topics.
  analytic hierarchy processes, 501-502
  balance scales, 499
  examples of, 503f-505f
  feeling thermometers, 499-501, 500f
  formal utility assessments, 499-501
  overviews and summaries of, 498-499
  standard gambles, 501
  threshold techniques, 501
  time trade-offs, 501
  visual analogue scales, 499-501, 500f
Impact analyses and tests, 361-362, 367-369
  accuracy rates, 368

Impact analyses and tests *(Continued)*
  meta-analyses and, 367-368
  overviews and summaries of, 361-362,
      367-368
  steps of, 361-362
Implementation components and processes, 170,
    188-190, 194t-197t
Inclusiveness, 159-160, 293-295
Incorporation bias, 342
Incremental costs, 308-310, 309t
Independent associations, 226
Independent *vs.* dependent variables, 459-466
Indexing (electronic databases), 375t
Indirect evidence support, 260
Individual characteristics, 184, 185b
Individual patient care applications, 481-489.
    See also Patient care applications.
Informed decision-making, 23
Innovation characteristics, 180, 184b-185b
Inquiry directions, 75t
Institutional/ethics review board approval, 375t
Instruments (measurement). *See* Measurement
    instruments.
Intention to treat principle, 245-250
  future perspectives of, 250
  intention-to-treat analyses and, 249-250
  misleading use of, 249-250
  overviews and summaries of, 245
  RCTs and, 246-249, 247f-249f
    examples for, 246-249, 247f-249f
    overviews and summaries of, 246
  reference resources for, 250
Interactive education, 192t
Interactive workshops, 189
Internal *vs.* external validity, 269-270
Interobservers/interraters, 447
Interpretation guidelines, 254-260, 254t
  between-study *vs.* within-study differences,
      254-255
  hypothesized effects
    consistency of, 259-260
    magnitudes of, 255-257
    statistical significance of, 257-259, 258f
  indirect evidence support, 260
  overviews and summaries of, 254, 254t
  post hoc analyses, 255
  a priori analyses, 255
Interpreting systems, 321t
Interraters/interobservers, 447
Interrupted time-series studies, 272-273
Intervals (confidence), 432-445. *See also* CIs
    (confidence intervals).
Intervention-related topics. *See* Health care
    intervention topics.
Interviewer bias, 79
Interviews, 126-128, 126f
Investigator triangulation, 129
Irwig, Les, 526

J

Jaeschke, Roman, 20, 205, 407, 423, 432, 455
Joanna Briggs Institute, 36t
Johnston, Linda, 154, 172, 481
Journal selections, 375t
Judgmental sampling, 125-126
Jull, Andrew, 48, 137, 222, 339-370, 432, 446-454, 455, 469, 490
　　agreement beyond chance measures and, 446-454
　　clinical manifestations of disease topics and, 339-348
　　clinical prediction rules and, 359-370
　　differential diagnoses topics and, 349-358
Juniper, Elizabeth, 205

K

Kappa (chance-corrected agreement), 447-454. *See also* Agreement beyond chance measures.
　　calculations for, 448-451, 449f, 451t, 545
　　limitations of, 452-453
　　ORs and, 453-454, 453f
　　overviews and summaries of, 447-448, 448f
　　vs. phi, 453-454, 453f
　　with three or more raters or categories, 451-452, 452f
　　weighted kappa statistics, 452
Kessenich, Cathy, 3, 172, 222, 245, 423-431, 432, 469
Knowledge components, 174, 175f
Knowledge enhancement, 134
Knowledge Finder, 40
Koyama, Mariko, 508

L

Lacchetti, Christina, 235, 469, 490
Lay press reports, 375t
Leading hypotheses, 89
Lee, Hui, 71
Leung, Raymond, 542-546
Levels, 474t-476t, 526-541. *See also under individual topics.*
　　of evidence, 526-541
　　of risk, 474t-476t
Levine, Mitchell, 71, 298
Life-years (disability-adjusted *vs.* quality-adjusted), 214-215
Lijmer, Jeroen, 87, 349
Likelihood ratios, 95-102, 96f, 98f, 99t-102t
　　LR+, 97
　　LR−, 97
　　overviews and summaries of, 95-102, 98f, 99t-102t
Literature use methods, 21-23, 22f
　　background *vs.* foreground questions, 21-23, 22f
　　for informed decision-making, 23
　　novice *vs.* expert questions, 21-23, 22f
　　overviews and summaries of, 21
　　research currency, 23

Literature use principles (basic concepts). *See also under individual topics.*
　　clinical practice guidelines-related topics, 154-171
　　diagnoses-related topics, 87-107
　　evidence discovery factors, 20-43
　　fundamental topics, 3-19
　　harm-related topics, 44-47, 71-86
　　health care intervention topics, 48-70
　　literature use methods, 21-23
　　organizational practice change topics, 172-200
　　prognoses-related topics, 108-119
　　qualitative research topics, 120-136
　　systematic review and summarization topics, 137-153
Lock, Sharon, 235, 349, 407
Loss (follow-up), 401
LR− (likelihood ratio for negative test results), 97
LR+ (likelihood ratio for positive test results), 97

M

Management applicability, 118
Manifestations-related topics, 339-348. *See also* Clinical manifestations of disease topics.
Marks, Susan, 3, 137, 407, 526
Marshall, Deborah, 298-317
Masking, 52-54
McAlister, Finlay, 222, 407, 481, 490
McCaughan, Dorothy, 3, 154, 172, 481
McKibbon, Ann, 20
McGinn, Thomas, 359, 446
Meade, Maureen, 48, 446
Measurement instruments, 209-217. *See also under individual topics.*
　　Braden Scale for Predicting Pressure Sore Risk, 210-211
　　Chronic Heart Failure Questionnaire, 304
　　Diabetes Life Satisfaction Scale, 216b
　　Diabetes Quality of Life for Youth Measure, 209b-213b
　　Disease Impact Scale, 216b
　　Disease-Related Worries Scale, 216b-217b
　　Health Utilities Index, 310
　　measurement properties and, 210-212
　　Medical Outcomes Study, 213
　　New York Heart Association functional classification, 216
　　Owestry Back-Disability Index, 215-217
　　for patient-derived assessments, 209-210
　　Sickness Impact Profile, 213
Measures-related topics. *See also under individual topics; individual topics.*
　　agreement beyond chance measures, 446-454
　　association measures, 407-422
　　differential measures, 401
　　measurement instruments. *See* Measurement instruments.
　　utility measures, 214-215
Medical Outcomes Study, 213

MEDLINE, 35t, 38-41, 92, 142
Melnyk, Bernadette, 3
Meta-analyses, 12, 139-140, 145-149, 148f, 367-368, 382-385, 383f-384f
Meta-syntheses, 140
Methodological quality, 143-144, 305-306, 306t
Mirroring (target populations), 340-342, 351-352
Mixed method studies, 275
Models. *See also under individual topics.*
  ARIMA, 291
  costs as outcomes, 301-302
  Cox regression, 419-420
  decision, 300-302
  fixed-effects, 147, 388-393
  random-effects, 147, 388-393
Mohide, Ann, 423
Montori, Victor, 137, 373, 381, 388
Moyer, Virginia, 71, 339
Multifaceted interventions, 191t-192t
Multivariate analyses, 280
Multivariate regression equations, 461-464

N
Narrative reviews, 375t
Narrow budgetary viewpoints, 305
National Guidelines Clearinghouse, 36t, 42, 527
Naylor, David, 205, 339, 359
Negative trials (apparent), 438-440
Negative *vs.* positive studies, 374
Nelson, Andrea, 108, 222, 245, 490, 526
New York Heart Association functional classification, 216
New Zealand Guidelines Group, 517, 518t
Newman, Mark, 3, 48, 120, 154, 172, 481, 526
NNH (number needed to harm), 409, 486-487.
  See also Harm-related topics.
NNT (number needed to treat) factors, 469-480.
  See also under individual topics.
  association measures and, 409, 414-416, 415f
  benefit-risk ratios and, 486-487
  benefits summarizations for, 470
  examples of, 472t
  future perspectives of, 478-479
  harm-benefit factors, 470-479
    ARR, 470-479
    baseline risks, 471-473, 477t
    CIs, 473-477
    dichotomous outcomes, 471
    follow-up times, 477
    NNH, 477-479
    overviews and summaries of, 470-471
    precision, 473-477
    risk levels, 474t-476t
    RRR, 470-479
    RRs, 470-479
  HRQL topics and, 216-219, 217t
  overviews and summaries of, 469

NNT (number needed to treat) factors *(Continued)*
  patient care applications for, 486-487
  reference resources for, 479-480
  risk summarizations, 470
No-test *vs.* test thresholds, 90
Noise-signal relationships, 210-211
Nomograms, 97-99, 98f
Non-adherent patients, 54
Nonrandomized cohort studies, 273-274, 288-289
Novice *vs.* expert questions, 21-23, 22f
Null hypotheses, 374, 433, 458
Number needed to harm (NNH), 409, 486-487.
  See also Harm-related topics.
Number needed to treat (NNT), 469-480. *See also* NNT (number needed to treat) factors.
Nursing literature use principles (basic concepts).
  See also under individual topics.
  clinical practice guidelines-related topics, 154-171
  diagnoses-related topics, 87-107
  evidence discovery factors, 20-43
  fundamental topics, 3-19
  harm-related topics, 44-46, 71-86
  health care intervention topics, 44-70
  organizational practice change topics, 172-200
  prognoses-related topics, 108-119
  qualitative research topics, 120-136
  systematic review and summarization topics, 137-153
NZCG (New Zealand Guidelines Group), 517, 518t

O
Objectives consistency, 168
O'Brien, Bernie, 298-317
Observability characteristics, 180
Observational designs, 236-243, 271-275. *See also* Designs (research).
  before-and-after studies (controlled), 271-272
  case-control studies, 274-275
  cohort studies, 273-274
    historical *vs.* nonrandomized, 274
    overviews and summaries of, 273-274
  CQI processes and, 272
  overviews and summaries of, 271-275
  surprising results of, 236-243, 238t-242t
  time-series studies (interrupted), 272-273
O'Connor, Annette, 490-507
Odds ratios, 77-78, 81, 409-413, 438
Omissions (aspect), 212-213
Operational construct sampling, 125-126
Opinion leaders, 189
Opportunistic sampling, 125-126
Opportunity costs, 313
Organizational characteristics, 180, 185b
Organizational practice change topics, 172-200
  academic detailing, 189, 191t

Organizational practice change topics *(Continued)*
  action plans, 178f-179f
  Adult Asthma Care Guidelines for Nurses, 173,
    176b-177b, 185b
  audit and feedback, 189
  characteristics, 177, 185
    compatibility, 180
    complexity, 180
    environmental, 180, 185b
    individual, 184, 185b
    innovation, 180, 184b-185b
    observability, 180
    organizational, 180, 185b
    overviews and summaries of, 181t-183t
    trialability, 180
  clinical scenarios and resolutions for, 173b
  Diffusion of Innovations theory, 174
  education outreach visits, 189, 191t
  frameworks, 173-198
    confirmation components, 190-198, 191t-192t
    decision components, 186-188
    evaluation components, 194t-197t
    implementation components, 188-190,
      194t-197t
    knowledge components, 174-177
    overviews and summaries of, 173-174
    persuasion components, 177-186, 178f-179f,
      181t-183t
  hierarchies (evidence), 174
  interactive education, 192t
  interactive workshops, 189
  multifaceted interventions, 191t-192t
  opinion leaders, 189
  overviews and summaries of, 172-174, 175f
  process evaluations, 190, 192
  reference resources for, 198-200
  reminder systems, 189
  reminders, 191t
  structure evaluations, 190
  users' guides for, 176b-177b, 184b-190b, 193b
  workshops, 192t
ORs (odds ratios), 77-78, 81, 409-413, 438
Ottawa ankle rules, 360b, 361f, 362, 365-369, 369b
Ottawa Decision Support Framework, 495-497, 496t
Outcomes-related topics. *See also under individual*
  topics.
  comprehensiveness of, 151
  continuous outcomes, 409
  determinants, 399-400
  dichotomous outcomes, 60, 409, 471
  inclusivity, 293-294
  matrices, 311-313, 312f
  measurement instruments, 209-217. *See also*
    Measurement instruments.
  occurrences over time, 115
  patient-important outcomes, 224
  surrogate outcomes, 222-234
  target outcomes, 158-160, 225-229, 399-400

Outreach visits, 189, 191t
Overall results, 146-149
Overviews and summaries, 3. *See also under*
  individual topics.
  of advanced concepts (education- and
    application-related principles)
    agreement beyond chance measures, 446-447
    association measures, 407-409, 408f
    bias- and random error-related topics, 397-399
    CDSS, 318
    CIs, 432-433, 444
    clinical manifestations of disease topics,
      339-340
    clinical prediction rules, 359-362, 361f
    differences evaluations (results), 381
    differential diagnoses topics, 349
    economic evaluations, 298-299
    health services interventions, 265, 267-268
    HRQL topics, 205-207
    hypotheses and hypotheses testing topics,
      423-424
    intention to treat principle, 245
    NNT factors, 469
    patient care applications, 481-482, 487-488
    patient values incorporation topics, 490
    publication bias, 373
    regression and correlation topics, 455-456, 466
    screening recommendations, 526
    subgroup analyses topics, 251-252, 260-261
    surprising results-related topics, 235, 243
    surrogate outcomes topics, 222
  of basic concepts (nursing literature use
    principles)
    diagnoses-related topics, 87-88
    evidence discovery, 20-21
    evidence sources, 33
    fundamental topics, 3, 17
    harm-related topics, 44-45, 71
    health care intervention topics, 48
    organizational practice change topics,
      172-173, 175f
    patient values incorporation topics, 490
    prognoses-related topics, 108
    qualitative research topics, 120
    systematic review and summarization topics,
      137
Owestry Back-Disability Index, 215-217
Oxman, Andrew, 137, 251, 388

P
P values, 425-427
  alpha levels, 425
  statistical significance, 426-427
  type I errors, 425
Patient care applications, 481-489. *See also under*
  individual topics.
  for advanced concepts (education- and
    application-related principles)

Patient care applications *(Continued)*
  CDSS, 329-333
  clinical manifestations of disease topics,
    346-347
  differential diagnoses topics, 347, 356-357
  economic evaluations, 311-315, 312f
  health services interventions, 292-294
  HRQL topics, 217-219
  screening recommendations, 536-539
  surrogate outcomes topics, 229-231
  applicability, 103
  for basic concepts (nursing literature use
    principles)
    clinical practice guidelines-related topics, 168-169
    diagnoses-related topics, 102-106
    harm-related topics, 45-46, 82-84
    health care intervention topics, 65-68
    prognoses-related topics, 117-118
    qualitative research topics, 133-134
    systematic review and summarization topics,
      150-151
  benefit-harm ratios, 105-106
  benefit-risk ratios, 485-487
    adverse effects risks and, 485-487
    NNH and, 486-487
    NNT and, 486-487
    RRR and, 486-487
  biologic issues of, 482-484
  cost-benefit ratios, 151
  cost expectation transferability, 314-315
  cost-risk ratios, 151
  diagnostic test reproducibility, 102
  differential diagnoses generation, 347
  disease probability changes over time, 356-357
  epidemiologic issues, 485
  follow-up durations, 117
  future perspectives of, 488
  health care personnel influences, 485
  knowledge enhancement, 134
  management applicability, 118
  manifestation changes over time, 346-347
  opportunity costs, 313
  outcomes comprehensiveness, 151
  outcomes matrices for, 311-313, 312f
  overviews and summaries of, 481-482, 487-488
  patient care contexts, 133-134
  primary objectives consistency, 167
  provider adherence, 485
  recommendation applicability, 168-169
  reference resources for, 488-489
  relevancy, 133
  results interpretations, 150-151
  socioeconomic issues of, 484-485
  study-clinical setting patients similarities, 65-66,
    82, 117, 346, 356
  treatment benefits *vs.* risks and costs,
    311-313, 312f
  users' guides for, 483t

Patient-derived assessments, 209
Patient enrollments, 351-352
Patient-important outcomes, 224
Patient sample homogeneity, 112-113
Patient values incorporation topics, 490-507
  clinical scenarios and resolutions for,
    491b, 502b
  decision aids, 494-498
    advantages of, 497
    CREDIBLE criteria, 498
    Ottawa Decision Support Framework, 495-497,
      497t
    overviews and summaries of, 494
    success of, 497-498
  evidence discovery, 491-493
  identification (values), 498-505
    analytic hierarchy processes, 501-502
    balance scales, 499
    examples of, 503f-505f
    feeling thermometers, 499-501, 500f
    formal utility assessments, 499-501
    overviews and summaries of, 498-499
    standard gambles, 501
    threshold techniques, 501
    time trade-offs, 501
    visual analogue scales, 499-501, 500f
  overviews and summaries of, 490
  reference resources for, 506-507
  strategies for, 493-494
    decision-making processes, 494
    explicit strategies, 494
    implicit strategies, 493-494
    overviews and summaries of, 493
    patient participation, 494
Peer reviews, 162, 375t
Personnel influences, 485
Persuasion components, 177-186, 178f-179f,
  181t-183t
Phi *vs.* kappa (chance-corrected agreement),
  453-454, 453f
Pilot studies, 375t
Pinelli, Janet, 137
Placebo effect, 400
Plausible explanations, 288-289
Ploeg, Jenny, 48, 120-136, 265, 455
Policy decision-making, 303-304
Pooling, 382-387, 389
Portability-related issues, 330
Positive trials (apparent), 440-442, 441t
Positive *vs.* negative studies, 374
Post hoc analyses, 255
Posttest *vs.* pretest probabilities, 88
Power and false-negative
  risks, 427-428
Practical and clinically important
  recommendations, 164
Practice-related topics. *See also under individual
  topics.*

Practice-related topics *(Continued)*
  application-related topics, 467-541
    evidence level interpretations and health care
      grade recommendations, 508-525
    NNT factors, 469-480
    patient care applications, 481-489. *See also*
      Patient care applications.
    patient values incorporation topics, 490-507
    screening recommendations, 508-525
  clinical practice guidelines-related topics, 154-171
  organizational practice change topics, 172-200
Precision-related topics, 61-64, 115-116, 149, 345,
    355-356, 377-379, 473-477
  estimate precision, 115-116
  formulae for, 355
  funnel plots (magnitude *vs.* precision), 377-379,
    378f-379f
  harm-benefit factors and, 473-477
  NNT and, 473-477
  systematic review and summarization topics and,
    149
Predicting systems, 321t
Prediction rules, 359-370. *See also* Clinical
    prediction rules.
Preliminary studies, 375t
Preprocessed sources, 34-39, 34f, 35t
Press reports, 375t
Pretest *vs.* posttest probabilities, 88
Primary objectives consistency, 167
Probability, 88, 320, 355-357
  changes over time, 356-357
  conditional, 320
  estimates, 355-356
  pretest *vs.* posttest, 88
Process evaluations, 190
Profiles (health), 213
Prognoses-related topics, 108-119
  bias and, 399-400. *See also* Bias-related topics.
  clinical scenarios and resolutions for, 109b, 118b
  evidence discovery, 109-111
  evidence sources, 109-111
  future perspectives of, 118
  identification factors (results), 115-117
    CIs, 115-116
    estimate precision, 115-116
    outcomes occurrences over time, 115
    survival curves, 115-116, 116f
  overviews and summaries of, 108
  patient care applications, 117-118
    follow-up durations, 117
    management applicability, 118
    study patients-clinical setting patients
      similarities, 117
  reference resources for, 119
  surrogate outcomes, 226
  users' guides, 110t, 114b-115b, 117b
  validity factors (results), 111-115
    bias, 111

Prognoses-related topics *(Continued)*
  follow-ups completeness, 113
  outcomes criteria bias, 113-114
  patient sample homogeneity, 112-113
  representative patient samples, 111
Properties (measurement), 210-212
Provider adherence issues, 485
PsycINFO, 142
Publication bias, 373-380. *See also* Bias-related
    topics.
  future perspectives of, 379
  identification strategies for, 377-379, 378f-379f
    asymmetry and, 377
    funnel plots (magnitude *vs.* precision) for,
      377-379, 378f-379f
    overviews and summaries of, 377-379
    trim-and-fill methods and, 378
  negative *vs.* positive studies and, 374
  null hypotheses and, 374
  overviews and summaries of, 373
  reduction strategies for, 379
  reference resources for, 379-380
  researcher contributions to, 374-377
  sources of, 374, 375t-376t, 376f
    author revisions and resubmissions, 375t
    decision-maker retrieval, 375t
    editorial considerations, 375t
    electronic database indexing, 375t
    funding and funding opportunities, 375t-376t
    further trial evidence, 375t
    institutional/ethics review board approval, 375t
    journal selections, 375t
    lay press reports, 375t
    narrative reviews, 375t
    overviews and summaries of, 374, 376-377
    peer reviews, 375t
    pilot studies, 375t
    practice guidelines, 376t
    preliminary studies, 375t
    report completions, 375t
    report publications, 375t
    study completions, 375t
    systematic review submissions, 376t
    trial designs, 375t
    trial organization, 375t
  in systematic reviews, 374
  trial magnitudes and, 374
PubMed, 34-39, 34f, 35t, 92, 109,
    319, 350
Purposeful sampling, 125-126

Q
QALYs (quality-adjusted life-years), 214-215, 303
Qualitative research topics, 120-136
  clinical scenarios and resolutions, 121b, 134b
  evidence discovery, 121-122
  evidence sources, 121-122
  identification factors (results), 131

Qualitative research topics *(Continued)*
    cautious detachment, 131
    thoroughness, 131
    overviews and summaries of, 120
    patient care applications, 133-134
        knowledge enhancement, 134
        patient care contexts, 133
        relevancy, 133
    validity factors (results), 122-131, 126f
        constant comparative methods, 124
        convenience samples, 124-125
        design appropriateness, 123-125
        document analyses, 126-129, 126f
        ethnographies, 123
        field observations, 126-127, 126f
        grounded theories, 123-124
        information redundancy, 129
        information sources, 126-128, 126f
        interviews, 126-128, 126f
        investigator triangulation, 129
        judgmental sampling, 125-126
        opportunistic sampling, 125-126
        overviews and summaries of, 122-123
        purposeful sampling, 125-126
        question clarity and adequateness, 123
        sampling appropriateness, 125-126
        saturation, 129
        symbolic interactionism, 123-124
        systematic data collection and management,
            126-128
        theoretical sampling, 124
        theory-based operational construct sampling,
            125-126
        theory triangulation, 129
Qualitative studies, 32
Quality of life topics, 205-221. *See also* HRQL
    (health-related quality of life) topics.
    applications (patient care), 217-219
    clinical scenarios and resolutions for,
        206b, 219b
    definitions of, 206-207
    future perspectives of, 219
    identification factors (results), 215-216
    importance of, 207-208
    overviews and summaries of, 205-207
    reference resources for, 219-221
    users' guides for, 207t, 208b-213b, 215b-219b
    validity factors (results), 209-215
Quantitative studies, 28-32, 28f-31f
Quantity-quality of life trade-offs, 213-215, 214f
Question-related topics, 21-28, 123, 141-142
    background *vs.* foreground questions,
        21-23, 22f
    clarity and adequateness, 123
    explicitness and sensibility, 141-142
    novice *vs.* expert questions, 21-23, 22f
    question framing methods, 23-27
    question type determinations, 28

R
Raffle, Angela, 526
Randolph, Adrienne, 108, 318
Random-effects models, 147, 388-393
Random error topics, 397-406
Randomization, 51-54, 271, 276-279, 428-429
Randomized controlled trials (RCTs), 46, 52-59, 72-79,
    236-243, 238t-242t, 246-250, 247f-249f, 270-271
Ratios. *See also under individual topics.*
    benefit-harm ratios, 105-106
    benefit-risk ratios, 485-487, 523-524, 528t
        adverse effects risks and, 485-487
        NNH and, 486-487
        NNT and, 486-487
        RRR and, 486-487
    cost-benefit ratios, 151
    cost-risk ratios, 151
    cost-to-charge ratios, 307
    hazard ratios, 60
    likelihood ratios, 95-102, 96t, 98t, 99t-102t
        LR+, 97
        LR–, 97
    ORs, 409-413, 438
Raynor, Pauline, 3
RBI (relative benefit increase), 532-536
RCTs (randomized controlled trials), 46, 52-59, 72-79,
    236-243, 238t-242t, 246-250, 247f-249f, 270-271
RDs (risk differences), 409
Recent developments inclusion, 162
Recommendations (screening), 526-541
Records reviews, 283-285, 283t
Reduction strategies, 379, 404-406, 404t
    for bias (general), 404-406, 404t
    for publication bias, 379
Reference resources. *See also under individual topics.*
    for advanced concepts (education- and
        application-related principles)
        agreement beyond chance measures, 454
        association measures, 422
        bias- and random error-related topics, 406
        CDSS, 334-335
        CIs, 444-445
        clinical manifestations of disease topics, 348
        clinical prediction rules, 369-370
        differences evaluations (results), 387
        differential diagnoses topics, 357-358
        economic evaluations, 315-317
        health services interventions, 294-297
        HRQL topics, 219-221
        hypotheses and hypotheses testing topics, 431
        intention to treat principle, 250
        NNT factors, 479-480
        patient care applications, 488-489
        patient values incorporation topics, 506-507
        regression and correlation topics, 466
        screening recommendations, 540-541
        subgroup analyses topics, 261-262
        surprising results-related topics, 243-244

Reference resources *(Continued)*
  surrogate outcomes topics, 231-234
  for basic concepts (nursing literature use
      principles)
  clinical practice guidelines-related topics,
      170-171
  diagnoses-related topics, 106-107
  evidence discovery, 42-43
  fundamental topics, 17-19
  harm-related topics, 47, 85-86
  health care intervention topics, 69-70
  organizational practice change topics, 198-200
  prognoses-related topics, 119
  publication bias, 379-380
  systematic review and summarization topics,
      152-153
Reference standard tests, 342
Regression and correlation topics, 455-466
  coefficients (correlation), 457
  correlation examples, 456-458, 457f
  future perspectives of, 466
  multivariate regression equations, 461-464
  null hypotheses, 458
  overviews and summaries of, 455-456, 466
  reference resources for, 466
  regression examples, 458-466, 459f-460f,
      462f-463f, 465t
  univariate/simple regression, 460
  variables, 459-466
    continuous variables, 461
    dependent *vs.* independent variables, 459-466
    dichotomous variables, 461
Regression techniques, 291
Relative benefit increase, 532-536
Relative risk reduction, 58-64, 63f, 253-254, 408,
    411, 470-479, 486-487, 532-536
Relative risks, 410-411, 413-414, 470-479
Relevancy, 11t, 133
Reliability, 331
Reminder systems, 189, 321-322, 321t
Reminders, 191t
Rennie, Drummond (users' guides), 20, 48, 71, 87,
    108, 120, 137, 154, 205, 222, 235, 245, 251, 298,
    318, 339, 349, 359, 373, 381, 388, 407, 423, 432,
    446, 455, 469, 481, 490, 508, 526. *See also* Users'
    guides.
Report completions and publication, 375t
Representative patient samples, 111, 340-342,
    351-352
Reproducibility, 144, 352-353
Research-related topics. *See also under individual
    topics.*
  health services research topics, 263-335
    CDSS (computer decision support systems),
        318-335
    economic evaluations, 298-317
    health services interventions, 265-297
  qualitative research topics, 120-136

Research-related topics *(Continued)*
  reference resources. *See* Reference resources.
  research designs, 269-276
  systematic review and summarization topics,
      137-153
Researcher contributions (publication bias),
    374-377
Resource-intensive approaches, 303
Responsiveness factors, 211
Resubmissions and revisions, 375t
Results-related topics, 395-466. *See also under
    individual topics.*
  agreement beyond chance measures, 446-454
  association measures, 407-422
  bias and random error topics, 397-406
  CIs, 432-445
  differences evaluations (results), 381-387
  false-positive *vs.* false-negative results, 528-529
  hypothesis testing topics, 423-431
  identification factors. *See* Identification factors
      (results).
  overall results, 146-149
  patient care applications of. *See* Patient care
      applications.
  regression and correlation topics, 455-466
  true-negative results, 528-529
Review board approval, 375t
Revisions and resubmissions, 375t
Richardson, Scott, 20, 108, 154, 298, 339, 349,
    481, 508
Risk-related topics. *See also under individual topics.*
  absolute risk, 409-410
  adverse effects risks, 485-487
  ARR, 60, 253-254, 409-410, 413-414, 470-479,
      532, 532t
  association measures and, 407-422
  baseline risk reporting differences, 306-307
  benefit-risk ratios, 485-487, 523-524, 528t
  cost-risk ratios, 151
  false-negative result risks, 427-428
  NNH and, 486-487
  NNT and, 486-487
  RDs, 409
  relative risks, 410-411, 413-414
  risk levels, 474t-476t
  risk summarizations, 470
  RRR, 60-64, 63f, 253-254, 408, 411, 470-479,
      486-487, 532-536
  RRs, 470-479
  screening recommendations and, 531-536
  STRATIFY (risk assessment tool), 360
Rival plausible explanations, 288-289
RNAO Best Practice Guidelines Project, 34, 34f,
    36t, 42
RRR (relative risk reduction), 58-64, 63f, 253-254,
    408, 411, 470-479, 486-487, 532-536
RRs (relative risks), 410-411, 413-414, 470-479
Russell, Cynthia, 120-136

S

Sample homogeneity, 112-113
Sarah Cole Hirsh Institute, 36t
Saturation, 129
Scales (visual analogue), 499-501, 500f
Scientific Advisory Council of the Osteoporosis
    Society of Canada, 516t
Scottish Intercollegiate Guidelines Network, 516t
Screening recommendations, 526-541
    benefit-risk ratios, 528t
    clinical scenarios and resolutions for, 527b,
        539b-540b
    consequences of, 527-529, 528t
    evidence discovery for, 527
    evidence sources for, 527
    false-positive vs. false-negative results, 528-529
    identification of, 531-536
        ABI, 532
        ARR, 532
        clinical consequences, 534t
        overviews and summaries of, 531
        RBI, 532
        risks, 531-536
        RRR, 532
    overviews and summaries of, 526
    patient care applications and, 536-539
    reference resources for, 540-541
    true-negative results, 528-529
    users' guides for, 529t, 531b
    validity factors (results), 529-531
Search methods, 28-32, 28f-31f. See also Evidence
    discovery.
    overviews and summaries of, 28
    for qualitative studies, 32
    for quantitative studies, 28-32, 28f-31f
    question type determinations, 28
    for systematic reviews, 32
Seers, Kate, 3, 71
Self-reported data reviews, 285
Sensitivity, 99-102
Sensitivity analyses, 146-147, 310-311
Sentinel effects, 332-333
Sickness Impact Profile, 213
Signal-noise relationships, 210-211
Silo effects, 305
Silver Platter, 40
Simple/univariate regression, 460
Sinclair, Jack, 154, 490, 508
Smith, Karen, 20
Social responsibility, 6-7
Socieconomic issues, 484-485
Societal viewpoints, 305-306
Sources (evidence). See also under individual topics.
    ACP Journal Club, 23
    Adult Asthma Care Guideline for Nurses, 173,
        173b, 176b-177b, 185b
    for advanced concepts (education- and
        application-related principles)

Sources (evidence) (Continued)
    CDSS, 319-322
    differential diagnoses topics, 350
    economic evaluations, 299
    screening recommendations, 527
    AGA guidelines, 527-536
    AHRQ, 155
    for basic concepts (nursing literature use
        principles)
        clinical practice guidelines-related topics,
            155-159
        diagnoses-related topics, 92
        harm-related topics, 72
        health care intervention topics, 49-50, 56
        prognoses-related topics, 109-111
        qualitative research topics, 121-122
        systematic reviews, 138
    Centre for Evidence-Based Medicine
        (Oxford), 36t
    Centre for Evidence-Based Medicine
        (Toronto), 36t
    Centre for Evidence-Based Nursing, 36t
    CINAHL, 33, 35t, 39-40, 142
    Clinical Evidence, 16, 34, 37, 39, 34f, 35t, 157
    CMA Infobase, 223
    Cochrane Central Register of Controlled Trials,
        142-143
    Cochrane Database of Systematic Reviews, 39, 138,
        223, 527
    Cochrane Library, 16-17, 34-39, 34f, 35,
        49-50, 138, 223-224
    Dissertation Abstracts Online, 143
    EMBASE, 35t, 41, 142
    ERIC, 142
    Evidence-Based Cardiovascular Medicine, 23, 37
    Evidence-Based Mental Health, 23, 37
    Evidence-Based Nursing, 16-17, 23, 37, 49-50, 56, 121
    German Centre for Evidence-Based Nursing, 36t
    Google.com, 155
    Joanna Briggs Institute, 36t
    journal selections, 375t
    Knowledge Finder, 40
    MEDLINE, 35t, 38-41, 92, 142
    National Guidelines Clearinghouse, 36t, 42, 527
    overviews and summaries of, 33
    preprocessed sources, 34-39, 34f, 35t
    PsycINFO, 142
    PubMed, 34-39, 34f, 35t, 92, 109, 319, 350
    RNAO Best Practice Guidelines Project, 34,
        34f, 36t, 42
    Sarah Cole Hirsh Institute, 36t
    selection criteria for, 33-34
    Silver Platter, 40
    TRIP Database, 42
    Ulrich's Periodicals Directory, 21
    United Kingdom National Health Service
        Economic Evaluation Database, 299
    unprocessed sources, 35t

Sources (publication bias), 374, 375t-376t, 376f
Specificity, 99-102
Stacey, Dawn, 490-507
Standard gambles, 214-215, 214f, 501
Standard tests (reference), 342
Standards appropriateness, explicitness, and
    credibility, 352-353
Statistical significance, 257-259, 258f, 311, 426-427
Stiell, Ian, 359
Stone, Patricia, 298
STRATIFY (risk assessment tool), 360
Straus, Sharon, 48, 481, 490
Structure evaluations, 190
Study-clinical setting patients similarities, 65-66, 82,
    117, 346, 356
Subgroup analyses topics, 251-262
    definitions for, 252-253
        subgroups analyses, 252-253
        treatments effects, 252
    effects measures, 253-254, 254t
        ARR, 253-254
        guidelines for, 254t
        overviews and summaries of, 253, 254t
        RRR, 253-254
    future perspectives of, 260-261
    importance of, 252-253
    interpretation guidelines, 254-260, 254t
        between-study vs. within-study differences,
            254-255
        hypothesized effects consistency, 259-260
        hypothesized effects magnitudes, 255-256,
            255-257
        hypothesized effects statistical significance,
            257-259, 258f
        indirect evidence support, 260
        overviews and summaries of, 254, 254t
        post hoc analyses, 255
        a priori analyses, 255
    overviews and summaries of, 251-252, 260-261
    reference resources for, 261-262
Suggesting systems, 321t
Summarization-related topics, 137-153. See also
    Systematic review and summarization topics.
Support systems (computer decision), 318-335. See
    also CDSS (computer decision support
    systems).
Surprising results-related topics, 235-244
    case-control studies, 236-243, 238t-242t
    cohort studies, 236-243, 238t-242t
    future perspectives of, 243
    observational studies, 236-243, 238t-242t
    overviews and summaries of, 235, 243
    RCTs, 236-243, 238t-242t
    reference resources for, 243-244
    surrogate end points, 236-243, 238t-242t
Surrogate end points, 229, 236-243, 238t-242t
Surrogate outcomes topics, 222-234
    clinical scenarios and resolutions for, 223b, 231b

Surrogate outcomes topics (Continued)
    definition of, 224-225
    evidence discovery, 223-224
    evidence sources, 223-224
    future perspectives of, 231
    identification factors (results), 229-231
        intervention magnitudes, precision, and
            duration, 229
        surrogate end points, 229
    overviews and summaries of, 222-225
    patient care applications, 229-231
    reference resources for, 231-234
    users' guides, 226b, 226t, 228b-229b
    validity factors (results), 224-229, 226t
        in drug evaluations (phase II vs. phase II
            trials), 224-225
        independent associations, 226
        overviews and summaries of, 225, 226t
        patient-important outcomes, 224
        prognostic factors, 226
        target outcomes, 225-229
Surveillance bias, 79, 286
Survival analyses and curves, 60, 115-116, 116f
Symbolic interactionism, 123-124
Symptom temporal sequences (presenting,
    concurring, eventual), 345-346
Syndrome diagnoses, 342
Systematic data collection and management,
    126-128
Systematic review and summarization topics.
    See also under individual topics.
    advanced concepts (education- and application-
        related principles), 371-393
        differences evaluations (results), 381-387
        fixed-effects vs. random-effects models,
            388-393
        publication bias, 373-380
    basic concepts (nursing literature use principles),
        137-153
    clinical scenarios and resolutions for, 138b,
        151b-152b
    definitions for, 138-141
    differences evaluations and, 382
    evidence discovery for, 138
    evidence sources for, 138-142
        CINAHL, 142-143
        Cochrane Central Register of Controlled
            Trials, 142
        Cochrane Database of Systematic Reviews, 138
        Cochrane Library, 138
        Dissertation Abstracts Online, 143
        EMBASE, 142-143
        ERIC, 142
        MEDLINE, 142
        PsycINFO, 142
    identification factors (results), 145-150, 148f
        fixed-effects models, 147
        heterogeneity tests, 145-146

Systematic review and summarization topics
   (Continued)
      meta-analyses, 146-149, 148f
      overall results, 146-149
      precision, 149
      random-effects models, 147
      results similarities, 145-146
      sensitivity analyses, 146-147
   meta-analyses, 139-140, 145
   meta-syntheses, 140
   overviews and summaries of, 137-141
   patient care applications, 150-151
      cost-benefit ratios, 151
      cost-risk ratios, 151
      outcomes comprehensiveness, 151
      results interpretations, 150-151
   processes for, 140t
   publication bias and, 376t
   reference resources for, 152-153
   search methods for, 32
   vs. unsystematic reviews, 139
   validity factors (results), 141-145
      critical question explicitness and sensibility,
         141-142
      methodological quality, 143-144
      publication bias, 143
      reproducibility, 144

T

Tables (2 × 2), 409, 410t, 416-418
Target outcomes, 158-160, 225-229, 399-400
Target population mirroring, 340-342, 351-352
Temporal sequences (presenting, concurring,
   eventual), 345-346
Test *vs.* no-test thresholds, 90
Theoretical sampling, 124
Theory-based operational construct sampling,
   125-126
Theory triangulation, 129
Therapeutic thresholds, 89-90, 89f
Thompson, Carl, 3, 318-336
Thoroughness, 131
Thresholds, 89-90, 501
   no-test *vs.* test thresholds, 90
   techniques for, 501
   therapeutic, 89-90, 89f
Time-series regression techniques, 291
Time-series studies (interrupted), 272-273, 291
Time trade-offs, 501
Treatments effects, 252
Trial magnitudes, 374
Trialability characteristics, 180
Triangulation (investigator and theory), 129
Trim-and-fill methods, 378
TRIP Database, 42
True-negative results, 528-529
Tugwell, Peter, 108, 490-507
Two × two tables, 409, 410t, 416-418

Type I errors, 425
Type II errors, 427-428

U

Ulrich's Periodicals Directory, 21
Underdiagnosed patients, 354
UNIS (Urological Nursing Information Systems), 322
Unit/cluster assignment analyses adjustments,
   287-288
*United Kingdom National Health Service Economic
   Evaluation Database,* 299
United States Panel on Cost-Effectiveness in Health
   and Medicine, 308
Univariate/simple regression, 460
Unprocessed sources, 35t
Unsystematic reviews, 139
Up-front costs, 309
Urological Nursing Information Systems, 322
Users' guides. *See also under individual topics.*
   for advanced concepts (education- and
      application-related principles)
      CDSS, 323t, 326b-329b
      clinical manifestations of disease topics, 341t,
         343b-344b, 346b
      differential diagnoses topics, 351t, 354b-357b
      economic evaluations, 304t
      health services interventions, 277t, 289b-292b
      HRQL topics, 208b-213b, 215b-219b
      patient care applications, 483t
      screening recommendations, 529t, 531b
   for basic concepts (nursing literature use
      principles)
      clinical practice guidelines-related topics,
         158t, 163b-164b, 167b-168b
      diagnoses-related topics, 92t, 95b, 101b,
         103b-105b
      harm-related topics, 73t, 79b-80b
      health care intervention topics, 51t
      organizational practice change topics,
         176b-177b, 184b-190b, 193b
      prognoses-related topics, 110t, 114b-115b, 117b
   Guyatt (Gordon) and Rennie (Drummond) and,
      20, 48, 71, 87, 108, 120, 137, 154, 205, 222,
      235, 245, 251, 298, 318, 339, 349, 359, 373,
      381, 407, 423, 432, 446, 455, 469, 481, 508,
      526
Utilitarian approaches, 302-303
Utility assessments (formal), 499-501
Utility-cost analyses, 303
Utility measures, 214-215

V

Validation processes (clinical prediction rules),
   361-366, 362f, 363t. *See also* Clinical prediction
   rules.
   bootstrap techniques, 364
   derivation methodological standards, 364t
   overviews and summaries of, 361-362

Validity factors (results)
  for advanced concepts (education- and
      application-related principles)
    CDSS, 322-328, 323t
    clinical manifestations of disease topics,
        340-344
    differential diagnoses topics, 351-355
    economic evaluations, 304-308
    health services interventions, 276-290, 278t,
        280t, 282t-283t
    HRQL topics, 209-215, 214f
    screening recommendations, 529-531
    surrogate outcomes topics, 224-229, 226t
  allocation concealment, 52-54
  aspect omissions, 212-213
  baseline risk reporting differences, 306-307
  for basic concepts (nursing literature use
      principles)
    clinical practice guidelines-related topics,
        159-164
    diagnoses-related topics, 93-95
    health care intervention topics, 50-59
    prognoses-related topics, 111-115
    qualitative research topics, 122-131, 126f
    systematic review and summarization topics,
        141-145
  bias, 111
  blinding, 52-54
  channeling bias, 76-78
  cointerventions, 57
  concealed randomization, 52-54
  confounding variables, 75-76
  constant comparative methods, 124
  controls, 77-78
  convenience samples, 124
  cost-to-charge ratios, 307
  critical question explicitness and sensibility,
      141-142
  design appropriateness, 123-124
  detection bias, 79
  diagnoses, 342, 352-353
    reproducibility of, 352-353
    verification criteria credibility and
        independence of, 342
  document analyses, 126-128, 126f
  in drug evaluations (phase II vs. phase II trials),
      224-225
  ethnographies, 123
  evaluation and assessments, 93
  evidence identification, selection, and
      combination, 160-161
  expectation bias, 94
  exposed patient identification, 79
  face vs. construct validity, 211-212
  field observations, 126-127, 126f
  follow-ups, 57-59, 58t, 113, 354-355
    completeness of, 57-59, 58t, 113, 354
    durations of, 354

Validity factors (results) (Continued)
  grounded theories, 123-124
  health profiles, 213
  inclusiveness, 159-160
  independent associations, 226
  inquiry directions for, 75t
  internal vs. external validity, 269-270
  interviewer bias, 79
  interviews, 126-128, 126f
  investigator triangulation, 129
  judgmental sampling, 125-126
  manifestation classifications, 343
  masking, 52-54
  measurement properties, 210-212
  methodological quality, 143-144, 305-306, 306t
  narrow budgetary viewpoints, 305
  non-adherent patients, 54
  opportunistic sampling, 125-126
  ORs, 77-78, 81
  patient-derived assessments, 209
  patient enrollments, 351-352
  patient-important outcomes, 224
  patient sample homogeneity, 112-113
  patient values and preferences specification, 161
  peer review and testing, 162
  preferences, 158
  prognostic factors, 226
  publication bias, 143
  purposeful sampling, 125-126
  QALYs vs. DALYs, 214-215
  quantity-quality of life trade-offs, 213-215, 214f
  recent developments inclusion, 162
  representative patient samples, 111, 340-342,
      351-352
  reproducibility, 144
  responsiveness, 211
  RRR, 58
  sampling appropriateness, 125-126
  saturation, 129
  signal-noise relationships, 210-211
  silo effects, 305
  societal viewpoints, 305-306
  standard gambles, 214-215, 214f
  standards appropriateness, explicitness, and
      credibility, 352-353
  surveillance bias, 79
  symbolic interactionism, 123-124
  systematic data collection and management,
      126-128
  target outcomes, 158-160, 225-229
  target population mirroring, 340-342, 351-352
  test gold standards, 94-95
  theoretical sampling, 124
  theory-based operational construct sampling,
      125-126
  theory triangulation, 129
  underdiagnosed patients, 354
  utility measures, 214-215

Validity factors (results) *(Continued)*
  verification bias, 94-95
  viewpoint broadness, 304-306
  workup bias, 94-95
Values (patient), 490-507. *See also* Patient values
    incorporation topics.
Van Soeren Mary, 87, 222, 339, 359, 446
Variability, 382-385, 384f-385f
Variables, 459-466
  confounding variables, 75-76
  continuous variables, 428, 461
  dependent *vs.* independent variables, 459-466
  dichotomous variables, 461
Verification bias, 94-95
Verification criteria credibility and independence,
    342
Viewpoint broadness, 304-306

Visual analogue scales, 499-501, 500f
Voth, Tanya, 20-43

W
Wallace, Margaret, 3
Walter, Stephen, 71, 407, 423, 432, 455
Weighted kappa statistics, 452
Wells, George, 108
Williams, John, 339
Willman, Ania, 120, 154, 172, 349, 469, 481
Wilson, Mark, 20, 87, 154, 339, 349, 508
Within-study *vs.* between-study differences, 254-255
Working diagnoses, 89
Workshops, 189, 192t
Workup bias, 94-95
Wyatt, Jeremy, 318
Wyer, Peter, 20, 359